Cultural & Medical Centres of Historic Interest

Byzantium

Pergamos

Athens

Delos

Cos

Rhodes

Edessa
(Urfa)

Nineveh

Babylon

Jundi Shapur

Ur

Alexandria

A HISTORY OF MEDICINE

A HISTORY OF
MEDICINE

DOUGLAS GUTHRIE
M.D., F.R.C.S.Ed., F.R.S.E.

With Supplement

THOMAS NELSON AND SONS LTD
LONDON EDINBURGH PARIS MELBOURNE
TORONTO AND NEW YORK

THOMAS NELSON AND SONS LTD
Parkside Works Edinburgh 9
36 Park Street London WI
312 Flinders Street Melbourne C1

302–304 Barclays Bank Building
Commissioner and Kruis Streets
Johannesburg

THOMAS NELSON AND SONS (CANADA) LTD
91–93 Wellington Street West   Toronto 1

THOMAS NELSON AND SONS
19 East 47th Street New York 17

SOCIÉTÉ FRANÇAISE D'ÉDITIONS NELSON
97 rue Monge Paris 5

———

First published September 1945
Reprinted 1945, 1946, 1947
New and revised edition, with supplement, 1958
Reprinted 1960

PREFACE

" THE longer you can look back, the further you can look forward," said Mr. Winston Churchill, when addressing the Royal College of Physicians in March 1944. This truth provides ample justification for the appearance of this book. The past supplies the key to the present and the future. History forms the basis of all knowledge and is a convenient avenue of approach to any subject of study. It is therefore only natural to regard the evolution and progress of medicine from bygone times as an essential background to modern medical education. Unfortunately, however, the rapid advances and new discoveries of recent years have tended to eclipse the work of the early pioneers, and although due reverence is still accorded to the memory of such great figures as Harvey, Hunter, and Lister, the history of medicine in general has not received that recognition which the importance of the subject would appear to demand.

There is at present no systematic teaching of medical history in any medical school in this country, nor is there any British periodical devoted to this aspect of medicine, although the Section of the History of Medicine, Royal Society of Medicine, which has done so much to foster medical culture, has kept interest alive by publication of its *Proceedings*. Too often early medical practice has been regarded as merely quaint and sometimes amusing, now obsolete and of little value to the modern world. On the other hand it is encouraging to note, especially in the younger generation, a growing appreciation of the true purport of history in medicine and of its bearing upon the medical science of to-day.

The need for an historical background to modern medicine is securing recognition among those who regard the practice of medicine as something more than a mere technical accomplishment. Since no British text-book has been produced in recent years to meet this need, an attempt has been made in the following pages to construct an outline of the progress of medicine from the days of Imhotep to those of Sir William Osler. An outline does not aim at finality, and many worthy names have been omitted in order that the story may not lose interest by being overweighted with detail.

A history of medicine should not be simply a chaplet of

biographies nor yet a maze of dates and events, but rather a consecutive narrative, showing the progress of the healing art from the earliest times to the present day. The work of the leading scientists and practitioners, the fashions and sects in medicine throughout the ages, the geographical march of medicine from Greece to Salerno and Padua, and thence, by way of Leyden, to Britain and America, the epoch-making researches of Harvey and Claude Bernard, of Lister and of many another—these are but a few of the topics which the historian must fit into his mosaic of medical history, each detail as it falls into place revealing a steady and natural sequence. It is a noble theme, and it is hoped that the story, however imperfectly told, may stimulate interest in those achievements of the past which help us to solve the problems of the present, and which must constitute the foundation of all future progress in medical science.

As a guide to the reader who desires to pursue the study more deeply, references have been added, giving the authorities from which the author has drawn his information, and there is also a classified bibliography of works dealing with various aspects of this many-sided theme. In selecting the illustrations an effort has been made to avoid the commonplace and to secure pictures and portraits from original sources.

Geography is so closely related to history that a map is an essential complement to a work such as this. A simple outline, in which some of the important centres of medical learning are shown, has been regarded as sufficient. It is designed merely as a rough guide to the reader who may wish to pursue his investigations with the aid of a more detailed atlas.

It is obvious that a work of this nature cannot be undertaken without assistance, and the writer would like to pay tribute to the many friends who have assisted him in his task :

It was the late Dr. John D. Comrie who first led the author into the fascinating paths of early medicine, and it is only fitting to honour the memory of one who did so much by his lectures and writings to foster an interest in the subject among Edinburgh students and others.

To Mr. Alexander Miles, LL.D., F.R.C.S., his friend and teacher, the author is greatly indebted. Mr. Miles read the original manuscript and supplied much helpful criticism in the early stages of the work, and the aid of one so well-informed in history and so skilled in editorship proved invaluable.

Another generous collaborator was Mr. G. F. Home, Librarian of the Royal Society of Medicine, who made many valuable suggestions and responded to numerous requests for books and references with his customary alacrity and good nature.

Others to whom sincere thanks must be accorded for their expert assistance are the librarians and staffs of the National Library of Scotland, Edinburgh University Library, Hunterian Library of Glasgow University, Signet Library of Edinburgh, and the libraries of the Royal Colleges of Physicians and of Surgeons of Edinburgh. Grateful acknowledgement is also due to many friends and colleagues who have assisted by supplying references and by reading the proofs.

In every work of reference a good index is indispensable, and it was fortunate that the aid of one so skilled in indexing as Dr. J. C. Corson, Edinburgh University Library, was secured for this part of the task.

In conclusion, the author desires to thank the publishers most cordially for their unfailing courtesy and enthusiastic support at a time when publishing is attended by so many difficulties and restrictions.

D. G.

21 CLARENDON CRESCENT
EDINBURGH, *February 1945*

PREFACE TO REVISED EDITION, 1958

The very favourable reception of this work by reviewers and readers when first published in 1945, and the steady demand since then, not only for the British edition, but also for the American, Spanish, and German versions, seem to indicate a definite need for a one-volume history of medicine.

This edition contains much new material and many annotations. Most of those amendments have been incorporated in the text, but some of the more lengthy notes have been collected at the end of the book in the form of a Supplement. Many references to recent medico-historical research have been added, and it is hoped that this edition may prove of even greater interest to the general reader and of enhanced value to the more serious student of medical history.

D. G.

21 CLARENDON CRESCENT
EDINBURGH, *May 1958*

TO THE MEMORY OF MANY PRACTITIONERS
WHO, THOUGH UNKNOWN, HAVE ADVANCED
THE PROGRESS OF MEDICINE

Who knows whether the best of men be known, or
whether there be not more remarkable persons
forgot, than any that stand remembered in the
known account of time?

Sir Thomas Browne, *Hydriotaphia*

For the growing good of the world is partly dependent on unhistoric acts ; and that things are not so ill
with you and me as they might have been, is half
owing to the number who lived faithfully a hidden
life, and rest in unvisited tombs.

George Eliot, *Middlemarch*

And some there be, which have no memorial ;
   who are perished, as though they had never been ;
and are become as though they had never been born ;
   and their children after them.
But these were merciful men,
   whose righteousness hath not been forgotten. . . .
Their bodies are buried in peace ;
   but their name liveth for evermore.

Ecclesiasticus 44:9, 10, 14

CONTENTS

I THE GENESIS OF MEDICINE 1

Prehistoric Drawings, Tools, and Bones ; Primitive Man and His Concept of Disease ; The Problem of Death ; The Riddle of Disease ; Prehistoric Trephining or Trepanning ; Trephining as Practised by Modern Primitive Man ; The Motives for Trephining among Primitive Races ; Domestic Medicine or Folk Medicine ; Charms, Amulets, and Talismans ; The Powder of Sympathy ; The Origin of Medical Practice.

II THE FIRST KNOWN MEDICAL MEN 17

Medical Ethics in Babylonia ; Influence of Writing and the Calendar ; Sekhet'enanach and Imhotep ; The Medical Literature of Ancient Egypt ; Embalming and the Pathology of Mummies ; Medicine in the Bible ; Ancient Medicine of India ; China's Contribution to Medicine.

III EARLY GREEK MEDICINE 39

" Where Delos rose and Phoebus sprung " ; Apollo, and the Oracle of Delphi ; " Incubation " or Temple Sleep ; Homeric Medicine and Surgery ; Philosopher-Physicians of Ancient Greece.

IV HIPPOCRATIC MEDICINE 51

The Background to Hippocrates ; The Hippocratic Collection ; The Hippocratic Oath ; The Nature of Disease ; The Importance of Prognosis ; Hippocrates on Treatment ; The Aphorisms ; Aristotle and his Influence ; Medical Botanists.

V ALEXANDRIAN AND ROMAN MEDICINE 63

The Medical School of Alexandria ; Etruscans and Early Greek Settlers in Rome ; Roman Gibes at Greek Medicine, " Cito, tuto, et jucunde " ; Party Politics in Medicine ; Mithridaticum and Theriac ; A Follower of Hippocrates ; Celsus—*De re Medicina* ; Galen : the Medical Dictator ; Galen as Practitioner ; The First Experimental Physiologist ; The Blood in Motion, but not in Circulation ; Galen as Author ; The Byzantine Compilers ; Public Hygiene in Rome ; The State Medical Service of Ancient Rome ; The Roman Hospital System ; The Fall of Rome.

VI ARABIAN MEDICINE : THE SCHOOL OF SALERNO . 84

The Influence of Christianity upon Medicine ; The Dawn of Arabian Medicine ; The Nestorians and the School of Jundi-Shapur ; Rhazes and Avicenna ; Arabian Surgery in Spain ; Hospitals, and the End of the Moslem Empire ; Monastic Medicine; Patron Saints in Medicine ; St. Vitus's Dance and St. Anthony's Fire ; The School of Salerno ; The Medical Curriculum at Salerno ; Famous Graduates ; *Regimen Sanitatis Salernitatum.*

VII MEDIÆVAL MEDICINE 111

The Schools of Montpellier and Bologna ; Englishmen at Montpellier ; A Medical Pope ; Medicine and Surgery at Bologna ; Paris and Padua ; Roger Bacon and Albertus Magnus ; The Restoration of Anatomy ; Surgery also " Restored " ; English and German Surgeons ; The Black Death " ; Mediæval Hospitals ; Medical Illustrations ; The Herbal in Medical Literature.

VIII MEDICINE OF THE XV AND XVI CENTURIES. REFORMERS AND REVOLUTIONARIES 134

Art and Anatomy. Leonardo da Vinci ; The Truth about Anatomy. Andreas Vesalius ; The Pulmonary Circulation ; Fallopius and Eustachius ; Humane Surgery. Ambroise Paré ; *Journeys in Divers Places* ; " I Dressed Him and God Healed Him " ; Ambroise Paré at Court ; Itinerant Lithotomists ; Surgery in Italy and Germany ; English Surgery in . the Sixteenth Century. Early Scottish Physicians and Surgeons.

IX PHYSICIANS OF THE RENAISSANCE 156

The Enigma of Paracelsus ; Paracelsus as a Writer ; A Chemical View of Life ; The Mission of Paracelsus ; Astrology, Algebra, and Medicine ; A Consultation at Edinburgh ; The Versatile Physician ; The Origin of Syphilis ; Syphilis in Poetry ; The First Epidemiologist ; Early Physicians of England ; The Royal College of Physicians ; Oxford *v.* Cambridge ; The Sweating Sickness. Early English Medical Books ; *A Breviarie of Health* ; Pediatrics in England ; *The Byrth of Mankynde*.

X WILLIAM HARVEY AND HIS TIMES. XVII-CENTURY MEDICINE. 176

Philosophers and Scientists ; The Genius of William Harvey ; *De Motu Cordis et Sanguinis* ; Lacteals, Lymphatics, and Capillaries ; The Early Microscopists ; Societies and Journals ; Leyden, the Medical Centre.

XI SCIENCE AND SUPERSTITION. THE QUEST FOR A NEW BASIS 196

The Human Body ; Machine or Test-tube ? ; Clinical Medicine in England ; The Return to Hippocrates ; Thomas Sydenham ; The History of Cinchona ; The Great Plague of London ; The King's Evil and the Royal Touch ; *Religio Medici*.

XII XVIII-CENTURY MEDICINE 215

Animism and Vitalism ; Doses Large and Small ; Clinical Medicine under Boerhaave ; Pupils of Boerhaave ; The Old Vienna School ; Leyden and Edinburgh ; Influence of the Monros ; Foundation of the Edinburgh School ; The Teaching of Surgery ; Home, Whytt, and Gregory ; Medicine in the Army and Navy.

CONTENTS

XIII XVIII-CENTURY MEDICINE (*Continued*) 235
The Man-Midwife. Smellie and Hunter ; Eighteenth-Century Surgery ; "Why Think, Why not Try the Experiment? " ; Pupils and Contemporaries of John Hunter ; Applied Pathology ; Inoculation and Vaccination ; The Career of Edward Jenner ; Quaker and American Physicians ; *The Gold-headed Cane* ; Heberden and Withering ; Percussion and Auscultation ; Public Health and Hygiene ; Mesmerism, Phrenology, and Quackery.

XIV THE DAWN OF SCIENTIFIC MEDICINE IN THE XIX CENTURY 266
Sir Charles Bell and his Work ; The Tragedy of Robert Knox ; Anatomy under Henle and Hyrtl ; Physiology and Physics ; Pioneer British Physiologists ; The Genius of Claude Bernard ; Pathology and Bacteriology ; The Birth of a New Science.

XV XIX-CENTURY CLINICIANS 290
London and Edinburgh Physicians ; Clinical Medicine in Dublin, Paris, and Vienna ; Medical Pioneers in America ; A Bold First Ovariotomist ; The History of Anaesthesia ; Care of the Unborn Child.

XVI EARLY XIX-CENTURY SURGERY 307
Three Great London Surgeons ; Dupuytren, a Born Teacher ; Antecedents of the Antiseptic System ; The Tragedy of Puerperal Fever.

XVII LISTER AND HIS DISCIPLES 321
Early Life in Edinburgh and Glasgow ; The Antiseptic System ; Lister Returns to Edinburgh ; His Work and Later Years in London ; Disciples of Lister ; Abdominal Surgery Established ; Appendicitis Defined ; Surgery in America ; Specialism in Surgery.

XVIII MILITARY AND NAVAL SURGERY. CONQUEST OF TROPICAL DISEASE 337
Military Surgeons of Early Times ; Baron Larrey and the Practice of Military Surgery ; British Military Surgery ; Military Surgery in Germany and Russia ; The Teaching of Military Surgery ; The Royal Army Medical Corps ; Preventive Medicine in the Army ; The Surgery of Modern Warfare ; Medicine and Surgery in the Navy ; Medical Men as Explorers ; The Conquest of Tropical Disease.

XIX THE RISE OF SPECIALISM AND OF PREVENTIVE MEDICINE 363
Specialization in Medicine ; Disorders of Metabolism ; Diseases of the Heart ; Diseases of Children ; Neurology ; Psychiatry and Medical Psychology ; Ophthalmology ; Otology and Laryngology ; Dermatology and Venereal Diseases ; Radiology ; Medicine as a Career for Women ; The Growth of Preventive Medicine ; Philosophy and Health ; The Sanitary Idea ; Health as a National Problem ; Public Health in other Countries ; The Coming of Communal Medicine.

xi

CONTENTS

XX JOURNALISM, BIBLIOGRAPHY, AND MEDICAL
HISTORY 393
The Rise of Medical Journalism ; American Medical Journals ;
Medical Journals of France ; Medical Journalism in Germany
and other Countries ; Journals of Medical History ; Medical
Bibliography ; Medical Historians of Recent Times ; Osler
and Medical History ; Conclusion.

APPENDIX 412
A Classified Bibliography of Medical History.

GENERAL INDEX 421

SUPPLEMENT 449

xii

LIST OF PLATES

Facing page

I DISEASE IN ANCIENT TIMES 4
Fig. 1 from *The Antiquity of Disease*, by R. L. Moodie, 1923 ;
Fig. 2 from *Pithecanthropus Erectus*, by E. Dubois, 1894 ; Fig. 3
from *Studies in the Palaeopathology of Ancient Egypt*, by Sir Armand
Ruffer, 1921. (Figs. 1, 3 by courtesy of the Chicago University
Press)

II PREHISTORIC AND PRIMITIVE TREPHINING . . 5
Figs. 1, 2 from Muniz Collection (by courtesy of Smithsonian
Institution) ; Fig. 3 by courtesy of Royal Anthropological
Institute ; Fig. 4 from *Arab Medicine and Surgery* by Hilton-Simpson,
1922 (by courtesy of The Clarendon Press) ; Fig. 5 from London
Museum ; Fig. 6 from National Museum of Antiquities of Scotland

III TECHNIQUE OF PREHISTORIC TREPHINING . . 12
Figs. 1 to 4 by courtesy of Dr. T. Wilson Parry and the Editor of
Man

IV CHARMS, AMULETS, AND TALISMANS 13
Fig. 1 from *Amulets* by W. M. Flinders Petrie, 1914 (by courtesy
of Messrs. Constable) ; Figs. 2, 5, 6 from the Wellcome Historical Medical Museum ; Figs. 3, 4 by courtesy of the Society
of Antiquaries of Scotland

V MEDICAL LITERATURE IN BABYLON AND EGYPT 20
Fig. 1 from *The Seal Cylinders of Western Asia*, by W. Hayes Ward,
1910 (by courtesy of the Carnegie Institute of Washington) ;
Fig. 2 from *The Edwin Smith Surgical Papyrus*, ed. by J. H. Breasted,
1930 (by courtesy of the University of Chicago Press)

VI THE LIVER IN DIVINATION 21
Fig. 1 from the British Museum ; Fig. 2 from Museum of
Piacenza

VII THE FIRST KNOWN MEDICAL MAN : IMHOTEP . . 28
By courtesy of the Wellcome Historical Medical Museum

VIII DISEASE IN EGYPTIAN MUMMIES 29
Figs. 1, 2 from *Egyptian Mummies*, by Elliott Smith and
W. R. Dawson, 1924 ; Figs. 3, 4 from *Studies in the Palaeopathology
of Ancient Egypt* by Sir Armand Ruffer, 1921 (by courtesy of the
University of Chicago Press)

IX RELICS OF APOLLO, GOD OF HEALING . . . 32
Photographs by the Author

X EPIDAURUS, A CENTRE OF AESCULAPIAN HEALING 33
Photographs by the Author

XI THE ISLAND OF COS 48
Photographs by the Author

XII THE FATHER OF MEDICINE : HIPPOCRATES . . . 49
Statue found at Cos

XIII EARLY ROMAN SURGICAL INSTRUMENTS . . 84
From Naples Museum

XIV PUBLIC HEALTH IN THE ROMAN EMPIRE . . 85
Pont du Gard (photograph by the Author) ; Imperial Baths of
Caracalla, from *The Architecture of Greece and Rome* by Anderson
and Spiers, 1907 (by courtesy of Messrs. Batsford)

xiii

LIST OF PLATES

Facing page

XV EARLY ARABIAN SURGERY 92
From Avicenna's *Canon of Medicine* (Latin ed. 1608)

XVI CORDOVA, CENTRE OF ARABIAN CULTURE IN
WEST 93
From *Spain* by Albert F. Calvert, 1911

XVII ARABIAN SURGICAL INSTRUMENTS 96
From *Chirurgia* of Albucasis (Arabic and Latin ed., 1778)

XVIII THE PATRON SAINTS OF SURGERY: 97
By courtesy of Professor Charles Singer

XIX SURGICAL PRACTICE AT SALERNO 112
From Sloane MS. 1977 in the British Museum

XX A MEDIEVAL SPA: PLOMBIÈRES 113
Woodcut from *De Balneis*, Venice, 1553 (from the National
Library of Turin)

XXI THE LEGEND OF MANDRAGORA 116
Figs. 3, 4 from *English Medicine in Anglo-Saxon Times* by
J. F. Payne, 1904 (Clarendon Press)

XXII ANATOMY IN MEDIEVAL TIMES 117
From *Chirurgia Magna* by Guy de Chauliac (a 14th cent. MS.)

XXIII A MEDIEVAL HOSPITAL: RHODES 124
Photograph by the Author

XXIV THE KNIGHTS OF ST. JOHN AT RHODES . . 125
Photographs by the Author

XXV ZODIAC MAN 128
From *Fasciculus Medicinae* by Johannes de Ketham, 1491

XXVI MECHANICAL AIDS TO MEDICINE AND SURGERY 129
Fig. 1 from *Cirurgia* by Brunschwig, 1497 ; Fig. 2 from
Feldtbuch der Wundartzney by Gersdorff, 1517

XXVII VESALIUS TEACHING ANATOMY 144
Title-page of *Fabrica* by Vesalius, 1543

XXVIII SURGERY UNDER AMBROISE PARÉ 145
Fig. 1 from a miniature in a contemporary MS. at the Hôtel-
Dieu, Paris ; Fig. 2 from *The Works of that famous chirurgeon,
Ambrose Parey* (Eng. trans., 1678)

XXIX SIXTEENTH-CENTURY SURGERY 148
From *A Discourse of the Whole Art of Chyrurgery* by Peter Lowe,
1654

XXX THE BARBER-SURGEONS RECEIVE THEIR
CHARTER 149
Painting in the Royal College of Surgeons of England (by
courtesy of Professor A. J. Cave and the Royal College of
Surgeons of England)

XXXI MEDICINE AND MATHEMATICS: JEROME CARDAN 156
From *De Subtilitate* by Cardan, 1551

XXXII CAIUS COLLEGE, CAMBRIDGE: THE GATE OF
HONOUR 157
From *Cambridge* by John Steegman (Batsford) ; photograph
by permission of A. F. Kersting

XXXIII "THE BREVIARIE OF HEALTH" 176
Title-page from a copy of the book (1557 edition) in the
Hunterian Library, Glasgow University

xiv

Facing page

XXXIV BIRTH SCENE IN THE SIXTEENTH CENTURY . 177
From a copy of *De Conceptu et Generatione Hominis* by Rueff,
1554, in Edinburgh University Library

XXXV THE PHYSICIAN'S VISIT 180
From the Stephenson Clarke Collection (by courtesy of
Colonel Stephenson Clarke)

XXXVI THE VALVES OF THE VEINS 181
Fig. 1 from *De Venarum Ostiolis* by Fabricius, 1603; Figs. 2, 3
from *De Motu Cordis* by Harvey, 1628

XXXVII HARVEY AND THE KING 188
From a painting by R. Hannah in the Royal College of
Physicians of London

XXXVIII EARLY MICROSCOPES 189
Fig. 1 from *Antony van Leeuwenhoek and his " Little Animals "*
by Clifford Dobell, 1932 (John Bale & Sons) ; Fig. 2 from
Micrographia by Robert Hooke, 1665

XXXIX DECORATIVE ANATOMY 192
From *Thesaurus Anatomicus* by Ruysch, 1701

XL AN EARLY EXPONENT OF METABOLISM:
SANCTORIUS 193
From *Medicina Statica* by Sanctorius, 1614.

XLI THE ANATOMY OF THE BRAIN 208
Fig. 1 from *Cerebri Anatome* by Thomas Willis, 1664 ; Fig. 2
from *De Homine* by Descartes, 1662

XLII THE GREAT PLAGUE OF LONDON 209
From *Loimotomia* by George Thomson, 1666

XLIII THE ROYAL GIFT OF HEALING 224
From *Adenochoiradelogia* by John Browne, 1684

XLIV A MEDICAL LECTURE AT LEYDEN . . . 225
Title-page of *De Comparando Certo in Physicis* by Boerhaave,
1715

XLV THE FOUNDER OF THE GLASGOW SCHOOL:
WILLIAM CULLEN 228
From an engraving by T. Sommers in the National Portrait
Gallery of Scotland of the painting by W. Cochrane

XLVI THE FOUNDER OF THE EDINBURGH SCHOOL:
ALEXANDER MONRO 229
From engraving by J. Basire of the painting by Allan Ramsay

XLVII EDINBURGH DOCTORS OF THE EIGHTEENTH
CENTURY 236
From Kay's *Edinburgh Portraits*

XLVIII ARTISTIC OSTEOLOGY 237
From *Osteographia* by Cheselden, 1733

XLIX THE MASTER OF BRITISH MIDWIFERY: WILLIAM
SMELLIE 240
From a painting in the Royal College of Surgeons of Edin-
burgh

L EARLY PATTERNS OF OBSTETRIC FORCEPS . 241

LI THE WORK OF JOHN HUNTER 256

LII THE MEDICAL SOCIETY OF LONDON . . . 257
From a painting by Samuel Medley in the Society's house

Facing page

LIII EIGHTEENTH-CENTURY PHYSICIANS AND QUACKS 260
From a cartoon by Hogarth

LIV A STUDENT'S CLASS CARDS, EARLY NINE-
TEENTH CENTURY. 261

LV CERTIFICATE OF SIR CHARLES BELL'S CLASS . 268
Original in the Royal College of Surgeons of Edinburgh

LVI LAËNNEC'S STETHOSCOPE. 269
From *Traité de l'Auscultation Médiate*, 1818

LVII THE CONQUEST OF RABIES 276
Statue in courtyard of Pasteur Institute of Paris

LVIII PATIENT AND DOCTOR IN THE NINETEENTH
CENTURY 277
Fig. 1, Rahere Ward, St. Bartholomew's Hospital, by courtesy
of Mr. Sidney Scott ; Fig. 2, Dr. Joseph Bell, by courtesy of
Mrs. Cecil Shisted

LIX BRIGHT AND BRIGHT'S DISEASE 284
From *Reports of Medical Cases* by Bright, 1827

LX AMERICAN PIONEERS: DANIEL DRAKE, EPHRAIM
McDOWELL 285

LXI THE FIRST USE OF ETHER ANAESTHESIA IN
BRITAIN 304
From a painting formerly in the Wellcome Historical Medical
Museum, London

LXII A LECTURE ON SURGERY: JAMES SYME . . . 305
From a sketch in the Museum of the Royal College of Surgeons
of Edinburgh

LXIII LISTER AND HIS FELLOW HOUSE-SURGEONS . 320
From *Looking Back* by John Chiene (1907), by courtesy of
Messrs. Oliver & Boyd

LXIV LISTER'S EXPERIMENT 321
Facsimile page from W. S. Anderson's notebook

LXV AN OPERATION AT ABERDEEN IN LISTER'S DAY 324
Photograph supplied by Charles A. Wilson, Aberdeen

LXVI THE MAYO CLINIC 325
By courtesy of Dr. Donald C. Balfour and the Mayo Foundation

LXVII NAPOLEON'S CHIEF SURGEON: BARON LARREY . 332

LXVIII A DIRECTOR-GENERAL OF MEDICAL SERVICES:
SIR JAMES McGRIGOR 333

LXIX THE INVENTOR OF THE LARYNGOSCOPE : MANUEL
GARCIA 384
From a painting by John F. Sargent, by courtesy of Rhode
Island School of Design

LXXX A NEW KIND OF RAY 385
Radiogram taken by Roentgen

LXXI THE EARLIEST MEDICAL JOURNAL IN ENGLISH : 400
Medicina Curiosa, 1684, by courtesy of the Wellcome Historical
Medical Museum

LXXII OSLER WRITING HIS TEXT-BOOK 401
From *The Life of Sir William Osler*, by permission of Sir
Humphrey Milford

A HISTORY OF MEDICINE

CHAPTER I

THE GENESIS OF MEDICINE

" NOTHING more difficult than a beginning," wrote Byron of Poetry, and his remark may be fitly applied to the History of Medicine, for it is no easy task to describe the means by which our primitive ancestors discovered and developed the art of healing. Indeed, the whole vast subject of beginnings in Medicine is largely a matter of conjecture. There are, of course, no written records, and even such prehistoric drawings as have survived represent a relatively late phase in the evolution of Stone Age man ; moreover, they are liable to be misinterpreted.

Prehistoric Drawings, Tools, and Bones

Magicians or medicine men constitute the oldest professional class in the evolution of society.[1] On the wall of the Trois Frères Cave in the Pyrenees is a drawing which is probably the oldest known portrait of a " medical man," or, rather, of a " medicine man " or sorcerer.[2] Arrayed in the skin of some animal, his limbs adorned with stripes of paint and his head with a pair of large antlers, this terrifying personage closely resembles the African " witch doctor " of recent times. Artist and model are said to have been members of the Aurignacian race, living about 15,000 B.C., a relatively recent date for the Stone Age epoch, which is said to have lasted for some 500,000 years. Dates in prehistory can never be regarded as exact, and are, at best, merely rough estimates.

Numerous stone and flint implements have been found and described as the tools and weapons of prehistoric man. Some of them may well have been employed as surgical instruments, just as the Australian aboriginal still uses a flint knife in ritual circumcision.

[1] R. A. S. Macalister, *Textbook of European Archæology*, 1921, vol. i. p. 133
[2] W. J. Sollas, *Ancient Hunters*, 1911, p. 400 ; M. C. Burkitt, *Pre-history : A Study of Early Cultures in Europe and the Mediterranean Basin*, Cambridge, 1921, p. 257

More informative than any other relics are the skeletal remains of prehistoric man. Bones of palæolithic and of neolithic dates have shown definite evidence of osteo-arthritis and of tuberculosis, while the femur of the ape-like Pithecanthropus erectus, discovered in Java by Dr. Dubois in 1891,[1] bears a large bony tumour or exostosis near its upper end (Plate 1). Pithecanthropus was a member of a very primitive race of ape-men which became extinct about 400,000 years ago. Disease is much older than man himself, as Professor Roy Moodie has proved by his discovery in Wyoming of a dinosaur (Apatosaurus) with a bony tumour in the caudal vertebrae (Plate 1). The age of such a pathological specimen must be measured in millions of years.

Still more remarkable are the numerous prehistoric skulls which bear unmistakable evidence of the operation of trephining. Prehistoric trephining was performed long before any other surgical procedure was contemplated, and it deserves special consideration. It may be convenient, however, to defer further reference to the subject until the motives which prompted its performance have been mentioned. To this question—the attitude of primitive man towards disease—let us now turn our attention.

We have seen that the direct sources of information on the prehistory of medicine are scanty. Nevertheless, there remain certain indirect lines of investigation which deserve careful study. These are, firstly, the beliefs and customs of primitive man as he still exists, the miscalled " savage " of modern times ; and secondly, the folk medicine which has passed from generation to generation down the centuries, and which is still practised to-day in many parts of the world.

Primitive Man and His Concept of Disease

Although it seems perfectly legitimate to argue that prehistoric man in ancient times behaved in the same manner as primitive man to-day, one must bear in mind two possible errors in such an argument.

Man's evolution is not always in an upward direction, consequently primitive man of modern times may represent a degenerate type, even less intelligent than his prehistoric ancestor.

[1] E. Dubois, *Pithecanthropus Erectus, eine menschenaenliche Uebergangsform aus Java*, Batavia, 1894; M. Boule, *Fossil Men: Elements of Human Palæontology*, trans. by J. Ritchie, Edinburgh, 1923, Chap. IV

Again, there must be very few primitive native-communities to-day which have not reacted for better or worse to the impact of modern civilization, and there is therefore a limited field for anthropological research. The field is steadily narrowing, and little can be learned from the native races segregated in " reserves," as in a sort of human zoo.

Nevertheless, much valuable information regarding primitive medicine has been collected during recent times, in spite of the difficulties imposed by the march of time in a rapidly shrinking world, and, by analogy, one is justified in concluding that the manners and customs of primitive man to-day (or at all events until quite recently) closely resemble those of his prehistoric prototype.

The Problem of Death

At a very early stage in his evolution prehistoric man must have sought a solution for the age-long problem of death. No doubt he believed, as does primitive man of modern times, that man was at first destined to be immortal.[1] Death came as a punishment for man's disobedience. According to a Central African (Bantu) legend, man was at one time capable of renewing his youth by casting his skin each time he grew old, but it was essential that the process should take place in secret. One old man indiscreetly allowed his granddaughter to witness the operation, and thus so aroused the wrath of the gods that the boon was for ever withdrawn.[2] The well-known Biblical version of the tradition is that the eating of the forbidden fruit in the Garden of Eden " brought Death into the world, and all our woe."

Even a brief consideration of the innumerable beliefs connected with death would take us far from our present subject. Rather let us study the attitude of primitive man towards disease.

The Riddle of Disease

In whatever part of the world we investigate the matter we shall find the same result, namely, that primitive man does not admit the existence of disease from what we call natural causes.

[1] Sir J. G. Frazer, The Golden Bough, 3rd ed. 1890–1915, vol. ii. p. 95
[2] W. R. Dawson, Magician and Leech : a Study in the Beginnings of Medicine, 1929, p. 3 ; R. H. Codrington, The Melanesians, 1891, p. 260 ; T. Besterman, " The Belief in Re-birth among the Natives of Africa," Folk-lore, 1930, vol. xli. pp. 42–94

Invariably disease is viewed as the result of malevolent influence exercised by a god or supernatural being or by another human being, alive or dead. In other words, disease is a magical or magico-religious rather than a natural phenomenon.

W. H. R. Rivers, whose researches in Melanesia are well known, tells us that " a case of snake bite is not ascribed to the act which according to our ideas is natural to a venomous animal, but it is believed that the snake has been put in the path of the victim by a sorcerer, or has been endowed with special powers by a sorcerer, or it may even be held that the animal which has bitten the victim is no ordinary snake, but the sorcerer himself in snake-like form." [1]

Reasoning in this fashion, primitive man ascribes disease to two possible causes : (a) the projection of some morbid material or influence into the victim ; and (b) the abstraction of the soul from the body of the victim. As an example of the first cause there may be mentioned the custom of " pointing the bone," which prevails to this day in Australia. The aboriginal of Central Australia is universally admitted to be the most primitive type of man in the world to-day, and to this race the attention of many able anthropologists has been directed. [2] The "bone," which is used with malevolent intent, is a long slender stick marked with rings to indicate the number of victims. It is held in a special way and pointed towards the victim, the ritual being accompanied by a song appropriate to the occasion. [3] The bone is then buried, and the aggressor awaits the illness of his enemy. The latter, learning that he has been " boned," is not slow to respond to the suggestion, and has been known even to die of sheer fright. In other cases, the onset of illness is the first indication to the sick man that a bone has been pointed at him. In any event, the friends of the patient search for the bone, and if they find it recovery is rapid. They also seek retribution from the aggressor, who receives a severe mauling or may even be killed.

As for the actual treatment of the sick, this is carried out by the medicine man, who proceeds to extract the evil influence by suction. He then expectorates into his hand, and lo, the victim beholds in the palm of the doctor a small rock crystal, the cause of all his trouble. Needless to add, the patient then

[1] W. H. R. Rivers, *Medicine, Magic, and Religion*, 1924, p. 10
[2] W. B. Spencer and F. J. Gillen, *The Native Tribes of Central Australia*, 1899
[3] A. W. Howitt, *The Native Tribes of South-east Australia*, 1904, p. 359 ; Sir Baldwin Spencer, *Wanderings in Wild Australia*, 1928, vol. i. p. 251

PLATE I   DISEASE IN ANCIENT TIMES

Bone tumour of caudal vertebrae of a large dinosaur, Apatosaurus (page 2)

Femur of Pithecanthropus Erectus, showing a bony outgrowth (page 2)

Spondylitis deformans in an ancient Nubian of pre-Dynastic times.   Several
lumbar vertebrae are fused into a solid mass by osteo-arthritis (page 29)

PLATE II   PREHISTORIC AND PRIMITIVE TREPHINING

Ancient Peruvian skull ;
cross-cut trephining (page 7)

Ancient Peruvian skull ; multiple
trephining at different dates

Skull of modern Melanesian, trephined by native method (page 8)

Skull from Aures Mountains,
Algeria, trephined by modern
native surgeon (page 9)

The " Thames " skull, probably of
Neolithic Age, showing trephined
opening (page 7)

Skull of Early Bronze Age, found
in Bute. Opening may be result
of trephining (page 8)

feels better, and soon recovers. In Melanesia, disease is believed to be produced in a manner very similar to bone-pointing, by a weapon called the "tamatetikwa," or ghost-shooter. It consists of a hollow bamboo containing fragments of a dead man's bones. When the enemy is sighted, the open end of the tube is uncovered, and the evil spirit leaps out upon the victim.[1]

The second widely held belief is that disease is caused by the separation of the soul from the body. In Borneo, where this idea prevails, the dayong or professional soul-catcher is called to treat the patient. Dr. Charles Hose has described the technique of soul-catching in his fascinating book.[2] The ceremony is conducted by torch-light, the patient lying in the centre of a large circle of friends and onlookers. The dayong falls into a trance, and sends out his own soul to find that of the patient, and to persuade it to return. With closed eyes he chants an account of the journey in search of the soul. At last, emerging from his hypnotic state, the soul-catcher, like the Australian medicine man, exhibits a pebble or bead containing the soul. This is rubbed on the head of the patient, and then the soul, restored to its habitat, is prevented from escaping again by tying a strip of palm-leaf round the wrist. The dayong also undertakes to extract pain from the human body by suction through a tube, from which, in the true fashion of the conjurer, he produces small black pellets of wax to show that his efforts have been successful.

Such observations would appear to show that to primitive man in modern times, and probably also in prehistoric times, disease is, and was, attributed to supernatural causes, and treated by methods resembling those employed by the psycho-therapist to-day. Truly there is nothing new under the sun, and although the details vary, the underlying principle has persisted through the centuries.

Prehistoric Trephining or Trepanning

Let us now consider this strange surgical operation of which we find such definite evidence in skulls of prehistoric date from various parts of the world, and which is still practised by certain primitive people.

[1] Sir J. G. Frazer, *The Fear of the Dead in Primitive Religion*, 1933, p. 155 ; W. H. R. Rivers, *Medicine, Magic, and Religion*, 1924, p. 13
[2] Charles Hose, *Natural Man, a Record from Borneo*, 1926, pp. 215, 239

In 1865 Dr. Prunières of Marvejols, near the Cevennes, a general practitioner interested in archæology, discovered in a dolmen at Aiguières in Central France a skull bearing in the occipital region a large artificial opening with smooth edges. Along with the skull he found a number of rounded or irregular pieces of bone, which appeared to have been cut from another skull. He concluded that the skull had been perforated so that it might be used as a drinking cup, a custom not uncommon in primitive races, and one which might well have obtained in neolithic times.[1] Shortly afterwards a number of other holed skulls were found in Brittany and other parts of France, and Professor Paul Broca of Paris in 1876 [2] showed that Dr. Prunières had been mistaken in his conclusions, and that the openings in the skulls were the result of the operation of trepanning or trephining, which, he stated, was often performed upon the children of the dolmen people (late neolithic). The instrument employed was a flint scraper. Furthermore, Broca suggested that those who survived this operation were endowed with mystical powers, and that, when these individuals died, portions of their skulls, preferably including a part of the edge of the artificial opening, were greatly in demand as charms or amulets against epilepsy or mental disease. Thus he explained the fragments of skull which Prunières had found, and to these pieces of bone, usually of circular form and often pierced so as to be worn as a necklace, there was applied the name " rondelles." [3] The entire margin of the trephined aperture was not removed. Sufficient was left for the needs of the owner of the skull in the next world, and in some cases the abstracted portions were replaced by pieces of bone from other skulls (Plate III).

Further discoveries followed, and it soon became apparent that the operation had not been performed upon children only, as Broca had suggested. Indeed, the trephined skulls were all those of adults ; not a single trephined child's skull was ever found. It was also noted that the majority of them showed unmistakable evidence of healing ; in other words, the edges of the opening were rounded and smooth, showing that the patient had survived the ordeal, and had lived for some years afterwards.

[1] P.-B. Prunières, " Sur les crânes artificiellement perforés et les rondelles crâniennes à l'époque des dolmens," *Bull. Soc. d'Anthrop. de Paris*, 1874, vol. ix. p. 185
[2] P. Broca, " Sur l'âge des sujets à la trépanation chirurgicale néolithique," *Bull. Soc. d'Anthrop. de Paris*, 1876, vol. xi. p. 572
[3] J. Dechelette, *Manuel d'Archéologie Préhistorique*, Paris, 1924, p. 476

In rare cases, more than one trephining has been performed and a skull showing five distinct perforations has been found in Peru. Dr. Muniz, who in 1894 examined 1,000 skulls, probably of pre-Incan age, found that nineteen of them had been trephined.[1] Three of these showed two, and one showed three, distinct operations (Plate II). In some of the Peruvian skulls the opening is not oval, but quadrilateral. The instrument used was the T-shaped knife or " tumi," which has been adopted as the emblem of the Peruvian Academy of Surgery.

Since the publication of Broca's paper numerous specimens of trephined skulls of neolithic man have been found in France, and also, though in smaller numbers, in Austria, Poland, Russia, Germany, and Spain. Until recently, only two authentic specimens had been found in Britain. One of them, an adult male skull, was dredged from the bed of the Thames in 1864 close to the present Hammersmith Bridge. At this place, there appears to have been a number of pile-dwellings, as the discovery of various objects of stone and bronze indicates. The skull, which is probably of neolithic period, shows an opening in the centre of the vertex, an unusual site, and the subject of the trephining was indeed fortunate to escape death by injury to his superior longitudinal venous sinus (Plate II).

The second British specimen was found in 1863 in a dolmen near Bisley, in Gloucestershire, by Dr. W. H. Paine. In this skull the operation is incomplete ; a circular groove has been made in the frontal area, but the disc of bone is not separated. The patient may have died during the procedure or the surgeon may have failed, for some reason, to complete his task.

Several other holed skulls have come to light in Britain, and Dr. T. Wilson Parry, who has given much attention to the subject, has described two other specimens, both found in Dorset. From each skull a large disc of bone had been removed, probably with the aid of a flint saw or scraper. As the cut margin showed no sign of healing, death had probably resulted from the operation [2] (Plate III).

Among the doubtful British specimens is the skull of a young

[1] M. A. Muniz and W. J. McGee, " Primitive Trephining in Peru," *Report Bureau Ethnol.*, *1894-95*, Washington, 1897, vol. xvi. pp. 1–72
[2] T. Wilson Parry, " The Prehistoric Trephined Skulls of Great Britain," *Proc. Roy. Soc. Med.* (Sect. Hist.), vol. xiv. p. 1 ; " Trephination of the Living Skull in Prehistoric Times," *B.M.J.*, 1923, vol. i. p. 457 ; " Two Prehistoric Skulls, lately excavated in the county of Dorset," *Man*, 1940, No. 46, p. 33

woman which was found in a cist at Mount Stuart, Isle of Bute, together with a jet necklace, an urn, and a small fragment of bronze. The skull, which shows a hole in the left frontal bone an inch above the outer angle of the orbit, surrounded by a dense thickened rim of bone, was described by Dr. Robert Munro in 1891,[1] and is now in the museum of the Society of Antiquaries of Scotland. (Plate II.) It is uncertain whether the aperture was produced by trephining or by disease of the bone.

Trephining as Practised by Modern Primitive Man

Our knowledge of prehistoric trephining would be very meagre indeed were it not for the fact that the operation is still performed, or was performed until very recent times, by primitive races in some widely separated parts of the world, such as the South Pacific Islands, Caucasia, and Algeria.[2]

From Melanesia many skulls have been collected which show perforations closely resembling those found in neolithic specimens. They have been found in New Guinea and the neighbouring Bismarck Archipelago, and also in New Caledonia and the adjoining islands of the Loyalty Group.[3] All the trephined openings show healed edges, suggesting that recovery from the operation was the rule. The Rev. J. A. Crump[4] stated that in New Britain the operation was practised solely in cases of fracture, a common occurrence in tribal fights. The instrument employed was a piece of shell or obsidian (volcanic natural glass), and the wound was dressed with strips of banana stalk, which is very absorbent. The mortality was about twenty per cent., but many deaths resulted from the original injury rather than from the operation (Plate II).

In certain other islands of the South Pacific the operation is (or was until recently) performed to cure epilepsy, headache, and insanity ; while it is stated that in New Ireland, an island north of New Guinea, a large number of natives had undergone trephining in youth as an aid to longevity.

The practice of trephining in Asia is described by a writer

[1] R. Munro, *Prehistoric Scotland and its Place in European Civilization* (1899), p. 213
[2] F. Terrier and M. Péraire, *L'Opération du Trépan*, Paris, 1895
[3] I. Brodsky, " The Trephiners of Blanche Bay, New Britain," *Brit. Journ. Surg.*, 1938–39, vol. xxvi. p. 1.
[4] J. A. Crump, " Trephining in the South Seas," *Jour. Anthrop. Inst. London*, 1901, vol. xxxi. p. 167

to *The Lancet* in 1888,[1] who tells us that the inhabitants of the Caucasian province of Daghestan, bordering on the Caspian Sea, employ it for all head injuries, and that the aggressor is obliged to pay the " surgeon " for his services.

The best recent account of trephining by primitive man in modern times is given by Hilton-Simpson, in his book on Arab medicine and surgery.[2] The author visited the Aures Mountains, north-east of Biskra in Algeria, on four occasions. Gaining the confidence of the native practitioners, he was able to study their methods at first hand. One wishes that there had been more expeditions of this nature, as the literature on primitive medicine in modern times is far too scanty. The art of medicine in the Aures is hereditary, the knowledge being passed on from father to son. Its origin is obscure. It might be argued that here we find a degenerate form of Greek or classical medicine, and such a possibility cannot be denied, although of course the argument could not apply to the primitive medicine and surgery of Melanesia which so closely resembles that of North Africa. Hilton-Simpson describes the use of drugs collected and prepared from various local plants. He also attributes to those Arab doctors a sound acquaintance with the principles of surgery. Splints are used for fractures, dislocations are reduced, circumcisions and litho-tomy are practised, and even the operations of bone grafting to replace a bone destroyed by injury or disease. The bone of a freshly killed dog or sheep is employed, and the results are very successful.

One is not surprised to learn that trephining is also commonly performed by these people, always as a treatment of some form of head injury, usually a fracture, the result of a blow (Plate II). In operating, two rules are carefully observed, namely, the opening must not involve any of the sutures, and the dura mater must be carefully preserved from injury. The operation consists in removing a circular portion of scalp with a cylindrical iron punch, heated red-hot, and then cutting the opening in the bone by the confined use of a small drill and a metal saw. The instruments, which are hafted in wooden handles, are of various shapes. One of them closely resembles the more modern " Hey's saw." Hilton-Simpson's offer of a modern trephine was declined by those Arab surgeons, who preferred to use their own

[1] Krivyakin, " Trephining in Daghestan," *Lancet*, 1888, vol. i. p. 138
[2] M. W. Hilton-Simpson, *Arab Medicine and Surgery*, 1922

tools, cast by the local native jewellers. The set acquired by Hilton-Simpson may be seen in the Pitt-Rivers Museum at Oxford. The results of the operation are said to be very satisfactory.

The Motives for Trephining among Primitive Races

It is not surprising that the problem of primitive trephining has engaged the attention of many distinguished archæologists, and many theories have been advanced to explain the motives which induced neolithic man to practise this serious operation.[1] Attempts have been made to classify the indications as (*a*) a ritual or magical rite, and (*b*) a therapeutic measure. Such a classification ignores the fact that no clear-cut distinction can be drawn between these two motives. All who have studied the early history of medicine have noted that the physician was at first a priest, and that the religious and medical duties were intimately intermingled.

Mention has already been made of the concept of disease in the mind of prehistoric man, and it seems reasonable to accept the notion, to which many authorities subscribe, that trephining was originally performed in order to cast out a demon which had taken possession of the individual. The absence of any sign of cranial injury in the holed skulls of neolithic origin lends support to this view. Such cases of devil possession would to-day be diagnosed as epilepsy, mental disease, cerebral tumour, tic douloureux, migraine, etc. No one can read in the New Testament the account of the epileptic boy without admitting that, to one ignorant of neurology, a logical explanation was that the youth was in the grip of a demon. Further, what treatment could be more obvious than to make an opening in his head so that the evil spirit could escape ? It also seemed reasonable to attribute magical powers to those who survived the operation, and to use as charms or talismans pieces of bone (rondelles) cut from the edge of the trephined opening, when at length the patients died from some other cause.

As time went on trephining was employed in cases of fracture of the cranial vault, which must have been very common in the

[1] J. F. Horne, *Trephining in its Ancient and Modern Aspect*, 1894 ; M. Braune, *Die Geschichte der Trepanation*, Berlin, 1875 ; M. A. Ruffer, "Studies in Paleopathology : some recent researches on prehistoric trephining," *Jour. Path. and Bact.*, 1918, vol. xxii. p. 90

Stone Age, and thus we find evidence of fracture in many of the skulls discovered in Peru, where the Inca civilization persisted as late as the sixteenth century.

Among the Melanesians of comparatively recent times the reasons for trephining appear to have been headache, vertigo, epilepsy, and like disorders, as well as cranial injury, while the Arab surgeons of Algeria only a few years ago still practised trephining solely for injury resulting from a blow on the head.

Considering those facts, one cannot accept the view of Dr. Guiard that trephining was originally a treatment for head injuries, and was gradually extended to cases of migraine, neuralgia, and epilepsy.[1]

Primitive trephining illustrates one of the leading facts of medical history, namely, that medicine was at first in the hands of the priests, and that not until the days of Hippocrates did the healing art take its rightful place, and was no longer merely a branch of magic or of religion.

Domestic Medicine or Folk Medicine

As has been already remarked, the " medicine " of prehistoric man was probably based upon an animistic attitude towards disease. In his view, disease was caused by the evil influence of an enemy, a demon, a god, or even an animal, and it must accordingly be treated by means calculated to dislodge the malevolent cause from the body of the patient. Like the present-day native of Borneo, early man may have attributed disease to a separation of soul and body. In any case, there doubtless arose a class of men who claimed skill in the art of healing, and whose methods of treatment included exorcism, incantations, dancing, grimacing, sleight of hand, and all the tricks of the magician.

In some cases it was deemed necessary to combine physical with psychical methods ; of this we have an excellent example in trephining, which originated as a means of permitting the escape of an evil spirit from the head of the victim, and which gradually became a method of treating fractures of the skull and various intracranial lesions.

Massage, another means of inducing the evil spirit to leave

[1] E. Guiard, *La Trépanation crânienne chez les Néolithiques et chez les primitifs modernes*, Paris, 1930

the body, consisted in stroking the limbs in a centrifugal direction
—that is, towards the extremities.[1]   Later, as devil possession
gave place to more enlightened pathology, the direction of the
massage changed and was applied in a centripetal direction.
The unpleasant taste and disgusting nature of many of the older
prescriptions may also indicate a determination to dislodge from
the body of the patient the supernatural intruder causing the
disease.

Another curious and ancient method of treating disease, and
one still in use to-day, was based on the belief that the disease
might be transferred from the patient to another individual, to
an animal, or even to a plant.[2]   Not so very many years ago
a touch from the hand of a corpse was regarded as a cure for
many diseases, which the dead man then took with him on his
long journey.   Best of all was the touch of an executed criminal,
and many a fee did the hangman receive for granting this boon
to the sick.

In Lancashire, warts were treated by touching each wart
with a pebble.   The pebbles were then placed in a bag, which
was intentionally " lost " as the patient proceeded on his way
to church.   Whoever found the bag acquired the warts.   From
Cheshire came a remedy for aphthous ulcers of the mouth, consisting in holding a live frog in the mouth for a few moments,
and then allowing it to escape.   A somewhat similar treatment,
this time for whooping cough, was until lately practised in
Cumberland.[3]   The head of a freshly caught fish was introduced for a minute or so into the child's mouth, and the fish was
then returned to the river, " taking the whooping cough with it."

To cure toothache, according to a widespread belief, it was
merely necessary to scarify the gum with a nail, and then drive
the nail into an oak tree.   A somewhat similar belief may have
inspired those inhabitants of Selborne, who, according to Gilbert
White (Letter LXX), cleft young ash trees asunder in order that
naked children suffering from rupture might be passed through
the gap.   The ceremony over, the tree was bound together, and
as it grew together and healed, so also did the child become cured
of rupture.   From all these examples it would appear that " casting
out " or " transference " was the dominant factor in the primitive

[1] M. Bartels, *Die Medizin der Naturvölker*, Leipzig, 1893, p. 145
[2] D. McKenzie, *The Infancy of Medicine*, 1927, p. 84
[3] W. G. Black, *Folk Medicine* (Folk-lore Society publication), 1883, pp. 36, 41, 100

PLATE III TECHNIQUE OF PREHISTORIC TREPHINING

Skull of Early Bronze Age, with large trephined opening, found in Crichel Down, Dorset, in 1938. Fig. on right shows excised bone replaced (page 7)

Experiments to illustrate trephining by means of a flint scraper, showing two stages of the operation (page 7)

Cranial amulets from dolmens in France. (*l.*) An irregular fragment with margin of trephined hole in centre of the lower margin ($\frac{1}{2}$ natural size). The other two specimens (natural size) are " rondelles," one of them perforated for use as a charm (page 6)

PLATE IV   CHARMS, AMULETS, AND TALISMANS

(*l.*) Ancient Egyptian enamel charm, representing the eye of Horus (page 20).
(*r.*) Amulet inscribed *Richardson's Magneto-Galvanic Battery*, and on the reverse
Pat. in U.S. 1880.   Sold as cure for rheumatism

The Lee Penny, or Talisman, described by Sir Walter Scott (page 14)

(*l.*) Wart-like stone, from Ottery St. Mary, Devon, 1910, used for curing
warts (page 12).   (*r.*) Stone resembling a tooth, used to cure toothache

treatment of disease. In the bed of the River Dee near Aberdeen there is a large stone, perforated by the action of the water, and known locally as " The Deil's Needle." It was believed that to crawl through the opening was a cure for sterility in women.[1]

Nevertheless primitive man became gradually convinced that not all diseases were caused by supernatural agents. There were minor maladies which could be simply cured by homely remedies, and in such cases it was unnecessary to call in the sorcerer or medicine man. Few persons to-day consult a doctor for a common cold ; so also did prehistoric man employ his witch doctor only when ordinary domestic remedies had proved unavailing.

The discovery of these remedies must have been a very gradual process. Just as cats and dogs eat grasses as their medicines, so did primitive man discover the therapeutic value of certain plants. By painful experience he distinguished between the poisonous and the harmless, and although his methods of treatment included much magic and superstition he evolved a system of domestic medicine of which traces remain in every nation to this day. To mention a very simple example : early man, finding that contact with a nettle caused itching and burning, found that this was relieved by applying the nearest cool broad leaf available, which happened to be a dock or sorrel leaf, a treatment still employed by some country children to-day.

The best remedies of folk medicine still form the basis of modern herbalism, and there is a good deal of sound teaching in the art, although unfortunately there is also much charlatanism.

Charms, Amulets, and Talismans

A study of folk medicine reveals many curious beliefs, yet it is worthy of study and forms an important part of medical history. The remedies were not always taken internally ; some of them were worn or carried as charms or talismans. Who has not met some friend who keeps his rheumatism in check by carrying in his pocket a raw potato, or the right forefoot of a hare ? Belief in such mascots is almost universal. The skin of a snake, the patella of a sheep, the nail of a coffin, and all manner of other charms have been, and still are, in daily use. The bezoar stone,[2]

[1] D. Rorie, " The Stone in Scottish Folk-medicine," *Caledonian Med. Jour.*, 1911, vol. viii. No. 9, p. 410

[2] C. Elgood, " A Treatise on the Bezoar Stone," *Ann. Med. Hist.*, 1935, vol. vii. p. 73

found in the intestine of a goat, was an infallible proof against poison, and since the introduction of writing and printing, phylacteries, or small tablets or papers bearing words of the Koran or the Bible, have been said to endow the wearer with immunity from many ills.

One of the most famous charms was the talisman from which Sir Walter Scott named his novel, which was in the possession of the Lockharts of Lee, near Lanark (Plate IV). The Lee Penny, as it is called, is a dark red stone set in a silver coin of Edward IV.[1] At one time it had great reputation, and water in which it had been dipped became highly curative for many disorders. In the reign of Charles I the city of Newcastle, attacked by an epidemic, borrowed this talisman, depositing £6,000 as surety. The Church viewed this proceeding with disapproval, and admonished the Laird of Lee to "tak heid that it [the talisman] be used hereafter with the least scandal that possiblie may be."

Another curious aspect of folk medicine is the importance ascribed to colour.[2] Red, for example, the colour of the blood, was closely associated with healing, and to this day red wine is sometimes advised in the treatment of anaemia. Mummies were painted with red ochre to restore a life-like appearance, red hangings in the sick-room prevented marking in smallpox, red flannel is believed to ward off sore throats, and a red thread worn round the neck, and tied in front with nine knots, would prevent nose bleeding. Red pills were used in ancient China.[3] Blue is a colour much less in favour than red, but green has recently been used as a distinctive mark.

The Powder of Sympathy

No account of folk medicine would be complete without some reference to the so-called sympathy cure, perpetuated by the familiar saying, "Take a hair of the dog that bit you." The application of dog's hair to heal a dog bite is an ancient and

[1] T. Reid, "The Lee Penny," *Proc. Soc. Antiq. Scot.*, 1922–23, vol. lvii. p. 112 ; G. F. Black, "Scottish Charms and Amulets," *Proc. Soc. Antiq. Scot.*, 1892–93, vol. xxvii. p. 477 ; J. G. Lockhart, *Curses, Lucks, and Talismans*, 1938, p. 119 ; Sir J. Y. Simpson, *Archæological Essays*, 1872, vol. i. p. 199
[2] W. G. Black, *loc. cit.*, p. 108 ; J. G. Dalyell, *The Darker Superstitions of Scotland*, Edinburgh, 1934, p. 138
[3] N. B. Dennys, *The Folk-lore of China*, 1876, p. 54

world-wide method, for it is practised in China as well as in Britain. A variation consists in the internal administration of the heart or liver of the dog.

Perhaps the most fantastic remedy based upon this reasoning was the " powder of sympathy," which was applied, not to the wound but to the weapon which caused it, or to some clothing or first-dressing, which had been in contact with the wound. The powder, which was simply copper sulphate, was warmly recommended by the courtly Sir Kenelm Digby,[1] who, though not a medical man, was wont to dabble in the sciences. Nevertheless, the idea of the sympathy cure was no invention of his, as it is not unlikely that it originated in prehistoric times. The reason for the success of the method of Sir Kenelm Digby lay probably in the fact that the wound was left to nature, being simply bound up and allowed to heal.

The whole subject of folk medicine is full of quaint superstition, but perhaps enough has been said to illustrate the part which it has played in the evolution of medicine. It may be noted that folk medicine is not confined to remote country districts. Even in cities one may discover its existence, usually in hereditary form by word of mouth. Some of it dates from remote antiquity, and little of it has been transmitted by the printed word.

Folk-lore has been called " the archæology of the mind," and it is an important guide to man's intellectual history. In studying the history of mankind one may gain more information from tales, charms, superstitions, and proverbs than from politics, religions, and food habits, because the former are innate in man, while the latter have been imposed upon him from without.

The Origin of Medical Practice

In seeking to learn how the healing art arose in prehistoric times, we can draw no positive conclusion from the scanty evidence at our disposal. Nevertheless, it is not unreasonable to conclude that the cures of injuries or diseases followed two distinct lines.

The first, based upon magical or religious beliefs, consisted in dealing with the " soul " of the patient or in persuading or forcing the evil spirit which had entered the body of the patient to depart.

[1] Sir Kenelm Digby, *A late discourse made in a Solemn Assembly of Nobles and learned men, at Montpellier in France, touching the cure of wounds by the powder of Sympathy*, 3rd. ed., 1660.

The second, at first applied only to minor disorders, was of the nature of domestic or folk medicine, much of which has persisted to the present day even in civilized communities.[1]

The two methods became intermingled in course of time. The operation of trephining, for example, originally practised to allow a demon to escape, was ultimately applied to cases of depressed fractures, and still later to many other intracranial lesions. It is noteworthy also, that while folk medicine includes many remedies, some rational, others most irrational, it is closely bound up with superstitions, incantations, and other forms of magic, showing that the original conception of disease as a supernatural phenomenon has persisted throughout the centuries since Neolithic times.

[1] J. D. Rolleston, " Folk-lore and Medicine," *West London Med. Jour.*, 1939, vol. xxxiv. No. 2, p. 44 ; " The Folk-lore of Children's Diseases," *Folk-lore*, 1943, vol. liv. p. 287 ; " Otology and Folk-lore " and " Laryngology and Folk-lore," *Jour. of Laryng. and Otol.*, 1942, vol. lvii. p. 311

BOOKS FOR FURTHER READING

BALDWIN BROWN, G. *The Art of the Cave-dweller*, 1928

BLACK, W. G. *Folk Medicine*, 1883

BOULE, M. *Fossil Men*, trans. J. Ritchie, Edinburgh, 1923

BUDGE, Sir E. WALLIS. *Amulets and Superstitions*, 1930

BURKITT, M. C. *Pre-History : A Study of Early Cultures in Europe and the Mediterranean Basin*, Cambridge, 1921

CHILDE, V. GORDON. *Man makes Himself*, 1936

FRAZER, Sir J. G. *The Golden Bough*, 1911

GUIARD, E. *La Trépanation crânienne*, Paris, 1930

HILTON-SIMPSON, M. W. *Arab Medicine and Surgery*, 1922

HORNE, J. F. *Trephining in its Ancient and Modern Aspect*, 1894

HOSE, C. *Natural Man : a Record from Borneo*, 1926

HOVORKA, O., and KRONFELD, A. *Vergleichende Volksmedizin*, Berlin, 1908-9

KEITH, Sir ARTHUR. *The Antiquity of Man*, 2nd ed., 1921

LOCKHART, J. G. *Curses, Lucks, and Talismans*, 1938

MACALISTER, R. A. S. *Textbook of European Archæology*, 1921

McKENZIE, D. *The Infancy of Medicine*, 1927

MOODIE, R. L. *The Antiquity of Disease*, Chicago, 1923

OSBORN, H. F. *Men of the Old Stone Age*, 1916

RIVERS, W. H. R. *Medicine, Magic, and Religion*, 1924

SOLLAS, W. J. *Ancient Hunters*, 1911

SPENCER, Sir B. *Wanderings in Wild Australia*, 1928

CHAPTER II

THE FIRST KNOWN MEDICAL MEN

AFTER that long prehistoric epoch, of which we have such shadowy and indefinite records, came the invention of writing, the establishment of the calendar, and, in consequence, the dawn of recorded history.

The scene was laid in Mesopotamia, the " cradle of mankind," and in the adjacent land of Egypt. Between the northern boundary of the Arabian Desert and the mountains of Asia Minor there lies a semi-circular belt of country well watered by the great rivers Euphrates and Tigris, and known as the Fertile Crescent. Here, at a very early period, probably from 4000 B.C., arose the great civilization known at first as Sumerian, and later as that of the kingdoms of Sumer and Akkad.[1]

The greatness of the Sumerian civilization, which lasted for about two thousand years, has only recently been revealed by the excavation of the ancient city of Ur.[2] This magnificent capital was situated at the eastern end of the Fertile Crescent, on the Euphrates, and about one hundred miles from the Persian Gulf.

Agriculture and cattle-breeding were the chief sources of revenue of the Sumerians. Systems of irrigation and of transport by land and water had been evolved, and many of the houses at Ur were provided with bathrooms and drains. Art and craftsmanship attained a high standard. Wheeled vehicles were in use, and tools and utensils of copper. A number of small knives of hardened copper have been found, and are believed to be surgical instruments. A method of writing upon clay tablets in cuneiform signs had been invented. There can be no doubt of the existence of a Sumerian medical profession, as some of the tablets which have been discovered have a bearing on medicine, and there is in the Wellcome Museum the seal of a Sumerian physician who lived about 3000 B.C. There is a similar seal of a Babylonian medical man, dated about 2300 B.C., in the Louvre Museum (Plate v). Sumerian culture, therefore, appears to

[1] Sidney Smith, *Early History of Assyria to 1000 B.C.*, 1928
[2] C. Leonard Woolley, *Ur of the Chaldees*, 1929

have rivalled and perhaps even to have preceded the better known culture of Egypt. It is not unlikely that there was a commercial and cultural link between the two great nations, while the intervening country of Palestine, home of the Hebrews, acted as a buffer state, and derived benefit from both neighbours. The kingdom of Sumer and Akkad came to an end about 2000 B.C., and the country, with its glorious civilization, passed into the hands of two great nations, the south to the Babylonians, who built their renowned capital city of Babylon, and the north to the Assyrians, who had their capital first at Assur and later at Nineveh.

Medical Ethics in Babylonia

One of the earliest kings of Babylon was an able ruler named Hammurabi (1948–1905 B.C.)[1]. He drew up a Code of Laws which was engraved on a pillar of hard stone and set up in the temple at Babylon. This code, the oldest in existence,[2] now preserved in the Louvre, treats of property, of criminal offences, of marriage laws, and, what is of great interest to us, of laws relating to medical practice.

It is stated,[3] for example, that " if the doctor shall treat a gentleman and shall open an abscess with a bronze knife and shall preserve the eye of the patient, he shall receive ten shekels of silver. If the patient is a slave, his master shall pay two shekels of silver." That there might be a debit account for the unfortunate doctor is shown by the following rule : " If the doctor shall open an abscess with a bronze knife and shall kill the patient or shall destroy the sight of the eye, his hands shall be cut off." In the case of a slave the penalty is less drastic : " He shall replace the slave with another slave."

If the eye of a slave was destroyed as a result of operation, the operator was to pay to the master half the value of the slave.[4]

Reprisals such as these might well have deterred the ambitious surgeon of Babylon, yet there appears to have been a well-organized medical profession in those ancient times. It is true that magic entered largely into the treatment, and the lists of remedies which

[1] L. W. King, *A History of Babylon*, 1915, p. 162
[2] *The Oldest Code of Laws in the World*, trans. by C. H. W. Johns, Edinburgh, 1905
[3] J. D. Comrie, " Medicine among the Assyrians and Egyptians in 1500 B.C." *Edin. Med. Jour.* 1909, New Series, vol. ii. p. 101
[4] R. F. Harper, *The Code of Hammurabi, King of Babylon*, 2nd edition, Chicago, 1904

have been deciphered from clay tablets are liberally interspersed with incantations and charms.[1]

Herodotus,[2] who wrote his history about 430 B.C., tells us that every Babylonian was an amateur physician, as it was the custom to lay the sick in the street so that any passers-by " if they have ever had his disease themselves, or have known of any who has suffered from it, may give him advice . . . and no one is allowed to pass the sick man in silence." Yet the existence of a medical profession is implied in the Code Hammurabi. The physicians were probably of the priestly class, and medical concepts were dominated by primitive magical and religious ideas. From the appearance of clay models of the liver, found in Babylon, it has been shown that divination was widely practised.[3] The model of the sheep's liver, carefully mapped out in squares, each with a hole for a wooden peg, was inspected along with the fresh liver of a sacrificed animal. Any alteration on the surface of the fresh specimen was carefully pegged out on the model, and a deduction was drawn from the result (Plate VI). We may read of such divination in the Bible : " The King of Babylon stood at the parting of the ways . . . to use divination, . . . he consulted with images, he looked in the liver " (Ezekiel, xxi. 21).

We know little of Babylonian medicine.[4] Not a single name of a physician has survived. Nevertheless, the background which we have attempted to sketch is an essential link in the chain of medical history, and forms a suitable introduction to the more familiar medicine of ancient Egypt.[5]

Influence of Writing and the Calendar

The influence of the Sumerian civilization upon that of Egypt is a debatable problem which need not concern us here. Certain it is that in Egypt, as early as 4000 B.C., there was a well-

---

[1] R. C. Thomson, " Assyrian Medical Texts," *Proc. Roy. Soc. Med.* (Sect. Hist.), 1924, vol. xxvii. p. 1, and 1926, vol. xix. p. 29
[2] *Herodotus*, trans. H. Cary, Bohn Library, 1848, p. 86 (Book 1, § 197, p. 86), and trans. A. D. Godley, Loeb Library, 4 vols., 1921, vol. i. p. 250
[3] M. Jastrow, " The Signs and Names for the Liver in Babylonia," *Zeitsch. f. Assyriol.*, 1906, Bd. 20, p. 105
[4] M. Jastrow, " The Medicine of the Babylonians and Assyrians," *Proc. Roy. Soc. Med.* (Sect. Hist.), 1914, vol. vii, p. 109
[5] O. Temki, " Egyptian and Babylonian Medicine," *Bull. Hist. Med.*, 1936, vol. iv. p. 247 ; M. B. Gordon, " Popular Medicine in Sasanian Babylonia," *Ann. Med. Hist.*, 1942, 3rd Ser., vol. iv. p. 241

organized government for several millions of people, a system of pictorial writing from which the modern alphabet was evolved, and a means of recording time which with very few alterations remains as our calendar to-day. Professor Breasted remarks in his fascinating volume, *Ancient Times*,[1] that " the invention of writing has had a greater influence in uplifting the human race than any other achievement in the life of man." The introduction of writing naturally exercised a profound effect on the progress of medicine. Picture writing, or hieroglyphic, gave place to sign writing or hieratic, and the earliest alphabet came into use about 3500 B.C. Writing materials, too, were invented, and papyrus was found more convenient than clay bricks.

As for the calendar, it has been computed, by the aid of astronomy, that the date of its introduction was the year 4236 B.C. According to Breasted this is " the earliest dated event in human history." [2]

Unfortunately we know very little about the condition of medical practice in Egypt at this early date. There were various gods who presided over the arts and sciences.[3] Ra was the Sun god, with the head of a falcon ; Thoth, the ibis-headed god of Wisdom, was said to be the author of treatises on medicine, while the lion-headed Sekhmet was the deity of childbirth. Horus, god of health, engaged in a fight with Set, the demon of evil, and lost an eye, which, however, was restored by miraculous means. The eye of Horus formed the design for a charm or amulet which was second only to the scarab or sacred beetle as a mascot of ancient Egypt. It is said to be the origin of the recipe (℞) sign which preceded medical prescriptions.[4] Originally an elaborate design, the eye of Horus passed through various phases until it became conventionalized as something resembling a capital R, and it was placed on all objects associated with danger, such as ships, chariots—and prescriptions (Plate IV).

The galaxy of gods to which reference has been made was later augmented by the addition of the famous god of medicine, Imhotep, who was originally a mortal.

[1] J. H. Breasted, *Ancient Times, A History of the Early World*, 2nd ed., Chicago, 1935, p. 66
[2] J. H. Breasted, *loc. cit.*, p. 59
[3] E. A. Budge, *Gods of Egypt*, 1904, vol. i. pp. 514, 525
[4] J. D. Comrie, " Medicine among the Assyrians and Egyptians in 1500 B.C.," *Edin. Med. Jour.*, 1909, New Series, vol. ii. p. 101

PLATE V   MEDICAL LITERATURE IN BABYLON AND EGYPT

Description of a case of tetanus following a wound of the head—
from the *Edwin Smith Papyrus* (page 26)

Inscription on Seal :

Edina-mu-gi
The messenger
The god Girra
Ama-gan-sa-du
Ur-Lugal-Edina,
the physician, his
servant.

Seal of a Babylonian physician.   Some of the signs may represent the
knives, cups, and needles used by the physician (page 17)

PLATE VI THE LIVER IN DIVINATION

Clay model of sheep's liver, used in Babylonia about 2000 B.C. Original
in British Museum (page 19)

Bronze model of liver found at Piacenza bearing inscription in Etruscan;
probably third century B.C. (page 65)

Sekhet'enanach and Imhotep

We have so little definite information regarding the state of medicine in ancient Egypt that we cannot tell who the greatest physicians were. There are, however, two names which deserve to be mentioned, though it would be futile to discuss whether Sekhet'enanach or Imhotep has the better claim to be regarded as the first medical man known to us by name.

According to Dr. Withington,[1] SEKHET'ENANACH was chief physician to one of the Pharaohs who lived about 3000 B.C. In his tomb he is depicted dressed in a leopard skin and carrying two sceptres, while behind him stands his wife, her hand resting on his shoulder. Of Sekhet'enanach it is briefly recorded that " he healed the king's nostrils." The royal patient was willing to mark this service by any desired reward, but the physician chose to have his portrait fashioned in stone, together with a record of the case, and suggested that this should be set up in a prominent position in the palace, and should afterwards mark his tomb.[2] By making this choice, Sekhet'enanach has established a claim to be the first physician of history.

The second name, much better known to medical historians, is that of IMHOTEP, a name which means " he who cometh in peace," truly a good name for a physician. Osler[3] states that Imhotep was the first figure of a physician to emerge from the mists of antiquity. Yet we have even less evidence of his prowess as a physician than we have of the rival claimant Sekhet'enanach. It is true that for long after his death he was worshipped as the god of medicine, until well on in the Christian era, and that, as Imonthes, he was identified by the Greeks as identical with their own Aesculapius. During his lifetime, however, so far as our present knowledge goes, Imhotep was better known as vizier and as architect than as physician, and it is difficult to justify the suggestion which has been made by Dr. J. B. Hurry[4] and others, that Imhotep, rather than Hippocrates, should be regarded as the Father of Medicine, or that he should supplant Aesculapius as the God of the Healing

[1] E. T. Withington, *Medical History from the Earliest Times*, 1894, p. 14
[2] E. Meyer, *Geschichte des alten Aegyptens*, Berlin, 1885, vol. ii. p. 95 ; E. M. Guest, " Ancient Egyptian Physicians," *Brit. Med. Jour.*, 1926, vol. i. p. 706
[3] W. Osler, *The Evolution of Modern Medicine*, 1922
[4] J. B. Hurry, *Imhotep : The Vizier and Physician of King Zoser and afterwards the Egyptian God of Medicine*, 1928

Art. Imhotep was grand vizier to King Zoser, who lived from about 2980 to 2900 B.C.[1] The vizier was the leading official, and presided, like Joseph, over the various state departments. Not only did Imhotep achieve notable success as a politician, he also distinguished himself as one of the greatest architects of all time.[2] He designed the Step Pyramid of Sakkarah, a familiar sight to every tourist who ascends the Nile or visits Memphis.[3]

This magnificent tomb, which Imhotep built for his royal master, is not only the oldest surviving stone building in the world, but is interesting as a transition between the simple stone-fronted tombs of earlier times and the conventional smooth-sided pyramids which followed, and which culminated in the building of the Great Pyramid at Gizeh, the largest of the pyramids, and the greatest stone edifice of ancient times.

As Professor Breasted[4] remarks, the rapidity of the decline of barbarism and the growth of civilization in ancient Egypt was truly remarkable. Less than a century and a quarter elapsed from the earliest example of stonemasonry to the Great Pyramid (begun about 2885 B.C.), a solid mass of blocks, more than two millions of them, each weighing about $2\frac{1}{2}$ tons.

The Step Pyramid which Imhotep[5] built was therefore a magnificent achievement. It is 200 feet high, and consists of six gigantic steps. The task of organizing the labour for such a building must have been enormous.

It is unfortunate that we know nothing of Imhotep as physician.[6] Yet he must have been at least as distinguished in medicine as in architecture and politics, for he was worshipped for many centuries after his death as the god of medicine, at first as demigod, and eventually (about 500 B.C.) as a full deity. Numerous statuettes have been found, most of them of solid bronze, representing Imhotep seated, reading a papyrus which rests on his knees. The British Museum possesses ten such statuettes and the Wellcome Historical Medical Museum has thirty-one, including two standing figures (Plate VII).

Three temples are known to have been built in honour of

[1] K. Sethe, *Imhotep, der Asklepios der Aegypter*, Berlin, 1902, vol. ii. p. 134
[2] G. Maspero, *Études de Mythologie et d'Archéologie Egyptiennes*, Paris, 1916
[3] R. J. Forbes, "Imhotep," *Proc. Roy. Soc. Med.* (Sect. Hist.), 1940, vol. xxxiii. p. 769; C. M. Firth and J. C. Quibell, *The Step-pyramid*, Cairo, 1936, 2 vols.
[4] J. H. Breasted, *loc. cit.*, p. 113
[5] J. B. Hurry, *loc. cit.*, p. 10
[6] W. A. Jayne, *The Healing Gods of Ancient Civilization*, 1925, p. 138

Imhotep, at Memphis, Thebes, and Philæ.[1] There and elsewhere Imhotep was worshipped, and there is reason to believe that the practice of incubation, or temple-sleep (see p. 43), was followed in Egypt as in Greece. Of those three temples only one survived, on the island of Philæ, far up the Nile, but this has been submerged since the construction of the great dam at Assuan close by. It was a fine specimen of Egyptian architecture.

Imhotep is buried near the city of Memphis, but his tomb has not yet been found. Perhaps one day it may be discovered, and the claim for recognition of this great sage as " the first known medical man " may thus be substantiated.

The Medical Literature of Ancient Egypt

Mention has been made of the invention of writing, and of the use of papyrus in ancient Egypt,[2] so that it might be expected that a study of the existing papyri would yield full information regarding the medical knowledge of the time. Such an expectation has not been fulfilled as yet. The available papyri are mere fragments of a great literature which began with the so-called Hermetic books of the god Thoth. Those books, thirty-two in number, of which six dealt with medicine, were kept for reference in the temples and were carried in the sacred processions. All of them have been lost, although the medical papyri which are still available appear to have been compiled from those earlier lost works.[3] So highly were the Hermetic books esteemed that no blame was incurred if the patient died, so long as the physicians adhered closely to their teaching. If, however, the physician departed in the least from the accredited methods of treatment, and the case ended fatally, his own life was forfeited. Thus the Egyptian code of medical ethics meted out punishments for malpractices even more severe than those of the Babylonian code.

It is perhaps unfair to judge the condition of medicine in ancient Egypt from the papyri at our disposal, as these contain, for the most part, merely a series of notes and abstracts from the lost Hermetic books. Nevertheless they contain much informa-

[1] A. E. Weigall, Guide to the Antiquities of Upper Egypt, 1913, p. 298
[2] A. S. Hunt, article " Papyrology " in Ency. Brit., 14th ed., 1929–37
[3] H. Ranke, " Medicine and Surgery in Ancient Egypt," Bull. Hist. Med., 1933, vol. i. 7, p. 237

tion of interest to the student of medical history.[1]   The Ebers Papyrus is the best known of the medical papyri.   It was found in a tomb of Thebes in 1862 by Professor Georg Ebers,[2] and is now preserved in the University of Leipzig.   Not only is it the oldest complete medical book in existence,[3] it is said to be the most ancient existing book of any kind.   It consists of 110 pages, and contains about 900 recipes or prescriptions.   As it is in almost perfect condition, and as a calendar has been written on the back of the manuscript, the date of writing may be fixed with fair accuracy at about 1500 B.C.

There is abundant evidence to show that much of it has been copied from other works many centuries older,[4] and its value is enhanced by the marginal notes by its first owner, such as, " Good, I have often used it," or, " An excellent remedy." [5]   Like the other medical papyri to which we shall presently refer, the Ebers Papyrus is plentifully sprinkled with spells and incantations, which suggest that the remedies were given with the intention of driving out or banishing the demon of disease.[6]   The primitive idea of devil possession was still the keystone of Egyptian pathology. The " directions for use " in these days were, to repeat, while taking the medicine, such words as, " Welcome, remedy !   Welcome !   that dost drive away that which is in this my heart and in these my limbs."   This is only one of the many magical spells recommended in the papyrus.   Amulets, too, are advised, consisting of images of the gods or other objects, to be hung round the neck or tied to the foot or to the great toe.   Sometimes merely a knotted cord was to be used, with a specified number of knots, usually seven, a form of amulet which has survived in folk-lore to this day.

The greater part of the writing, however, consists of lists of prescriptions, giving, in each case, the remedy, with its dosage and quantity, the disease for which it is to be used, and often also the appropriate spell or incantation.   Among the drugs

[1] J. Finlayson, " Ancient Egyptian Medicine," *Brit. Med. Jour.*, 1893, vol. ii. pp. 748, 1014, and 1061
[2] G. Ebers, *Papyros Ebers, das hermetische Buch über die Arztneimittel der alten Aegypter in hieratischer Schrift*, Leipzig, 1875
[3] J. Joachim, trans. into German : *Papyros Ebers, das älteste Buch über Heilkunde*, Berlin, 1890
[4] C. H. von Klein, " The Medical Features of the Ebers Papyrus," *Journ. Amer. Med. Assn.*, 1905, vol. xlv. No. 26
[5] R. H. Major, " The Papyrus Ebers," *Ann. Med. Hist.*, 1930, vol. ii. p. 347
[6] C. P. Bryan, *The Papyrus Ebers*, trans. from German version, 1930

mentioned are castor oil, which was used as a purgative, also as a fuel for lamps. The seeds were chewed and swallowed with beer as an internal remedy, and the oil was applied externally for septic wounds and for burns. Another drug was hartshorn, which has had a long career in pharmacy. It was applied externally " to drive out painful swellings," or used as a fumigation " to expel demons."

One strange remedy was bile from various animals ; pig bile was applied to the eyes. Other animal substances were used, some of them of disgusting nature, while the fat of various animals was greatly favoured. Among the prescriptions for baldness was one consisting of equal parts of the fat of the hippopotamus, the lion, the crocodile, the goose, the snake, and the ibex.[1] Apparently the pharmacist of those days was also a good hunter.

There is very little reference to symptoms or to diagnosis in the Ebers Papyrus. One interesting section deals with the action of the heart, which was regarded as the principal vital organ, the brain being only of minor importance. The heart was carefully left in position during the process of embalming, although all the other viscera were removed.

It is noted that the pulse may be felt in many parts of the body, and that it is synchronous with the heart beat.[2] There were described three vessels for each arm and leg, four for the head, four for the liver, and four for the lungs.

The ears were believed to be organs of respiration as well as of hearing, and the statement is made that " the breath of life enters by the right ear and the breath of death by the left ear." This rather confused series of observations shows that at least some attempt was being made to understand the mechanism of the human body, although the medicine of the period appears to have been mainly blind empiricism. We learn, too, from the papyrus, that the Egyptian habitually employed enemata, for three successive days each month. This hygienic measure was later applied in the treatment of disease.

Among the diseases mentioned in the papyrus affections of the stomach and intestines figure prominently, as also do fevers and diseases of the eyes, showing that there has probably been little change in the incidence of these maladies from those early times

[1] W. R. Dawson, *Magician and Leech*, 1929, p. 91 (one of the best concise accounts)
[2] W. R. Dawson, article on Medicine in *The Legacy of Egypt*, ed. S. R. K. Glanville, 1942, p. 189

until the present day. Copper sulphate was largely used for eye diseases.[1]

A study of the Ebers Papyrus alone would suggest that the medicine of ancient Egypt was of the empirical or magical variety.

Indeed, the standard of Egyptian medicine was regarded as rather low, in comparison with the general cultural level, until a few years ago, when the translation of another papyrus revealed a more logical and scientific outlook. This was the Edwin Smith Papyrus (Plate v). Discovered at the same time and place as the Ebers Papyrus, it remained the property of the private collector whose name it bears, until at his death it was presented to the Historical Society of New York. Recently it has been studied and described by Professor Breasted.[2] He has shown that it is of slightly earlier date than the Ebers Papyrus. It is a sort of handbook on the treatment of wounds and bruises, commencing with those of the head, and passing downwards. Unfortunately the description ends with the thorax, as the book is incomplete.[3] There is evidence to show that surgical instruments were used, and that fractures were treated with splints.[4] Wounds were treated by fresh flesh, kept in place by a bandage, for the first day, an idea still favoured in some quarters, and afterwards dressings of fat and honey were used.

The following description of a case of dislocated jaw, from the papyrus, is surprisingly modern : " If you examine a man having a dislocation of his mandible, should you find his mouth open, and his mouth cannot close for him, you should put your two thumbs upon the ends of the two rami of the mandible inside his mouth and your fingers under his chin and you should cause them to fall back so that they rest in their places."

The other medical papyri which have come to light are smaller and more fragmentary than those just mentioned. The Hearst Papyrus, found in Upper Egypt in 1899, is now in the University of California.[5] The contents are very similar to those of the Ebers Papyrus, and it is of later date (1400 B.C.). Another docu-

[1] A. C. Krause, "Ancient Egyptian Ophthalmology," Bull. Hist. Med., 1933, vol. i. p. 258
[2] J. H. Breasted, The Edwin Smith Surgical Papyrus, Chicago, 1930, 2 vols.
[3] J. C. de Lint, " Le verso de Papyrus Edwin Smith," Bull. Soc. de l'Hist. de Méd., 1935, vol. xxix. p. 49
[4] G. Elliot Smith, "The Most Ancient Splints," Brit. Med. Jour., 1908, vol. i. p. 732
[5] Papyrus Hearst, ed. G. A. Reisner, Univ. of Cal. Publ. Egypt. Archaeol., 1903, vol. v. p. 1

ment, known as the Kahun Papyrus, was discovered in 1889 by Sir Flinders Petrie. Written about 1850 B.C., it is in fragmentary condition, but appears to deal with the treatment of vaginal and uterine disorders, in effect a textbook of gynæcology.

In the British Museum there is another fragmentary papyrus, largely composed of incantations, and probably of very early date. It is sometimes called the London Medical Papyrus.

There are two medical papyri in the Berlin Museum (Berlin Papyri). One is a poor production, but the contents are similar to those of the Ebers Papyrus. The other is a short but interesting document, written about 1450 B.C., and consisting of prescriptions and incantations for the protection of mothers and babies, and for the treatment of diseases of children. Apparently it is the oldest known work on pediatrics.

Many other medical papyri have been found, mostly of much more recent date, all of them consisting of prescriptions and charms, while there is preserved at Cairo a Coptic manuscript of the tenth century. Like the older papyri, it is made up of lists of drugs, with no reference to diagnosis.

Embalming and the Pathology of Mummies

No account of the medicine of ancient Egypt would be complete without some reference to the strange custom of preserving the human body after death. The fact that dead bodies, buried in the dry hot sands of the desert, remained for many years in a remarkable state of preservation, may have suggested to the Egyptians that the natural preservation might be favoured by artificial means, and that this would assist that physical survival after death in which they believed. As burial customs changed this became the more necessary, because the corpse which was placed in a tomb chamber or pyramid cell was no longer subjected to the desiccating effect of the desert grave. Embalming was practised in Egypt from about 4000 B.C. to A.D. 600, and it is estimated that about seven hundred million bodies were so treated. Herodotus gives a graphic description of the process.[1] He writes : " They take first a crooked piece of metal, and with it they draw out the brain through the nostrils, thus getting rid of a portion, while the skull is cleared of the rest by rinsing with

---

[1] *Herodotus*, trans. H. Cary, Bohn Library, Bk. ii., 1848, § 86, p. 126 ; trans. A. D. Godley, Loeb Library, 1921, 4 vols., vol. i, Bk. ii, §86, p. 371

drugs ; next they make a cut along the flank with a sharp stone, and take out the whole contents of the abdomen. After this they fill the cavity with myrrh, cassia, and other spices, and the body is placed in natron for seventy days. Then it is washed, and wrapped from head to foot in fine linen bandages smeared with gum . . . it is given back to the relations, who enclose it in a wooden case, shaped in the figure of a man. The case is fastened and placed upright in the sepulchral chamber. Such is the most costly way of embalming the dead."

Less expensive methods consisted in the injection of cedar oil into the body cavities, or in the simple pickling of the cadaver in a salt bath. The incision in the abdomen was made by the " paracentetai " (παρακεντηται), who were much despised, and who, indeed, were obliged to fly for their lives on completing the task. The " taricheutai " (ταριχευται) who removed the organs, were held in greater esteem. The heart was carefully preserved intact in its original position ; all other viscera were removed, treated by some preservative, wrapped in parcels, and returned to the body. Mr. Warren Dawson [1] believes that the body was dried or desiccated by heat, as many mummies show signs of fire. During this process of heating resin was freely applied, and the bandages were also soaked in heated resin.

It seems rather surprising that in spite of the post-mortem examination which was part of the process of embalming, the Egyptians showed no great interest in anatomy or physiology, nor were they concerned to ascertain the cause of death. Yet this curious custom of embalming has had this advantage, it has provided the modern investigator with a rich field for investigation into the pathology of mummies. Interesting facts have been reported. It has been shown, for example, that osteo-arthritis was extremely common, and dental caries rare. Gouty concretions, urinary calculi, and gall-stones have been found, and the existence of tuberculous disease of the spine, with its characteristic deformities, has been seen in mummies dating as far back as 3400 B.C., and has also been depicted in tomb portraits. Elliot Smith and Derry [2] have described the mummy of Nesperehan, a high civic dignitary of the 21st Dynasty, which showed kyphosis of the thoracic region resulting from disease

[1] W. R. Dawson, *Magician and Leech*, 1929, p. 43
[2] G. Elliot Smith and D. E. Derry, *Bull. of Archaeological Survey of Nubia*, No. 5, Cairo, 1910, p. 21

PLATE VII THE FIRST KNOWN MEDICAL MAN

Statuette of Imhotep, physician and vizier to King Zoser about 2980 B.C.
(page 21)

PLATE VIII   DISEASE IN EGYPTIAN MUMMIES

Mummy of the priest Nesperehan (*c.* 1000 B.C.), showing tuberculous disease of the spine and a large psoas abscess on the right side (pages 28–29)

(*l.*) Jaws of a Gizeh pyramid builder (*c.* 2800 B.C.) showing absorption of alveolar margin caused by pyorrhoea alveolaris (page 29).   (*r.*) Lower end of femur of ancient Nubian, with advanced osteo-arthritis of knee-joint (page 29) and collapse of the vertebrae and also a large psoas abscess [1] (Plate VIII). In other mummies pleural adhesions have been seen, and even appendicitis has been recognized. Bilharzia eggs have been discovered in the kidney of mummies, showing that this disease, still so common in Egypt, is of very ancient date.[2]

Two other diseases of widespread incidence in Ancient Egypt were chronic suppurative periodontitis (pyorrhoea alveolaris) and chronic osteo-arthritis, and they may have been intimately associated (Plate VIII). No evidence of syphilis or of rickets was found in the skeletons examined by Sir MARK ARMAND RUFFER (1859–1917), but a number of statuettes and incised representations of achondroplasic and (?) rickety dwarfs are figured in his work, a noteworthy contribution to palaeontology.[3]

The Egyptians do not appear to have possessed that spirit of inquiry and that thirst for knowledge which characterized the Greeks, and in the light of the existing evidence we are hardly justified in dethroning Aesculapius from his time-honoured position as god of Medicine and setting Imhotep in his place, as some writers have suggested (p. 21). Also, as far as mortals are concerned, Hippocrates must remain the Father of Medicine. Nevertheless, let us honour the physician Imhotep, who came in peace and showed the way. He was the first medical man whose name we know. (See also Supplement, page 453.)

Medicine in the Bible

In our search for medical knowledge of ancient times, we are inclined, very naturally, to turn to the Bible for information.[4] Unfortunately the quest is disappointing. In the Old Testament there is little place for the physician, if indeed he existed at all, because God alone was regarded as the healer. He was the source of life and health, sending disease and disaster as a punishment for sin, and healing it only if the sufferers were worthy of cure. " If thou wilt diligently hearken unto the voice of the Lord thy God . . . and wilt give ear to his commandments, and keep all his statutes, I will put none of these diseases upon thee which I

[1] A. J. E. Cave, " The Evidence for the Incidence of Tuberculosis in Ancient Egypt," *Brit. Jour. of Tuberculosis*, 1939, vol. xxxiii., p. 142 and *The Surgery of Ancient Egypt*
[2] M. A. Ruffer, " Note on the Presence of Bilharzia Haematobium in Egyptian Mummies," *Brit. Med. Jour.*, 1910, vol. i. p. 16
[3] M. A. Ruffer, *Studies in the Paleopathology of Ancient Egypt*, Chicago, 1921 ; statuettes showing evidence of spinal tuberculosis (Pott's disease) have also been found in Peru
[4] C. J. Brim, *Medicine in the Bible*, 1936

have brought upon the Egyptians : for I am the Lord that healeth thee " (Exod. xv. 26).

Any human knowledge of healing was regarded with disfavour, lest it should detract from a power which ought to belong to God alone. Few remedies are mentioned in the Old Testament, and in every case the treatment is recommended by a " man of God." Naaman, the leper, is told by Elisha (2 Kings v. 10) to wash himself seven times in the River Jordan ; King Hezekiah, " sick unto death " from a boil (the exact diagnosis is obscure), is bidden by Isaiah to apply a lump of figs (2 Kings xx. 7) ; while Elijah restored to life the son of the widow of Zarephath, apparently by performing artificial respiration (1 Kings xvii. 17–23).

There were midwives in those days, and birth stools or obstetric chairs were in use (Exod. i. 15–20) (Plate xxxiv). The only surgical operation mentioned is circumcision, performed by the priest as a ritual procedure (Gen. xvii. 10–14 ; Exod. iv. 25). Isaiah (i. 6) speaks of wounds which " have not been closed, neither bound up, neither mollified with ointment," showing that the Jews knew something about first aid, and they could also treat fractures (Ezek. xxx. 21).

If physicians did exist among the Jews when the Old Testament was written, there is surprisingly little reference to them in the sacred writings. The oft-quoted eulogy commencing " Honour a physician with the honour due to him for the uses which ye may have of him : for the Lord hath created him," is from a book which, strangely enough, was not included in the Canon, " The Wisdom of Jesus, the son of Sirach, or, Ecclesiasticus." It is a noble testimonial to the medical profession, although the last verse, " He that sinneth before his Maker, let him fall into the hand of the physician "—is capable of more than one interpretation.

In spite of this disappointing absence of references to medicine and surgery, the Bible is a mine of information on personal and social hygiene, and might even be regarded as the first textbook of public health. The thirteenth and fourteenth chapters of Leviticus contain explicit instructions to be observed by the priest in cases of leprosy. The isolation of the patient, the washing or burning of infected clothing, and the disinfection of houses, involving, if necessary, complete destruction, are all described in detail.

Plague is frequently mentioned in the Old Testament.[1] We are told that twenty and four thousand died of plague at Baal-peor (Numbers xxv. 9). There appears to be little doubt that the " emerods " with which the Lord smote the Philistines were the buboes of plague, and the belief is strengthened by the fact that the trespass offering which " priests and the diviners " recommended to stay the epidemic consisted of five golden emerods and five golden mice, " images of your emerods, and images of your mice that mar the land " (1 Sam. vi. 4, 5). This is probably the first reference to the rat as a disseminator of bubonic plague.

The Old Testament contains many references to personal hygiene.[2] One example may be given, showing that every soldier was obliged to carry an implement to facilitate the disposal of his excreta. " And thou shalt have a paddle upon thy weapon ; and it shall be, when thou wilt ease thyself abroad, thou shalt dig therewith, and shalt turn back and cover that which cometh from thee " (Deut. xxiii. 13). Physical purity was complementary to moral purity and cleanliness was literally next to godliness. For the first time in history the individual was subordinated to the community. Personal comfort or convenience must be sacrificed if that is necessary for the good of the greater number. A social conscience had awakened, and the Jews were the pioneers of public health.

Not only in the Bible but also in the Talmud [3] (fifth century A.D.), there is to be found much information on personal and social hygiene. The Talmud is mainly a book of regulations and laws, but it contains some details regarding Jewish medicine which are not to be found in the Old Testament. Human anatomy is described in considerable detail. Especially interesting is the reference to the bone Luz, which, situated in some ill-defined part of the vertebral column, was the permanent nucleus of the body which persisted after death.[4] This belief held throughout the Middle Ages, and was not exploded until Vesalius so startlingly disposed of this and many other anatomical myths.

The Talmud refers to blood-letting, cupping, and the use of splints and bandages, and although there was apparently no

[1] S. B. Blakely, " The Medicine of the Old Testament," *Med. Record*, 1915, vol. lxxxvii. No. 23, p. 934
[2] E. Hagemann, " Zur Hygiene der alten Israeliten," *Janus*, 1903, vol. xii. pp. 309, 449
[3] J. Preuss, *Biblische-Talmudische Medizin*, Berlin, 1911
[4] F. H. Garrison, " The bone called ' Luz,' " *N.Y. Med. Jour.*, 1910, p. 149

organized medical education, the standard of "domestic medicine" was fairly high.

A study of ancient Hebrew literature,[1] therefore, leads us to the conclusion that although no great physician appeared among the Jews, nor indeed any medical men at all, they did nevertheless contribute very materially to the progress of medical science by promoting a social conscience among the people, and by instituting valuable measures for the prevention of epidemic disease and the promotion of the health of the community.

Ancient Medicine of India

No account of the first known medical men would be complete without some reference to the early medical practice of the East.[2]

Our knowledge of Hindu medicine in ancient times is incomplete and inaccurate, owing largely to the difficulty of separating fact from fiction in oriental writings. The earliest Sanskrit document, the Rig-Veda[3] (about 1500 B.C.), indicates that the treatment of disease at that time consisted mainly of spells and incantations. A later work, or series of works, dated about 700 B.C., called the Atharva-Veda, contains much medical information. Some of the writing is attributed to CHARAKA and SUSRUTA, although the original Atharva-Veda is of much earlier date than either of those great Hindu physicians.

Charaka[4] lived at the beginning of the Christian era, and Susruta[5] about the fifth century A.D. The works of the latter are the more noteworthy. He wrote on many subjects: on malaria, which was known to be caused by mosquitoes; on plague, which followed when many dead rats were seen; on phthisis, which showed itself by hæmoptysis, cough, and fever; and on smallpox, which was also very common. Hindu medicine was

[1] B. L. Gordon, " Medicine among the Ancient Hebrews," Ann. Med. Hist., 1942, p. 219
[2] Sir B. S. Jee, A Short History of Aryan Medical Science, 1896 ; T. A. Wise, The Hindu System in Medicine, 1845 ; D. C. Muthu, " A Short Review of the History of Ancient Hindu Medicine," Proc. Roy. Soc. Med., 1913, vol. vi. p. 177, also The Antiquity of Hindu Medicine, 3rd. ed. 1930 ; A. F. R. Hoernle, Studies in the Medicine of Ancient India, 1907 ; S. N. Dasgupta, " Die Medizin der alten Hindus," Arch. f. Gesch. d. Med., 1928, vol. xx. p. 80
[3] D. Liétard, " La Doctrine humorale des Hindous et le Rig-Veda," Janus, vol. viii. p. 17
[4] Works of Charaka, trans. A. C. Kaviratna, Calcutta, 1912
[5] Works of Susruta Samhita, trans. K. L. Bhishagratna, 3 vols., Calcutta, 1907–16

PLATE IX   RELICS OF APOLLO, GOD OF HEALING

The Grotto on the island of Delos, alleged birthplace of Apollo (page 40)

The Omphalos at Delphi, beside the Sacred Way leading to the Temple of Apollo (page 41)

PLATE X   EPIDAURUS, A CENTRE OF AESCULAPIAN HEALING

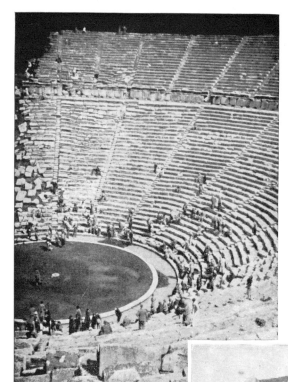

The Theatre. Beautifully situated on the hillside near the Temple, with accommodation for 20,000 persons (page 45)

The stone of Hermodikes, the story of which is inscribed on one of the stelæ at Epidaurus (page 44) rich in drugs, and Susruta mentions seven hundred and sixty medicinal plants. External applications were largely used, as ointments, baths, sneezing powders, and inhalations.

Some of the general information is of great interest. One of the remarks, " He who knows only one branch of his art is like a bird with one wing," might well be pondered by the modern specialist.

The duties of the army surgeon were indicated in the following terms, quoted by Withington [1] : " When the king goeth with his army . . . he shall take with him a skilful physician who . . . must see to the food, water, wood, and places of encampment. If he find poison he must remove it, and so save the army from death and destruction. His tent shall be near the king's tent, and there shall be a flag over his tent, so that the sick, poisoned, or wounded may find him quickly."

It was in surgery above all that the ancient Hindus excelled.[2] Susruta described more than a hundred surgical instruments.[3] This was their greatest contribution to the art of healing, and the work was bold and distinctive. It is not unlikely, though difficult to prove, that some of it was of Greek origin. Some, indeed, state that the Greeks drew much of their knowledge from the Hindus.[4] Operative procedures were taught, using as models for practice the hollow stems of plants, as well as leaves and gourds. This pioneer work in surgery is all the more remarkable because the knowledge of anatomy was so slight.[5] The nerves and blood-vessels were believed to originate from the umbilicus, and many other anatomical facts were distorted and fanciful.

Nevertheless the Hindus treated fractures with bamboo splints, and performed many operations including Cæsarean section, the excision of tumours, and lithotomy. The performance of the last-mentioned operation was continued through the ages, and was undertaken by native trained surgeons until recent times. Of peculiar interest and of very ancient date is the operation of rhinoplasty, which originated in India. It was frequently

[1] E. T. Withington, *Medical History from the Earliest Times*, 1894, p. 27
[2] G. N. Mukhopadhyav, *The Surgical Instruments of the Hindus*, Calcutta, 1913
[3] R. F. G. Müller, " Indische chirurgische Instrumente," *Arch. f. Gesch. d. Med.*, 1937, vol. xxx. p. 91
[4] F. S. Hammett, " The Anatomical Knowledge of the Ancient Hindus," *Ann. Med. Hist.*, 1929, vol. i. p. 325
[5] P. J. Sarma, " Hindu Medicine and its Antiquity," *Ann. Med. Hist.*, 1931, vol. iii. p. 318

required, as adulterers were punished by having their noses cut off. The leaf of a tree, cut to the desired shape and size, was used as a pattern, and a piece of skin from the cheek or forehead, fashioned to form the new nose, was sutured in position. Thus were the Hindus the pioneers of modern plastic surgery.

China's Contribution to Medicine

Let us now turn our thoughts still farther east, and seek to ascertain the scope and extent of China's contribution to Medicine.[1] Many inventions have been attributed to China, although they may have been re-invented in Europe at later dates. In medicine, the Chinese have shown originality and enterprise although, to quote one of themselves, Dr. Chi Min Wong (1932)[2]: ". . . they have never pursued a single subject in a way calculated to lead them to final success." Nevertheless, as we shall presently seek to prove, the history of Chinese medicine is well worthy of investigation.

It is not accurately known who was the originator of Chinese medicine, yet none can have a better claim to the title, "Father of Medicine," than SHEN NUNG, who lived about 3000 B.C. This Emperor of China was a man of great ability who not only devised methods of cultivation and of raising stock, but also, experimenting upon himself for many years, discovered a large number of drugs and of poisons. This knowledge he set forth in *Pen Tsao* (the Great Herbal, or Chinese Materia Medica). There were many subsequent editions of this book, which contains descriptions of over a thousand drugs, and is still in use in China. An English edition was published as recently as 1911.[3] Five thousand years is truly a wonderful record of longevity for a medical work. Many of the drugs described are now obsolete, many are inert and useless, but some, such as opium, rhubarb, aconite, croton—to mention only a few examples—are in use to this day.[4] Inorganic remedies such as iron, arsenic, and sulphur were also used. Scientific investigation of certain old Chinese drugs has been undertaken in recent years and has already

[1] W. R. Morse, *Chinese Medicine* (Clio Medica), New York, 1934; Hübotter, *Die chinesische Medizin*, Leipzig, 1929
[2] Chi Min Wong and Lien-Teh Wu, *History of Chinese Medicine*, Tientsin, 1932, (2nd. ed. 1936)
[3] G. A. Stuart, *A Chinese Materia Medica*, Shanghai, 1911
[4] K. K. Chen, "Chinese Drug Stores," *Ann. Med. Hist.*, 1925, vol. vii. pp. 2, 103

yielded valuable results.[1] One of the discoveries made in this way was that of ephedrine, an alkaloid isolated from the Chinese herb *Ma Huang* ; it is not unlikely that other useful substances in the Chinese Herbal await discovery, or rather rediscovery.

At a slightly later date another noteworthy medical work was written by another Chinese emperor. HWANG TI (2650 B.C.) is believed to be the author of *Nei Ching*. the Book of Medicine which is the foundation of all Chinese medical literature ; an English translation of this is now available.[2] It contains a statement which is often quoted in support of the contention that the Chinese discovered the circulation of the blood many centuries before Harvey. " All the blood in the body is under the control of the heart. . . . The blood current flows continuously in a circle and never stops." The statement is the more remarkable when we remember that, owing to religious scruples, the Chinese seldom practised dissection, and their ideas of anatomy and physiology were grossly inaccurate.

As time went on, medicine in China gradually escaped from the control of magic and sorcery, and a theory was evolved which served as a basis for all subsequent practices.[3] Two fundamental principles were involved, Yang and Yin. These two opposing forces were believed to dominate everything. They were ebb and flow, male and female, life and death, sun and moon, heat and cold, strength and weakness, and so on. Everything in the universe depended upon the adjustment of balance between the two forces, and naturally the principle was applied to health and disease. Another doctrine was that of the five elements—earth, fire, water, wood, and metal—of which the human body was composed. The magical figure five was also applied to the organs (heart, liver, spleen, lung, and kidney), to colours, climate, and heavenly bodies. Health was believed to consist in a harmonious balance between the various elements. This theory was independently evolved in somewhat similar fashion by the Greeks, when they attributed diseases to ill-balanced " humours."

Among the methods of treatment which have been used in China from very ancient times are massage and acupuncture.

[1] B. E. Read, " Gleanings from old Chinese Medicine," *Ann. Med. Hist.*, 1926, viii. 16
[2] Ilza Veith, *Huang Ti Nei Ching Su Wen*—The Yellow Emperor's Classic of Internal Medicine, Baltimore, 1949
[3] E. H. Hume, " The Square Kettle," *Bull. Hist. Med.*, 1934, vol. ii. p. 547, and *The Chinese Way in Medicine*, 1940

Blind masseurs were there employed for the first time. Acupuncture consisted of the introduction of long fine needles at various specified points in the body. More than 300 such points are described.[1] The procedure probably did more harm than good, though it survives in the treatment of sciatica and fibrositis. Another therapeutic measure was the use of the " moxa," a small cone of combustible material which was applied at various points and then ignited. It must have demanded considerable self-control on the part of the patient. Inoculation against small-pox was practised in China from ancient times ; dried crusts from a smallpox patient were insufflated into the nose. Organo-therapy was also practised in China, cretins being fed on sheep's thyroid gland.[2]

Early in the Christian era there appeared two famous Chinese medical men, Chang Chung-King and Hua Tu. CHANG CHUNG-KING, who lived about A.D. 195, is sometimes called the Chinese Hippocrates. His book on fevers is one of the classics of Chinese medical literature, and he was probably the first to treat certain fevers by cold baths. He also inaugurated a study of disease which was based upon observations of the patient rather than upon theories, the true Hippocratic outlook. Furthermore, he was revered on account of his noble aims and high ideals.

HUA TU (A.D. 115–205)[3] was the most famous surgeon of ancient China. To him is attributed the discovery of anaesthesia, as he gave his patients a narcotic draught, believed to be *Cannabis indica*, before operating upon them. His operations included laparotomy and excision of the spleen, but we know nothing of his methods, as none of his books have survived. Hua Tu had a great reputation, which continued after his death, and even in recent times effigies of him might be seen in certain temples. He was one of those who made a profound study of the pulse, a method of examination which is very prominent in Chinese medicine. Two hundred varieties of pulse have been described, and it is believed that any internal disease may be diagnosed from the pulse alone. Several hours may be spent in the investigation, the pulse being felt in many different places.

[1] E. W. Cowdry, "Taoist Ideas of Human Anatomy," *Ann. Med. Hist.*, 1921, vol. iii. p. 301
[2] J. Regnault, *Médecine et Pharmacie chez les Chinois*, Paris, 1902
[3] K. K. Chen and A. S. H. Ling, "Fragments of Chinese Medical History," *Ann. Med. Hist.*, 1926, vol. viii. p. 185

The Chinese have always felt a profound reverence for the past, and their ancient medical classics are more highly regarded by them than are the more modern works.

In 1744 the Emperor Kien Lung, a great patron of literature, conceived the idea of gathering together all the medical knowledge then available and publishing it as an encyclopædia of medicine and surgery. The work was undertaken by a committee of experts, and *The Golden Mirror of Medicine*, in forty volumes, was the result. It is still regarded as a standard work. Shortly after this time the pioneers of modern medicine began to reach China and to influence the traditional beliefs. One of the first to introduce European medicine into the East was THOMAS R. COLLEDGE, a young surgeon in the service of the East India Company, who, in 1827, opened a hospital for diseases of the eye at Macao. A few years later (1835), Colledge collaborated with an American medical missionary, PETER PARKER, in the establishment of a general hospital at Canton. One of the main objects of this hospital was " to educate Chinese youths in Western medicine." Among those youths was SUN YAT SEN (1867–1925), first President of the Chinese Republic, who graduated at Hong-kong, but continued to take an active interest in the hospital and school at Canton which now bears his name[1].

The first Chinese to study medicine abroad was WONG FOON, who graduated at Edinburgh in 1855 and then practised at Canton until his death in 1878.

The pioneer work at Canton was followed by the foundation of hospitals and medical schools in many other parts of China. Originally staffed mainly by British and American doctors, all those institutions have now come under the management of the Chinese, who are well fitted for the task, although the need for well-trained medical men is enormous. Although some of the ancient ideas and methods still hold their own, China is gradually evolving a system of medical practice which follows Western teaching and yet retains all that is best in the old and venerated Chinese tradition.

Medicine in Japan followed the adopted Chinese lines until 1867, when the influence of Germany became prominent. Many of the leaders of Japanese medicine were trained in Germany,

[1] W. W. Cadbury and M. H. Jones, *At the Point of a Lancet* (*One Hundred Years of the Canton Hospital*, 1835–1935), Shanghai, 1935

and German was adopted as the language of scientific periodicals. Japan has made some noteworthy contributions to progress, especially in bacteriology. Among those who led the way were such men as Kitasato (p. 287) and Noguchi (p. 359).

To sum up what has been described in this chapter, it may be said that the Babylonians and Egyptians practised an empirical and magical kind of medicine, regulated by a strict code but not inspired by any deep spirit of inquiry into the causes of disease. The Hebrews laid great stress on personal and social hygiene, and were the founders of epidemiology and public health. The Hindus contributed materially to the art of surgery, while the Chinese were the originators of many discoveries in medicine which came to full fruition at later dates.

BOOKS FOR FURTHER READING

BREASTED, J. H. *Ancient Times, a History of the Early World*, Chicago, 1935

BRIM, C. J. *Medicine in the Bible*, New York, 1936

DAWSON, W. R. *Magician and Leech*, 1929

EBBELL, B. Trans. of *The Papyrus Ebers: The Greatest Egyptian Medical Document*, Copenhagen, 1937

GLANVILLE, S. R. K. Ed. *The Legacy of Egypt*, 1942

GODLEY, A. D. Trans. of *Herodotus*, Loeb Library, 4 vols. 1921

HOERNLE, A. F. R. *Studies in the Medicine of Ancient India*, 1907

HUME, E. H. *The Chinese Way in Medicine*, Baltimore, 1940

HURRY, J. B. *Imhotep: the Vizier and Physician of King Zoser*, 1928

JEE, Sir B. S. *A Short History of Aryan Medical Science*, 1896

JOHNS, C. H. W. *The Oldest Code of Law in the World*, 1905

MOODIE, R. L. *Palæopathology: An Introduction to the Study of Ancient Evidences of Disease*, Illinois, 1923

PREUSS, J. *Biblische-Talmudische Medizin*, Berlin, 1911

RUFFER, Sir M. A. *Studies in the Palaeopathology of Egypt*, Chicago, 1921

WONG, C. M., and WU, LIEN-TEH. *History of Chinese Medicine*, Tientsin, 1932

WOOLLEY, C. L. *Ur of the Chaldees*, 1929

CHAPTER III

EARLY GREEK MEDICINE

MODERN civilization owes an immense debt to Ancient Greece. Almost everything that contributes to the interest and happiness of life originated in Greece. Philosophy and history, poetry and drama, sculpture and architecture, mathematics and astronomy, science and medicine ; all had their roots there, and indeed attained in some instances a level of excellence which has never since been equalled.

Medicine, separated from magic, became inspired by the spirit of scientific inquiry which dominated all the work of Hippocrates, the Father of Medicine, whose leadership, undimmed throughout the centuries, remains unchallenged to this day.[1]

It is interesting to study the manner in which Greek medicine arose,[2] and the steps by which it progressed towards the golden Hippocratic Age. In pursuing such a study we are confronted by the difficulty of separating fact from fiction, history from legend, and gods from men. Nevertheless we may trace through the maze the thread of thought which led by devious ways to the foundation of medicine.[3]

By this time the practice of medicine, though dominated by empiricism and superstition, had already attained a high standard. There can be no doubt that Babylonia and Egypt, and even Persia and India, handed on to Greece the torch of learning. Herodotus himself furnishes proof of this.

It was in the Greek Islands that this knowledge was collected and amplified in the pre-Hellenic period. Only within comparatively recent times, thanks to the labours of Sir Arthur Evans and others, has the importance of the Minoan Civilization been established. The Minoans, a race of obscure origin, had their headquarters in Crete, and the beautiful frescoes and statuary which adorned the Palace of Knossos show that their arts had

[1] W. Langdon-Brown, G. E. Gask, J. D. Comrie, and J. A. Nixon, " What Medicine owes to Greek Culture," *Lancet*, 1939, vol. ii. p. 90
[2] C. G. Cumston, *An Introduction to the History of Medicine*, 1926, p. 72
[3] A. P. Cawadias, " From Epidauros to Galenos. The Principal Currents of Greek Medical Thought," *Ann. Med. Hist.*, 1921, vol. iii. p. 501

progressed far.[1] Unfortunately we have no records of the condition of medicine at the epoch which extended from 4000 to 2000 B.C., but the serpent, symbol of healing, is depicted on the statuary and baths, and sanitary arrangements have been brought to light. Many inscriptions remain undeciphered, so that the future may show the stage at which medicine had arrived in Minoan times.

" Where Delos rose and Phœbus sprung "

On another Ægean island we may still find records of the sources of the healing art in Ancient Greece.[2] The island of Delos, in the Cyclades group, was the reputed birthplace of Apollo, the god of health, from whom arose the current of medical thought which passed on through the oracle of Delphi and the cult of Aesculapius, through the Homeric heroes and the philosopher-physicians of Greece, to reach at last yet another island, that of Cos, where Hippocrates, the master physician, was born.

From Greek mythology we learn that Delos, once a floating island, was raised from the bed of the sea and anchored by Zeus to provide a resting-place for the goddess Leto, who there gave birth to the twins, Apollo (Phœbus) and Artemis (Diana).

Delos, still a lovely isle set in a clear azure sea, is crowned by Mount Cynthus, on whose slope, near the summit, there is a grotto, consisting of a cleft in the rock roofed by a double row of huge stone slabs forming a primitive arch (Plate IX). This, we are told, was the birthplace of Apollo. There can be few lovelier spots in the Ægean archipelago. Delos became not only a place of pilgrimage but the centre of government of the Delian league, a great city and an international market, the chief merchandise being wheat and slaves. One may still discern the floor of the market, where 15,000 slaves were sold in a single day.

Delos is now an uninhabited isle, and even in the time of Ovid it had become " Delos, the desolate, where once men prayed." Only a few ruined pillars mark the place of the temple, only a few of the subterranean water cisterns show the position of the mansion-houses of the classic period. Close by is the little islet of Rheneia, which served both as cemetery and as maternity hospital for the community, because neither death nor birth was permitted on the holy ground of Delos.

[1] Sir A. Evans, *The Palace of Minos at Knossos*, 4 vols., 1921
[2] W. MacNeile Dixon, *Hellas Revisited*, 1929, p. 51

EARLY GREEK MEDICINE

Apollo, and the Oracle of Delphi

Apollo, tradition tells us, did not long remain on Delos. He must have been very young when he was transported to Delphi, because it was then that his umbilical cord separated, a fact commemorated by the "omphalos," a large sugar-loaf stone which may still be seen near the temple (Plate IX). According to another tradition the omphalos is said to have been set up to mark the centre or navel of the earth. The exact position of this spot had been determined by Zeus, who had released at opposite ends of the earth (as then known) two eagles, which flew towards each other, and met at Delphi.[1] There is another omphalos, probably of more recent date. This is preserved in the local museum at Kastri, a village which occupied the site of Delphi and which was bodily transplanted half a mile eastwards by the French excavators before they unearthed the ruins which may now be seen.[2] High up on the side of Mount Parnassus, approached by a steep and winding road from the port of Itea on the Gulf of Corinth, twelve miles distant, Delphi is a most eerie and awesome place even to-day, and one may readily understand why it occupied the central point in maps of Greece, just as Jerusalem was placed in the centre in the later days of Christendom.

The first act of the infant Apollo, on his arrival at Delphi, was to slay a python or monster, which had rendered the site untenable. Delphi thereupon leapt into fame, and for centuries it remained a shrine for the worship of Apollo, the most sacred spot in all Greece. Here arose the famous oracle which made Delphi a household word.[3]

Beside the marble-paved Sacred Way, by which the tourist now ascends the hill towards the Temple of Apollo, there stands a circular platform.[4] Close by, though it has long since disappeared, there was a chasm or cleft in the rock from which issued intoxicating fumes. Over it was a tripod on which the priestess sat, chewing laurel leaves, and uttering her raving replies to questions. These, however incoherent, were cleverly transcribed

[1] Sir William Smith, *A Classical Dictionary of Biography, Mythology, and Geography*, 1891, 21st ed.
[2] Sir J. G. Frazer, *Studies in Greek Scenery, Legend, and History*, 1931, p. 374
[3] H. W. Parke, *A History of the Delphic Oracle*, Oxford 1939
[4] E. A. Gardner, *Greece and the Ægean*, 1938, p. 116

into hexameter verse which usually conveyed an ambiguous meaning. Clearly the " sibyl " performed the function of a spiritualistic medium. Her " ego," under the influence of fumes or laurel, became " submerged," and a " dissociated personality " replied to inquirers. The staff of interpreters was in close touch with all the events of the day, constituting a Ministry of Information, well qualified to advise, and protected from failure by their non-committal answers. King Crœsus, for example,[1] inquiring of the oracle whether he should go to war against the Persians, was told that if he did so he would destroy a mighty empire. That empire turned out to be his own !

Again, the inhabitants of Camarina wished to drain a lake near their city which they regarded as a source of malaria. The idea was doubtless correct, but the oracle, on being consulted, replied that Lake Camarina was better left undisturbed. The advice was flouted, the lake was emptied, and the city was captured by an enemy advancing over the dried bed.[2]

The services of the oracle were well rewarded ; indeed, so numerous and so valuable were the gifts to Delphi that treasuries or safe deposits were built by the donors, and some of these, in ruins or partially restored, to-day adorn the sacred precinct. One of the finest of the offerings, discovered only a few years ago, is the life-size bronze figure of a charioteer, amazingly natural, and complete even to the painted ivory eyes and delicate bronze eyelashes.

There can be no doubt that among the many problems submitted to the Delphian Oracle there were some concerned with health and sickness. In those days prognosis was quite as important as treatment, a principle elaborated by Hippocrates, and respected even to-day, when a patient desires reassurance even more than he desires treatment. Yet therapeutic advice may have been given at Delphi, as one cannot imagine that the astute " brains trust " established there would neglect so obvious an opportunity of raising their prestige as that afforded by the treatment of disease. The Oracle of Delphi was almost certainly a centre for medical advice, although its influence has been neglected by medical historians.

---

[1] T. Dempsey, *The Delphic Oracle, its Early History, Influence, and Fall*, Oxford, 1918, p. 69
[2] J. D. Rolleston, "The Medical Aspects of the Greek Anthology," *Janus*, 1914, vol. xix. p. 105

" Incubation," or Temple Sleep

It is only a step from Apollo and the Delphic Oracle to Aesculapius and the cult of " temple healing " associated with his name.[1] Apollo taught the healing art to Chiron, the gifted centaur, who is sometimes regarded as the god of Surgery, and Chiron in his turn instructed Jason, Achilles, and Aesculapius.[2] Aesculapius (Asklepios) is a shadowy figure, who may have had a human existence about 1250 B.C.[3] At all events, it was at Delphi that he performed miracles of healing, even restoring the dead to life. So many patients did he cure that Pluto, the ruler of the Underworld, fearing that the supply of souls might thereby be decreased, appealed to the supreme god Zeus, who promptly slew Aesculapius with a thunderbolt. Nevertheless, Aesculapius reaped his posthumous reward, for he became a god and was worshipped in hundreds of temples throughout Greece.[4] Ruins of these temples, or Asklepieia, may still be seen. One of the most famous was at Epidaurus ; there were others at Cos, Athens, Pergamos, and many other places.

To the Asklepieia came many sick persons for the healing ritual known as " incubation," or temple sleep.[5] On arrival the patient was expected to make a sacrificial offering, and to purify himself by bathing. Then he lay down to sleep in the *abaton*, a long colonnade open to the air at each side. During the night Aesculapius appeared in a dream and gave advice, or in certain cases performed an operation, and in the morning the patient departed cured.

Snakes, of the harmless variety still found in Greece, assisted in the treatment by licking the eyes or sores of the patient. The significance of the serpent in medicine has never been satisfactorily explained. It has been suggested that the snake was originally kept to rid buildings of rats, and it was esteemed in Greece in much the same fashion as the cat was in Egypt. Close to each temple was the *tholos*, a small building consisting of two concentric

[1] R. Caton, "Health Temples in Ancient Greece and the Work Carried on in Them," *Proc. Roy. Soc. Med.* (Sect. Hist.), 1914, vol. vii. p. 57
[2] J. D. Gilruth, "Chiron and his Pupil Asclepius," *Ann. Med. Hist.*, 1939, 3rd. Ser., vol. i. p. 158
[3] E. M. Bick, " The Cult of Asklepios," *Ann. Med. Hist.*, 1927, vol. ix. p. 327
[4] R. Caton, *The Temples and Ritual of Asklepios*, 1900 ; I. S. Wile, " The Worship of Asklepios," *Ann. Med. Hist.*, 1920, vol. viii. p. 419
[5] Mary Hamilton, *Incubation, or the Cure of Disease in Pagan Temples and Christian Churches*, St. Andrews, 1906

walls of stone, enclosing a paved pit or well, and it has been suggested that the snakes were housed there. On the other hand, the *tholos* may have been a sacrificial altar. The revelation which came to the sleeping patient consisted of a vision of Aesculapius surrounded by dazzling lights, or only the voice of the god. Incubation apparently depended upon the methods adopted by the Delphian Oracle, and both phenomena could doubtless be explained as forms of psychotherapy.

Our knowledge of incubation is largely derived from inscriptions on the stone *stelæ*, or tablets, found at Epidaurus. Forty-four cases are described, and among them are the following :

1. Kleo was with child for five years. After these five years of pregnancy she came as a suppliant to the god and slept in the *abaton*. As soon as she left it and got outside the temple precincts she bore a son, who immediately after birth washed himself at the fountain and walked about with his mother.

5. A dumb boy came as a suppliant to the temple to recover his voice. When he had performed the sacrifices and fulfilled the rites, the temple priest who bore the sacrificial fire turned to the boy's father and said, " Do you promise to pay within a year the fees for the cure, if you obtain that for which you have come ? " Suddenly the boy answered, " I do." His father was greatly astonished at this, and told his son to speak again. The boy repeated the words and so was cured.

12. Euippos had had for six years the point of a spear in his cheek. As he was sleeping the god extracted the spear-head and gave it to him into his hands. When day came Euippos departed cured, and he held the spear-head in his hands.

15. Hermodikes of Lampsakos was paralysed in body. In his sleep he was healed by the god, who ordered him to bring to the temple as large a stone as he could, when he left the *abaton*. The man brought the stone, which now lies before the *abaton* (Plate x).

29. Agestratos suffered from insomnia on account of head-aches. As soon as he came to the *abaton* he fell asleep and had a dream. He thought that the god cured him of his headache and, making him stand up, taught him wrestling. When day came he departed cured, and after a short time he competed at the Nemean games and was victor in wrestling.

In reading those records of temple treatment one is impressed by two facts. All cases without exception were cured, and the cure appeared to be miraculous, as many had been regarded as incurable. Failures were not recorded and deaths were never mentioned. How different, as we shall see, were the records of Hippocrates, who faithfully recorded his observations, whatever the issue.

Another source of information on incubation is to be found in the " Ploutos " of Aristophanes. In an amusing and satirical account of a night at the *abaton*, he describes how the blind Ploutos had his sight restored by two prodigious serpents which licked his eyelids while he slept. Aristides, who lived in the second century A.D., describes in his " Sacred Orations " his experiences as a patient at various temples of Aesculapius. At Pergamos the treatment was vigorous, but one must remember that Aristides was a hypochondriac, and would respond only to strong measures. He tells us that " the god ordered him to rub himself over with mud, to wash in the well, and to run three times round the temple." It was a north wind and a keen frost, yet he did as he was told, and found himself in fine condition. Another description of temple healing, from the patient's point of view, may be found in Chapter III of Walter Pater's romance, *Marius the Epicurean* (1885).

Although in the early days of the cult of incubation the methods employed were mystical and supernatural, physical therapy, comprising diet, bathing, and exercise, played an increasingly important part in the cure. Instead of being cured, as by a miracle, in a single night, the patient sometimes remained for days or weeks taking the waters and baths, and following a routine of diet and exercise as at any modern spa. The Asklepieia were usually in healthy places, with natural springs and fine scenery. Even in its present ruined state Epidaurus is a lovely place, and in spring the abundant anemones and other gay flowers enhance its attractiveness. Amusements were provided for the patients and their friends. The theatre at Epidaurus, in a remarkably good state of preservation, is one of the finest in Greece, seating about 20,000 persons (Plate x). One may also visit the stadium or sports ground, and may use the massive stone seats provided for patients in the temple grounds.

Incubation was practised as early as the eighth century B.C. It was continued far into the Christian era, and even to-day, in

Greece and the Ægean Islands, in Asia Minor and in Italy, traces of this ancient cult may still be found. In the churches of Palermo, Naples, Sardinia, and Styria, the custom survives to this day. On the sacred island of Tenos, close to Delos, a great religious festival is held twice a year, and many sick persons sleep in the church in expectation of a cure. Each year miracles are reported. Incubation is also still practised on a small scale in Cyprus, in Rhodes, and at many country churches on the mainland of Greece and in Asia Minor.

The subject is worthy of careful study, and has been discussed at length by Mary Hamilton in a most interesting monograph, now rather a rare book, published at St. Andrews in 1906.[1]

Before we pass from the early Greek period to the Hippocratic era, two further sources of information must be examined, because both illustrate how medicine, shaking off the bonds of magic and of empiricism, emerged at last as a subject of scientific study.

No description of the medicine of Ancient Greece is complete without some reference to her greatest poet, and to the philosophers, who included medicine in their comprehensive survey of knowledge.

Homeric Medicine and Surgery [2]

The reader of Homer, in search of information bearing upon medicine, may well be bewildered by the difficulty of distinguishing between gods and men in the characters, and between historical fact and poetic fancy in the narrative. Dr. Schliemann, by his excavations at Troy and at Mycenæ, about 1876, did much to infuse reality into the epic tales of the *Iliad* and the *Odyssey*. As a result, the modern traveller in Greece and adjacent lands may visualize the Trojan war and may follow the wanderings of Odysseus. Nor can he remain unmoved as he enters the citadel of Mycenæ through the Lion Gate, one of the most famous sights of Greece, with its gigantic hundred-ton lintel stone, surmounted by two carved lions ; that gate through which Agamemnon marched forth to aid his brother Menelaos in the siege of Troy, and through which he returned victorious ten years later, only to be murdered

---

[1] Mary Hamilton, *Incubation, or the Cure of Disease in Pagan Temples and Christian Churches*, St. Andrews, 1906
[2] C. W. Daremberg, *La Médecine dans Homère*, Paris, 1865 ; O. Körner, *Die ärztlichen Kenntnisse in Ilias und Odyssee*, Munich, 1929

on his bathroom floor by his unfaithful wife, Clytemnestra. The history of the campaign is well known. From the *Iliad* [1] we learn that the army was supplied with surgeons. There is this description of a dressing station : " Wounded is Odysseus, spearman renowned, and Agamemnon ; and smitten is Eurypylos on the thigh with an arrow. And about them the leeches skilled in medicine are busy, healing their wounds " (xvi. 28). A wounded soldier is told : " Sit where thou art, and drink the bright wine, till Hekamede of the fair tresses shall heat warm water for the bath, and wash away the clotted blood " (xiv. 6). Two of the surgeons are well known as sons of Aesculapius, and they appear to have taken part in the fighting. We are introduced to them thus : " Of them that possessed Trikke and that possessed Oichalia. . . . Asklepios' two sons were leaders, the cunning leeches Podalarius and Machaon.[2] And with them were arrayed thirty hollow ships " (ii. 732).

We are also informed that Agamemnon commanded his herald that he should " with all speed call Machaon hither, the hero son of Asklepios, the noble leech, to see Menelaos, whom one skilled in archery hath wounded with a bow shot, to his glory and our grief. . . . The god-like hero came and drew forth the arrow, and as it was drawn forth the keen barbs were broken backwards . . . and when he saw the wound where the arrow had lighted, he sucked out the blood and cunningly spread thereon soothing drugs, such as Cheiron of his good will had imparted to his sire " (iv. 190).

There are many descriptions of wounds in the *Iliad*. The following suggests that the writer was familiar with the acetabulum, though it is uncertain to what " sinews " he refers : " Then Tydeides grasped in his hand a stone . . . therewith he smote Aineias on the hip where the thigh turneth in the hip joint, and this men call the ' cup bone.' So he crushed his cup bone, and brake both sinews withal, and the jagged stone tore apart the skin. Then the hero stayed fallen upon his knees . . . and the darkness of night veiled his eyes " (v. 294). Other mortal wounds are described. For instance, " Achilles, smiting the neck [of Deukalion] with his sword, swept far both head and helm, and the marrow rose out of the backbone and the corpse lay stretched

---

[1] Homer, *The Iliad*, trans. by A. Lang, W. Leaf, and E. Myers, 1883
[2] S. Wood, " Homer's Surgeons ; Machaon and Podalarius," *Lancet*, 1931, vol. i. pp. 892, 947

on the earth." (xx. 479). Or again, " Idomeneus . . . smote him with a spear in the throat below the chin and drove the point straight through, and he fell as an oak falls, or a tall pine tree . . . so he lay stretched out, groaning and clutching the bloody dust " (xiii. 387).

The existence of those military " leeches " or surgeons shows that, in the army at least, medicine was not entirely in the hands of the priests. Surgery naturally lends itself less readily to magical methods of cure than does medicine, but it is not unreasonable to infer, regarding priestly physicians and lay " leeches," that each practised his art at the same epoch, and each, being consulted by a different class of patient, was probably quite independent of the other. As we shall presently note, the medical work of Hippocrates had little in common with that of the priests of the Asklepieia in his native island of Cos. Even in the days of Homer, about 1000 B.C., there was a movement towards scientific medicine guided by observation and reason rather than by magic and superstition.

The *Odyssey*,[1] though it does not tell of bloody battles like the *Iliad*, supplies interesting facts on the medical lore of the time. We read that " Odysseus had come on his swift ship to seek a deadly drug, that he might have wherewithal to smear his bronze-shod arrows " (i. 260).

There is also the famous " nepenthe " used by Helen, and the hint that in medicine the Greeks may have learned from the Egyptians : " Then Helen, daughter of Zeus . . . cast a drug into the wine whereof they drank, a drug to lull all pain and anger, and bring forgetfulness of every sorrow. . . . Medicines of such virtue had the daughter of Zeus, which Polydamna, the wife of Thon, had given her, a woman of Egypt, where earth yields herbs in greatest plenty, many that are healing in the cup, and many baneful. There each man is a leech skilled beyond all human kind " (iv. 220).

The Philosopher-Physicians of Ancient Greece

It is to the work of the early Greek philosophers,[2] however, five hundred years after Homer's day, that Greek medicine is indebted for that impetus which led men to refuse to be blindly guided by

[1] Homer, *The Odyssey*, trans. by S. H. Butcher and A. Lang, 1887
[2] J. Burnet, *Early Greek Philosophy*, 1908

PLATE XI   THE ISLAND OF COS

The so-called " Tree of Hippocrates " (36 ft. in circumference).   It is surrounded by a marble wall, one face of which bears the inscription illustrated in Plate XII
(page 52)

Castle of the Knights of St. John, of an earlier date than the more famous headquarters at Rhodes (see Plates XXIII and XXIV)

PLATE XII   THE FATHER OF MEDICINE

IPPOCRATE DI COO
ALL'OMBRA DI QVESTO PLATANO
ISTRVENDO ED EDVCANDO I GIOVANI
ALL'ARTE ED AL SACERDOZIO DELLA MEDICINA
ISTITVIVA QVESTO GIVRAMENTO
NEL SECOLO IV A. C.

MCMXXX - VIII - E.J.

Upper.   Statue found on the island of Cos, believed to be that of Hippocrates
(page 52)

Lower.   Modern Italian inscription at the base of the "Tree of Hippocrates"
in Cos (see Plate XI)

supernatural influences or by rule-of-thumb, and impelled them rather to seek out for themselves the causes and reasons of all the phenomena of Nature. The philosophers, indeed, determined the course which Greek medicine was to take in the hands of Hippocrates and his followers.[1] We know little of the lives of those philosophers ; and their writings, apart from a few fragments, have all perished, so that the story is soon told, though it is none the less important. One of the greatest was PYTHAGORAS (580–498 B.C.). Save that he was a native of Samos and an extensive traveller, and that he lived for many years at Croton in Southern Italy, we know nothing of his life. His chief claim to fame was his discovery of the theory of numbers. He may be said to have founded Arithmetic. He showed that the pitch of a note produced by a stretched string depended upon the length of the string, and that there was a numerical ratio between the lengths which gave forth the concordant notes of the octave. He was the first to believe that the earth was a sphere. He believed in immortality and in the transmigration of souls, and he contended that animals also possessed souls. Pythagoras and the school which he founded exercised a profound influence upon medicine ; their ideas were a stimulus to critical thought, and taught men to inquire into causes for the sake of knowledge alone, whether such knowledge could yield immediate practical results or not. The doctrine of numbers suggested to Hippocrates the idea of critical days in illness, and of the four elements and humours.

More closely identified with medicine was ALCMÆON of Croton, a pupil of Pythagoras, who lived about 500 B.C. We know that he dissected animals, for he described the optic nerves and the Eustachian tubes, and he enunciated the strange theory that goats breathe by their ears (*cf.* p. 25). He distinguished between veins and arteries, although he subscribed to the current view that the arteries contained air, as they appeared empty when opened after death. Alcmæon noted that the brain, and not the heart, was the seat of the senses and the intellect. He stated, too, that disease was a discord or disharmony of the elements composing the body, and that health was dependent upon harmony.

It may be sufficient for our purpose to mention one more philosopher of the Pythagorean school. EMPEDOCLES of Agri-

---

[1] J. Wright, "A Medical History on the Timaeus," *Ann. Med. Hist.*, 1925, vol. viii. p. 116 ; J. D. Rolleston, " The Medical Aspects of the Greek Anthology," *Janus*, 1914, vol. xix.

gentum, in Sicily, lived from 504 to 443 B.C.[1] His life was surrounded by an aura of mystery. Various miracles were attributed to him, and he was said to have ended his days by leaping into the crater of Mt. Etna, so that he might become a god. He regarded the universe and everything in it as composed of four elements— fire, air, earth, and water. In this idea we have the nucleus of the theory of humours which was to dominate medical practice for centuries. Empedocles also held that the heart was the organ by which the " pneuma," which was identified with life and breath, was distributed throughout the body. He believed that breathing took place through the pores of the skin, as well as through the lungs. " All beings," he wrote,[2] " have bloodless tubes of flesh spread over the outside of the body, and at the openings of these the outer layers of the skin are pierced all over with close set ducts, so that the blood remains within, while a facile opening is cut for the air to pass through." The conception of the pneuma was later to find its way into the doctrines of Galen and his followers. That Empedocles was a practical physician is shown by the report that he checked an epidemic in his town of Agrigentum by draining a swamp and fumigating the houses.

[1] J. Burnet, *Early Greek Philosophy*, 1908, p. 234
[2] *Ibid*, p. 253

BOOKS FOR FURTHER READING

BURNET, J.   *Early Greek Philosophy*, 1908
CATON, R.   *The Temples and Ritual of Asklepios*, 1900
DAREMBERG, C.   *La Médecine dans Homère*, Paris, 1865
DEMPSEY, T.   *The Delphic Oracle, its Early History, Influence, and Fall*, Oxford, 1918
FRAZER, Sir J. G.   *Studies in Greek Scenery, Legend, and History*, 1931
GARDNER, E. A.   *Greece and the Ægean*, 1938
HAMILTON, MARY.   *Incubation, or the Cure of Disease in Pagan Temples and Christian Churches*, St. Andrews, 1906
HOMER.   *The Iliad*, trans. by A. Lang, W. Leaf, and E. Myers, 1883 ; *The Odyssey*, trans. by S. H. Butcher and A. Lang, 1887
KÖRNER, O.   *Die ärztlichen Kenntnisse in Ilias und Odyssee*, Munich, 1929
PARKE, H. W.   *A History of the Delphic Oracle*, Oxford, 1939

CHAPTER IV

HIPPOCRATIC MEDICINE

THE age of Pericles, who died in 429 B.C., followed the decisive Greek victories over the Persians, and witnessed one of the greatest uprisings of the human spirit that the world has ever known. Aeschylus, the father of Greek tragedy, was followed by Sophocles and Euripides, and later by Aristophanes, the greatest of Greek writers of comedy. The Parthenon was being adorned by the sculptures of Pheidias, Socrates brought new life to philosophy, to be succeeded by Plato and Aristotle. Herodotus was writing his history, and geography, astronomy, and mathematics shared in the general advance. It was an opportune moment for the birth of scientific medicine, and for the entry upon the stage of history of the greatest physician of all time.

The Background to Hippocrates

In the little island of Cos, close to the coast of Asia Minor, HIPPOCRATES was born in 460 B.C.[1] He is said to have been a direct descendant of Aesculapius, who had two daughters, Hygieia and Panacea, whose names have become household words. It has also been stated that Hippocrates was a member of a guild of Asklepeiads, and was in some way connected with the Asklepieion, the ruins of which, partially reconstructed, stand on a beautiful hillside some three miles inland from the town of Cos.[2] Recent authorities have disproved this statement, and have stated that the Aesculapian cult of temple healing did not reach Cos until after the death of Hippocrates. Moreover, it is obvious to the most casual inquirer, as we have already remarked, that the methods and the records of the Hippocratic school were entirely different from those of the priests of Aesculapius.[3] The only relic of Hippocrates which remains in Cos is the gigantic tree, an Oriental

[1] J. Finlayson, "Hippocrates," *Glas. Med. Jour.*, 1892, vol. xxxvii. No. 4 ; H. Sigerist, "Notes and Comments on Hippocrates," *Bull. Hist. Med.*, 1934, vol. ii. p. 190
[2] G. E. Gask, "Early Medical Schools ; the Cult of Aesculapius and the Origin of Hippocratic Medicine," *Ann. Med. Hist.*, 1939, 3rd Series, vol. i. p. 128, and 1940, vol. ii. p. 383
[3] E. T. Withington, "The Asclepiadae and the Priests of Asclepios," in Singer's *Studies in the History and Method of Science*, 1921, vol. ii. p. 192

Plane, which stands in the centre of the town of Cos (Plate xɪ). Under the shade of its branches, now so carefully supported by props of wood and pillars of stone, Hippocrates is reputed to have taught his pupils, holding an open-air clinic. Two thousand five hundred years is a great age for a tree, yet one would fain believe that this is a genuine living memento of the great teacher, a vital link between him and those who learn from him even to-day. At all events it is, as it should be, a place of pious pilgrimage for all physicians. Hippocrates lived a long life, and although the date of his death is not known with accuracy, it was probably 355 B.C. Although he lived mainly at Cos, he was a great traveller, like the other wise men of his day, and he practised in Thessaly, Athens, and other places, and eventually died at Larissa.

None of the busts and statues of Hippocrates which still exist can be regarded as an authentic portrait, but all depict a dignified, thoughtful, and gracious figure, and one can well imagine him as an inspiring teacher and an ideal physician (Plate xɪɪ).

The Hippocratic Collection

Although we know very little of the man himself, we have in the Hippocratic Collection, or *Corpus Hippocraticum*, a complete exposition of his methods. Hippocrates was not the sole author of the hundred or more books which make up the collection, but that does not detract from their value as he certainly inspired them all. It would serve no useful purpose to discuss, as has so often been done, which of the works were genuinely those of Hippocrates, or whether there was more than one physician and author named Hippocrates. It will be more profitable to illustrate, by quotation from the books which are generally acknowledged to be most truly Hippocratic, what were the ideas and ideals, the methods and procedures, which inspired the Father of Medicine.

In studying the works of Hippocrates no one can fail to remark his high standard of ethical conduct, his insistence on prognosis, his accuracy of observation, and his clarity in recording cases.

A knowledge of Greek is no longer essential for such a study, as the works of Hippocrates have been translated into many languages, and have been the subject of innumerable commentaries. Some of the works, notably the *Aphorisms*, were used as textbooks until the beginning of the nineteenth century, and it is perhaps unfortunate that they have not remained in use until the present day. Although they contain much that is obsolete, they also embody a code of teaching and principles that are surprisingly modern. The first complete Greek edition of the works of Hippocrates was printed by Aldo Manuzio of Venice in 1526. A Latin edition had been issued from the press of Calvus in Rome the previous year. The most extensive translation is in French, in ten volumes, which appeared in 1839–61, by E. Littré (*Œuvres complètes d'Hippocrate*). Of English translations the best known is that of Dr. Francis Adams, the country practitioner and scholar who practised at Banchory, in Aberdeenshire, and who is the subject of a charming essay in Dr. John Brown's *Horae Subsecivae*. Adams' translation of Hippocrates appeared in 1849.[1] More recent translations are by W. H. S. Jones (which gives the original Greek alongside the translation), and by John Chadwick and W. N. Mann.[2]

Let us briefly glance at the contents of the works. Hippocrates, the first to separate Medicine from Philosophy, set a high standard for all who wished to follow what he called " The Art."

The Hippocratic Oath

The " Hippocratic Oath," has been adopted as a pattern by medical men throughout the ages.

In this noble code of ethics the disciple or graduand is shown the dignity and responsibility of his calling, and there is urged upon him the duty of respect for his school or university, of making freely available any new discovery, of maintaining professional secrecy, and refraining from gossip, of seeking above all the benefit of the patient, and of taking no mean advantage of the position of medical adviser. Some controversy has arisen regarding the promise not to perform lithotomy.[3] Whatever this may imply, it is clear that surgery, in certain cases, was regarded as unworthy of the physician. Even at that early date surgery was to be referred to a specialist class of craftsmen.

---

[1] *The Genuine Works of Hippocrates*, trans. by F. Adams for Sydenham Society, 1849, 2 vols. ; C. Singer, " A Great Country Doctor : Francis Adams of Banchory, 1796–1861," *Bull. Hist. Med.*, 1942, vol. xii. p. 1
[2] *Hippocrates*, trans. by W. H. S. Jones and E. T. Withington, Loeb Library, 4 vols., 1923–31 ; J. Chadwick and W. N. Mann, *The Medical Works of Hippocrates*, 1950
[3] S. Nittis, " The Hippocratic Oath in Reference to Lithotomy," *Bull. Hist. Med.*, 1939, vol. vii. p. 719 ; L. Edelstein, *The Hippocratic Oath*, Baltimore, 1943

The Oath is worth quoting in its entirety in one of the numerous English renderings :

" *I swear by Apollo the Physician, by Aesculapius, by Hygieia, by Panacea, and by all the gods and goddesses, making them my witnesses, that I will carry out according to my ability and judgment, this oath and this indenture. To hold my teacher in this art equal to my own parents; to make him partner in my livelihood; when he is in need of money to share mine with him; to consider his family as my own brothers, and to teach them this art, if they want to learn it, without fee or indenture; to impart precept, oral instruction, and all other instruction to my own sons, the sons of my teacher, and to pupils who have taken the physicians' Oath, but to nobody else. I will use treatment to help the sick according to my ability and judgment, but never with a view to injury and wrong-doing. Neither will I administer a poison to anybody when asked to do so, nor will I suggest such a course. Similarly I will not give to a woman a pessary to cause abortion. But I will keep pure and holy both my life and my art. I will not use the knife, not even, verily, on sufferers from stone, but I will give place to such as are craftsmen therein. Into what-soever houses I enter, I will enter to help the sick, and I will abstain from all intentional wrongdoing and harm, especially from abusing the bodies of man or woman, bond or free. And whatsoever I shall see or hear in the course of my profession, as well as outside my profession in my inter-course with men, if it be what should not be published abroad, I will never divulge, holding such things to be holy secrets. Now if I carry out this oath, and break it not, may I gain for ever reputation among all men for my life and for my art ; but if I transgress it and forswear myself, may the opposite befall me.*"

Various embellishments of the oath and hints on professional conduct are to be found in other Hippocratic writings.[1] The book entitled *Precepts*, generally believed to be of later date than Hippocrates, but the work of one of his school, gives the following advice : " I urge you not to be too grasping, but to consider carefully your patient's means. Sometimes give your services for nothing . . . and if there be an opportunity of serving one who is a stranger in financial straits, give full assistance to all such. *For where there is the love of man, there is also love of the art.*" (*Prec.* vi.) The same writer is even more personal when he advises the physician to " avoid adopting, in order to gain a patient, luxurious

[1] S. Nittis, " Hippocratic Ethics and Present-day Trends in Medicine," *Bull. Hist Med.*, 1942, vol. xii. p. 336 ; W. H. S. Jones, *The Doctor's Oath*, 1924

headgear or elaborate perfume." "Yet," he adds, "I do not forbid your trying to please, for it is not unworthy of a physician's dignity."

The Nature of Disease

Hippocrates knew little of anatomy or physiology, and he possessed neither clinical thermometer nor stethoscope. It is true that he employed auscultation, placing his ear to the chest of the patient and describing, for example, the friction sound of pleurisy, which he aptly likened to the creaking of leather. But although he had no scientific apparatus, he had scientific method, and his writings are full of sound observation and logical reasoning. He had no patience with the idea that disease was a punishment sent by the gods.[1] His book on *The Sacred Disease* (believed to be epilepsy [2]) begins : " It is not in my opinion, any more divine or more sacred than other diseases, but has a natural cause, and its supposed divine origin is due to man's inexperience . . . fevers, tertians, and quartans, seem to me to be no less sacred and god-sent than this disease, but nobody wonders at them." " Every disease," he continues, " has its own nature and arises from external causes, from cold, from the sun, or from changing winds." Hippocrates noted the effect of food, of occupation, and, especially, of climate in causing disease. One of his most interesting books deals with *Airs, Waters, and Places*. He advises the physician about to set up practice in an unfamiliar town, to observe the exposure, the prevailing winds, the water supply, the nature of the soil and the habits of the people. From this information he will be able to deduce what diseases are the most prevalent, and will thus " achieve the greatest triumphs in the practice of his art." The writer is much impressed by the influence of climate upon mind and body. " When the land is oppressed by winter's storms and burned by the sun, men are hard, stubborn, and independent, with more than average intelligence in the arts, and in war of more than average courage."

[1] H. O. Taylor, *Greek Biology and Medicine*, 1922, p. 23 ; R. O. Moon, *Hippocrates and his Successors in Relation to the Philosophy of their Times* (Fitzpatrick Lectures), 1923
[2] O. Temkin, " The Doctrine of Epilepsy in the Hippocratic Writings," *Bull. Hist. Med.*, 1933, vol. i. p. 277

The Importance of Prognosis

From a study of the natural history of disease, Hippocrates was able to forecast how the symptoms would develop, and whether a fatal issue was likely to result. Perhaps his own long life was conducive to his study of prognosis. Sir James Mackenzie used to remark, " No doctor lives long enough to write a reliable book on prognosis." One of the greatest works of Hippocrates is entitled *Prognostic*. Here is an extract from the preface : " I hold that it is an excellent thing for the physician to practice forecasting . . . he will carry out treatment best if he knows beforehand from the present symptoms what will take place later." The routine method of examination is described thus : " First, he must examine the face of the patient." Then follows the classical description of the " Hippocratic facies," which denotes impending death—" Nose sharp, eyes hollow, temples shrunken, ears cold and with their lobes turned outward, the skin of the face parched and tense, the colour yellow or very dusky." The description is closely mirrored by Shakespeare in his account of the death of Falstaff : " . . . his nose was as sharp as a pen, and a' babbled of green fields."

In *Prognostic* the physician's attention is also directed to the position assumed by the patient in bed, the nature of the respirations, the appearance of the sputum, and to many other signs upon which prognosis may be based. The concluding paragraph runs, " Do not regret the omission, from my account, of the name of any disease. For it is by the same symptoms in all cases that you will know the diseases that come to a crisis at the time I have stated."

The school of Hippocrates was not without its rivals. On the mainland close to the island of Cos there was the school of Cnidos, and the Cnidian physicians classified all symptoms as diseases, and produced a remedy for each.[1] For them diagnosis and treatment were everything. They were not concerned with causes, nor with prognosis. Hippocrates, on the other hand, was essentially an observer. He knew how to record a case clearly and concisely. Not for him were the boastful cures of the Aesculapian temples. Success and failure he recorded without partiality. His case mortality was high, 60 per cent. in the 42 cases described

---

[1] C. Singer, " Medicine " in *The Legacy of Greece*, ed. R. W. Livingstone, 1921, p. 206

in the books of *Epidemics*, but one must remember that most of the cases were of acute and serious disease.

Malaria was very common and fatal, so was dysentery. The following may be a case of blackwater fever. " Philliscus lived by the wall. He took to his bed with acute fever on the first day and sweating ; night uncomfortable. Third day—until midday he appeared to have lost the fever, but towards evening acute fever, sweating, thirst, dry tongue, black urine. Sleepless ; completely out of his mind. Fifth day—distressing night, irrational talk, black urine, cold sweat. About midday on the sixth day he died. The breathing throughout, as though he were recollecting to do it, was rare and large." The last sentence describes what we now call Cheyne-Stokes respiration.

One other case may be quoted, a head injury followed by otitis and meningitis. " The daughter of Nerios, a beautiful maiden aged twenty, was playing with a girl friend, who struck her with the open hand on the top of the head. She saw a blackness before her eyes and lost her breath, and on getting home was taken with severe fever, with headache, and redness of the face. On the seventh day there issued from the right ear more than a cupful of fœtid reddish pus, and she seemed a little relieved. But the fever returned, she became comatose and speechless ; the right side of her face was drawn ; spasms ; tremor and breathlessness followed ; her tongue and eyes became paralyzed ; she died on the ninth day."

Hippocrates on Treatment

Hippocrates made little use of drugs in treatment. He watched the course of the disease and did not interfere with nature.[1] He knew that there was in most diseases a tendency to natural cure, the principle of *Vis Medicatrix Naturæ*. " Our natures," he said, " are the physicians of our diseases." We must refrain from meddlesome interference. Yet he gave sound advice, employed baths and fomentations when indicated, and prescribed a simple diet. His methods may be studied in his *Regimen in Acute Diseases*. The favourite diet was barley gruel, and sometimes no other food was given. This was no great

[1] E. W. Goodall, " On Infectious Diseases and Epidemiology in the Hippocratic Collection," *Proc. Roy. Soc. Med.* (Sect. Hist.), 1934, vol. xxvii. p. 524 ; W. A. Heidel, *Hippocratic Medicine : Its Spirit and Method*, New York, 1943

hardship to the Greeks, who were simple livers, taking two meals a day, or even one meal only. Honey was also favoured. " The drink to be employed should there be any pain, is oxymel [vinegar and honey]. If there be great thirst, give hydromel [water and honey]." At the present day glucose would take the place of honey.

Hippocrates did not confine his practice to medicine. He was a good surgeon. He drained pus, set fractures, and reduced dislocations (using a special bench or table), and even trephined the skull, as he clearly describes in the work, *On Wounds in the Head* (xxi). His use of tar for wounds is a surprising forerunner of the antiseptic method. Even more remarkable is the advice which he gives in his short notebook entitled, *In the Surgery*. The following is an extract which might have been written to-day : " The nails neither to exceed nor come short of the finger tips. Good formation of fingers, with thumb well opposed to forefinger. Practice all the operations, with each hand and with both together." Details are also given regarding the use of boiled water, the position of the light, the instruments, and the assistants, and stress is laid upon the need for " ability, speed, painlessness, elegance, and readiness."

The " Aphorisms "

No account of Hippocrates is complete without some reference to his famous *Aphorisms*.[1] The first of these is almost hackneyed. " Life is short, and the Art long ; opportunity fleeting ; experiment dangerous, and judgment difficult," he writes, and he goes on to advise the doctor to be prepared to do the right thing at the right time, in which " patient, attendants, and external circumstances must co-operate."

A few of the other aphorisms may be quoted, as they illustrate so well the teaching of the great master :

I. 6. For extreme diseases extreme strictness of treatment is most efficacious.

I. 13. Old men endure fasting most easily, the man of middle age, youths very badly, and worst of all children, especially those of a liveliness greater than the ordinary.

[1] K. Deichgraber, " Goethe und Hippocrates," *Arch. f. Gesch. d. Med.*, 1936, vol. xxix. p. 27 ; B. Chance, " On Hippocrates and the Aphorisms," *Ann. Med. Hist.*, 1930, vol. ii. p. 31

I. 20. Do not disturb a patient either during or just after a crisis, and try no experiments, neither with purges nor with other irritants, but leave him alone.

II. 2. When sleep puts an end to delirium it is a good sign.

II. 16. When on starvation diet, a patient should not be fatigued.

II. 33. In every disease it is a good sign when the patient's intellect is sound and he enjoys his food ; the opposite is a bad sign.

II. 39. Old men generally have less illness than young men, but such complaints as become chronic in old men generally last until death.

III. 16. The diseases which generally arise in rainy weather are protracted fevers, fluxes of the bowels, mortifications, epilepsy, apoplexy, and angina. In dry weather occur consumption, eye diseases, diseases of the joints, strangury and dysentery.

III. 19. All diseases occur at all seasons, but some diseases are more apt to occur and to be aggravated at certain seasons.

III. 23. In winter occur pleurisy, pneumonia, colds, sore throat, headache, dizziness, apoplexy.

III. 24. In the different ages the following complaints occur : to little children and babies, aphthae, vomiting, coughs, sleeplessness, terrors, watery discharges from the ears.

III. 31. Old men suffer from difficulty in breathing, catarrh accompanied by coughing, difficult micturition, pains at the joints, dizziness, apoplexy, pruritus, watery discharges from the bowels, ears, and nostrils, dullness of sight, hardness of hearing.

V. 6. Those who are attacked by tetanus either die in four days, or, if they survive these, recover.

V. 9. Consumption occurs chiefly between the ages of eighteen and thirty-five.

V. 14. If diarrhœa attack a consumptive patient it is a fatal symptom.

VI. 38. It is better to give no treatment in cases of hidden cancer : treatment causes speedy death, but to omit treatment is to prolong life.

VII. 34. When bubbles form in the urine it is a sign that the kidneys are affected, and that the disease will be protracted.

VII. 72. Both sleep and sleeplessness, when beyond due measure, constitute disease.

VII. 87. Those diseases that medicines do not cure are cured by the knife. Those that the knife does not cure are cured by fire. Those that fire does not cure must be considered incurable.

Only a few of the aphorisms have been quoted, but they may suffice to illustrate the good sense and astute observation of the writer. Commentary is needless, though hundreds of commentaries upon the aphorisms have been published.[1] The originals deserve to be read and re-read by every practitioner of medicine and surgery. The work of Hippocrates is not a mere matter of historic interest. The idea of focusing full attention on the patient, rather than on scientific theories of disease or elaborate laboratory tests, was revived by Sydenham and Boerhaave, and to-day it is again engaging the attention of some of the best minds in medicine.[2] We cannot be too frequently or too forcefully reminded of the fact that " our natures are the physicians of our diseases." The physician and the specialist, whatever his field, should study the entire patient and his environment, and should view disease with the eye of the naturalist. That is the message of Hippocrates, as fresh to-day as it was 2400 years ago.

Aristotle and His Influence

Closely following Hippocrates in point of time was one who, though not himself a physician, exercised a profound influence upon the practice of medicine. ARISTOTLE (384–322 B.C.) was probably the greatest scientific genius the world has ever seen.[3] He was not only a profound philosopher ; his work, as the first great biologist, was of inestimable value to medicine.[4] His home was in Athens, where he was a pupil of Plato, and later he was tutor to the son of Philip of Macedon, Alexander the Great, who

[1] J. Wright, " Modern Commentaries on Hippocrates," *Ann. Med. Hist.*, 1919, vol. ii. p. 34

[2] B. Aschner, "Neo-Hippocratism in Everyday Practice," *Bull. Hist. Med.*, 1941, vol. x. No. 2, p. 260; A. P. Cawadias, " Neo-Hippocratism," *Proc. Roy. Soc. Med.* (Sect. Hist.), 1938, vol. xxxi. p. 27

[3] D'Arcy W. Thompson, "Aristotle the Naturalist," in *Science and the Classics*, 1940, p. 37 ; C. Singer, *A Short History of Biology*, 1931, p. 9

[4] J. Wright, " The Evolution and Thought of Aristotle," *Ann. Med. Hist.*, 1927, vol. ix. p. 144

in his brief meteoric career was destined to alter the world's history. Aristotle laid the foundations of comparative anatomy and of embryology.[1] He dissected innumerable animals, and was especially interested in fishes and molluscs. His account of the curious placental dog-fish was not confirmed until early in the nineteenth century, when it excited the interest and admiration of the great physiologist, Johannes Müller. He also gave an accurate description of the life of bees, of their "ruler" as he called the queen, not knowing her sex, and he noted how they swarm, gather honey, and build the comb. Aristotle encompassed the entire world of living things, and many of his descriptions and classifications remain sound to-day. In his conception of the Ladder of Nature there may be seen the first faint glimmer of a theory of evolution. He followed Hippocrates and others of his predecessors in believing that the human body possessed four fundamental qualities, the hot and the cold, the dry and the moist, and that it was composed of four "humours"—blood, phlegm, yellow bile, and black bile. Disturbance of the relative predominance of the humours constituted disease. To-day, this would be interpreted as a disturbance of endocrine balance. His investigation of the development of the chick within the egg was the first of many similar investigations, although no further progress was made until the days of Fabricius and Harvey (pp. 140, 183).[2]

Medical Botanists

Aristotle was followed by THEOPHRASTUS (370–287 B.C.), another biologist, who was, above all, a botanist. By his great work, *Historia Plantarum*, he laid the foundation of modern scientific botany.[3] It was the standard botanical textbook for many centuries, and is of medical interest, as the writer described not only the morphology and natural history of plants, but also their use in therapeutics.[4] He explains how frankincense and myrrh were collected, incisions being made in the stems of the plants in order to extract the gum. He also described the process of germination of seeds, and he was the first to distinguish monocotyledons and dicotyledons.

[1] C. Singer, "Greek Biology in Relation to the Rise of Modern Biology," in *Studies in the History and Method of Science*, 1921, vol. ii.
[2] J. Needham, *A History of Embryology*, 1934, p. 20
[3] Theophrastus. *De Historia Plantarum*, ed. by Sir A. Hort, Loeb Library, 2 vols. 1916
[4] C. Singer, "Greek Biology" in *Studies in the History and Method of Science*, 1921, p. 56

It remained for DIOSCORIDES (*fl.* A.D. 60), a Greek surgeon to the army of Nero, more than three hundred years later, to establish the science of Materia Medica.[1] His work on the subject, *De universa medicina*, which includes mineral remedies such as salts of lead and copper, was for centuries used as the standard authority.[2]

Theophrastus was one of the last great scholars of the high classical period. Greece was no longer to be the centre of intellectual supremacy. The period of decline had begun. Yet the torch of Greek medicine, which burned so brightly in the hands of Hippocrates and his immediate followers, was to be kept alight by other distinguished men, not only in the great empire of Alexander, but for four centuries in the still greater Roman Empire.

[1] R. T. Gunther, *The Greek Herbal of Dioscorides*, 1934
[2] A. C. Wootton, *Chronicles of Pharmacy*, 2 vols., 1910, vol. i. p. 206

BOOKS FOR FURTHER READING

CLEMOW, F. C.   *The Geography of Disease*, 1903

DICKINSON, G. LOWES.   *The Greek View of Life*, 1896

GUNTHER, R. T.   *The Greek Herbal of Dioscorides*, 1934

HEIDEL, W. A.   *Hippocratic Medicine ; Its Spirit and Method*, New York, 1943 ; *The Genuine Works of Hippocrates*, trans. by F. Adams, Sydenham Society, 2 vols., 1849 ; *The Works of Hippocrates*, trans. by W. H. S. Jones and E. T. Withington, Loeb Library, 4 vols., 1923–31

HUNTINGDON, E.   *Civilization and the Climate*, 1924

LIVINGSTONE, R. W.   *The Legacy of Greece* (article on Medicine by C. Singer), 1921

MOON, R. O.   *Hippocrates and his Successors in Relation to the Philosophy of their Times*, 1923

SINGER, C.   *A Short History of Biology*, 1931

TAYLOR, H. O.   *Greek Biology and Medicine*, 1922

THEOPHRASTUS.   *De Historia Plantarum*, ed. Sir A. Hort, 2 vols., Loeb Library, 1916

THOMPSON, D'ARCY.   *Science and the Classics* (chapter on Aristotle), 1940

Chapter V

ALEXANDRIAN AND ROMAN MEDICINE

THE brilliant epoch in Greece was now passing, and the country which had produced so many scholars and artists was now to give place to other lands. Nevertheless, though Greek culture was fading in the land of its birth, it was by no means dying. Its mission was not yet accomplished, for it was destined to exercise a far-reaching influence, and in some respects to attain further eminence. Athens was to give place to Alexandria, and then to Rome. It was natural that, at Alexandria, medicine should remain in Greek hands, but it is remarkable that all the great physicians of the Roman Empire were Greeks, and that their practice and teaching remained predominant throughout mediæval times, until the Renaissance brought new ideas and more enlightened teaching.

The Medical School of Alexandria

Before considering the rise of Greek medicine in Rome, however, which really began a new epoch, let us round off the Hippocratic period by a brief reference to the Medical School of Alexandria. Unfortunately our sources of information are very small. Of course we know that Alexander the Great, sweeping all before him in his astounding march of progress, conquered not only Greece and Asia Minor and Egypt, but marched eastward over Persia as far as India, and established a vast empire, which might have been even larger but for his untimely death at the age of thirty-three years. With a vision far ahead of his time, he took with him on his campaigns a number of scientists, who added greatly to the knowledge of the countries conquered. Alexandria was founded in 332 B.C., nine years before Alexander's death, and here was established a home of learning and a vast library, which eventually contained some 700,000 books. The loss to posterity which resulted from the burning of the library by a mob of fanatics, who were intent on getting rid of the past so as to found a " New Order," was a disaster almost too great to realize. Of the medical school at Alexandria we know little, save that work was established and led by two great men, Herophilus and Erasistratus, both of whom were born about 300 B.C. Their writings have perished, but we know something of their work from the pages of Galen and other authors.

HEROPHILUS was essentially an anatomist, and he may have been the first to practise public dissection of the human body.[1] His name survives in one of the venous sinuses of the brain, the *torcular Herophili* (wine-press of Herophilus), and he was the first to name the duodenum and to count the pulse. His treatise on anatomy was undoubtedly an amazing piece of work for its time.

ERASISTRATUS, regarded by some as the founder of physiology,[2] distinguished the cerebrum from the cerebellum, and noted the difference between sensory and motor nerves. He regarded the nerves as hollow tubes filled with fluid. His experiments marked a new development in Greek medicine, and led him to reject the accepted view that disease was due to maladjusted humours. Instead, he attributed disease to plethora, or an excessive blood supply.[3] He believed that the air entered the lungs and then the heart, where it was changed into the Vital Spirit, and then carried throughout the body by the arteries. This idea was elaborated and altered by Galen, as we shall see, but Galen severely criticized the ideas of Erasistratus. It is somewhat gruesome to record that both of those distinguished Alexandrians may have practised human vivisection. According to Celsus, they " procured criminals from prison by royal permission, and dissected them alive. This," adds Celsus, " was by far the best method for attaining knowledge."

As time went on the fame of Alexandria declined and the empire of Alexander was superseded by that of Rome. This opened a new field for Greek medicine.

Etruscans and Early Greek Settlers in Rome

Rome was not built in a day, nor was the medical system of Greece transferred to Rome with any haste, but rather by a gradual process of infiltration, which had begun while Greece was still the intellectual centre of the world. In science, as in

[1] J. F. Dobson, " Herophilus of Alexandria," *Proc. Roy. Soc. Med.* (Sect. Hist.), 1925, vol. xviii. p. 19
[2] J. F. Dobson, " Erasistratus," *Proc. Roy. Soc. Med.* (Sect. Hist.), 1927, vol. xx. p. 825
[3] E. T. Withington, *Medical History from the Earliest Times*, 1894, p. 63

art, Rome was a borrower. The origin of the Etruscans [1] is obscure, but that they were the founders of Rome we must admit, unless we prefer to accept the legend of Romulus and Remus. Like other primitive peoples they had their folk-lore, and it is known that they practised divination, foretelling the future by inspection of the liver of an animal slain for sacrifice. Bronze models of the liver, the reference textbooks, so to speak, have been found, resembling the clay models which, as we have noted (p. 19), were used in Babylon (Plate VI). Rough and ready methods of healing were doubtless practised, but as time went on there was no appearance of a native system of medicine. Roman medicine did not exist as a separate entity. Medicine as a profession was beneath the dignity of the Roman citizen. The ancient Roman doctored himself and doctored his household, invoking the aid of the gods, and there were no physicians before the advent of the Greeks. Everyone was his own physician. As Daremberg remarks,[2] they were " sans médecins, mais non pas sans médecine." Rome, therefore, was an attractive field for the itinerant Greek practitioner, and Rome was, moreover, a near neighbour, as Sicily and the southern half of Italy were still parts of Greece (Magna Græcia). Many of those early Greek physicians were slaves in Roman families. The status of the profession was low, and so it remained until 46 B.C., when Julius Cæsar accorded to physicians the full rights of Roman citizenship.[3]

Roman gibes at Greek Medicine

Apparently Greek medicine was of rather low standard in those early days of Rome. That the Greek immigrants had forsaken the noble precepts of Hippocrates, and that they were not slow to exploit the wealthy Romans, is obvious from many contemporary writings.[4]

Cato the Censor (234–149 B.C.), the first Latin prose writer of any importance, who hated the Greeks and all their works, wrote in his maxims of advice to his son (*Præcepta ad Filium*) : " They have sworn to kill all barbarians with their drugs, and they call

---

[1] A. Castiglioni, *A History of Medicine*, trans. E. B. Krumbhaar, Chicago, 1941, p. 189
[2] C. Daremberg, *La Médecine, Histoire et Doctrines*, 1865
[3] H. Barnes, " On Roman Medicine and Roman Medical Inscriptions Found in Britain," *Proc. Roy. Soc. Med.* (Sect. Hist.), 1914, vol. viii. p. 71
[4] T. Clifford Allbutt, *Greek Medicine in Rome* (Fitzpatrick Lectures), 1929

us barbarians. Remember that I forbid physicians for you."
Cato lived to the age of eighty-five years, and if we are to believe
Horace, his favourite prescription for himself and his household
was cabbage, applied externally, or eaten and washed down with
good wine. This was his panacea for all ills, and many Romans
followed his example.

The prejudice against Greek doctors appears to have continued
until the Christian era. Pliny the Elder (A.D. 23–79) wrote a
monumental natural history in thirty-seven books, in which he
dealt not only with unicorns and winged horses and other strange
beasts, but also with the medicine of the day. " It is unfortunate,"
he remarks, " that there is no law to punish ignorant physicians,
and that capital punishment is never inflicted on them. Yet they
learn by our suffering and they experiment by putting us to
death." Pliny, always a close observer, approached too closely to
investigate the eruption of Vesuvius when it overwhelmed the
town of Pompeii, and thus he met his death. To Pliny we are
indebted for the information that the first Greek practitioner to
come to Rome in 219 B.C. was Archagathus, a man who at first
acquired a good name and was called *Vulnarius* (Wound-curer).
Later, however, he fell from grace, and he was then named
Carnifex (Executioner).

Some of the Latin poets, too, found in the Greek physicians
a good target for their taunts.[1] One of the epigrams of Martial
(A.D. 40–102) relates to an eye specialist who had become a
gladiator.[2] It is best appreciated in the original, which shows
the play on the words :

> Hoplomachus nunc es : fueras ophthalmicus ante :
> Fecisti medicus quod facis hoplomachus.

> (You are now a gladiator, formerly you were an oculist ;
> As a medical man you did what you now do as a gladiator.)

Another of Martial's epigrams is of interest, as it shows that
clinical teaching was practised in Rome. The translation runs :

> I'm ill. I send for Symmachus ; he's here,
> A hundred students following in the rear :
> All paw my chest, with hands as cold as snow :
> I had no fever, but I have it now.

[1] P. Ménière, *Études médicales sur les poètes latins*, Paris, 1858
[2] Martial. *The Epigrams of Martial*, Bohn's Library, 1881, Bk. viii., No. lxxiv ;
R. Crawford, " Martial and Medicine," *Proc. Roy. Soc. Med.* (Sect. Hist.), 1914, vol. vii.
p. 15

" *Cito, Tuto, et Jucunde* "

Among the first Greek physicians to arrive in Rome was one who deserves to be remembered. ASCLEPIADES, the " Prince of Physicians," as he has been called, though the title is disputed by Avicenna, was born at Prusa in Bithynia on the southern shores of the Black Sea in 124 B.C.[1] Educated at Athens and at Alexandria, he eventually settled in Rome, where his sagacity and strong personality soon led him to become the fashionable physician of the day and the friend of Cicero and of Mark Antony. It is said that one day while walking in Rome, he met a funeral procession. The bearers had laid down the corpse and were resting, when Asclepiades, as he passed by, noticed signs of life in the dead man. He persuaded the relatives to delay the funeral and to convey the body to a neighbouring house, where after some manipulation by the physician they were astounded to see the dead restored to life. News of the incident spread rapidly in Rome, and, as may be imagined, Asclepiades did not lack patients, though his ability had already brought him success.[2] Although he was a worthy follower of the Father of Medicine, and has been called " The Hippocrates of chronic disease," he did not follow the Hippocratic rules, and indeed he denied the healing power of Nature, which he stigmatized as " merely a meditation on death." He believed in active measures by the physician, though he preferred dietetic and physical therapy (baths, massage, etc.) to treatment by drugs. It was he who originated the idea that disease should be treated speedily, safely, and agreeably (*Cito, tuto, et jucunde*). He held that disease depended upon the condition of the " pores " which permeated all the tissues of the body. If these were too contracted or too relaxed, ill-health was the result. Health was the balance between tension and relaxation. This theory, known as " Methodism," was elaborated by THEMISON (123–43 B.C.), the pupil of Asclepiades, who practised in Rome during the reign of Augustus, and in much more recent times it formed the basis of similar ideas, advanced by Broussais (theory of irritation) and by Brown (" Brunonian " theory of sthenic and asthenic states), and there have even been semblances of it in modern days.

[1] C. G. Cumston, *History of Medicine*, 1926, p. 119
[2] M. Neuburger, *History of Medicine*, trans. E. Playfair, 1910, vol. i. p. 201

Asclepiades is said to be the first writer to mention tracheotomy, though it is not known whether he ever practised it. His works have for the most part disappeared, but they are partly preserved for us in the quotations of other writers.[1]

Party Politics in Medicine

It may be convenient at this point to interpolate a note on the sects and cults which so largely dominated medical practice in the post-Hippocratic era. Instead of following the master in his reliance upon Nature and his observation at the bedside, various theories of disease were constructed, and an endeavour was made to explain all pathological phenomena by fitting them into the given theory. Medicine has suffered much at the hands of theorists, especially when the theory is allowed to supplant clinical observation.

In Græco-Roman times there arose the Dogmatists, the Empirics, the Methodists, the Pneumatists, and the Eclectics, names which have puzzled many a student of medical history. Some of them have been mentioned ; the others need not detain us long. The Dogmatists, or, as Galen preferred to call them, the Rationalists, were " the truest sons of Hippocrates." They believed that medicine must be founded in physiology, and their only mistake was that they erected a complete superstructure upon an insufficient foundation. The Empirics were not concerned with causes, but relied upon experience alone, labelling the disease and the corresponding remedy, and reducing medical practice to rule of thumb. For the Pneumatists, all disease was due to disturbance of the airy spirit or pneuma, which was detected by feeling the pulse. This pneuma or breath was the vehicle of the mind, and the mind governed all the organs of the body. Such a conception has ever been a favourite theme with poets and philosophers. Pneumatism was revived in the seventeenth century by Stahl, who called it animism, and a similar vogue was introduced by Van Helmont. Mention has already been made of Themison as a Methodist, and as for the remaining sect, that of the Eclectics, these were free lances who might adopt any or every theory to meet the current need. Parties and sects similar to those outlined above, and often difficult to define, may

[1] R. R. von Welz, *Asclepiades von Bithunia : Gesundheitsvorschriften,* 1842. (Includes Greek, Latin, and German texts).

be found at all epochs in the history of medicine. Before leaving this unprofitable subject, mention must be made of another " Methodist," because he may almost be regarded as the founder of obstetrical science.

SORANUS (A.D. 78–117), though a native of Asia Minor, practised in Rome because it offered great scope for his activities. A man of high status and a good clinician, he must be regarded as the leading authority on obstetrics, gynæcology, and pediatrics among the ancients.[1] His treatise remained the only authority on the subject for fourteen centuries, and became the chief source of information for Roesslin's *Rosgarten* (1513) and Raynalde's *Byrth of Mankynde* (1545) (p. 174). Soranus describes podalic version and the obstetric chair, shows how the umbilical cord should be ligated, and advises bathing the eyes of the new-born child. Only boiled water and honey should be given for two days, and on the third day nursing should commence. Soranus is said to be the first writer to refer to rickets. Dealing with " How the child should practise walking," he states that this should not be attempted too soon, because " the limbs may yield as the bones are not yet become firm."

Mithridaticum and Theriac

In dealing with the epoch of medical history between the death of Hippocrates and the birth of Christ, mention must be made of the king whose name was for many centuries perpetuated in an antidote to poisons. Mithridates VI, king of Pontus, who was wont to amuse himself by experimenting upon unfortunate criminals, claimed that he had thus discovered " an antidote for every venomous reptile and every poisonous substance." The drugs, known as *mithridaticum* (or *mithridatium*) and *theriac*, engaged the attention of pharmacists until William Heberden (p. 256), in 1745, wrote a counterblast to their use, which led to their expulsion from the various pharmacopœias.[2] The original *mithridaticum* contained about fifty ingredients, including vipers' flesh and all manner of vegetable products. The recipe underwent modification in course of time. Galen's prescription had no less than seventy-three ingredients, and he ordered it in the form of pills

[1] J. Pinoff, " Die Geburtshilfe des Soranus Ephesius," *Janus*, 1847, vol. ii. p. 217; T. Meyer-Steineg and K. Sudhoff, *Geschichte der Medizin*, Jena, 1921, p. 121
[2] W. Heberden, *An Essay on Mithridatium and Theriaka*, 1745

as large as grapes, of which ten were to be taken before and after food. To give King Mithridates his due, we must remember that it was he, so it is said, who discovered that he could immunize himself against certain poisons by gradually increasing doses.[1] *Theriac* was of different composition, although the two antidotes are often confused.[2] The basis of *theriac* was Venice treacle, but it was also an example of polypharmacy ; indeed, the Pharmacopœia of the Royal College of Physicians of London, dated 1724, mentions sixty-two ingredients. Apparently *theriac* was widely used, even as late as the eighteenth century, not only for the bites of venomous animals, but for the effects of poisons, in which case it was to be taken twice a day for seven years, but also for numerous other diseases. It was, in fact, a universal remedy, although, as one writer has said, " Never has a medicine containing so much cured so little."

A Follower of Hippocrates

It must not be inferred, however, that all the physicians of the Græco-Roman era were of the class who relied upon theories and *theriac*. Of ARETAEUS, the Cappadocian, we know nothing save that he lived in Alexandria about the second century A.D. A certain mystery surrounds Aretaeus, and it seems strange that his classical descriptions of disease should have been so little known or quoted during more than a thousand years. He may have been contemporary with Galen, yet neither writer mentions the other. Aretaeus quotes no medical authority except Hippocrates, not even Celsus, who probably preceded him. The first record of the work of Aretaeus is found in the writings of Aetius

[1] The methods of King Mithridates are described in A. E. Housman's well-known poem, *A Shropshire Lad* :

He gathered all that springs to birth
From the many-venomed earth ;
First a little, thence to more,
He sampled all her killing store :
    * * *
They put arsenic in his meat
And stared aghast to watch him eat,
They poured strychnine in his cup
And shook to see him drink it up.
They shook, they stared as white's their shirt ;
Them it was their poison hurt.
I tell the tale that I heard told.
Mithridates, he died old.

[2] C. E. Daniels, " Observations sur la Thériaque," *Janus*, 1911, vol. xvi. pp. 371, 457

of Amida (p. 79), who lived in the sixth century. At all events Aretaeus' valuable contributions to medicine passed unnoticed, and by the earlier historians he was regarded as a frank copyist who borrowed from the writings of one Archigenes (*c.* A.D. 100), whose original works are lost. Aretaeus was a close follower of Hippocrates and an accurate observer, although his work attracted little attention until comparatively recent times.[1] A beautiful edition by Wigan was published by the Clarendon Press in 1723, based upon two manuscripts, in the Vatican Library and the Bodleian Library, and a more recent translation, along with the Greek text, was prepared for the Sydenham Society in 1858 by the scholarly Francis Adams.[2] Aretaeus was a talented physician who wrote in a clear and attractive style, and his word pictures of disease resemble those of Hippocrates.[3] He divides his material into (1) acute diseases, and (2) chronic diseases. The former includes descriptions of pneumonia, pleurisy, tetanus, and diphtheria, while among the latter are accounts of insanity, paralysis, and phthisis. Of phthisis he writes that " most prone to phthisis are the slender, those whose scapulæ are like wings or folding doors, those who have prominent throats, who are pale, and have narrow chests." He was the first to distinguish between spinal and cerebral paralysis. " If the affection be in the spinal marrow, the parts homonymous with it are paralysed. But if the head be primarily affected on the right side, the left side of the body will be paralysed [and *vice versa*]. The cause of this is the interchange in the origins of the nerves . . . each passes over to the other side, decussating each other in the form of the letter X." It was Aretaeus who gave its name to the disease diabetes ; διαβήτης (" a passer through "), as he called it.[4] This disease, " fortunately rather rare," consisted in " a liquefaction of the flesh and bones into urine." " The kidneys and bladder do not cease emitting urine . . . as though the aqueducts were opened wide." " No matter what quantity of fluid the patient drinks, satisfaction never occurs . . . he cannot be stopped

[1] J. H. Couch, " The Literary Illustrations of Aretaeus of Cappadocia," *Canad. Med. Assoc. Jour.*, 1935, vol. xxxiii. p. 556 ; G. Didsbury, " Considérations sur la Migraine d'après Aretée de Cappadoce," *Bull. d'Hist. Med.*, 1936, vol. xxx. p. 260
[2] F. Adams, trans. *The Extant Works of Aretaeus the Cappadocian*, Sydenham Soc., 1860
[3] E. F. Cordell, " Aretaeus the Cappadocian," *Johns Hopk. Hosp. Bull.*, 1909, p. 371
[4] J. H. Barach, " Historical Facts in Diabetes," *Ann. Med. Hist.*, 1928, vol. x. p. 387 ; E. J. Leopold, " Aretaeus the Cappadocian and his Contribution to Diabetes Mellitus," *Ann. Med. Hist.*, 1930, vol. ii. p. 424

from drinking or from urinating. . . . For fluids do not remain in the body, but use the body only as a channel through which they may flow out. Life lasts only for a time, but not very long." Although Aretaeus was a frank copyist, he showed originality in his clinical descriptions, and his work is well worth reading even to-day. It reveals the true disciple of Hippocrates, the bedside observer disdainful of theory and preconceived ideas, and above all, eager to be of assistance to the patient.

Celsus—" De Medicina "

We now come to a writer who although not a Greek and probably not even a medical man, has imprinted his name indelibly upon the pages of medical history.[1] Although the Romans scorned to soil their hands in the practice of medicine, a calling only fit for slaves and foreigners, they were interested in the subject, and indeed some acquaintance with the art of healing became part of the equipment of every well-educated gentleman. CELSUS, a member of the noble family of the Cornelii, was the author of a great encyclopædia dealing with philosophy, military strategy, law, medicine, and probably other subjects.[2] It was written about A.D. 30, but the only part which has survived are the eight books entitled De Medicina. Written in Latin, and the work of a Roman, it is not surprising that it was hardly noticed by the Greek practitioners, but even in the Middle Ages it was overlooked. At last the manuscript was brought to light by Pope Nicholas V (1397–1455), and at Florence, in 1478, it was one of the first medical books to be printed. Celsus then attained a long delayed but well-merited fame. Written in excellent and elegant Latin, his work commanded the admiration of scholars ; as a clear and unbiased description of the medical knowledge of his time, it is unequalled and may still be read with profit. Many editions have been printed. A good English translation by J. Grieve appeared in 1756, and the most recent, giving Latin and English, is that of W. G. Spencer.[3] Celsus ingeniously bridges the gap between his work on agriculture and that on medicine by the introductory sentence of the latter

[1] J. Finlayson, " Celsus," Glas. Med. Jour., 1892, vol. xxxvii., 5, p. 321
[2] A. Castiglioni, " Aulus Cornelius Celsus as a Historian of Medicine," Bull. Hist. Med., 1940, vol. viii. p. 857
[3] W. G. Spencer, trans. Works of Celsus, Loeb Library, 1935, 3 vols.

work : " As agriculture promises food to the healthy, so medicine promises health to the sick." He prefaces his treatise by an impartial account of Greek medicine. The first two books deal with the digestibility and effects of many forms of food and drink ; a lengthy list, for the Roman kept a good table with great variety of dishes. Dietetic treatment is discussed, and the technique of blood-letting is described—" very easy to one who has experience, yet very difficult to one that is ignorant. For the vein lies close to the arteries, and to these the nerves." The third book treats of fevers (evidently malarial), of madness, of cardiac disorders, of lethargy, of dropsy, of consumption, of jaundice, and of palsy, and it is an interesting exercise, in reading the descriptions, to conjecture what the modern diagnosis would have been. In this book are mentioned the four cardinal signs of inflammation familiar to the medical student to-day—*calor*, *rubor*, *tumor*, *dolor* : heat, redness, swelling, and pain.

Internal diseases form the subject of the fourth book, the writer commencing with the head, passing to the throat, thorax, and abdomen, and ending with the feet. The first disease mentioned is hydrocephalus, the last, gout.

Book V includes an account of drugs and their uses, and the treatment of wounds. Among the drugs in common use were myrrh, nitre, saffron, and iris. Mandrake and poppy were employed to relieve pain ; they were the earliest anæsthetics.

Book VI is devoted to the " special subjects " skin, eye, ears, teeth, and venereal diseases. A quaint means of removing a foreign body from the ear is noted. The patient is bound to a board, lying on the affected side, and the board is struck with a hammer. " Thus, by shaking the ear, what is within it drops out."

The two remaining books deal with surgery. Book VII is concerned with operative procedures, such as the removal of arrow-heads, operations for goitre and for hernia, lithotomy, and various eye operations, including couching for cataract.[1] The last-mentioned is accomplished with a needle, which is " inserted through the two coats of the eye until it meets resistance, and then the cataract is pressed down so that it may settle in the lower part." The operation of tonsillectomy described by Celsus is the " modern " method of enucleation. " Tonsils," he writes,

[1] J. S. Milne, *Surgical Instruments in Greek and Roman Times*, Aberdeen, 1907

" that are indurated after an inflammation, since they are enclosed in a thin tunic, should be disengaged all round by the finger and pulled out."

It is in this book that the attributes of the surgeon are defined. He "should be youthful or in early middle age, with a strong and steady hand, as expert with the left hand as with the right, with vision sharp and clear, and spirit undaunted ; so far void of pity that while he wishes only to cure his patient, yet is not moved by his cries to go too fast, or cut less than is necessary." The eighth and last book gives precise direction for the treatment of fractures and dislocations. Splints were used, and were fixed by bandages stiffened with starch.

The *De Medicina* of Celsus is a medical classic with a modern flavour, and it would be a good thing for medicine if its popularity could be revived. Celsus states the facts, and wisely refrains from indulging in theory or argument. The surgical instruments which he describes correspond to those found in the house of the surgeon at Pompeii (destroyed A.D. 79), which are still on view in the Naples museum (Plate XIII).

Galen : the Medical Dictator

The Græco-Roman period reached its climax with the appearance of a man whose teaching dominated medicine for the next 1200 years.[1] Throughout the dull-witted early Middle Ages his views were not only accepted without question, but anyone who dared to differ was treated as a heretic. It is easy to understand why this was so. Galen regarded the body as the mere vehicle of the soul, a view which naturally met with the approval of Christian and Moslem alike in the new age of monotheism. Moreover, his teaching was imparted in so dogmatic a fashion as to carry conviction and disarm criticism, for Galen had an answer to every question and a solution to every problem, and although he was not nearly so great a man as Hippocrates, he acknowledged the authority of the Father of Medicine and incorporated much of his teaching in his own. In principle he followed both Hippocrates and Aristotle, believing, like the

[1] J. Walsh, " Galen's Writings, and the Influences Inspiring Them," *Ann. Med. Hist.*, 1934, vol. vi. pp. 1, 143 ; 1936, vol. viii. p. 65 ; 1937, vol. ix. p. 34; 1939, 3rd Ser., vol. i. p. 525. (A valuable and comprehensive study of the life and work of Galen)

former, in the healing power of the φύσις, or Nature, and like the latter, in the purposive creative power of Nature, or God, always working towards a definite end and leaving nothing to chance.

GALEN (*c.* A.D. 131–200) was born at Pergamos in Asia Minor. This city, now called Bergamum, is some fifty miles north of Smyrna (Izmir), and may be approached from that city by a very rough road (1939). One may inspect, on a hillside with a commanding view, the ruins of the theatre and of the Asklepieion, which ranked next to that of Epidaurus in fame, but the lovely temple was bodily removed by German archæologists last century, to be reconstructed at Berlin, where in the specially built " Per-gamon Museum " it became one of the greatest art treasures of Germany. Galen was the son of Nicon, a talented and wealthy architect.[1] " My father," he tells us, " was amiable, just, and benevolent. My mother, on the other hand, had a very bad temper ; she used to bite her serving maids, and was perpetually shouting at my father." Apparently, then, Galen inherited the brilliant intellect of his father, and the quarrelsome nature of his mother. To Nicon it was revealed in a dream that his son would become a distinguished physician, and he therefore gave him a good education, first in philosophy at Pergamos and Smyrna, and then in medicine at Alexandria.[2] After some further study and wandering in Greece, Italy, and Palestine, Galen returned to Pergamos at the age of twenty-eight, and was appointed surgeon to the school of gladiators, a post which naturally gave him ample experience in the treatment of injuries. His fame increased, and four years later he determined to seek further fortune in Rome. There he practised, taught, and conducted experiments, soon acquiring a large clientele and a vast reputation. After a few years, however, he returned to Pergamos. It was said that he did so to escape the plague, but a more likely explanation is that his successes had so aroused the enmity of his colleagues that life in Rome was becoming unpleasant and even dangerous. Later, the Emperor, Marcus Aurelius, needed him, saying that " we have but one physician, Galen." So he was summoned back to Rome, and there he remained until his death, thirty years later.

[1] J. S. Prendergast, " The Background to Galen's Life and Activities and its Influence on his Achievement," *Proc. Roy. Soc. Med.* (Sect. Hist.), 1930, vol. xxiii. p. 1131
[2] J. Walsh, " Galen's Studies at the Alexandrian School," *Ann. Med. Hist.*, 1927, vol. ix. p. 132

Galen as Practitioner

In practice Galen followed the Hippocratic method, accepting the doctrine of the " humours," which regarded the body as composed of blood, phlegm, yellow bile, and black bile. In mediæval times the humours were changed to " temperaments "—sanguine, phlegmatic, melancholy, and choleric, a nomenclature which persists to this day. There were four elements : air, fire, earth, and water, and four qualities : heat, cold, moisture, and dryness ; and treatment was based upon the preponderance and interaction of the elements and qualities. Galen recognized the exciting and predisposing causes of disease, terms which are still used. He supported the theory of " coction," introduced by Hippocrates ; and applying this to the healing of wounds, he regarded pus as " laudable," an error which greatly retarded the progress of surgery. Galen employed diet, massage, and exercises in treatment, and he also used many drugs, his simple vegetable products being still known as " galenicals." That he was a clever diagnostician is shown by the case of Eudamus the philosopher. This man complained of a loss of sensation in the fourth and fifth fingers of one hand, which other physicians had failed to cure by local treatment. Galen ascertained that the patient had recently fallen from a chariot, and had struck his neck against a sharp stone. Applying his physiological knowledge, the physician regarded the brachial plexus as the seat of the trouble, and by applying counter-irritants to the region he was successful in achieving a cure. This success is related by Galen in no modest fashion, for he was a forceful and opinionative man. Professor Singer remarks, " Galen was, at one and the same time, the last of the ancients and the first of the moderns." [1]

The First Experimental Physiologist

The lasting fame of Galen is based, not upon his clinical work but rather upon his investigations, which laid the foundation of experimental physiology. He recognized the value of anatomy in medicine, stating that a physician without anatomical knowledge was like an architect without a plan. His anatomy, however, was based on a study of apes and pigs, and he unhesitatingly transferred his discoveries to human anatomy, thus perpetuating

[1] Charles Singer, " Galen as a Modern," *Proc. Roy. Soc. Med.*, xlii. pp. 563–70, 1949

many errors. Dissection of the human body had become illegal, and although he had studied the human skeleton, Galen's anatomy was founded upon investigation of the Barbary ape, then easily obtainable in Europe, but now found only upon the Rock of Gibraltar. Galen gives a good description of the muscles in the ape, the facts being supplemented from his dissections of other animals.[1] He was familiar with all the gross structures of the brain, and he recognized seven pairs of cranial nerves, the first pair being the optic nerves, and the fifth the facial and auditory together. One of the first to distinguish between the sensory and motor nerves, he also discovered the sympathetic nervous system.

His experiments, conducted for the most part on pigs, revealed the effects of division or of hemisection of the spinal cord at various levels, and he showed that loss of voice was produced by division of the recurrent laryngeal nerve. He also demonstrated the position of the ureters by animal experiment.

The Blood in Motion, but not in Circulation

In the opinion of Galen the vital principle was the " pneuma," which entered the lung in the act of breathing and there mingled with the blood. The blood was formed in the liver from the foodstuff or chyle, brought thence from the intestine by the portal vein.[2] In the liver the blood, endowed with Natural Spirit, passed to the right ventricle, whence it was distributed to nourish all the tissues and organs, and also to the lungs, in order that the impurities might be exhaled in the breath. Part of the venous blood, on reaching the heart, passed through minute and invisible pores in the interventricular septum, and mingling with the blood which arrived from the lungs by the " arterial vein " (as he calls the pulmonary artery), became charged with a second variety of pneuma, the Vital Spirit. From the heart it passed throughout the body, to confer power upon the organs and tissues. The blood which reached the brain became charged with the pneuma of the soul, the Animal Spirit, and was carried forth by the nerves, believed to be hollow during life, to endow the body with sensa-

[1] C. Singer, *The Evolution of Anatomy*, 1925, p. 57
[2] J. Prendergast, "Galen's View of the Vascular System in Relation to that of Harvey," *Proc. Roy. Soc. Med.* (Sect. Hist.), 1928, vol. xxi. p. 1839 ; E. Wenkebach, " Galenos von Pergamon," *Arch. f. Gesch. d. Med.*, 1938, vol. xxxi. 4, p. 254 ; J. F. Payne, " The Relation of Harvey to his Predecessors and Especially to Galen," *Lancet*, 1896, p. 1136

tion and motion. Galen recognized that the arteries contained
blood, and not merely air, as had been believed before his day.
Furthermore, he recognized that it was the heart that set the
blood in motion. But he had no idea that the blood circulated ;
he imagined that it ebbed and flowed in the vessels, and his idea
of a porous septum in the heart was one of these fallacies which
was blindly accepted and followed for centuries.

Galen as Author

, Galen was truly a voluminous writer. More than five hundred
books were attributed to him, but many of his manuscripts were
destroyed by a fire at his house in Rome while others were lost,
and only about eighty remain extant. They were copied and
recopied many times during the Middle Ages, and there have
been numerous printed editions.[1] One of the earliest of the latter,
a book which is now extremely rare, was that edited by no less
a person than Rabelais (1537).[2] Some of Galen's works have
been translated into many languages. There is an excellent
French edition by Daremberg (1856),[3] and although no edition
so comprehensive exists in English, one of the best-known and
most characteristic of the works, *On the Natural Faculties*, has been
translated (1917) by A. J. Brock for the Loeb Classical Library.[4]
Additional interest has been focused on the anatomy of Galen by
the work of Max Simon,[5] and in 1944 Galen's *Treatise on Medical
Experience* was translated into English by R. Walzer from a ninth-
century Arabic manuscript found at Constantinople in 1931.
Galen's achievement was the high-water mark of Græco-Roman
medicine. That he remained for centuries the undisputed
authority from whom none dared to differ was not his fault.
Galen, and not Hippocrates, was the chief guide of the mediæval
physician ; forceful, dogmatic, and infallible, until Paracelsus had
the audacity to preface his lectures by publicly burning Galen's
volumes, and Vesalius disposed of many anatomical myths by
dissecting the human body, and Ambroise Paré used simple
dressings in place of boiling oil, and admitted the possibility of
healing by first intention.

[1] A. Malloch, " Galen," *Ann. Med. Hist.*, 1926, vol. viii. p. 61
[2] D. Slaughter, " Medicine in the Life of François Rabelais," *Ann. Med. Hist.*, 1939,
3rd Ser., vol. i. pp. 396, 438
[3] C. Daremberg, *Œuvres anatomiques physiologiques et médicales de Galen*, Paris, 1856
[4] A. J. Brock, trans. *Galen : On the Natural Faculties*, Loeb Library, 1917
[5] M. Simon, *Sieben Bücher Anatomie des Galens*, Leipzig, 1906

The Byzantine Compilers

According to Gibbon the second century, in which Galen lived, was the most happy and prosperous period in the history of the world. Nevertheless, after two centuries of peace, the Roman Empire was already heading for a fall. Barbarian invaders were appearing on every side : the Goths, the Vandals, and the Huns. Although the noble and enlightened emperor Marcus Aurelius delayed the period of decline and fall by fighting and by diplomacy, and although Constantine postponed the final dissolution of the empire by transferring his capital from Rome to Byzantium (Constantinople), the final crash in the fifth century was inevitable. During the years which elapsed between the death of Galen and the collapse of Roman authority, medicine was kept alive by a series of learned physicians who, although possessed of little originality, earned the gratitude of posterity by collecting and transcribing much of the work of their predecessors which might otherwise have been irretrievably lost.[1]

One of the first of these compilers was ORIBASIUS (A.D. 325–403), physician to the much-maligned Emperor Julian (the Apostate). Julian was the last of the Roman emperors to oppose Christianity and to uphold the old world of Greek civilization. Oribasius, like Galen, was a native of Pergamos. An industrious scholar, he wrote a digest of medicine and surgery in seventy books, of which twenty-five remain. These are well preserved in the French translation of Daremberg (1860), in six volumes. Oribasius was careful to quote the exact sources of his information, and this gives his work a special value as the mirror of a literature which might easily have been lost. He also prepared a synopsis for the use of his son, and a popular treatise, the *Euporista*, containing medical advice and hints on first-aid. To Oribasius we are indebted for our knowledge of ANTYLLUS (second century), who treated aneurysm by ligation above and below the lesion, and who described tracheotomy.

Another Byzantine writer, who lived in the sixth century, was AËTIUS, of Amida, a city on the River Tigris, and, like two other authors to whom we shall presently refer, he was of the Christian faith. This is reflected in his teaching, as he did not hesitate to

[1] E. T. Withington, *Medical History from the Earliest Times*, 1894, p. 129

employ incantations based upon the Bible. For example, in order to remove a bone impacted in the throat, the patient's neck is grasped, and the physician commands, " As Lazarus came forth from the grave, and Jonah out of the whale, bone, come up or go down."

The work of Aëtius is in sixteen books named the *Tetrabiblion*, and although less accurate than that of Oribasius, it was highly esteemed by the physicians of the Renaissance and later by Boerhaave. Particularly interesting and valuable is his account of poisons. His are said to be the best classical descriptions of disease of the eyes, ears, nose, and throat. There is as yet no complete modern edition of his work, although the Latin version of the sixteenth century is available.

ALEXANDER OF TRALLES (A.D. 525–605) also deserves mention, as his work is often quoted by later writers. John Freind, whose *History of Physick* is still worth reading, discusses at some length the writings of Alexander and of Aëtius.[1] Alexander is said to have travelled widely, and to have taught and practised in Rome. An experienced physician, he is the only Byzantine author whose writings show some originality. His accurate clinical picture of pleurisy is regarded as a classic, and he appears to have been the first to differentiate the intestinal parasites—ascaris, taenia, and oxyuris—which he treated with fern and pomegranate. He was also the first to define the uses of rhubarb and colchicum. His works were largely used in the school of Salerno. A number of Greek and Latin editions have appeared. A German translation by Puschmann was published in 1879, and a French version in four volumes by Brunet in 1933–37.

The last physician of the classical tradition was PAUL OF ÆGINA (A.D. 607–690).[2] His work, which he called the *Epitome*, consisted of seven books. The sixth book, devoted to surgery and still regarded as the best of his writings, was highly valued by the Arabs who, as we shall see, preserved and perpetuated the knowledge of Greek medicine during the ensuing centuries. The teaching of Paul of Ægina is available for English readers in the Sydenham Society translation,[3] by Francis Adams (1847).

[1] J. Freind, *History of Physick*, 1725, vol. i. p. 79
[2] J. Berendes, " Des Paulos von Ægina," *Janus*, 1907, vol. xvi. pp. 153, 381, 492, 548 ; also 1913, vol. xxiii. pp. 24, 120, 210, 282
[3] F. Adams, trans., *The Seven Books of Paulus Ægineta*, Sydenham Society, 1844–47, 3 vols.

Public Hygiene in Rome

Before passing on from the Græco-Roman epoch of medical history let us turn back for a moment to consider what the Roman Empire did for medicine. Measured in terms of the diagnosis and treatment of disease the Roman contribution was negligible, because, as we have noted, medical practice was in the hands of Greeks. But if a wider survey be taken, so as to include measures likely to benefit the public health, we must admit that Rome gave to the world a great example. The Roman system of sanitation and water supply is unequalled in history (Plate xiv). The surrounding marshes were drained during Etruscan times. The Cloaca Maxima, or main sewer, was constructed only a little later in the age of the Tarquins (sixth century B.C.).[1] Until the third century the Tiber was the only source of water supply for the city of Rome, but the construction of the famous aqueducts was then commenced, conveying a liberal supply of pure water from sources many miles distant.[2] By the beginning of the Christian era, when the empire was nearing its grandest phase, no less than fourteen aqueducts had been built, and the water supply of Rome amounted to more than 100 gallons per head, an allowance which has never been approached to this day by any other city. Roman houses were provided with plumbing and sanitation. Magnificent public baths were available, with dressings rooms, hot and cold baths, gymnasia, and swimming pools. Many were built by various emperors and wealthy citizens, the baths of Diocletian, of which a plan has survived, and those of Caracalla, being especially imposing (Plate xiv). Natural healing springs were patronised in later times (Plate xx).

The State Medical Service of Ancient Rome

Although the Romans were content to leave the practice of medicine and surgery to the Greeks, they were not slow to realize the value of organization of medical teaching and of medical services for the poor and for the army and navy. Under the Emperor Vespasian (A.D. 69–79), teachers of medicine were provided at public expense, probably in order to ensure a supply of doctors for the fighting services. In the army, medical men

[1] C. Singer, " Medicine," *The Legacy of Rome*, ed. C. Bailey, 1923, p. 289
[2] C. D. Leake, " Roman Architectural Hygiene," *Ann. Med. Hist.*, 1930, vol. ii. p. 135

were part of the establishment, and although they ranked only as non-commissioned officers, they were exempt from taxation and from combatant duty.[1] There were legionary surgeons and cohort surgeons, working in unison, and each ship of the line had its surgeon. On Trajan's column there is sculptured a scene showing the work of what might be called a first-aid dressing station.

Early in the history of the empire, public physicians or *archiatri* were appointed to attend the poor, and to supervise medical practice within their area. They were well paid, and were distributed to various towns and districts in proportion to the population. Those of Rome, the court physicians, were invested with a special dignity and had a voice in the government. Among them was Andromachus, who invented the poison antidote, *theriac*, to which reference has been made.

The Roman Hospital System

The legend of the origin of the first hospital in Rome has often been told. Plague or some other pestilence having broken out in the city in 293 B.C., a mission was sent to seek help from Epidaurus. A sacred serpent was entrusted with the task of healing, and as the ship sailed up the Tiber, the serpent swam ashore and landed on the island of St. Bartholomew.[2] The plague was stayed, and on the island, which is shaped like a ship, and bears a serpent and staff carved on the " prow," there was established the hospital from which, many years later (A.D. 1123), came Rahere the monk, to found St. Bartholomew's Hospital in London.[3] To the island hospital of Rome, in the days of the Republic, men sent their sick slaves, so as to avoid the trouble of caring for them at home. Thus it became a haven for the sick poor. Later, in the first and second centuries A.D., there is mentioned by various writers the existence of *valetudinaria* which appear to have been private hospitals or " nursing homes." They may have developed, eventually, into public institutions. It was only to be expected that in the well-organized Roman army there should be hospital accommodation for sick and

[1] Sir J. Y. Simpson, " Was the Roman Army Provided with Medical Officers?" *Archæological Essays*, Edinburgh, 1872, vol. ii. p. 197
[2] C. Singer, " Medicine," *The Legacy of Rome*, 1923, p. 304
[3] Sir N. Moore, *History of St. Bartholomew's Hospital*, 1918, 2 vols.

wounded soldiers. These were established at various strategic points, and the sites of several of them have been excavated. One of the most perfect examples is at Novaesium near Düsseldorf.[1] It dates from about A.D. 100, and, constructed on the corridor system, is strangely modern.

The Fall of Rome

In conclusion it may be said that while Rome, apart from Greek aid, contributed little to the advance of scientific medicine, she set a great example to the world by the inauguration of a system of public hygiene which in some of its aspects has never since been excelled.

The causes of the collapse of the mighty Roman Empire were many and various, and the problem has exercised the minds of numerous historians. Undoubtedly it was the result of moral and political corruption, the decline of farming, and the burden of taxation. But there was also another factor of peculiar interest to the medical historian. A severe form of malaria was rampant. This disease destroyed many thousands of persons, and undermined the mental and physical condition of many others. It has been regarded by some authorities as one of the main factors which led to the final collapse of Rome.[2] The plague of A.D. 542, which wiped out more than half the inhabitants of Constantinople, produced in the Byzantine Empire results similar to those caused by malaria in the West. (See Supplement, page 453.)

[1] C. Singer, " Medicine," *The Legacy of Rome*, 1923, p. 294
[2] W. H. S. Jones, *Malaria and Greek History*, Manchester, 1909

BOOKS FOR FURTHER READING

ADAMS, F. Trans. *The Extant Works of Aretaeus the Cappadocian*, Sydenham Society, 1860. Trans. *The Seven Books of Paulus Ægineta*, 3 vols., 1844–47
ALLBUTT, T. CLIFFORD. *Greek Medicine in Rome* (Fitzpatrick Lectures), 1929
BAILEY, C. Ed. of *The Legacy of Rome*, 1923. (" Medicine," by C. Singer)
BROCK, A. J. Trans. *Galen : On the Natural Faculties*, Loeb Library, 1917
DAREMBERG, C. *La Médecine, Histoire et Doctrines*, 1865. *Œuvres anatomiques, physiologiques et médicales de Galen*, Paris, 1856
JONES, W. H. S. *Malaria and Greek History*, Manchester, 1909
MÉNIÈRE, P. *Études médicales sur les poètes latins*, Paris, 1858
MILNE, J. S. *Surgical Instruments in Greek and Roman Times*, Aberdeen, 1907
MOORE, Sir N. *History of St. Bartholomew's Hospital*, 2 vols., 1918
SPENCER, W. G. Trans. *Works of Celsus*, 3 vols., Loeb Library, 1935

CHAPTER VI

ARABIAN MEDICINE; THE SCHOOL OF SALERNO

THE Byzantine copyists were, as we have seen, the last to contribute a few bricks to the immense edifice of Græco-Roman medicine. Faded was the glory that was Greece; gone was the grandeur that was Rome. Ahead lay the Dark Ages, the thousand odd years during which learning was no longer held in high esteem, experiment was discouraged, and originality was a dangerous asset. Medicine entered a long period of bondage and slavish convention which continued until it was broken by those bold spirits of the Renaissance who dared to break away from tradition.

It is sometimes said that the dogmatic assertions and forceful teaching of Galen actually retarded the progress of medicine. Nevertheless Galen, with his monotheistic outlook and his acceptance of the soul as more lasting and important than the body, was held in favour by the Christian Church. Had his views been rejected, there is no doubt that the Dark Ages, so far as medicine is concerned, would have been even darker. But was this age so very dark after all? If contrasted with the preceding and the succeeding eras it certainly had little of their brilliance, yet it not only preserved the accumulated store of Greek medicine for the benefit of succeeding generations, but it also made its own contribution.

Medicine now passed into the hands of two very different classes of mankind—the Christian Church and the Arab scholars. Let us see what they made of it.

The Influence of Christianity upon Medicine

It cannot be denied the early Christian Church retarded the progress of medical science.[1] It is true that Christ bade his followers "heal the sick," and gave many practical illustrations of His own healing power. Yet the early Christians interpreted this teaching too literally when they denied to physicians the power of healing. Nothing, they alleged, must detract from the

---

[1] J. R. Russell, *History and Heroes of the Art of Medicine*, 1861, p. 97

PLATE XIII   EARLY ROMAN SURGICAL INSTRUMENTS
FOUND AT POMPEII

1. Scalpel with leaf-shaped double-edged blade.   2. Spring tenaculum forceps.
3. Sharp hook or tenaculum.   4. Scissor-action forceps with serrated blades.
5. Shears with spring handle.   (All are ⅔ natural size, and are bronze, except
the scalpel blade, which is steel.)   (Page 74)

PLATE XIV PUBLIC HEALTH IN THE ROMAN EMPIRE

Pont du Gard, the Roman aqueduct which conveyed water to Nîmes from springs 25 miles distant. The water channel is above the highest series of arches (page 81)

Interior of the Tepidarium of the Imperial Baths of Caracalla at Rome (Reconstruction by R. Phené Spiers)

pre-eminence of the one Great Physician. Prayer and fasting were above all other remedies. Medicine must give place to the Church. The Christian view of disease, too, was a retrograde step. Even St. Basil of Caesarea,[1] who in A.D. 372 established one of the first known hospitals, denied that all disease was of natural origin. Many diseases, he alleged, were sent as punishments for sin, and such chastening demanded only prayer and repentance. The sensible views of Hippocrates were denied ; men returned to ideas analogous to those which prevailed in the days of the Æsculapian temples. Miracles of healing were witnessed in the churches, and doubtless took place, as they still do. But in the early days no other method of healing was admitted or permitted by the bigoted Christians.

Furthermore, the human body was held sacred, and its dissection was prohibited, a veto imposed also by the Moslems. Anatomy and physiology became dead sciences which might not be studied at first hand, but only in the pages of Galen. Such restrictions naturally deterred students from entering the medical profession, and the best brains were attracted to the Church, where an increasing mass of theological dogma afforded ample scope for many scholars.

The antagonism to " secular " learning reached its climax in A.D. 391, when a mob of Christian fanatics set fire to the great library of Alexandria and destroyed many priceless treasures of learning. Such, then, were the blows levelled at the science of medicine by the early Christians ; such were the adverse influences of the Church.

Nevertheless, when all the evidence is weighed, it must be admitted that Christianity has generally favoured the advance of medicine.[2] The infinite pity and patience expended by the Church upon the care of the sick far outweighs any temporary intolerance shown towards medicine. In addition, it must not be forgotten that we are indebted to the mediæval monks for the very existence of those ancient works which influenced, and still influence, the trend of medicine. By day and night the monk in his cell engaged in the work of translation and transcription, until, eventually, the invention of printing made learning available for all.

[1] J. J. Walsh, *Medieval Medicine*, 1920, p. 170
[2] E. T. Withington, *Medical History from the Earliest Times*, 1894, p. 119

The Dawn of Arabian Medicine

The second great reservoir of medical knowledge during the early Middle Ages was provided by the Arabs.[1] Their influence was greater than that of the Christian Church, because Arabian physicians not only approved of the views of their predecessors, and indeed even revered them, but they added much original work of their own which has become incorporated into the medical science of to-day.[2] It must be explained at once that the words "Arab" and "Arabian" are applied solely in respect of the language which these physicians spoke and wrote. All were not natives of Arabia; very few were genuine Arabs. Some were Syrian, some Persian, some, as the Moslem Empire extended, were Spaniards. Nor were all of them Mohammedan. Many were Christians; some were Jews. In those early times the Moslem was as tolerant and favourable towards learning as the Christian was intolerant and antagonistic. Had not the Prophet himself written : "O servant of God, use medicine, because God hath not created a pain without a remedy for it"? There was then a brotherhood of scholars in the Moslem Empire; wise men were highly respected. The Arab was by no means an uncultured savage, and, as Dr. Withington remarks, a Byzantine emperor was astonished to find that the right of collecting Greek manuscripts was among the terms dictated by the victorious Arab, and that an illustrated copy of Dioscorides was the most acceptable present he could offer to a friendly chief.

The Arabs constructed their system of medicine in a logical and regular manner. They began by translating the works of the Greeks into Arabic. Later, they added original observations of their own. Many facts were discovered regarding epidemic fevers. Diseases of the eye, so common in the East, also claimed their attention. The greatest contribution to medicine was in materia medica, which emerged in the nineteenth century as pharmacology. Many new drugs were introduced by the Arabs and their uses described. The word "drug" itself is of Arabic origin; so are the words "alcohol," "alkali," "syrup," "sugar," "jujube," and "spinach," to name only a few. As for the actual

[1] M. Meyerhof, "Science and Medicine," *The Legacy of Islam*, ed. Sir T. Arnold and A. Guillaume, 1931
[2] D. Campbell, *Arabian Medicine*, 1926, 2 vols. ; L. Leclerc, *Histoire de la Médecine arabe*, Paris, 1876, 2 vols.

Arab drugs, these include benzoin, camphor, saffron, myrrh, musk, laudanum, naphtha, senna, and many others.

Intimately associated with materia medica is chemistry, or alchemy, as it was called. The Arabs excelled in chemistry. They invented methods of distillation, sublimation, and crystallization, and perfected many of the processes familiar to chemists to-day. Although the science of alchemy was often misdirected into useless channels, such as the search for " potable gold," " the elixir of life," and the influence of the stars upon the metals, much useful work was also done. The " Father of Arabic Alchemy " was Jabir ibn Hayyan, sometimes called Jebir or Geber,[1] who lived about the tenth century and wrote many books, some of which survive. Such, then, was the contribution of the Arab to medicine. Let us now glance at the lives and work of some of the Arabian physicians.

The Nestorians and the School of Jundi-shapur

The Prophet Mohammed was born in A.D. 570, and the Moslem Empire which he founded, and which eventually stretched from Spain to Samarkand, lasted from the seventh to the thirteenth century, i.e. from the life-time of the Prophet to the sack of Baghdad by the Tartars. Before the birth of Mohammed, however, the roots of Arabian medicine had been planted ; planted, moreover, by an unorthodox but liberal-minded Christian. Nestorius, patriarch of Constantinople, was banished for heresy in A.D. 431. With a band of followers he fled to Edessa (now Urfa) in Asia Minor, and there established a school of medicine. Thence, under further persecution, he proceeded to Jundi-shapur (Gondisapor, Jondisabur) in south-west Persia, where the Sassanian king Chosroes, whose capital was at Ctesiphon, had founded a university.[2] The Arch of Ctesiphon is still a familiar landmark, but of the great city of Jundi-shapur not a trace remains, although Rawlinson claimed to have located it in 1890, at what was then a native village midway between the towns of Dizful and Shustar (see end map). There, for two centuries, the Nestorians laboured

[1] E. J. Holmyard, "Jabir ibn Hayyan," *Proc. Roy. Soc. Med.* (Sect. Hist.), 1923, vol. xxvi. p. 46
[2] C. Elgood, "Jundi-shapur. A Sassanian University," *Proc. Roy. Soc. Med.* (Sect. Hist.), 1939, vol. xxxii. p. 1033

at the work of translating Greek medical texts into Arabic.[1]
Sometimes the translation passed through the medium of Syriac,
and Professor E. G. Browne states that some of the Syriac translations are " so literal as to be quite devoid of sense." If the
translator did not understand the meaning of a Greek word, he
transcribed it into Syriac characters and left the reader to conjecture the sense.[2] The direct Arabic translations, on the other
hand, were well rendered. Among the works translated were
those of Hippocrates, Galen, Dioscorides, Oribasius, and Paul
of Ægina.

The chief physician to the great hospital of Jundi-shapur was
JÚRJÍS BUKHT-YISHÚ (George Bachtishua). He was the first of a
dynasty of six generations of pre-eminent doctors. A still more
famous member of this family of Syrian Christians was Jibra-il
or Gabriel, grandson of George and physician to the court of
Haroun al Raschid, of *Arabian Nights* fame. He must have been
one of the wealthiest medical men in history, as he accumulated
a fortune from fees representing three million pounds in our
coinage. On one occasion he received for curing a caliph a fee
computed to be equivalent to £25,000, while his salary was £1,000
per month, with a present of £1,250 each New Year's Day.

Another Christian physician of Jundi-shapur was HUNAYN IBN
ISÁQ, better known as Honain or Johannitus, who lived early in
the ninth century.[3] He was responsible for many translations
of the Greek masters, and so excellent was his work that he is
said to have received for his manuscripts their weight in gold.
That he showed some originality is evident from his original
work, *Questions on Medicine*, and from his *Ten Treatises on the Eye*,
which is probably the earliest known textbook of ophthalmology.
By this time papyrus and parchment had been supplanted by
paper invented in China, and a paper factory had been established
in Baghdad (A.D. 794).

Rhazes and Avicenna

Arabic medicine now entered upon a period of intense
activity, and there appeared one of the greatest, if not the

[1] A. O. Whipple, " Rôle of the Nestorians as the Connecting Link between Greek
and Arabic Medicine," *Ann. Med. Hist.*, 1936, vol. viii. p. 313
[2] E. G. Browne, *Arabian Medicine* (Fitzpatrick Lectures), 1921, p. 28. (Probably the
best and most concise account of the subject by an acknowledged authority.)
[3] L. M. Sa'di, "A Bio-bibliographical Study of Hunayn Ibn Is-Haq Al-Ibadi
(Johannitus), A.D. 809–877," *Bull. Hist. Med.*, 1934, vol. ii. p. 409

greatest, of Moslem physicians. Abú Bakr Muhammad ibn Zakariyýa (A.D. 860–932) was born at Rai, in Persia, near the modern Teheran, and is therefore commonly known as RHAZES.[1]

Originally a philosopher and musician, he did not commence the study of medicine until he was forty years of age, but that he made good use of the remainder of his long life is evident from the volume of his work. The folio edition, in Latin, dated 1486, of his *Liber Continens*, is said to weigh twenty-two lbs. Rhazes practised in the town of his birth and afterwards at Baghdad. It is said that when he was asked to choose a site for the hospital there, he hung pieces of meat at various points in the city, and selected the place at which putrefaction was longest delayed. To this hospital he became chief physician. At an early stage of his career he unfortunately quarrelled with the ruler of Bokhara, who ordered him to be struck on the head with his own book until either his head or his book was broken. The head was the first to give way, and the injury is said to have caused blindness in later life. When in old age it was suggested to him that his sight might be improved by operation, he declined on the grounds that he had seen enough of this world's sorrow and misery. Yet Rhazes did not allow physical infirmity to interfere with his life mission. He was the author of about a hundred and fifty works, some of which have been lost. His most famous book deals with his most noteworthy contribution to medicine, the distinction between smallpox and measles. Apparently these were the only two endemic infectious diseases known to the Arabs. Rhazes gives a clear picture of each, in a passage which must be regarded as a medical classic. Only one sentence need be quoted : " Excitement, nausea, and unrest are more prominent in measles than in smallpox, whilst the aching in the back is more severe in smallpox than in measles." An English translation of the volume, *On Smallpox and Measles*, undertaken for the Sydenham Society by Greenhill, appeared in 1848.[2] The most important of Rhazes' works, however, is the encyclopædia of medicine known as *El Hâwi*, or in Latin *Liber Continens*. The Latin version, published in 1486 at Brescia, is extremely rare, and no complete manuscript of the original

---

[1] P. Ménétrier, " Le Millénaire de Razès," *Bull. d'Hist. Méd.*, 1931, vol. xxv. p. 191 ; L. M. Sa'di, " The Millenium of Ar-Razi (Rhazes), A.D. 850–932," *Ann. Med. Hist.*, 1935, vol. vii. p. 62

[2] W. A. Greenhill, trans. of *A Treatise on the Smallpox and Measles*, by Rhazes, Sydenham Society, 1848

exists. Professor Browne,[1] who has translated such fragments of the work as are still in the Bodleian Library, " doubts if more than half of this immense work exists at all at the present day."

Rhazes adopts the characteristically Arabic method of prefacing his own views by those of other writers.[2] " So-and-so says," he writes, and finally " but I say," etc. On the subject of asthma he tells us that " Ben Mesue said, ' Let persons troubled with asthma take two drachms of dried and powdered fox lung in their drink.' Galen said that many cure asthma with owls' blood given in wine. I say that owls' blood is not to be given, for I have seen it administered, and it was useless." *El Hâwi* contains many case histories, well recorded, for Rhazes was a close follower of Hippocratic methods. He discountenanced the claim, then so often affirmed, that disease could be diagnosed simply by inspection of the urine, and he was strongly opposed to all magic and quackery. His encyclopædia comprises not only medicine, but also philosophy, astronomy, and mathematics, for like many other sages Rhazes was a man of wide interests. Much smaller, but no less interesting, is the small textbook of medicine, dedicated to the ruler Mansúr ibn Isháq, and called *Mansúri* or " Liber Almansoris." It deals with such subjects as " Physiognomy, with Advice on Slave-buying." " Medical Hints for Travellers," and " Bites of Venomous Beasts."

A contemporary of Rhazes who lived in another part of the Moslem Empire deserves mention as a writer of note. ISAAC JUDÆUS (A.D. *c.* 845–*c.* 940), an Egyptian Jew and physician to the rulers of Tunisia, was the author of books on diet, on fevers, on simple drugs, and on the urine. His collected works, printed in 1515, were greatly in demand as late as the seventeenth century, and he is quoted by Robert Burton (1577–1640) in the *Anatomy of Melancholy.* A number of pithy aphorisms are included in his *Guide for Physicians.*[3] For example : " Ask thy reward when the sickness is at its height, for being cured the patient will surely forget what thou didst for him." Another maxim is : " Should adversity befall a physician, open not thy mouth to condemn, for each hath his hour." A third runs thus : " Treating the sick is like boring holes in pearls, and the physician must act with caution lest he destroy the pearl committed to his charge."

[1] E. G. Browne, *Arabian Medicine*, 1921, p. 48
[2] E. T. Withington, *Medical History from the Earliest Times*, 1894, p. 146
[3] E. G. Browne, *loc. cit.*

The summit of excellence in Arabian medicine was reached by Abú Alí al Hussein ibn Abdalláh ibn Síná, a name which has fortunately been contracted into AVICENNA (A.D. 980–1037). Like Rhazes, he was a Persian, born near Bokhara, and he has been called, with some justification, the Prince of Physicians.[1] He appears to have been something of an infant prodigy, as he knew the Koran by heart before he was ten years old. Turning his attention to medicine, he soon achieved a great reputation, as is evident from his appointment as Court Physician at the age of eighteen years. The perquisite of this office which he most highly prized was free access to the royal library, which contained many priceless manuscripts. Avicenna appears to have been a wanderer ; we find him at Khiva, at Jurjan, at Isfahan, and at Hamadan, where he died after many vicissitudes. His tomb is still a place of pilgrimage. Engaged in the care of others, he took little count of his own health, and though he worked hard he also loved wine and minstrelsy. This reputation has led certain writers to identify him with the poet Omar Khayyám. Omar, however, was never highly esteemed in Persia as a poet, and was popularized only in England by Edward Fitzgerald in his classic translation. One stanza may well apply to Avicenna :

> Up from Earth's Centre through the Seventh Gate
> I rose, and on the Throne of Saturn sate,
> And many a knot unravelled by the Road,
> But not the Master-knot of Human Fate.

Certainly the personality of Avicenna resembled that of Omar. It may be that alcohol shortened his life, for he died at the age of fifty-seven, but his literary output was great, and his work exercised a profound effect upon European medicine. As a philosopher, he was at one time renowned ; as a physician, his influence still lives. Professor Browne ranks him as equal to Aristotle. Dr. Max Meyerhof [2] writes of Avicenna's great book, the *Canon of Medicine*, " Probably no medical work ever written has been so much studied, and is still in current use in the East." In the five books which compose his Canon, or *Q ānūn*, Avicenna endeavours to reconcile the teaching of Galen with that of Aristotle. It is a lengthy work, and probably on that

[1] J. A. Chatard, " Avicenna," *Johns Hopk. Hosp. Bull.*, 1908, vol. xix. p. 157
[2] M. Meyerhof, " Science and Medicine " in *The Legacy of Islam*, ed. Sir T. Arnold 1931 ; Cyril Elgood, *A Medical History of Persia and the Eastern Caliphate*, 1951

account it was regarded by Arnold of Villanova as " scribblings " and by Avenzoar as " wastepaper." Nevertheless, the Canon was highly prized in the later Middle Ages, was used as a text-book in many medical schools, even in that of Montpellier as late as 1650, was eventually printed in numerous editions, and was the subject of many commentaries. An English translation of Book I, in 1921, was undertaken by O. C. Gruner.[1] Avicenna introduced many aphorisms into his work. " The body, to be in a healthy state, must have the heart warm, the nerves cold, and the bones dry." " Extreme pain in the abdomen, with fever, is serious." " If a patient makes movements with his hands as if picking things off himself, it is a sign of death." In the Canon, pulmonary tuberculosis is for the first time regarded as a con-tagious disease. The fifth book of the Canon is devoted to drugs, to the methods of preparing them, and to their action. It was accepted as the most authoritative text up to the time of the Renaissance (Plate xv).

The Canon of Avicenna supplied a great deal of information outside the scope of the modern textbook of medicine. Discussing the choice of a residence, Avicenna gives valuable hints which may still apply. He notes the effect upon health of water supply, climate, the seasons, bathing, sleep, and emotional disturbance, and he makes some interesting remarks on the therapeutic value of music. Advice to travellers is included, and there is a chapter on the care of the aged. In his confident and dogmatic method of expressing himself he resembles Galen, and it is perhaps largely on that account that his teaching was, like that of Galen, regarded as authoritative for many years after his death.

Arabian Surgery in Spain [2]

The Arabs were not well versed in the art of surgery. During the time of the Moslem Empire, and indeed throughout all history until recent times, surgery was regarded as inferior to medicine, and its practice was relegated to craftsmen rather than to scholars. At the time of which we speak there existed a still more powerful drag upon surgical progress, the neglect of anatomy and

[1] O. C. Gruner, *The Canon of Avicenna*, Book I., 1921
[2] Zaki Aly, " Chirurgie arabe en Espagne," *Bull. Soc. de l'Hist. de Méd.*, 1932, vol. xxvi. p. 236 ; H. P. J. Renaud, " Les Origines de la Médecine arabe en Espagne," *Bull. d'Hist. Méd.*, 1935, vol. xxix. p. 321

PLATE XV EARLY ARABIAN SURGERY

Treating a fracture-dislocation (? tuberculosis) of the spinal column (from *Canon* of Avicenna).   *Upper.* Direct pressure by a board hinged on the wall, the operator throwing his weight on the other end.   *Centre.* Direct pressure or pounding with a heavy instrument.   *Lower.* Extension above and below the seat of injury, combined with local manipulation (page 92)

PLATE XVI CORDOVA, CENTRE OF ARABIAN CULTURE
IN THE WEST

Tower of the Cathedral,
formerly the Mosque
(page 93)

Chapel of the Maksurrah,
originally a sanctuary for
the Ruler

physiology, those two great sciences which were the first to revive at the Renaissance. It is therefore all the more interesting to find that towards the end of the period under discussion, an Arab surgeon did appear with ideas ahead of his time.[1] ALBUCASIS (A.D. 936–1013) (sometimes written Abulcasis) was born near Cordova (or Córdoba) (Plate XVI). The centre of interest, in medicine at least, had shifted by this time to the Western Caliphate. Cordova, a large and important city, with a population of over a million, had become a centre of commerce and of culture.[2] The facts that the library contained 200,000 volumes, that there were fifty hospitals in the city, and that the university was founded in the eighth century, suggest that during the lifetime of Albucasis, Cordova stood high as a seat of medical learning. Albucasis did much to raise the status of surgery which, he tells us, " had passed into the hands of vulgar and uncultivated minds and had fallen into contempt." His chief work was called the Collection, or *Tasrif*, and was a complete account of surgery and medicine. The surgical portion, produced separately, was the first illustrated work on surgery (Plate XVII). It was repeatedly translated into Latin, one of the earliest translations being that of Guy de Chauliac, the great mediæval surgeon. The work contains many illustrations of surgical instruments and appliances.[3] " Surgical operations," remarks Albucasis, " are of two kinds, those which benefit the patient and those which usually kill him." That he was a conservative surgeon is evident from the motto " Caution," with which he begins and ends his book. The cautery was the favourite instrument, and to its use the first book is devoted. The second book is virtually a compilation from Paul of Ægina, and deals with lithotomy and other operations, while the third book is devoted to fractures and dislocations. It is interesting to compare the surgical methods of Albucasis with those of the Arabian surgeons of to-day, as described in Hilton-Simpson's work (cf. p. 9).

Spain was the home of several other Arabian physicians of the twelfth century. Little is known of the life of AVENZOAR (A.D. *c.* 1091–1162), but his treatise, entitled *Thesir* (or "Assistance") had a far-reaching influence in Europe, and exists in many

[1] M. S. Spink, "Arabian Gynæcological and Obstetrical Practice Illustrated from Albucasis," *Proc. Roy. Soc. Med.* (Sect. Hist.), 1937, vol. xxx. p. 653
[2] J. W. Draper, *History of the Intellectual Development of Europe*, 2 vols., 1864, vol. ii. p. 29
[3] T. Meyer-Steineg and K. Sudhoff, *Geschichte der Medizin*, Jena, 1921, p. 161

Latin versions. He is credited with having discovered the itch mite (*acarus scabiei*), " a very small beast, so small that he is hardly visible."

A careful observer, Avenzoar records a number of interesting cases, as, for example, a case of rupture cured by rest. " I told him to eat nothing but baked bread and boiled sparrows and to rest quietly on his back for two months, so that he could not even say his prayers, save in his heart. He got perfectly well." Avenzoar is said to have been the first to suggest that a patient suffering from œsophageal stricture might be fed by nutrient enemata.

AVERROES (A.D. 1126–1198) was a friend and pupil of Avenzoar, a free-thinking philosopher of the Aristotelian school, whose unorthodox opinions involved him in trouble, for he died in prison in Morocco after spending most of his life at Cordova.[1] Although his medical work, the *Colliget* (or " Universals ") was translated into Latin, his influence was mainly that of a philosopher.[2] Another distinguished philosopher was the Jew, Moses ben Maimon, or MAIMONIDES (A.D. 1135–1204).[3] He was born in Cordova, and grew up at a time when the sun of Arabic culture was setting. Doomed to banishment because he would not accept the Moslem faith, he wandered to Morocco, and then to Cairo, where laws were more lenient and where he acquired so great a reputation that, despite his religion, he was appointed physician to Saladin, the Saracen leader who so frequently met the Crusaders in battle. It is said that Richard Cœur de Lion also desired Maimonides as personal physician but that he declined this offer. He is said to have been the original of the physician El Hakim, who figures in Sir Walter Scott's *Talisman*.[4] For the benefit of the eldest son of Saladin he wrote a guide to personal health, or *Book of Counsel*. It includes a talk on the worthlessness of riches and the importance of character. True happiness was to be found only in things of the spirit.[5] Another work dealt with poisons, including those introduced by the bites of snakes, scorpions, dogs, and,

[1] I. Abraham, E. R. Bevan, and C. Singer, *The Legacy of Israel*, 1927, p. 190
[2] G. G. Coulton, " Averrhoism," *Studies in Medieval Thought*, 1940, p. 121
[3] W. Mendelson, " Maimonides, a Twelfth-century Physician." *Ann. Med. Hist.*, 1923, vol. v. p. 250 ; W. M. Feldman, " The Life and Medical Work of Maimonides," *Proc. Roy. Soc. Med.* (Sect. Hist.), 1935, vol. xxviii. p. 1544
[4] G. K. Tallmadge, " The Character of El Hakim in *The Talisman*," *Ann. Med. Hist.*, 1938, vol. x. p. 318
[5] H. A. Savitz, " Maimonides' Hygiene of the Soul," *Ann. Med. Hist.*, 1932, vol. iv. p. 80

" worst of all," he tells us, the bite of a fasting man. Treatment should consist in keeping the wound open, and abstracting the poison by sucking, cupping, scarification, cauterization, and the application of a tight bandage above the wound, if situated in a limb. The long incubation period of rabies is noted. In this work, as also in the work, *On Causes and Nature of Disease*, Maimonides shows his wisdom by advising simple drugs rather than complicated mixtures and by his opposition to all forms of magic and astrology. This search for causes suggests that he was far ahead of his time, as does also his advocacy of fresh air, and his belief in the close relationship between mental and physical health. *Aphorisms according to Galen* is the title of his most valued work. In the 1,500 aphorisms, arranged under twenty-five headings, there is embodied all that was best in Galen's teaching, stated with praiseworthy brevity.[1] To the busy practitioner who had no time to search for information in the immense labyrinth of Galen's original works, this synopsis must have been invaluable. Maimonides had a very large practice in Cairo, and the fact that his literary output was of such high quality reveals him as a keen scholar and a tireless worker. The *Aphorisms* is carefully annotated, and the source of every statement is quoted. Not only was Maimonides a distinguished physician, he was a talented philosopher. In his *Guide for the Perplexed* he reconciled religion with medicine, and showed how each might assist the other. For him the patient was always a human being, not merely a case.

The tomb of Maimonides at Tiberias is still a place of pilgrimage, which is not surprising, as he was held in great esteem by his colleagues and is still regarded as one of the greatest of the many great Jewish physicians. All his works were written in Arabic. A few were translated and printed in Latin in the fifteenth and sixteenth centuries, but no English translation is available, with the exception of the *Guide for the Perplexed*.

Hospitals, and the End of the Moslem Empire

Mention has already been made of the great teaching hospitals at Jundi-shapur and at Baghdad. Even more magnificent were the hospitals of Damascus, of Cordova, and of Cairo. The Mansur hospital at Cairo, for example, had male and female

[1] D. J. Macht, " Moses Maimonides, Physician and Scientist: The William Osler of Medieval Arabic and Hebrew Medicine," *Bull. Hist. Med.*, 1935, vol. iii. p. 585

wards for general cases, also wards reserved for wounds, for eye diseases, and for fevers, the last-mentioned being cooled by fountains. There were courtyards for lectures, a botanical (or herbal) garden, a dispensary, and a library with six librarians. Fifty speakers recited the Koran day and night without ceasing, while at night soft music was played to lull the sleepless, and there were story-tellers to amuse all. Each patient, on departure, was given a sum of money, sufficient to tide him over convalescence, until he should be fit to resume work. Withington [1] tells us that this hospital was completed in A.D. 1284. Masons and carpenters were brought from all parts of Egypt. Loiterers in the street, and passers-by, whatever their rank, were obliged to assist in the holy work, insomuch that " most people avoided going that way."

When this great hospital was opened the day of Arabian medicine was already far spent. The Moslem Empire had been subjected to hard blows from the east and from the west. Cordova had fallen in 1236, though Granada resisted conquest for 200 years longer. Baghdad was sacked by the Mongols in 1258. The lands of Islam had become too unsettled to provide a suitable field of learning for scholars, and in any case the famous medical school of Salerno was already well established. Europe was once again to provide the intellectual centre to the known world.

So ended the bright epoch of Arabian medicine. Further research may show that the Arabs have contributed to medical progress a share even greater than can at present be claimed. That it was a great contribution is certain, for not only did they preserve the Greek learning, but they also added much of their own. To quote Dr. Meyerhof [2] : " Islamic medicine reflected the light of the Hellenic sun, when its day had fled, and shone like a moon in the Dark Ages. Some bright stars lent their own light, and the moon and stars alike faded at the dawn of the Renaissance, though their influence remains to this day."

Monastic Medicine

After the downfall of the Roman Empire, medicine followed two distinct and divergent paths, which went their separate ways

[1] E. T. Withington, *Medical History from the Earliest Times*, 1894, p. 166
[2] M. Meyerhof, in *The Legacy of Islam*, ed. Sir T. Arnold, 1931, p. 354

96

PLATE XVII ARABIAN SURGICAL INSTRUMENTS

الـفـصـل الخـامـس والـعـشـرون ـفي كيِّ الابط ،

اذا انخلع رأس العضد بسبب رطوبات مزلقة او لم يتبث ـفي حيں رده
بعد انخلعه حتي يصبر له ذلك عادةً برد ثم يتخلع عند ادني حركة كما
شاهدنا مـراراً فلينبغي اں يرد الفك اولاً نم تستلقي العليل ـعلي ظهره
او ـعلي الجانب الصحيح ثم ترفع الجلد الذي ـفي داخل الابط الي فوتـ
باصبعك من يدك البسري اں كاں المفصل انخلع الي داخل ثم تحم
المكواة ذات السفودين التي هذه صورتهـا

ثم تكوي بها الجلد حتي تنغدها الي الجانب الاخر وباني شكل الكي اربع
كبـات وقـد تكو بمكواة ذات السفانيد الثلاث فيكوں شكـل
الـكي حينبد ست كبـات ويكوں السفانيد رقة المرود وهذه صورة
المكواة ذات السـفـانيد الثلاث

صـورة اجـري

وقد تزاد ـعلي هذة العدد واحدة فيكوں الكبات تمانية ثم تحمل
علي الكي الكراث المدقوق مع الملح ثم تلزم العليل الدعة ولا تحرك
الـعـضـو زمـانـاً حـتـي تقوي ،

Page from the 1778 Oxford edition of Albucasis' *De Chirurgia* (Tasrif),
printed in Arabic and Latin. The text is illustrated by various patterns
of cautery, a favourite instrument with the early Arabian surgeons
(page 93)

PLATE XVIII   THE   PATRON   SAINTS   OF   SURGERY

Miniature painting ascribed to Mantegna, showing the twin saints, Cosmas and Damian, cleaning their instruments after having amputated a cancerous leg and having grafted in its place the leg of a Moor recently deceased. The amputated limb is on the floor at their feet. The patient, now having one leg white and the other black, lies in bed as the spectators regard the miracle with amazement. In the panel on the right may be seen another group around the coffin of the dead Moor at the door of a church (page 97)

until they fused five hundred years later in the school of **Salerno.** One path, that of Arabian medicine, we have just traced in its long journey. The other, hidden in cell and cloister, and on that account sometimes called monastic medicine, is not so easy to follow.[1] It was no path of progress, yet it served a useful function in transmitting to the more enlightened time which followed part of the great heritage of Greek medicine which might otherwise have been lost. The relapse of medicine into the hands of a priestly class is not surprising. One of the first principles of Christianity was the healing of the sick, and the quiet retreat from the world's strife which the monastery offered was attractive to those of scholarly bent. The manuscript works of the Greek masters of medicine were now safe in the keeping of the Church. Many an unknown monk toiled for years copying, illuminating, and translating the classic authors. Adjoining the monastery there was often a herb garden, where simple vegetable remedies were grown, and another adjunct was the hospice, in which the sick were nursed back to health.

Nevertheless the physical means of healing were regarded as a mere adjunct to the spiritual cure. The early Christians, if they did not actually view disease as a punishment for sin, as did their pagan ancestors, at least regarded it as a discipline to be patiently borne and endured. Any investigation into the natural causes of sickness was out of the question. The means of healing adopted by the Church were strangely like those of the Aesculapian temples. Prayers, litanies, and paternosters took precedence over drugs, and the churches dedicated to certain saints and martyrs, were places of pilgrimage for the sick. Votive offerings were revived, and so was temple-sleep or incubation, although now in Christian churches in place of pagan temples.

Among the earliest Christian saints to be associated with the healing art were the twin brothers Cosmas and Damian. They were Arabian physicians, who travelled far and wide, preaching Christianity and curing the sick (Plate xviii). Condemned to death by drowning, they were rescued by an angel, after which, when burning and stoning had failed to disrupt body and soul, they were beheaded in a.d. 303. They became the patron saints of surgery, and miracles such as they performed during life were continued after their death in churches at Byzantium and

[1] L. Thorndike, *History of Magic and Experimental Science*, New York, 1923-41, vol. i. pp. 481, 616

elsewhere.[1] In those days the unorthodox were liable to suffer at the hands of their fellow Christians, and it is not surprising to learn that Priscillian, a Spanish monk, was burned alive in A.D. 385 for suggesting that the signs of the zodiac might preside over the various organs of the body, a view which became widely adopted at a later date. Saint Patrick, who had carried the work of evangelization as far as Ireland, established there a centre of missionary enterprise. Among his followers were Saint Columba, Saint Gall, and Saint Cuthbert.

Saint Columba landed in the little Scottish island of Iona in A.D. 563, there to establish a monastery, which included a herb garden and a hospice.

Saint Gall (A.D. 614) travelled as far as Switzerland, where one of the cantons still bears his name.[2] There still exists a plan of his monastery and of the garden, the latter showing fields devoted to various medicinal plants : lily, sage, rue, fennel, pennyroyal, mint, rosemary, cumin, and other herbs.

Saint Cuthbert (b. A.D. 635) was associated with Lindisfarne on the Northumbrian coast. An illustrated manuscript of the twelfth century, in the Bodleian Library, describes many of his miraculous cures.

Patron Saints in Medicine

In the Middle Ages there were many saints, besides Saint Cosmas and Saint Damian and the others just mentioned, whose names were associated with the art of healing.

As the Christian Church of early times became more powerful, an effort was made to replace the signs of the zodiac, allotted to organs and members of the human body, by patron saints, who were believed to dominate the various parts. Thus, Saint Blaise or Blasius dominated the throat ; Saint Bernardine the lungs ;

[1] K. Sudhoff, " Healing Miracles of SS. Cosmas-Damian and Cyrus-John," *Essays in the History of Medicine*, trans. F. H. Garrison, New York, 1926, p. 219 ; C. and D. Singer, " On a Miniature ascribed to Mantegna, of an Operation by Cosmas and Damian," *Contributions to Medical and Biological Research*, Osler's 70th Birthday volume, New York, 1919, p. 166 ; L. M. Zimmerman, " Cosmas and Damian, Patron Saints of Surgery," *Amer. Jour. Surg.*, 1936, vol. xxxiii. p. 160 ; L. Oliver, " Les Images de la Confrérie des Bienheureux Martyrs Saint Cosme et Saint Damien," *Bull. d'Hist. Méd.*, 1929, vol. xxiii, p. 184 ; C. G. Cumston, " A Note on St. Cosmas and St. Damian, the Patron Saints of the Confraternity of the Surgeons of France," *Proc. Roy. Soc. Med.*, 1918, vol. xi. p. 70
[2] D. Riesman, *The Story of Medicine in the Middle Ages*, New York, 1933, p. 19 ; E. M. Holmes, " Horticulture in Relation to Medicine," *Jour. Roy. Hort. Soc.*, 1906, vol. xxx. p. 42

Saint Apollonia the teeth ; Saint Lawrence the back ; and Saint Erasmus the abdomen.[1] Sometimes more than one saint held sway over the part. For example, the patron saints of the eyes were Saint Bridget, Saint Triduana, or Saint Lucia,[2] according to the country. Frequently the association arose during the life of the saint. For example, Saint Triduana of Scotland, admired by a Pictish chief on account of her eyes, is said to have plucked them out and presented them to her lover impaled on a skewer. Pictures of Saint Triduana illustrate this incident. That belief in tradition dies hard is proved by the fact that as recently as 1927, according to Comrie,[3] persons with eye disorders still visited Saint Triduana's well at Holyrood, Edinburgh, although the well house had been removed from its original site (Restalrig) to another well about a mile distant.

To other saints was accredited the power to cause or to cure certain diseases. Saint Dymphna, a martyr of the seventh century, was one of the saints invoked in cases of insanity. In vertigo and epilepsy prayers were offered to Saint Avertin, while diseases of the rectum, such as hæmorrhoids or fistula, apparently common in mediæval times, were healed by the intervention of Saint Fiacre. The effigy of this saint adorned the inn at Paris where carriages were first offered for hire, a circumstance which led to the introduction of the French word *fiacre*, to signify a horse cab.

One of the best known of the patron saints, as might be expected, was Saint Roch, who presided over plague.[4] Born in Montpellier, of noble parents, about the beginning of the fourteenth century, he devoted his energy and his wealth to the care of the stricken people while the Black Death was devastating Europe. After he had visited many cities on his mission of mercy, he was himself a victim of plague at Piacenza, where he crawled outside the walls to die. Each day his dog brought him a loaf of bread, none knew from whence. Then an angel appeared one night, and healed his sore so that he recovered. Returning to his native Montpellier, he was not recognized, but was arrested as a spy and cast into prison, where he died, leaving this message : "All

[1] M. Bortarel, " Les Saints guérisseurs," *Paris Méd.*, 1921, vol. xiii. p. 166 ; 1922, vol. xiv. p. 127 ; G. Gordon-Taylor, " Abdominal Injuries," *Brit. Jour. Surg.*, 1938, vol. xxvi. p. 217 (contains reference to St. Erasmus)

[2] R. Greff, " Santa Lucia, die Schutzheilige Hilferin und Retterin der Augenkranken," *Klin. Monatsbl f. Augenheilkunde*, 1938, vol. c. p. 97

[3] J. D. Comrie, *History of Scottish Medicine*, 1932, 2 vols., vol. i. p. 45

[4] Raymond Crawford, *Plague and Pestilence in Literature and Art*, Oxford, 1914, p. 105

A HISTORY OF MEDICINE

those stricken by plague who pray for and through the merit and intercession of Saint Roch shall be healed." The cult of Saint Roch did not appear immediately, but it became widespread during the fifteenth century, when his effigy was often carried in processions in order to check an epidemic.

Other saints associated with plague are Saint Sebastian and Saint Cyprian.

St. Vitus's Dance and St. Anthony's Fire

Certain saints have given their names to diseases.[1] A familiar example is St. Vitus's Dance, or chorea. Saint Vitus was a Sicilian youth who, just before he suffered martyrdom under the Emperor Diocletian in A.D. 303, prayed to God that all who should commemorate the day of his death might be protected from the dancing mania. The dance of Saint John or Saint Vitus, usually associated with the name of the latter saint, was characterized by a complete loss of control of the persons affected, who continued to dance in wild delirium until they fell to the ground exhausted. Although the last known epidemic of this nature occurred in Germany and the Netherlands in the fourteenth century, following close upon the Black Death, the mania dated from the tenth century or earlier, and it appeared at intervals during the Middle Ages.[2] In Italy, especially in Apulia, it was attributed to the bite of a venomous spider, the tarantula, and was accordingly called tarantism. It was said to be relieved by music of a lively and impassioned nature, the Tarantellas, some of which have been preserved. Tarantism was at its height in Italy in the seventeenth century, long after the St. Vitus's Dance of Germany had disappeared. The dancing mania of Germany was regarded as the work of the devil, curable only by the Church, until Paracelsus attempted to prove that it was really a disease, chorea. Diseases, Paracelsus affirmed, should not be named after saints, as all could be ascribed to natural causes. Hippocrates, it will be remembered, held a similar view regarding "the sacred disease," epilepsy.

Another saint whose name was linked with a disease was Saint Anthony.[3] There have been various interpretations of "St.

[1] R. Fletcher, " Some Diseases Bearing Names of Saints," *Bristol Med.-Chir. Jour.*, 1912, vol. xxx. p. 289
[2] J. F. K. Hecker, *The Epidemics of the Middle Ages*, trans. by B. G. Babington, Sydenham Society, 1844, p. 93
[3] D. H. Kerler, *Die Patronate der Heiligen*, Ulm, 1905

Anthony's Fire " a name sometimes applied to erysipelas even in modern times. Saint Anthony was born in Egypt in A.D. 251. The disease to which his name was applied was common in epidemic form throughout the Middle Ages when it was also termed *ignis sacer, feu sacré*, and *mal des ardents*.[1] The last-mentioned is now believed to have been bubonic plague, the other two were synonyms for St. Anthony's Fire. Some cases, or even epidemics, may have been erysipelas, but the accepted explanation identifies St. Anthony's Fire with ergotism, arising from the use of bread prepared from grain infected by *claviceps purpurea* or rye disease.[2] The victims suffered from severe burning pain and cramp in the limbs, followed by a long and painful stage of gangrene and separation. The disease was particularly severe in France during the tenth and eleventh centuries, but many epidemics have been reported since then, and in the nineteenth century epidemics of ergotism appeared in Russia.[3] St. Anthony is represented in art as a tall man, bearing a staff with bells attached, and accompanied by a hog with a bell fastened to one ear.

The pursuit of learning by the monks of those dark ages was encouraged by a number of wise and influential rulers. Theodoric, king of the Ostrogoths (A.D. 454–526), fostered the cultural life of the countries he had conquered, and encouraged the monks to undertake the care of the sick poor, a duty which had previously devolved upon the Roman *archiatri*. His chief minister, Cassiodorus (490–585) founded two monasteries at his ancestral home of Squillace in Calabria the " toe " of Italy, and encouraged the collection and copying of medical manuscripts.

Associated with Theodoric in his work of charity was St. Benedict of Nursia (480–547), who regarded the care of the sick as one of the leading objects of the order he founded. The rules of the Benedictine monks were less stringent and more hygienic than those of other orders. The hours of sleep and exercise were reasonable, and there was ample time for study and for the copying of manuscripts, a task favoured by those in authority. The monks were encouraged to study Greek, to read the works of Hippocrates and Galen and the Byzantine commentators, and above all to master the writings of Dioscorides on the nature and uses of herbs. On the summit of Monte Cassino, near Salerno,

[1] H. Chaumartin, *Le Mal des Ardents et le Feu Saint Antoine*, Paris, 1946
[2] E. Ehlers, *L'Ergotisme*, Paris, 1902
[3] F. G. Clemow, *The Geography of Disease*, Cambridge, 1903, p. 163

Benedict founded his monastery, destined to take an important part in the foundation of that famous first school of medicine.

Among the great rulers who favoured the literary efforts of the monks were Charlemagne (A.D. 768) and Alfred the Great (A.D. 871). The earliest surviving Saxon medical manuscript is the *Leech Book of Bald,* which was written in the tenth century.[1] It is a strange mixture of charms and incantations, with the names of many herbal remedies and indications for their use.[2]

Before leaving the rather arid subject of monastic medicine one other name must be mentioned, that of HILDEGARD OF BINGEN (A.D. 1098–1179), who is credited with many miraculous cures. This clever and learned woman, sometimes called Saint Hildegard, though she was never canonized, spent most of her long life as abbess of a Benedictine nunnery at Bingen on the Rhine.[3] She made no serious contribution to medicine, and the most interesting of her works are those in which she describes her visions, which revealed to her the structure of the universe and the nature of the soul. The *Scivias* is illustrated by most curious illuminations, resembling the drawings of William Blake. The fact that some of them show a series of fortification lines has suggested to Dr. Charles Singer that Hildegard was a victim of migraine.[4] Hildegard's *Physica* contained some curious remedies. For leprosy she recommended an ointment made from unicorn's liver and white of egg, and she even tells her readers how to capture a unicorn, using as the bait a virgin in whose lap the animal would innocently lay its head, while the hunter rushed up and slew it.

The School of Salerno

The charming seaside town of Salerno, some thirty-five miles south of Naples, will ever be remembered as the seat of the first organized medical school in Europe. At Salerno, after five centuries of comparative stagnation in the widely scattered monasteries of Christendom and in the cities of the vast Moslem

[1] T. O. Cockayne, *Leechdoms, Wortcunning, and Starcraft of Early England,* 1864–66, 3 vols.
[2] J. F. Payne, *English Medicine in Anglo-Saxon Times* (Fitzpatrick Lectures), 1904, p. 39
[3] G. M. Engbring, " Saint Hildegard, Twelfth-century Physician," *Bull. Hist. Med.,* 1940, vol. viii. p. 770
[4] C. Singer, " The Visions of Hildegard of Bingen," in *From Magic to Science,* 1928, chap. vi. ; " The Scientific Views and Visions of Saint Hildegard, 1098–1180," in *Studies in the History and Method of Science,* 1921, vol. i. p. 1

Empire, medical learning became established on a sound basis.[1] Although the School of Salerno produced no brilliant genius, nor any startling discovery, it may at least be claimed that here was planted the seed which was to come to full fruition in the brilliant epoch of the Renaissance a few centuries later. A famous health resort since early Roman times, easy of access from all directions, and close to the Greek-speaking lands of Sicily and southern Italy, it is not surprising that Salerno was chosen as a Civitas Hippocratica, a meeting place for physicians of every race and creed. " The flowering time of Salerno covered the period of the Crusades (1096–1270)." [2] Regarding the origin of the school, no accurate details are available. According to legend it was founded by " four masters "—Elinus the Jew, Pontus the Greek, Adale the Arab, and Salernus the Latin. Such a legend at least points to two conclusions : that the school was open to all, irrespective of language or nationality, and that it was a lay foundation, and not, as some have supposed, a product of the adjacent monastery of Monte Cassino. It is known, however, that friendly relations existed between the Benedictine monks and the Salernitans, and there can be little doubt that the valuable collection of medical manuscripts at Monte Cassino were available to the physicians of Salerno. Some contend that the school was founded by Charlemagne ; others that it was a direct outcome of Arabian medicine, but there is no strong evidence that either view is correct. It is now generally accepted that Salernitan medicine bears little or no trace of Arab influence. Indeed, to quote from Rashdall's famous work on mediæval universities, " so far from the rise of the fame of Salerno having been due to Oriental influences, it was these influences which brought about its fall. It was the increasing popularity of the Arabic medicine in the thirteenth century, combined with the growth of medical faculties elsewhere, which destroyed the popularity of the more conservative Civitas Hippocratica." [3] The only certain facts are that it came into being in a somewhat obscure fashion about the ninth century, that it reached the zenith of its fame in the tenth or eleventh century, that in the thirteenth century it gave way to the adjoin-

[1] G. W. Corner, "The Rise of Medicine at Salerno in the Twelfth Century," in *Lectures on the History of Medicine*, Mayo Foundation, 1937, p. 371

[2] K. Sudhoff, " Salerno, a Medieval Health Resort and Medical School " in *Essays in the History of Medicine*, 1926, trans. by F. H. Garrison, p. 245

[3] H. Rashdall, *The Universities of Europe in the Middle Ages*, new ed. by F. M. Powicke and A. B. Emden, 1936, 3 vols., vol. i, p. 75

ing school of Naples and to the newly established universities of Montpellier and Bologna, although it lingered on, in name at least, until it was finally closed by Napoleon in 1811. Not a trace of its existence is to be found in Salerno to-day.[1]

Salerno owed much to Duke Robert Guiscard, the Norman knight who captured the town in A.D. 1075, after a siege of eight months, and who made it his capital and a great centre of trade and of culture.

For our scanty knowledge of the teachers of Salerno we are indebted to the researches of De Renzi, who published all the available information and manuscripts.[2] One of the earliest Salernitan masters was GARIOPONTUS (d. 1050), of whose life little is known. His *Passionarius*, a textbook of medicine, enjoyed a wide vogue, though it was mainly derived from Greek writings. Rashdall calls it " a compilation with an earlier tradition behind it." Gariopontus disregarded mystical medicine, but he quotes freely from Hippocrates, whom he highly revered.

Another textbook was the *Practica* of BARTHOLOMEUS ANGLICUS, in which stress was laid upon the pulse and the urine in diagnosis, and upon venesection and diet as means of treatment.

BARTHOLOMEW the Englishman was the author of a popular encyclopædia, *De Proprietatibus Rerum*, which was a widely read book of popular information during the Middle Ages, and which gives a clear picture of the life and learning of the time (thirteenth century).[3] It was translated into English by John of Trevisa in 1397. The edition edited by Wynkyn de Worde, which appeared in 1495, was one of the finest and earliest books to be printed in England. A subsequent edition by Berthelet (1535), is well known to bibliophiles.[4]

Of greater interest are the women doctors who taught in this progressive school. Here again we enter the realm of legend, as it is not certain whether the " ladies of Salerno " were anything more than nurses and midwives.[5] Of them we know little more than their attractive names : Trotula, Abella, Rebecca, Con-

[1] C. Daremberg, "De l'école de Salerne," in *La Médecine, Histoire et Doctrines*, 1865, p. 123
[2] S. De Renzi, *Storia documentata della Scuola Medica di Salerno*, 1875, 2nd. ed., 5 vols.
[3] J. J. Walsh, *Medieval Medicine*, 1920, p. 192
[4] R. Steele, *Medieval Lore from Bartholomaeus Anglicus*, King's Classics, 1907
[5] H. P. Bayon, "Trotula and the Ladies of Salerno," *Proc. Roy. Soc. Med.* (Sect. Hist.), 1940, vol. xxxiii, p. 471 ; K. C. Hurd Mead, *A History of Women in Medicine*, Haddan, Conn., 1938, p. 127

stanza, and others. TROTULA is said to be the author of a work on obstetrics written about A.D. 1050, and she is still better known as the original of the " Dame Trot " of modern fairy tales. Anatomy was taught, not from human dissection, but from the pig, whose organs were believed to resemble closely those of man. A treatise on the anatomy of the pig, *Anatomia Porci*, by KOPHO (or Copho), is of great interest as the first textbook of anatomy.[1] Usually linked with the school of Salerno is the name of CON-STANTINE THE AFRICAN (1010–1087), who translated many Arabic works into Latin, and thus linked together the medicine of East and West. Born in Carthage, Constantine visited Persia and India, wandering and studying medicine for over thirty years. On his return to Carthage he was regarded with disfavour, as apparently he knew too much, and he was obliged to flee for his life. He sought refuge at Salerno, where his learning was recognized, and where he was made welcome at the Court of Robert Guiscard. Whether he taught in the school of Salerno is very doubtful, but his residence in the town was not long.[2] He soon retired to Monte Cassino, becoming a monk and devoting himself to translating into Latin the works of the Arabic physicians and the classical Greek medical writings which had been preserved through the Arabian route.[3] It is said that Constantine passed off many of those works as his own, and that he seldom acknowledged the source of his information. His *Pantegni*, the " Whole Art," is largely a compilation. Singer is of opinion that Constantine has been greatly overrated.[4] Be that as it may, he deserves credit for his assiduous work in making available for Latin readers the rich resources of Arabian medicine. Although it is agreed that Constantine did not confer an Arabian flavour upon Salerno, he had, according to Thorndike, " as good a right to be called Salernitan as most of the authors in De Renzi's collection." [5]

Surgery was not neglected at Salerno. Its principal exponent was ROGER OF PALERMO who in A.D. 1180 wrote his *Chirurgia*, or,

[1] R. Creutz, " Der Magister Copho und seine Stellung im Hoch-Salerno," *Arch. Gesch. f. Med.*, 1938, vol. xxxi. p. 51
[2] P. Capparoni, *Magistri Salernitani Nondum Cogniti*, 1923, p. 39 (English trans.)
[3] L. M. Sa'di, " Reflection of Arabian Medicine at Salerno and Montpellier," *Ann. Med. Hist.*, 1933, vol. v. p. 215
[4] C. Singer, *From Magic to Science*, 1928, chap. vii., " The School of Salerno and its Legends," p. 240
[5] L. Thorndike, *A History of Magic and Experimental Science*, New York, 1923–41, vol. i. p. 742

as it is sometimes called from its opening phrase, *Post fabricam mundi*. This work, which was for centuries regarded as a classic, was revised by ROLAND OF PARMA, a pupil of Roger. The surgery of Roger is, in the main, conservative and non-operative [1] (Plate XIX). He regarded suppuration as an essential process in the history of wounds, though he employed ligatures as well as styptics to check hæmorrhage. Skin diseases were included in the surgery of that day, and were treated for the most part with mercurial ointment.

Another interesting contribution to Salernitan literature was made by MUSANDINUS,[2] who wrote *De modo praeparandi cibos et potus infirmorum*; in other words, a textbook of sickroom cookery. More interesting still is the work on Medical Ethics entitled *De Adventu Medici*, or " The Doctor's Visit," written by ARCHIMATHEUS in 1140. The following quotation gives some idea of the nature of the advice [3] : " When called to a patient commend yourself to God and to the angel who guided Tobias. On the way, learn as much as possible from the messenger, so that, if you discover nothing from the patient's pulse, you may still astonish him and gain his confidence by your knowledge of the case. On arrival ask the friends whether the patient has confessed, for if you bid him do so after the examination you will frighten him. Then sit down, take a drink, and praise the beauty of the country and the house, if they deserve it, or extol the liberality of the family. Do not be in a hurry to give an opinion, for the friends will be more grateful for your judgment if they have to wait for it. If asked to dinner, do not hasten to take the first place unless is is offered to you. Send often to inquire for the patient, that he may see you do not neglect him for the pleasures of the table, and on leaving, express your thanks for the attentions shown you."

The Medical Curriculum at Salerno

The study of medicine at Salerno was no haphazard affair. Early in the twelfth century medical practice had been brought under official jurisdiction by King Roger II of Sicily, and later, the Emperor Frederick II, most able and enlightened of the

[1] A. Castiglioni, " The School of Salerno (Work of Roger)," *Bull. Hist. Med.*, 1938, vol. vi. p. 883
[2] C. Daremberg, *La Médecine, Histoire et Doctrines*, 1865, p. 154
[3] *Ibid.*, p. 148

House of Hohenstaufen, decreed in 1221 that no one should practise medicine until he had been publicly examined and approved by the masters of Salerno, " in order that the king's subjects should not incur danger through the inexperience of their physicians." Furthermore, no one could proceed to the study of medicine until he had attained the age of twenty-one years, had proved his legitimacy, and had studied logic for three years. The medical course lasted for five years, with an additional year of practice under the supervision of an older practitioner. The candidate, having passed the examinations, took the oath to uphold the school, to attend the poor gratis, to administer no noxious drug, to teach nothing false, and not to keep an apothecary's shop. He then received a ring, a laurel wreath, a book, and the kiss of peace, after which he was entitled to call himself Magister or Doctor, and to practise medicine.[1] It was at Salerno that the medical man was first called " Doctor." The School of Salerno was also the first attempt to co-ordinate the teaching of medicine without any restriction as to religion or nationality, and also the first to grant degrees after a definite course of study and examinations.

Famous Graduates

The fame of the Salerno school spread far, and among those who came to study was GILLES DE CORBEIL (Ægidius Corboliensis) (c. 1200),[2] a celebrated French physician who subsequently taught in the University of Paris, and who wrote, after the fashion of the time, two long poems in hexameter, De Pulsibus and De Urinis, which became widely known. Another famous pupil of Salerno was MICHAEL SCOT (A.D. 1175),[3] who had a great reputation as a practitioner, not only of medicine, but also of the magical art of astrology. One of Michael Scot's prescriptions casts an interesting light upon the early history of anaesthesia. " Take of opium, mandragora, and henbane equal parts, pound and mix them with water. When you want to saw or cut a man, dip a rag in this and put it to his nostrils. He will soon sleep

---

[1] L. Thorndike, *History of Magic and Experimental Science*, New York, 1934-41, vol. ii.
[2] S. D'Irsay, " The Life and Works of Gilles de Corbeil," *Ann. Med. Hist.*, 1925, vol. vii. p. 362
[3] J. W. Brown, *The Life and Legend of Michael Scot*, Edinburgh, 1897. (Michael Scot's best-known work, *De Phisionomie*, had a wide and long reputation.)

so deep that you may do what you wish." It is not easy to understand how such non-volatile substances were absorbed, but that they were used as anaesthetics appears certain. The *spongia somnifera* (or *soporifera*) are mentioned by Nicolas of Salerno in his *Antidotarium*, a large collection of formulæ, probably compiled in the eleventh century, and printed in Venice in 1471.[1] This work is sometimes called the *Antidotarium parvum*, to distinguish it from a later and more elaborate work, the *Antidotarium magnum*, which was compiled by another Nicolas, a Byzantine physician named Nicolas Myrepsos (Nicolas the ointment-maker), who lived in the second half of the thirteenth century.[2] A special study of *spongia somnifera* and of mediæval methods of surgical anaesthesia was made by Husemann some years ago.[3]

Regimen Sanitatis Salernitanum

No reference to Salerno is complete without some account of the poem which was the most famous literary product of the school, and which, as Castiglioni remarks,[4] " constituted the backbone of all practical medical literature up to the time of the Renaissance." The *Regimen Sanitatis Salernitanum*[5] is a work of composite authorship and uncertain date, probably of the thirteenth century, according to Sudhoff.[6] It exists in innumerable manuscripts, and was printed in almost three hundred different editions up to the year 1846. The most authentic manuscript, given in a commentary by ARNOLD OF VILLANOVA (1235–1312), contains 352 verses, but in subsequent editions this number has been multiplied at least ten times. It has been translated into many languages, and some of the phrases have become proverbs in common use. Indeed, it remains the most popular medical work ever written. The *Regimen* is a sort of handbook of domestic

[1] G. Sarton, *Introduction to the History of Science*, Washington, 1931, vol. ii. Pt. 1, pp. 135, 239
[2] G. Sarton, *loc. cit*, vol. ii. Pt. 2, p. 1094
[3] T. Husemann, " Die Schlafschwämme und andere Methoden der allgemeinen und örtlichen Anästhesie im Mittelalter," *Deutsch. Zeit. f. Chir.*, Leipzig, 1896, vol. xlii. pp. 517–596, and " Weitere Beiträge zur chirurgischen Anästhesie im Mittelalter," *Deutsch. Zeit. f. Chir.*, Leipzig, 1900, vol. liv. pp. 503–550
[4] A. Castiglioni, *A History of Medicine*, trans. E. Krumbhaar, Chicago, 1942, p. 309
[5] F. R. Packard, *The School of Salerno*, with Sir John Harington's trans. of *Regimen Sanitatis Salernitanum* (1607), Oxford, 1922
[6] K. Sudhoff, " Salerno," in *Essays in the History of Medicine*, trans. F. H. Garrison, New York, 1926

medicine, and is said to have been written for Robert, Duke of Normandy, son of William the Conqueror, who in returning from a crusade stayed at Salerno (*c.* 1100) for the treatment of his wound.[1] It was at Salerno that he met Sybilla, grand-niece of Robert Guiscard, who is said to have saved his life by sucking the wound while he slept, and who afterwards became his wife. Robert's absence at the crusades lost for him the throne of England and led him, through the treachery of his brother, to a long term of imprisonment which lasted until his death. Others allege that the poem was dedicated to the king of France.

One of the earliest English editions is the translation made for Queen Elizabeth by Sir John Harington and eventually published in 1607. More recent versions are by Sir Alexander Croke, 1830, and by Professor John Ordronaux, 1870.[2]

The nature of the " health hints " given in the *Regimen* may be appreciated from the following extracts from Sir A. Croke's version, but it is needless to add that the entire poem is worthy of study, and may be read with profit by every medical man. The dedication runs thus :

> The Salerne School doth by these lines impart
> All health to England's king, and doth advise
> From care his head to keep, from wrath his heart.
> Drink not much wine, sup light and soon arise.

Diet occupies a central place in the poem, for

> A King that cannot rule him in his diet,
> Will hardly rule his Realm in peace and quiet.

On milk, duck, and cheese, to select three foods at random, the following opinions are expressed :

> Cow's milk and Sheep's do well, but yet an Ass's
> Is best of all, and all the other passes.
>
>   *   *   *
>
> Good sport it is to see a Mallard killed,
> But with their flesh your flesh should not be fill'd.
>
>   *   *   *
>
> For healthy men may cheese be wholesome food
> But for the weak and sickly 'tis not good.

---

[1] P. Capparoni, *Magistri Salernitani Nondum Cogniti.* A contribution to the history of the Medical School of Salerno, 1923, p. 13
[2] Sir A. Croke, trans. of *Regimen Sanitatis Salernitanum*, 1830 ; J. Ordronaux, *The Code of Health of the School of Salernum*, Philadelphia, 1870

There is some quaint advice on the care of the eyes :

> Three things preserve the sight, glass, grass, and fountains.
> At even springs, at morning visit mountains.

A number of herbal remedies are mentioned, thus :

> Some affirm that they have found by trial
> The pain of gout is cured by Penny-royal.

> White pepper helps the cough, as flegme it riddeth,
> And Ague's fit to come it oft forbiddeth.

The doctrine of Humours is replaced by that of Elements, or as they are still called, Temperaments :

> Four Humours reign within our body wholly,
> And these compared to four Elements,
> The Sanguin, Choller, Flegme and Melancholy.

The technique of venesection is fully described, the time for the operation depending upon the moon :

> Three special months, September, April, May
> There are in which 'tis good to ope a vein.
> In these three months the moon bears greatest sway.

The poem appropriately concludes as follows :

> And here I cease to write, but will not cease
> To wish you live in health, and die in peace :
> And ye our Physic rules that friendly read,
> God grant that Physic you may never need.

BOOKS FOR FURTHER READING

ARNOLD, Sir T. and GUILLAUME, A., Ed. of *The Legacy of Islam.* (" Medicine,' M. Meyerhof), 1931

BROWN, J. W. *The Life and Legend of Michael Scot*, Edinburgh, 1897

BROWNE, E. R. G. *Arabian Medicine*, (Fitzpatrick Lectures,) 1921

CAMPBELL, D. *Arabian Medicine*, 2 vols., 1926

CAPPARONI, P. *Magistri Salernitani Nondum Cogniti*, English trans., 1923

COCKAYNE, T. O. *Leechdoms, Wortcunning, and Starcraft of Early England*, 3 vols., 1864–66

DE RENZI, S. *Storia Documentata della Scuola Medica di Salerno*, 5 vols., 2nd. ed. 1875

GREENHILL, W. A. *A Treatise on the Smallpox and Measles*, by Rhazes. Trans. Sydenham Society, 1848

ORDRONAUX, J. *The Code of Health of the School of Salernum*, Philadelphia, 1870

PACKARD, F. R. *The School of Salerno.* With Sir John Harington's trans. of *Regimen Sanitatis Salernitanum* (1607), Oxford, 1922

SINGER, C. *From Magic to Science* (chap. vi " Hildegard of Bingen "), 1928

SUDHOFF, K. *Essays in the History of Medicine* (" Salerno "). Trans. F. H. Garrison, 1926

Chapter VII

MEDIÆVAL MEDICINE

To write of the mediæval period imposes a severe test upon the critical faculties of the historian. It is usually regarded as an age of decadence and of stagnation, and the very name " mediæval " implies the negation of progress, and suggests backwardness, superstition, and sloth.[1]

It is true that at this stage of history medicine had sunk to a very low level indeed. The prevailing conception of disease was archaic ; diagnosis and prognosis were based on the state of the stars and on inspection of the urine ; treatment consisted of blood-letting and the use of herbs whose nature was ill understood ; anatomy was taught from ancient texts or at best from animal dissection ; alchemy was directed towards the discovery of an elixir of life ; and surgery was of the meddlesome type.[2] Under such circumstances, it does not surprise us to learn that in 1250 when a nobleman of Bologna had sustained an injury no one could be found to undertake the case for fear of fatal consequences. Eventually Hugh of Lucca treated him, but only after thirty of the friends and relations had taken an oath that in event of the patient's death no harm would befall the surgeon. Fortunately he recovered, and all ended happily.

Nevertheless, mediæval medicine does not present a picture of unrelieved gloom. Here and there a shaft of light appears to herald the coming brightness of the revival of learning. Schools of medicine were opening and methods of teaching improved. Anatomy, though still full of Galenic misconceptions, was recognized as the foundation of surgery, and some bold spirits even dared to hint that Galen might not be entirely reliable. In surgery some new methods were devised, and it was even suggested that suppuration was not an essential stage in the healing of wounds. Preventive measures, if somewhat crude, were introduced to prevent the spread of plague. Thus, the mediæval period made its small, yet important, contribution to medical science.

[1] H. O. Taylor, *The Medieval Mind*, 2nd. ed., 2 vols., 1914
[2] C. Singer, *From Magic to Science* (The Dark Ages and the Dawn of Science), 1928 ; H. E. Sigerist, " The Medieval Literature of the Early Middle Ages," *Bull. Hist. Med.*, 1934, ii. p. 26

Although the available information is scanty, the lives and works of the physicians and surgeons of the Middle Ages fill an important page in medical history.

The Schools of Montpellier and Bologna

The medical school of Salerno gave place to that of Montpellier.[1] As Rashdall states, it " may have been an offshoot of Salerno." [2] Somewhat later, Bologna, where there was a famous school of law, became well known also as a school of anatomy and surgery.

Montpellier, like Salerno, was a health resort. It was a district famous for its intellectual interests, and including a large Greek element. Furthermore, it was easily accessible from Spain and Italy, so that the appearance of a medical school in such a centre is not surprising. The date of the foundation of the school of Montpellier is uncertain ; probably it was during the twelfth century. It was renowned during the thirteenth and fourteenth centuries, when it was frequented by a number of famous men, to some of whom we shall presently refer. With the rise of the medical schools of Padua and of Paris and the departure of the Popes from Avignon, Montpellier was less frequented. Yet it did not share the fate of Salerno ; as a centre of medical learning it remains to this day, and in 1890 the sexcentenary of the university was celebrated. During the early days of the school of Montpellier the most distinguished teacher was ARNOLD OF VILLANOVA, whose name has already been mentioned as the writer of a commentary on the *Regimen* of Salerno. Arnold was born in Spain, but spent part of his life at Montpellier.[3] A graduate in theology and law as well as in medicine, he was highly esteemed at court, and among his patients were included two kings and three popes. When his unorthodox views brought him into conflict with the Church he sought the protection of Pope Boniface VIII, who advised him to leave theology alone and to stick to medicine. Fortunately, it was not until after his death that Arnold was regarded as a heretic in league

[1] S. Cooper, " The Medical School of Montpellier in the Fourteenth Century," *Ann. Med. Hist.*, 1930, vol. ii. p. 164
[2] H. Rashdall, *Universities of Europe in the Middle Ages*, 1936, vol. ii. p. 119
[3] L. Thorndike, *A History of Magic and Experimental Science*, 6 vols., New York, 1923–41, vol. ii. p. 841 ; vol. iii. p. 52

PLATE XIX   SURGICAL PRACTICE AT SALERNO

Illustration from a thirteenth-century MS. of Roger's *Cirurgia* in the British Museum, showing the treatment of a dislocated shoulder. Above are three figures from Our Lord's Passion, a reminder of the homage due to religion by surgery (p. 106)

PLATE XX   A MEDIÆVAL SPA: PLOMBIÈRES

Woodcut from *De Balneis*, Venice, 1553, showing a public bath in a health resort.
Some of the patients, including a man in the centre of the bath, are using crutches.
Another is being assisted down the steps into the water, while a woman bather,
immersed waist-deep, is drinking from a flask.   Signs on the surrounding
buildings may indicate that they are inns

with the devil, and some of his works were publicly burned.[1] Of the medical portion of his writings the best known is the *Breviarium Practicæ*, which was printed in a number of editions during the sixteenth century. That Arnold practised surgery as well as medicine is obvious from the following selections from his aphorisms : " To postpone opening an abscess is dangerous." " The bite of a mad dog should be enlarged and encouraged to bleed." He also gave advice not usually found in modern textbooks. For example : " To drive away mice, fumigate with pomegranate, hellebore, sulphur, and shells of shrimps. The mice will flee and never come back." His book on poisons begins : " In this book I propose, with God's help, to consider diseases of women, since women are poisonous creatures. I shall then treat of the bites of venomous beasts." As a physician and scientist, he was one of those who spent much time in the search for the Elixir of Life, and he did, in fact, apply to the brandy, which he made and prescribed, the name " aqua vitæ." In the course of this investigation he found that the virtues of herbs could be extracted by alcohol, and he was thus the inventor of the modern " tincture." Arnold must be credited with the desire to escape from dogma and empiricism, and with a reliance on his own observations. His was a spirit of investigation unusual at that time, he did not hesitate to criticize Galen and the Arabists.

Englishmen at Montpellier

Montpellier attracted students from many countries, including a number of enterprising Englishmen. There was GILBERTUS ANGLICUS (*d.* 1250), who wrote a compendium of medicine which contained nothing new, though the recipe for Gilbert's ointment for gout is worth quoting as an example of mediæval pharmacy. " Skin a fat puppy, and stuff him with cucumber, rue, pellitory, juniper, and fat of goose, fox, and bear, equal parts. Then boil him and add wax to the grease that floats on the top, to make an ointment."

A distinguished English student at Montpellier was JOHN OF GADDESDEN (1280–1361),[2] who studied and later taught at

---

[1] J. J. Walsh, *Medieval Medicine*, 1920, p. 66 ; M. Neuburger, *History of Medicine*, trans. E. Playfair, 1910–25, vol. ii. p. 75
[2] W. G. Lennox, " John of Gaddesden on Epilepsy," *Ann. Med. Hist.*, 1938, 3rd series, vol. i. p. 283

Merton College, Oxford, and whose book bears the curious title, *Rosa Anglica*. He treated his father for salivary calculus, and this is how he describes the case : " I saw a stone in my father's mouth under the tongue, the length of half a little finger, which I now carry about with me and exhibit in the schools. I extracted it with a fine knife, though at first I thought it was an inflammation. It was generated from milk foods, of which my father was very fond, and which had congealed by the heat of his choleric temperament." [1] John acquired a fashionable practice, and treated the son of Edward II for smallpox by wrapping him in a red cloth, and by having all the bed hangings and window curtains of red colour. Thus he cured him, without any vestiges of scarring. Freind [2] writes of John of Gaddesden : " Nothing came amiss to him. He could dissolve the Stone, draw out the humour of Gout with an ointment, conquer Epileptic fits with a necklace, and cure a Palsy with Aqua Vitae." Nevertheless, the *Rosa Anglica* [3] contains little that is new, and Guy de Chauliac, to whom we shall shortly refer, said that there had been sent to him " a foolish English rose which contained no sweetness but only a few old fables."

It is believed that Chaucer, a younger contemporary of John of Gaddesden, depicted him as the " Doctor of Physick " in *The Canterbury Tales*. The picture shows his reliance on astrology and on the pathology of " humours."

> Well coude he gesse the ascending of the star
> Wherein his patientes fortunes settled were.
> He knew the course of every maladye,
> Were it of cold or hete or moyst or drye,
> And where they engendered, and of what humour,
> He was a very parfit practisour.

BERNARD DE GORDON (*c.* 1285), another student or teacher of Montpellier, contributed to the garden of medicine by writing the *Lilium Medicinae*, which still exists in rare manuscript form. It contains the first description of a truss and the first mention of spectacles. Some historians have presumed, on account of his name, that Bernard was a Scot, but it is now generally believed that he was a native of the French town of Gourdon. [4]

[1] E. T. Withington, *Medical History from the Earliest Times*, 1894, p. 399
[2] J. Freind, *History of Physick*, 1725. (Full account of John Gaddesden, vol. ii. p. 287)
[3] A. C. Wootton, *Chronicles of Pharmacy*, 2 vols., 1910, vol. i. p. 134
[4] L. Thorndike, *A History of Magic and Experimental Science*, 6 vols., New York, 1923-1941, vol. ii., p. 488

A Medical Pope

Our list of distinguished Montpellier students may appropriately close with a brief mention of a physician who became Pope. Petrus Hispanus (c. 1277) was born at Lisbon, and after a brilliant career as a student of theology and medicine, was appointed physician to Pope Gregory X. A little later, owing to a series of unexpected events, he was elected to the papal chair as John XXI.[1] His best known work, *Thesaurus pauperum*, "Treasury of the Poor," was very popular. He met a violent death when the ceiling of his palace fell on him " as he was admiring himself," so the story goes. Yet he was the only Pope whom Dante met in Paradise.

Medicine and Surgery at Bologna [2]

One of the earliest teachers of medicine at Bologna was Taddeo Alderotti (1223–1303), sometimes called Thaddeus Florentinus, after his birthplace. Taddeo attracted many students, and Dante is said to have attended his lectures.[3] Although he wrote many commentaries, his chief claim to fame lies in his introduction of a new form of medical literature, called " consilia." These were discussions of clinical cases, giving a description of the symptoms and full details of treatment. Sometimes these notes were sent to unseen patients, or supplied to " practitioners " by " consultants." " Consilia " are essentially mediæval in character, and reflect the scholastic type of medical philosophy.[4]

There were also at Bologna two surgeons, father and son, who deservedly acquired high reputations. Of the father, Hugh of Lucca (Ugo Borgognoni), who died in 1252, little is known save that he was the leading surgeon of his day.[5] All his works have been lost. His son Theodoric (1205–98), combining theology with medicine in the fashion of the day, became Bishop of Cervia, and wrote a " Chyrurgia," which reveals him as one of the most original surgeons of all time. He

[1] D. Riesman, " A Physician in the Papal Chair," *Ann. Med. Hist.*, 1923, vol. v. p. 4
[2] G. Franchini, " The Origin of the University of Bologna, "*Ann. Med. Hist.*, 1932, vol. iv. p. 189
[3] H. Rashdall, *Universities of Europe in the Middle Ages*, 1936, vol. i. p. 285
[4] D. Riesman, *The Story of Medicine in the Middle Ages*, New York, 1935, p. 347
[5] L. Karl, " Théodoric, de l'Ordre des Prêcheurs, et sa Chirurgie," *Bull. d'Hist. Méd.*, 1929, vol. xxiii. p. 140

was one of the first to state that the formation of pus in wounds was unnecessary and undesirable, and he favoured simple dressings dipped in wine. He also used an anaesthetic sponge, impregnated with mandragora and opium, and soaked in hot water before being inhaled by the patient.

It may be convenient at this point to interpolate a note regarding mandragora, or mandrake, one of the most ancient of herbal remedies, which has already been mentioned as an ingredient of the so-called anaesthetic sponge (page 108). This plant, still common in the Mediterranean area, has a long tap-root, often bifid, and bearing some resemblance to the human figure (Plate XXI). Indeed, two varieties, male and female, were distinguished by the ancients, and are depicted in many herbals.[1]

As for its use in medicine, Dioscorides (first century A.D.) writes in his herbal that " the wine of the bark of the root " is to be given " to such as shall be cut or cauterised," and he notes that " they do not apprehend the pain because they are overborne with dead sleep." This is probably the earliest reference to surgical anaesthesia.[2] Mandrake was also regarded as a cure for sterility (Gen. xxx. 14).

Shakespeare refers repeatedly to mandragora and its effects :

Not poppy, nor mandragora,
Nor all the drowsy syrups of the world,
Shall ever medicine thee to that sweet sleep
Which thou ow'dst yesterday.

Othello, III. iii. 331

Give me to drink mandragora . . .
That I might sleep out this great gap of time
My Antony is away.

Antony and Cleopatra, I. v. 4

Or have we eaten on the insane root
That takes the reason prisoner ?

Macbeth, I. iii. 85

And shrieks like mandrakes' torn out of the earth,
That living mortals hearing them, run mad.

Romeo and Juliet, IV. iii. 47

The last-mentioned quotation refers to the widely shared belief that the gathering of the mandrake was not without danger, as the plant when uprooted uttered a shriek, which caused the death or insanity of those who heard it. The root was therefore

[1] *The Greek Herbal of Dioscorides*, ed. R. T. Gunther, Oxford, 1934, Book IV, p. 76
[2] C. J. S. Thompson, *The Mystic Mandrake* (1934)

PLATE XXI   THE LEGEND OF MANDRAGORA

Mandragora, or Mandrake, as represented in early herbals, showing the fancied resemblance of the plant to the human figure (pages 116–17)

(*l.*) Mandragora, with the dog used in gathering the root (from an early edition of the *Herbal* of Apuleius).   (*r.*) A more fanciful version of the mandragora legend, by an Anglo-Saxon artist of the thirteenth century.   (MS. in British Museum)

PLATE XXII   ANATOMY IN MEDIÆVAL TIMES

A teacher of anatomy in the fourteenth century demonstrating the skeleton to
his pupil. The bones are depicted according to pre-Vesalian ideas. Miniature
from a manuscript of Guy de Chauliac's *Chirurgia*, copied by Jean Tourtier
for the Duke of Bedford (page 123)

merely loosened by the digger, and then attached to a dog, which completed the process of uprooting, and then fell down dead. Explicit directions to be followed by the mandrake-gatherer are given in the *Herbarium* of Apuleius (fifth century A.D.) who writes, " When thou seest its hands and its feet, then tie thou it up. Take the other end, and tie it to a dog's neck, so that the hound be hungry ; next cast meat before him, so that he may not reach it, except he jerk up the wort with him." [1] Mediæval illustrations often represent the dog tethered to the mandrake root (Plate XXI).

Thus do we find in Theodoric of Bologna a pioneer, not only of antisepsis, but also of anaesthesia, the two great adjuncts to surgery which did not meet with general acceptance until six centuries later.

Another great teacher at Bologna was WILLIAM OF SALICET (Guglielmo Saliceti, 1210-77). William aimed at the reunion of medicine and surgery, and he contributed to both. He noted the association of dropsy with nephritis, and treated it by copious draughts of oxymel and barley water. Unlike the Arabs, he preferred the knife to the cautery. He distinguished between venous and arterial haemorrhage, and he emphasized the importance of a knowledge of anatomy, thus anticipating a much-needed reform. [2] In his sound words to physicians, he advised them to be " reflective, quiet, and with downcast countenance, giving an impression of wisdom," and he said that there should be little conversation with the patients' friends and relatives.

William of Salicet had two distinguished pupils, Henry de Mondeville and Lanfranc of Milan.

HENRI DE MONDEVILLE (1260-1320) was an advanced surgeon who, like his master, indicated the need for anatomical knowledge. [3] He advised the dry treatment of wounds, but he hesitated to adopt new operations because, to quote his own words, " it is dangerous for a surgeon, who is not of repute, to operate in any way different to that method in common use."

By this time the Church was losing its hold upon medicine. Some of the monks, finding that supernatural cures were sometimes unavailing, practised medicine for the sake of gain, and

[1] J. F. Payne, *English Medicine in Anglo-Saxon Times* (Fitzpatrick Lectures), 1904, p. 72
[2] W. T. Dempster, " European Anatomy before Vesalius," *Ann. Med. Hist.*, 1934, vol. vi. pp. 307, 448
[3] C. Singer, *The Evolution of Anatomy*, 1925

it was against such that Henri de Mondeville took his stand. Nevertheless, he himself did not fulfil the highest ethical rules when he suggested that in order to sustain the spirits of a patient, "false letters may be written telling of the death of his enemies, or if he is a canon of the Church, he should be told that the bishop is dead and that he is elected." He adds a more reputable means of cheer, namely, to "solace him by playing on a ten-stringed psaltery." Like the monks against whom he railed, he expected to be well paid for his services. He tells us that "when treating an accident, the friends should be excluded as they may faint and cause a disturbance ; nevertheless sometimes a higher fee may be obtained from persons fainting and breaking their heads than from the principal patient."[1] Perhaps it is best not to take Henri de Mondeville too seriously ; he may have been merely indulging his sense of humour. He certainly was doing so when he suggested that if a physician were attending a patient without result, he should say, " My business prevents me from attending you any longer, so I advise you to call in a surgeon." Obviously the rivalry between physicians and surgeons was keen, even in the Middle Ages. Although some amusing sayings of Henri de Mondeville have been quoted, he must be regarded as a sound surgeon and anatomist. His progressive outlook is indicated by his caustic remark that " God did not exhaust all his creative power in making Galen." One final quotation reveals Henri, or Henricus as he is often called in literature, as the far-seeing and broad-minded scholar. Speaking of the need for a close relationship between medicine and surgery, he states that "no surgeon can be expert who does not know medicine, just as no one can be a good physician if he is ignorant of surgery." His surgical works, translated into French by Nicaise, were published in an elegant edition in 1893.[2]

Paris and Padua

Montpellier did not long remain the most important medical school of Europe. Other centres of learning were coming into the picture. Paris and Padua [3] were about to take leading places

---

[1] E. T. Withington, *Medical History from the Earliest Times*, 1894, p. 214
[2] E. Nicaise, *La Chirurgie de Maître Henri de Mondeville*, Paris, 1893
[3] A. Castiglioni, " The Medical School at Padua," *Ann. Med. Hist.*, 1935, vol. vii. p. 214

in the history of medicine. It was Lanfranc, already mentioned as a pupil of Salicet, who became the leader of French surgery in those early days.[1]

GUIDO LANFRANCHI (d. 1315) spent the early part of his life at Milan, but becoming involved in the Guelph and Ghibelline controversy, he was obliged to flee from Italy to France.[2] Already a distinguished surgeon, he was well received in Paris, and in 1295 he became a member of the surgical school of St. Côme (St. Cosmas). Unlike his teacher, Salicet of Bologna, Lanfranc favoured the cautery, and he was a cautious surgeon who did not operate for stone or for hernia. Though he was acquainted with the ligature, he regarded pressure as the best means of arresting haemorrhage, and it is recorded of him that when a child fell with a knife in his hand and wounded a vein in the neck, Lanfranc held his finger to the spot for an hour, while an assistant fetched a styptic of frankincense, aloes, white of egg, and hare's fur. He had a high ideal of his calling, and he deplored the fact that venesection and minor surgery were still in the hands of barbers. Lanfranc was a popular teacher, who added largely to the reputation of Paris as a medical school. He held that a surgeon ought to be well versed in philosophy and logic, so that he may be able to state his views clearly and give good reasons for his beliefs. In his Chirurgia Magna, written in 1296 and printed in French in 1490, he treats of many things, including the importance of careful suture of the ends of divided nerves, a procedure which had been neglected by other surgeons,[3] and was not fully understood until the eighteenth century.

Meantime, at the University of Padua—a university which was destined to play so large a part in the renaissance of medical learning—there was a teacher whose advanced ideas helped to prepare the ground for that great movement. PETER OF ABANO (1250–1315)[4] had not only travelled far in search of knowledge before settling in Padua, but had also acquired a familiarity with Greek, an unusual accomplishment at that time. He was thus in a position to read the classic writings in the original tongue,

[1] J. J. Walsh, Medieval Medicine, 1920, p. 110
[2] G. Sarton, Introduction to the History of Science, 3 vols., Washington, 1931, vol. ii. Part 2, p. 1079
[3] Lanfrank's Science of Cirurgie, 1396, Early English Text Soc., No. 102, 1894 ; G. G. Coulton, Life in the Middle Ages, 4 vols., 1928–29, vol. iii. p. 69
[4] L. Thorndike, A History of Magic and Experimental Science, 6 vols., New York, 1923–41, vol. ii. p. 874

unaltered by the process of translation, and to interpret them to his students. His services were greatly in demand, and he had an enormous practice. Nevertheless, he devoted much time to the study of philosophy. His views were those of Aristotle and Averroes, and he sought to reconcile philosophy and medicine, as many had attempted before him, and as many have tried to do since. It is for this reason that his principal book, which deals with medicine and much else besides, is known as the " Conciliator." His discussions of fantastic problems and curious questions resemble those of Sir Thomas Browne. The problem of pain, how many meals a day should be eaten, and on which side should one sleep, are among the matters he debated.

It does not surprise us to learn that one of so inquiring a turn of mind should have found himself at variance with the Church, and when eventually he dared to suggest that certain miracles could be naturally explained, and that Lazarus might have been in a trance, his life was no longer safe. Indeed, it was only his death from illness that saved him from being burned alive, and his friends were obliged to hide his body. He was therefore burned in effigy, and his fortune was confiscated by the Church. Thus was the search for truth requited in the Middle Ages.[1]

Roger Bacon and Albertus Magnus

It is convenient at this point, in order to preserve the chronological sequence, to mention two great scholars, the one an English Franciscan, the other a German Dominican, each of whom exercised an influence upon the intellectual life of his time.

ROGER BACON (1214–94) was a scholar with ideas far ahead of his time ; so much so, indeed, that he seems a little out of place as a mediæval figure. The full significance of his work was not appreciated until many years after his death.[2] It is thus difficult to estimate his influence upon current thought. According to Neuburger, he is " one whose name can never be erased from the annals of the intellectual development of mankind, so long as the light of scientific freedom shall shine." Like so many other pioneers, he incurred the displeasure of the Church,

[1] D. Riesman, *The Story of Medicine in the Middle Ages*, New York, 1935, p. 75
[2] L. Thorndike, *loc. cit.*, vol. ii. p. 616. (Full discussion of work of Roger Bacon)

and was imprisoned for fourteen years towards the end of his career, which naturally limited his work. Many of his writings still remain unpublished, and the first edition of his *Opus Majus* was not printed until 1733. A student of Oxford, he taught in Paris for a time, earning there the title of " Doctor Mirabilis." Being a man of means, he was able to spend large sums of money on experiments, and he has been credited, rightly or wrongly, with the invention of the telescope, the microscope, the diving bell, spectacles, and gunpowder, and with the foretelling of aviation and mechanical transport.[1] Although he was not a physician, but rather a physicist, mathematician, and philosopher, he must have influenced medicine by his continual insistence on the value of experiment as opposed to argument. Medicine had strayed back into the paths of Aristotelian philosophy. Scholasticism, with its futile discussions that had no bearing on life and reality, was the philosophy of that day, and the salutary effect of a new outlook was sorely needed. This could only be supplied by one such as Roger Bacon, an active observer and tireless experimenter, who appears to have anticipated by many centuries the famous dictum of John Hunter, " Why think ? Why not try ? "

Associated with Roger Bacon in Paris was Albert von Bollstadt of Swabia, ALBERTUS MAGNUS (1192–1280), one of the most learned men of the Middle Ages, a Dominican monk who taught at Paris and at Cologne.[2] Unlike Bacon, he was a close follower and interpreter of Aristotle. A man of encyclopaedic knowledge, his writings include not only philosophy and theology but all the natural sciences, and though he dealt in magic and astrology [3] he was also an authority on the healing virtues of plants. His book on this subject, *De Vegetabilibus*, written about 1250, remained an authority for many years, containing as it did many original botanical observations. Singer, however, regards this work as " primarily a compilation," based on the work on plants by Nicolas of Damascus (first century B.C.).[4]

[1] R. Steele, " Roger Bacon and the State of Science in the Thirteenth Century," in Singer's *Studies in History and Method of Science*, 1921, vol. ii. p. 121
[2] C. Daremberg, " Albert le Grand et l'Histoire des Sciences au Moyen Âge," in *La Médecine : Histoire et Doctrine*, Paris, 1865
[3] H. Redgrove, *Alchemy, Ancient and Modern*, 1922, p. 44
[4] C. Singer, " Greek Biology," in *Studies in the History and Method of Science*, 1921, vol. ii. p. 73

The Restoration of Anatomy

Although the value of anatomy as the foundation of medicine gained recognition in the later Middle Ages, the teaching of the subject remained theoretical owing to the prevalent antipathy to dissection of the human body. In 1300 Pope Boniface VIII had issued a Bull forbidding the boiling and dismemberment of the bodies of dead Crusaders so that their bones might be sent back to their native lands. Post-mortem examination, for judicial reasons, was occasionally practised, and it is not easy to differentiate between such autopsies and public dissections. But it gradually became permissible to dissect in public the body of an executed criminal. This procedure, the *anatomia publica*, took place once a year, or even less frequently. At the University of Tübingen, for example, it was decreed that " every three years the body of a criminal shall be dissected. All who take part shall attend a mass for the subject's soul and shall afterwards attend the remains to the grave." The dissection was open to scholars and professional men, as well as to physicians and students. It consisted in a perfunctory examination of the contents of the abdomen and thorax, and lasted for only a few days. The actual work was performed by a menial, while the professor, seated on an elevated platform, pointed out from afar the various structures which had been exposed. The cranium was seldom opened, and there was no systematic dissection of the muscles, nerves, and vessels of the limbs.

The first attempt to remedy this condition of affairs and to introduce the systematic teaching of anatomy, " part " by " part," was made by Mondino de Luzzi, or MUNDINUS (*c.* 1275–1326), who was born and who taught at Bologna.[1] Interested in public affairs, he also took part in the government of the city. Under his guidance anatomy became recognized as the essential basis of the medical curriculum. His *Anothomia*, written in 1316, is the first practical manual of anatomy, and he is therefore entitled to be called the " restorer " of anatomy.[2] It is true that he perpetuated the errors of Galen, describing in his book the natural members or parts associated with digestion, the spiritual members or thoracic contents, and the animal members or parts within the head. The stomach is described as spheroid, the liver as

[1] C. Singer, *The Evolution of Anatomy*, 1925, p. 74
[2] C. Singer, trans. of *Anothomia of Mundinus* (*Mondino de Luzzi*, 1275–1326), 1925

possessing five lobes, the heart as having three ventricles, and the brain as under the control of a red worm (known to us now as the choroid plexus). To crown all, he depicted a seven-chambered uterus. He gives a most superficial account of the extremities ; and as for the bones, he remarks that these might be better studied if cleaned by boiling, but " to do so would be sinful." Many of his anatomical terms are Arabic. The abdominal wall is called *Mirach*, the peritoneum is *Siphac*, the omentum *Zirbus*. Arabic nomenclature remained in use for many years, until replaced by words of Greek or Latin origin. Yet, in spite of all its imperfections, the " Anatomy " of Mundinus remained the standard textbook for two hundred years or more.[1] It was eventually published in Pavia in 1478, and there were forty subsequent editions. Mundinus did not revolutionize anatomy, but he took the first step in this direction, that of leaving the professorial chair, and of casting aside his dignity in order to become his own demonstrator. He was wont to carry out the work of dissection with his own hand, assisted by his brilliant young girl pupil, Alexandra Galiani. Perhaps the time was not yet ripe for that complete reorganization of anatomical knowledge which was to be carried to a logical conclusion by the scalpel of Andreas Vesalius.

Surgery also " Restored "

The most famous surgeon of later mediæval times was a pupil of Mundinus. GUY DE CHAULIAC (1300–67), the son of a French peasant, studied medicine and theology at Montpellier and Bologna, and eventually became " physician and chaplain " to the Pope at Avignon, Clement VI, and to two of his successors.[2] Most of his life was spent at Avignon, where he gave devoted service during the terrible plague epidemic of 1348. Petrarch's Laura died then of plague, and Guy was himself a victim, though he fortunately recovered.[3] It was in his later years that he wrote the book which perpetuated his fame.[4] Guy was well qualified to write the *Chirurgia Magna*. He was a scholar of wide learning,

[1] C. Singer, " A Study in Early Renaissance Anatomy " in *Studies in the History and Method of Science*, 2 vols., 1917, vol. i. p. 79
[2] J. J. Walsh, *Medieval Medicine*, 1920, p. 118
[3] R. Crawfurd, *Plague and Pestilence in Literature and Art* (Fitzpatrick Lectures), 1914, pp. 115 and 120
[4] R. H. Major, *Classic Descriptions of Disease*, 1932, p. 73 ; D. Riesman, *The Story of Medicine in the Middle Ages*, New York, 1935, p. 258

a good physician as well as a surgeon, and no mere copyist, for he based his writing upon observation and experience. It is not surprising that his treatise was the authoritative text, and that Malgaigne wrote of it that never since Hippocrates had there been a surgical work so clearly written in so few words. The original manuscript was in Latin ; it was first printed, in French, in 1478, and was largely used until the sixteenth century.

In this classic text Guy gives an account of medical history, the first work of this kind since the time of Celsus. He reproaches his immediate predecessors for " following each other like cranes," though he himself rather closely followed Albucasis. By his dogmatic and forceful method of expression he perpetuated certain surgical methods which ought rather to have been improved, as, for example, the use of salves and plasters and of the cautery, in place of simple dressings.[1] Nevertheless, in other respects he was a reformer, and he well deserved the title of " The Restorer of Surgery." His noble ideal of his calling is shown in his remark, " A good surgeon should be courteous, sober, pious, and merciful, not greedy of gain, and with a sense of his own dignity." [2] He was interested in the radical cure of hernia, though he did not advise operation in every case, preferring the use of a truss whenever possible. When he did operate, he placed the patient in what we now call the Trendelenburg position, and he criticized the prevailing method of sacrificing the testicle in order to obliterate the canal. He may have been the first to employ extension in the treatment of fractures. Speaking of fractures of the thigh, he writes : " After the application of splints, I attach to the foot a mass of lead as a weight, taking care to pass the cord which supports the weight over a small pulley in such a manner that it shall pull on the leg in a horizontal direction."

He also suspended a rope above the bed of the patient so as to facilitate changes of position, a contrivance for which many thousands of patients have since been grateful. Guy insisted on the importance of anatomy, " without which one can do nothing in surgery" (Plate xxii). He deplored the fact that operations for hernia, stone, and cataract were still in the hands of the itinerant quack. He also made a noteworthy contribution to dentistry, giving rules for the care and cleansing of the teeth so as to prevent

[1] E. Gurlt, *Geschichte der Chirurgie*, 3 vols., Berlin, 1898, Bd. ii. p. 77
[2] L. Thorndike, *A History of Magic and Experimental Science*, New York, 1923-41, vol. iii. p. 518

PLATE XXIII A MEDIÆVAL HOSPITAL

The Street of the Knights at Rhodes. Just opposite the pedestrian figure is the gateway of the hospital, which is also illustrated in Plate XXIV (page 128)

PLATE XXIV   THE KNIGHTS OF ST. JOHN AT RHODES

Gateway of the hospital
(see Plate xxiii)

Courtyard of the hospital
(page 128)

Entrance to the harbour of Rhodes, formerly guarded by the Colossus decay, and advising the replacement of lost teeth by other human teeth or by artificial teeth made of bone.

English and German Surgeons

No doubt there were many surgeons in England about this time, but the only one of whom we have any clear record was JOHN OF ARDERNE (1307–90), who wrote an illustrated treatise on fistula in ano (edited in 1910 by Sir D'Arcy Power), which reveals him as a scholar and an expert surgeon.[1] Educated at Montpellier, he remained for some time in France as an army surgeon, and he was present at the battle of Creçy. On his return he practised at Newark, then an important centre and a meeting-place of Parliament ; later, he removed to London.

John of Arderne was a specialist in what is now called proctology, and he showed his originality by inventing a new operation for fistula, which consisted in boldly incising the wall and checking the bleeding by sponge pressure. He was careful to recognize cancer of the rectum, of which he gave a clear description, noting that treatment can only be palliative, that no operation should be attempted, and that friends should be warned of the fatal issue. John appears to have been an itinerant surgeon, travelling long distances to operate, and charging proportionately large fees, which were paid either at the time or in the form of an annuity, continuing as long as the patient lived. Apparently his practice was large, and included many persons of rank and distinction. He set a high moral standard for surgeons, counselling them to cultivate modesty, charitableness, and studious habits, and to be scrupulously clean in dress and in person, always with clean hands and well-trimmed nails. It is merely a sign of the times in which he lived that John mentioned the use of charms, as for instance, " the words Melchior, Jasper, and Balthazar to be written in blood from the little finger of the patient," as a cure for epilepsy. The patient was to wear for a month a sheet of paper bearing these words, and was to say daily three Paternosters and three Ave Marias. Apart from the edition just mentioned of the treatises on fistula in ano, hæmorrhoids, and clysters, most of the work of John of Arderne is still in manuscript form.

[1] Sir D'Arcy Power, " *De Arte Phisicale et De Cirurgia* " *of Master John Arderne, 1412*, 1922 ; John Arderne, *Treatises of Fistula in Ano, Haemorrhoids, and Clysters*, ed. by Sir D'Arcy Power, Early English Text Society, 1910

Although their work was of later date, it is here convenient to mention three German surgeons whose works, written in their own tongue, indicate how war promotes the art of surgery. HEINRICH VON PFOLSPEUNDT [1] was a Bavarian surgeon who wrote, in 1460, a manuscript on bandaging and the treatment of wounds, the *Bündth-Ertznei*, which was discovered and printed as recently as 1868. His main concern was with arrow wounds, though his work is interesting in containing a first brief reference to the extraction of bullets, and to plastic surgery of the face.

About the same time there lived another surgeon, an Alsatian named HIERONYMUS BRUNSCHWIG. [2] He wrote the *Buch der Cirurgia Hantwirckung der Wundartzny* in 1497, noteworthy as one of the first illustrated medical works, and now a rich prize for collectors. According to Garrison, Brunschwig gave " the first detailed account of gunshot wounds in medical literature." [3]

A still more extensive account of military surgery was given a little later by HANS VON GERSDORFF, who had for forty years served in various campaigns. His *Feldtbuch der Wundtartzney* appeared in 1517. He extracted bullets with special instruments, and dressed the wound with warm, but not boiling, oil. Amputation stumps he enclosed in the bladder of an animal, after checking the haemorrhage by pressure and styptics. His book, like Brunschwig's, contains some unique illustrations (Plate XXVI).

The Black Death

No account of mediæval medicine would be complete without some reference to the terrible and widespread epidemic of plague, the Black Death, which devastated the civilized world in the fourteenth century, causing the death of about a quarter of the population. [4] Half the people of London died. At Avignon the Pope consecrated the Rhône so that bodies might be cast into it. Ships without crews drifted helplessly in the North Sea and the Mediterranean, and spread the infection when driven ashore. Commencing in Central Asia, the plague spread along the trade

---

[1] Often misprinted Pfolsprundt. E. Gurlt, *Geschichte der Chirurgie*, 1898, vol. ii. 187
[2] A. Brunschwig, "Hieronymus Brunschwig of Strassburg," *Ann. Med. Hist.*, 1939, vol. i. p. 640. (Brunschwig's *Cirurgia* was reprinted in facsimile in 1911.)
[3] F. H. Garrison, *An Introduction to the History of Medicine*, 3rd ed., 1924, p. 194
[4] S. D'Irsay, " The Black Death and the Medieval Universities," *Ann. Med. Hist.*, 1925, vol. vii. p. 220 ; M. H. Allyn, " The Black Death," *Ann. Med. Hist.*, 1925, vol. vii. p. 226

routes to Europe, where it raged with great violence in the year 1348.[1] It spread through Italy and France to England and Germany, eventually reaching Russia in 1352, by which time the epidemic abated, though it returned in less violent form a few years later, and then at intervals up to the end of the seventeenth century. Boccaccio has given in his *Decameron* (1353) a dramatic account of the plague in Italy.[2] " The condition of the people was pitiable to behold . . . they sickened by the thousands daily and died unattended and unsuccoured. Many died in the open street ; others dying in their houses made it known that they were dead by the stench of their rotting bodies. Consecrated ground did not suffice for the burial of the vast multitude of bodies, which were heaped by the hundred in vast trenches, like goods aboard ship, and covered with a little earth." The Black Death showed itself in both pneumonic and bubonic forms. Haemoptysis betokened inevitable death, as did the black patches on the skin which followed the appearance of the swellings in groin or armpit. " How many valiant men, how many fair ladies," proceeds Boccaccio, " breakfasted with their kinsfolk and that same night supped with their ancestors in the other world." Treatment was unavailing and measures for prevention were adopted too late. Of the latter the most important was quarantine. Ships arriving from the Levant and Egypt were isolated at special ports, and travellers were detained at port for thirty, and later for forty, days ; hence the name *quaranta giorni*, or quarantine. This law was first enforced at Ragusa on the Adriatic in 1377.[3]

It is easy to understand how Europe was thrown into panic and demoralization by such a dreadful visitation. Jews were accused of poisoning the wells, and many of them were burned alive. Fields were left untilled, and flocks and herds wandered at large. Religious fanatics went about scourging themselves for their sins, which had brought such punishment upon mankind. Treatment was of little avail, although the " plague tracts," written for popular enlightenment, advised blood-letting and the drinking of vinegar.[4] It is interesting to note that a tract of this

[1] S. D'Irsay, " Defense Reactions against the Black Death, 1348–49," *Ann. Med. Hist.*, 1927, vol. ix. p. 169
[2] R. Crawfurd, *Plague and Pestilence in Literature and Art*, 1914, p. 115
[3] K. Sudhoff, " Epidemiological Rules from the Past " in *Essays in the History of Medicine*, trans. F. H. Garrison, New York, 1926, p. 152
[4] D. W. Singer, " Some Plague Tractates (Fourteenth and Fifteenth Centuries)," *Proc. Roy. Soc. Med.*, 1916, vol. ix. p. 159

nature may have been the first medical book to be printed in England (in 1485).[1] Preventive measures consisted in fumigating the house by burning juniper and other aromatic substances. The physician wore gloves, and a dress which covered him completely, with a " nose bag " containing a sponge soaked in vinegar, cloves, and cinnamon. Writers of the plague tracts advised the public to flee far and quickly, and to return slowly, advice which naturally spread the disease.

Mediæval Hospitals

The care of the sick poor was a duty incumbent upon Christians from the earliest times, and it is easy to understand how the first hospitals were of ecclesiastical foundation. Whatever obstacles the Church may have placed in the path of scientific medicine, there was no hindrance, but rather encouragement, in the provision of housing and nursing for sick and wounded persons. Many fine hospitals were built during the later Middle Ages, their spacious wards having tiled floors, large windows, and cubicles with beds for the patients. Each had an ample water supply, and arrangements for the disposal of sewage.

One of the first examples of those mediæval hospitals may still be seen on the island of Rhodes, where it was established during the Crusades by the Knights of St. John[2] (Plates XXII and XXIII). The Knights established themselves first at Jerusalem, then at Rhodes (1311) and eventually at Malta (1530). The organization, though vastly changed, has retained its ideal and exists to this day.

Some of the great hospitals of London were founded at the time, and were under the control of the Church : St. Bartholomew's in 1123,[2] and St. Thomas's in 1215. St. Bartholomews,[3] as Sir Norman Moore remarks, can claim to be the oldest British hospital of any great size, though there were various hospitals of earlier date throughout the country, some of them for the sick, others for pilgrims and travellers or for the aged. Gradually the administration of hospitals passed to the municipalities, and by the fourteenth century many of them were lay institutions.

[1] F. H. Garrison, *An Introduction to the History of Medicine*, 3rd ed., 1924, p. 195
[2] E. E. Hume, " The Medical Work of the Knights Hospitaller of Saint John of Jerusalem," *Bull. Hist. Med.*, 1938, vol. vi. pp. 398, 495, 677
[3] Sir N. Moore, *History of Saint Bartholomew's Hospital*, 2 vols., 1918 (*cf.* p. 82)
[4] F. G. Parsons, *The History of St Thomas's Hospital*, 3 vols., 1932

PLATE XXV ZODIAC MAN

Illustration from *Fasciculus Medicine* of Johannes de Ketham, 1491, of which a magnificent edition, translated by Sudhoff and Singer and edited by Sigerist, was printed at Milan in 1924 (*Cf.* " Wound Man," Plate xxvIII)
(p. 129)

PLATE XXVI MECHANICAL AIDS TO MEDICINE AND
SURGERY

Application of extension apparatus to a fractured arm. The procedure is surprisingly modern in principle. Woodcut from Gersdorff's *Feldtbuch der Wundartzney*, 1517 (page 126)

Method of expelling a worm from the body, described and illustrated by Brunschwig in his *Cirurgia*, 1497. By means of a winch the patient is suspended
head downwards over a basin of hot goat's milk. As the worm emerges to drink
the milk the winch is wound up until the entire worm is dislodged (page 126)

Besides hospitals there were institutions in which lepers could be segregated and nursed. Leprosy was a common disease in the Middle Ages, and numerous leper houses, or " lazar " houses, existed in Britain and throughout Europe.[1] When he walked abroad each leper was obliged to wear a distinctive dress, and to carry a bell or clapper to announce his presence, and thus warn all persons to avoid him. After the fourteenth century the number of lepers steadily declined, and by the seventeenth century the disease had almost disappeared in Europe.

Medical Illustrations

Much may be learned from the miniature paintings which adorn medical manuscripts and early printed books. Only crude efforts at anatomical illustration were made about the time of Mundinus, when it was customary to depict the bones, muscles, vessels, nerves, and viscera in a series of frog-like figures, usually five in number, the " five-figure series," in which the structures were shown in a very imperfect and unnatural fashion.[2] Our knowledge of those illustrations has been greatly extended by the researches of Professor K. Sudhoff.[3] The " Conciliator " of Peter of Abano, already mentioned, contains the first representation of a " muscle man," a full-length human figure showing the muscles dissected. Another very common illustration was the " zodiac man " (Plate xxv), showing the relation of the various heavenly bodies to the human frame, a belief widely held in the Middle Ages and still further developed during the sixteenth century.[4] For example, the constellation Taurus controlled the neck and throat, Scorpio was related to the genital organs, Capricornus to the knees, and Pisces to the feet. The best time for giving medicines or for drawing blood was ascertained by a study of those constellations and of the moon.[5] Indeed, the influence of the moon upon disease was a belief which held sway as late as the eighteenth century, and was the subject of a work by Dr.

[1] C. A. Mercier, *Leper Houses and Mediæval Hospitals* (Fitzpatrick Lectures), 1915
[2] C. Singer, *The Evolution of Anatomy*, 1925, p. 170
[3] K. Sudhoff, *Tradition und Naturbeobachtung in den Illustrationen Medizinischer Handschriften und Frühdrücke vornehmlich des 15 Jahrhunderts*, Leipzig, 1907 ; *Janus*, 1915, vol. xx. p. 443
[4] F. H. Garrison. *Introduction to the History of Medicine*, 3rd. ed., 1924, p. 190
[5] C. A. Mercier, *Astrology and Medicine* (Fitzpatrick Lectures), 1914

Richard Mead. Surgical works of mediæval times often illustrate a "wound man," showing the position of various wounds and the sites for ligation of arteries [1] (Plate XXVIII).

Another familiar illustration was the "vein man," showing some twenty-eight veins from which blood could be taken with the object of removing the *materia peccans*, or, as we now call it, the source of infection. The Arabs taught that blood should be taken from a vein at a distance from the diseased part, and from the opposite side of the body, the so-called method of "revulsion." It was PIERRE BRISSOT (1478–1522), of Paris, who pointed out that the contrary method of "derivation," used by Hippocrates, consisting in blood-letting near the lesion, and on the same side, was to be preferred.

In books and manuscripts of the period there are numerous other illustrations, from which much may be learned regarding mediæval medicine. [2] Representations of the anatomist engaged in dissecting and demonstrating were a favourite subject with the Dutch artists of the eighteenth century. [3] As already noted, the early drawings show that the actual work of dissection was not performed by the anatomist himself. [4] Finally, another common subject of illustration, which also persisted in more recent paintings, was the diagnosis of disease by uroscopy, or water casting. The physician, sometimes clad in his blue ermine cloak and velvet cap, and having his fingers adorned with rings, is shown holding up to the light the flask containing the patient's urine, and feeling the pulse at the same time, while the mother of the sufferer stands by, anxiously awaiting the verdict (Plate xxxv).

Many other miniature paintings and early woodcuts inform us of the medical life of the time. [5] We are shown what a pharmacy looked like, how operations were conducted, and many another interesting scene. Thus may one learn history without the trouble of reading or translating.

[1] G. W. Corner, *Anatomical Texts of the Earlier Middle Ages*, Washington, 1927
[2] P. M. L. Richer, *L'Art et la Médecine*, 1902
[3] H. E. Sigerist, ' The Historical Aspect of Art and Medicine," *Bull. Hist. Med.*, 1936, vol. iv. p. 271
[4] L. Choulant, *Geschichte und Bibliographie der anatomische Abbildung*, Leipzig, 1852, trans. by M. Frank as *History of Anatomic Illustration*, Chicago, 1920
F. Weindler, *Volksmedizin in den Wandmalereien des deutschen Mittelalters. Arch. f. Gesch. d. Med.*, 1937–38, vol. xxx. p. 78.

The Herbal in Medical Literature

A descriptive account of the plants used in medicine was essential to the physician in the days prior to the development of synthetic pharmacy. Among the earliest " herbals " is that of Dioscorides (p. 62), *De materia medica libri quinque*, of which the only surviving manuscript, now in the Imperial Library at Vienna, was made in A.D. 512 for Juliana Anicia, daughter of a Byzantine emperor, and usually known by her name. It was translated into English by John Goodyer of Petersfield in 1665, and reprinted at Oxford in 1934 under the editorship of R. T. Gunther. Of later date was the *Herbarium* of APULEIUS PLATONICUS (p. 117), to be distinguished from Apuleius, author of *The Golden Ass*. Printed at Rome about 1483, it was the first illustrated herbal to appear in print. A manuscript version of the ninth century was preserved, until recently, at Monte Cassino, and in the British Museum there is a Saxon translation, written about A.D. 1000, which was transcribed in Modern English by T. O. Cockayne in 1864 (*Leechdoms, Wortcunning and Starcraft of Early England* : Rolls Series). Mention has already been made (p. 102) of the *Leech Book of Bald*, in which infection is attributed to flying venom or " elf shot," a current belief in Saxon times. Soon after the publication of the Herbal of Apuleius, there were printed at Mainz, in Germany, three important works of undetermined authorship, based upon previous manuscripts and illustrated with crude and rather fanciful woodcuts. They were generally known as the *Latin Herbarius* (1484), the *German Herbarius* or *Gart der Gesundheit* (1485), and the *Hortus Sanitatis* (1491), sometimes spelled *Ortus Sanitatis*.

Of printed herbals, one of the earliest was this *Ortus sanitatis*, of uncertain authorship, printed in Germany in 1491 and containing many quaint woodcuts. The earliest English printed herbals are those of RYCHARDE BANCKES, whose *Herball* (1525) was very popular, and of PETER TREVERIS, who called his book *The grete herball* (1526), although neither work has any claim to originality. Banckes' Herbal is said to be a translation of the botanical part of the encyclopaedia of Bartholomaeus Anglicus (p. 104).

The most beautifully illustrated herbals of the sixteenth century were printed in Germany. A new and high standard of accuracy was set by OTTO BRUNFELS in his *Herbarium vivae eicones* (1530), while the year 1543, in which Vesalius and Copernicus published their epochal works, was also signalized by the appearance of the Flemish edition of LEONHARD FUCHS's *De historia stirpium* (Basel, 1542), with its accurate descriptions and fine coloured woodcuts. The name of Fuchs is commemorated in the plant "fuchsia." The pioneer of English herbalists is WILLIAM TURNER, sometimes called the "Father of British Botany," whose *New Herball* appeared in 1551 and was dedicated to Queen Elizabeth.[1] Turner was followed by JOHN GERARD, "herbarist" to James I, who cultivated more than a thousand different herbs in his garden at Holborn, London, including, it is said, the potato, recently introduced from Virginia. In his *Herball*, published in 1597, Gerard writes of bugloss growing in the ditches of Piccadilly and of marigolds in the marshes of Paddington.

During the following century there appeared the well-known work of JOHN PARKINSON, entitled *Paradisi in sole, Paradisus Terrestris* (1629), the title including an ingenious word-play upon his own name, Park-in-sun. The elaborate title-page of the *Paradisus* includes an illustration of the "Vegetable Lamb" which was believed to combine animal and vegetable in strange fashion. The lamb, attached to a stalk, fed upon the surrounding foliage, and when that was consumed the plant, and animal, died. The strange myth was believed for several centuries. Parkinson's famous Herbal, *Theatrum Botanicum*, was first published in 1640.

Parkinson was the last of the great English herbalists. Herbalism was becoming divorced from medicine ; and the rift was widened when NICHOLAS CULPEPER incurred the wrath of the College of Physicians by appropriating their Pharmacopoeia [2] as *A Physical Directory*, 1649, and by his diatribes against the College in *The English Phisitian*, 1652, which in its enlarged form had a wide circulation, and came to be known as Culpeper's Herbal. No longer a subject of scientific study, herbalism was kept alive, nevertheless, through the more genuine efforts of WILLIAM COLES, author of *The Art of Simpling*, 1656 ; of ELIZABETH BLACKWELL, who wrote *A Curious Herbal* in 1737 ; of JAMES NEWTON, whose *Compleat Herbal* is dated 1752, and of a number of other herbalists of repute. Even in our own day the latest phase of the subject

[1] C. E. Raven, *English Naturalists from Neckam to Ray*, 1947
[2] This first Pharmacopoeia in Britain was published in 1618 ; the College of Physicians of Edinburgh issued its own Pharmacopoeia in 1699. Many subsequent editions of both publications appeared until supplanted by the British Pharmacopoeia sponsored by the General Medical Council in 1864. (See also Supplement, p. 453.)

may be studied in *A Modern Herbal* by M. GRIEVE, published in 1931.

The above list is by no means complete, and the reader who desires to pursue the study will find complete information in the recent works by Agnes Arber [1] and by Eleanour Sinclair Rohde,[2] from which the present writer has derived most of the above data. The first-mentioned contains a number of beautiful woodcuts from some of the early herbals.[3]

Many of the remedies formerly derived from plants are now produced synthetically by chemical processes ; consequently the art of " simpling "—that is, of collecting plants, or " simples," and using them to prepare " compound " medicines—is now practised only by a few herbalists, and medical botany has assumed a position of minor importance. Indeed, the word " simpling " has become obsolete, although we still speak of the compounding of drugs. Herbs have come to occupy a sort of nondescript position between drugs and foods ; nevertheless, the lore of herbalism is not only of great interest to the medical historian, but is also of practical value to the pharmacologist, as it offers to the research worker a field which has not yet been fully explored. (See also Supplement, page 453.)

[1] A. Arber, *Herbals, Their Origin and Evolution*, Cambridge, 2nd. ed., 1938
[2] E. S. Rohde, *The Old English Herbals*, London, 1922
[3] E. G. Wheelwright, *The Physick Garden*, 1934

BOOKS FOR FURTHER READING

CHOULANT, L. *History of Anatomic Illustration*, trans. by M. Frank, Chicago, 1920

COULTON, G. G. *Life in the Middle Ages*, 4 vols., 1928–29

MERCIER, C. *Leper Houses and Mediæval Hospitals*, 1915

MERCIER, C. A. *Astrology and Medicine* (Fitzpatrick Lectures), 1914

MOORE, Sir N. *History of Saint Bartholomew's Hospital*, 2 vols., 1918

PARSONS, F. G. *The History of St. Thomas's Hospital*, 3 vols., 1932

PAYNE, J. F. *English Medicine in Anglo-Saxon Times*, 1904

POWER, Sir D'ARCY. " *De Arte Phisicale et De Cirurgia* " *of Master John Arderne*, 1922

RASHDALL, H. *The Universities of Europe in the Middle Ages*, 3 vols., 1936

RIESMAN, D. *The Story of Medicine in the Middle Ages*, 1935

SINGER, C. *Studies in the History and Method of Science*, 2 vols., 1921

SOUTH, J. F. *The Craft of Surgery in England*, 1886

TAYLOR, H. O. *The Medieval Mind*, 2 vols., 2nd ed., 1914

THORNDIKE, L. *A History of Magic and Experimental Science*, 6 vols., New York, 1923–41

WALSH, J. J. *Medieval Medicine*, 1920

CHAPTER VIII

MEDICINE OF THE XV AND XVI CENTURIES: REFORMERS AND REVOLUTIONARIES

THE wonderful phenomenon of the Renaissance, which began about the end of the fourteenth century and reached its climax some two hundred years later, did not consist merely in a revival of the ancient classic culture of Greece and Rome. It was also a change in the entire outlook of thinking men, who sought to escape from the tyranny of dogmatic scholasticism, and from the traditional limitations imposed by the Church. Italy was the birthplace of the movement, especially Florence, the city of Dante and of Petrarch, where a renewed appreciation of art and literature had been fostered by the powerful and wealthy ruler, Cosimo de' Medici, and by his grandson Lorenzo.[1] From Italy the enlightenment spread to other countries of Europe, and eventually to England, where it coincided with that noble period known as the Elizabethan Age. At first there arose a demand for freedom of thought, a new standard of human dignity, and a philosophy of living ; humanism in place of the dry and decadent scholasticism of the Middle Ages.

Attainment of the Renaissance ideal was facilitated by various discoveries. The invention of printing, the expansion of the known world by the discovery of America and of routes to the Indies, the alteration in methods of warfare which followed the invention of gunpowder—each exercised a profound influence upon the awakening and renewal of culture implied in the Renaissance. But more important than any discovery was the change of heart in the people, the appearance of a receptive and unbiased attitude towards innovations. Of course the change was not sudden, nor did it affect all mankind generally. A hard battle was to be fought, and the fight was to last for many years. It would be difficult to assign a definite date to a movement which began so quietly during the Middle Ages. We have already noted that in the field of medicine there was, here and there, a feeling of dissatisfaction with the ancient learning. Nevertheless it is generally agreed that the year

[1] Col. G. F. Young, *The Medicis*, 2 vols., 1910

134

1543 marks a peak in the history of medicine and of science,[1] because in that year Nicolaus Copernicus revolutionized astronomy by the publication of his treatise entitled, *De revolutionibus orbium coelestium,* and Andreas Vesalius rendered a similar service to medicine with his *De humani corporis fabrica.* Dr. J. M. Ball remarks, in his biography of Vesalius, that to turn from the writings of Galen, Mundinus, and others to the beauties of Vesalius' work is " like passing from darkness into sunlight." [2] Vesalius is chief among the great medical men of the Renaissance.

Art and Anatomy. Leonardo da Vinci

One of the results of the new outlook was an appreciation of the beauty of the human body. No longer was the body regarded as a sinful instrument which must be hidden, or as something so sacred that it must not even be investigated. Classical ideals were returning, and the artists were the first heralds of the new age. They looked to the anatomists for guidance, but the anatomists were still slaves of tradition, and their work was rendered difficult by the restrictions imposed upon dissection. Nevertheless these restrictions were gradually being overcome, and some of the bolder artists, eager for information, did not hesitate to use the scalpel so as to satisfy themselves regarding the structure of the human frame. Among the great artists who engaged in dissection were Michael Angelo, Raphael, and Albrecht Dürer. Greatest of all was LEONARDO DA VINCI (1452–1519). This gifted and versatile artist, a man centuries ahead of his time in original ideas, who visualized aviation and modern methods of warfare, and who discussed many problems of engineering which were later put into practice,[3] also made discoveries in anatomy, such as the maxillary sinus and the moderator band of the heart. He was the first to demonstrate the ventricles of the brain by wax injections, and to depict correctly the foetus and its membranes within the uterus.[4] Originally, he set out to study the bones and muscles in their relation to art, but his interest grew, and he pursued his investigation of the deeper parts, the viscera,

[1] L. Thorndike, *History of Magic and Experimental Science,* 6 vols., 1941, vol. v. p. 406
[2] J. M. Ball, *Andreas Vesalius, the Reformer of Anatomy,* St. Louis, 1910
[3] J. C. Hemmeter, " Leonardo da Vinci as a Scientist," *Ann. Med. Hist.,* 1921, vol. iii. p. 26
[4] E. Baumgarten, " Leonardo da Vinci as a Physiologist," *Ann. Med. Hist.,* 1932, vol. iv. p. 155

the brain, the blood vessels, and especially the heart.[1] He intended to publish a great work on anatomy in collaboration with Marco Antonio della Torre of Pavia, but this project was abandoned owing to the death of his co-worker. It is only within recent years that the value of Leonardo's contribution to anatomy has been fully appreciated. He made hundreds of sketches and manuscript notes, many of which are preserved in the Royal Library at Windsor, and have only recently appeared in print.[2] This apostle of naturalism in art must also be regarded as a leading pioneer in anatomy.

The Truth about Anatomy. Andreas Vesalius

The foremost anatomist of the Renaissance, and indeed of all time, was ANDREAS VESALIUS (1514–64).[3] A native of Brussels, he belonged to a medical family. His father was apothecary to the Emperor Charles V, and his grandfather, great-grandfather, and great-great-grandfather had all been medical men of good standing.[4]

Young Andreas, we are told, dissected dogs, mice, and other small animals, an approach to medicine which has been adopted by many a boy since then. He received a good education at the University of Louvain, learning not only Greek and Latin but also some Hebrew and Arabic. Thence he proceeded to Paris to study medicine. Among his teachers there were Sylvius and Guinther, anatomists of the old school, each with a great reputation. JACOBUS SYLVIUS (Jacques Dubois, 1478–1555), although an excellent teacher, was so close a follower of Galen that when he found any anatomical structure which did not conform to Galen's description, he alleged that the human body must have become changed since Galen's time. Cardan tells us that Sylvius taught from " fragments of dog's limbs," and that he omitted the difficult parts of anatomy from his lectures. (It was not he, but another of the same name, professor at Leyden a century later, who first

[1] H. Hopstock, "Leonardo as Anatomist," in *Studies in the History and Method of Science*, ed. C. Singer, 1921, p. 151 ; J. P. McMurrich, *Leonardo da Vinci the Anatomist*, Baltimore, 1930. (The most complete work on the subject)

[2] E. MacCurdy, *The Notebooks of Leonardo da Vinci*, 2 vols., 1938

[3] M. H. Spielmann, *The Iconography of Andreas Vesalius*, 1925 ; J. G. De Lint, "Les Portraits de Vesale," *Janus*, 1914, vol. xix. p. 416

[4] M. Roth, *Andreas Vesalius Bruxellensis*, Berlin, 1892 ; J. M. Ball, *Andreas Vesalius, the Reformer of Anatomy*, St. Louis, 1910 ; Harvey Cushing, *A Bio-bibliography of Andreas Vesalius*, New York, 1943

described the fissure of Sylvius in the brain.) Sylvius of Paris was not liberal in his judgments of the work of others. He strongly disapproved of the anatomical discoveries of his pupil, Vesalius, and even spoke of him, not as Vesalius, but as Vesanus (madman), " whose pestilential breath poisons Europe." Very different was JOHANNES GUINTHER (sometimes written Gunter or Winter) of Andernach (1487–1574), a man of humble birth, who was so poor a student that he was obliged to beg in the streets, but who nevertheless became Professor of Greek at Louvain. At the age of thirty-eight he turned to medicine as a career, was appointed Professor of Anatomy in Paris, where he attained eminence in practice and in teaching, and so rose in repute that he eventually became a nobleman of Strassburg, whence he had retired. Guinther made no great contribution to anatomy, but he was one of those who recognized and encouraged the work of the young Vesalius, to whose career let us now return.

Vesalius pursued his studies at Paris with great energy and enthusiasm. His search for material led him, at great personal risk, to undertake various " body-snatching " expeditions, and when owing to the outbreak of war he was obliged to return for a time to Louvain, he found on a gallows outside the city walls the skeleton of a criminal, almost complete and with ligaments intact. Aided by a friend, he secretly bore home his trophy, which proved of great value in his studies.

On the completion of his course at Paris, Vesalius travelled to Italy, and at Venice he met another Belgian, a student of art and pupil of Titian, named Jan Stephan van Calcar, who later drew many of the wonderful wood engravings which adorn the works of Vesalius.

Appointed Professor of Surgery and Anatomy at Padua in 1537, Vesalius now entered the most strenuous and productive years of his career. On two occasions he visited Bologna and held courses of instruction there. In Padua he lectured to a crowded classroom, seated for 500, and busied himself with the preparation of his great Anatomy.[1] Already he had translated the Ninth Book of Rhazes' " Almansor," a compendium of treatment which became a valuable textbook, but now he concentrated his attention on anatomy, as he continually found, in the course of his dissections, that the current teaching was full of errors

[1] J. B. de C. M. Saunders and C. D. O'Malley, *The Illustrations from the Works of Andreas Vesalius*, 1950

and that Galen could no longer be regarded as the final authority. After a year at Padua he published a series of six large plates for the use of students, *Tabulae Anatomicae Sex*, of which only two copies still exist. This, however, was only an introduction to the magnificent volume, *De Humani Corporis Fabrica* (On the Fabric of the Human Body), generally known as the *Fabrica*, a word best rendered in English as " mechanism " or " working," which appeared in June 1543, when Vesalius was twenty-eight years of age. An *Epitome* of the work, now extremely rare, was produced at the same time. No finer anatomical plates have ever been seen than those which adorn the *Fabrica*. The figures of the skeleton and of the muscles are of particularly high artistic merit, and have served as models for many generations of artists. It is no dead anatomy that is here represented. The subjects are full of life and expression, for the author sought to depict the body in action, and to teach physiology as well as anatomy. The frontispiece to the *Fabrica* shows Vesalius dissecting and demonstrating to a crowd of interested spectators (Plate xxvii). There are seven chapters or books in the volume, although the main interest centres in the plates. The description and delineation of the structures marks a great advance upon any previous work. Vesalius corrected Galen in showing that the lower jaw consisted of a single bone, and that the sternum was composed of only three parts, and not seven. He noted the existence of valves in the veins, but did not appreciate their significance. Observing that each artery supplying a viscus was accompanied by a vein, he deduced that this was simply an arrangement for the " mutual flux and reflux of materials." In the first edition of his work he admitted the existence of pores in the interventricular septum of the heart, but in the second edition, published in 1555, he states emphatically that there are no such openings, and that blood cannot possibly pass direct from one ventricle to the other. This was the first stage towards a complete denial of Galen's doctrine, and one of the fundamental data on which Harvey based his discovery of the circulation of the blood. Vesalius also helped to found the science of anthropology when he noted that the Germans had round heads, while the Belgian heads were long. The *Fabrica* was printed in Basel by Joannes Oporinus, and Vesalius went to Basel in order to superintend the production, which was carried out with the utmost care. Even the initial letters are works of art, showing cherubs engaged in dissection and other activities, a satirical representation of his students.[1] With the publication of the *Fabrica* and the *Epitome*, the brilliant career of Vesalius was virtually completed. One who had dared to revolutionize anatomy and to expose the mistakes of the ancients could not hope to escape criticism. His ideas were strongly opposed in certain quarters, and he found himself the subject of heated and bitter controversy. Perhaps it was on that account that he resigned his chair at Padua, and went to Madrid as physician to Emperor Charles V and then to his son Philip II. From both he received respect and honour, and his services were highly esteemed. But anatomy knew him no longer. His epoch-making work had been crowded into three short years, and now, at the age of thirty, he was finished.

Little is known of his life in Spain, or in the Netherlands, which he revisited. In 1564 he left Madrid to proceed on a pilgrimage to the Holy Sepulchre. The reason for such an action is uncertain. It is said that a nobleman whom he was attending having died, Vesalius was in the act of performing a post-mortem examination when the subject showed signs of life. The consequences were disastrous, as might well be imagined in those days of the Inquisition. The physician was pardoned only on condition that he would expiate his crime by a visit to Jerusalem. On the return journey his ship was wrecked on the island of Zante, at the entrance to the Gulf of Corinth, and there, in October 1564, Vesalius died.

The Pulmonary Circulation

The immediate successors and contemporaries of Vesalius were overshadowed by his greatness, but a few of them deserve mention, as their names are familiar to every student of anatomy.

Vesalius was succeeded at Padua by REALDUS COLUMBUS (Realdo Colombo, 1510–99), of Cremona, whose chief claim to fame rests in his discovery of the pulmonary, or lesser, circulation.[2] He demonstrated by experiment that blood passed from the lung into the pulmonary vein. " The blood," he said, " goes through the vena arteriosa to the lungs ; then, mixed with air, it goes through the arteria venosa to the left heart." In his book, *De Re Anatomica*, which appeared in 1559, long after he had left Padua for Rome, Columbus published these observations.

[1] K. Rosenkranz, " Die Initialen in Vesals Anatomie," *Arch. f. Gesch. d. Med.*, 1937–38, vol. xxx. p. 35
[2] A. Castiglioni, *History of Medicine*, New York, 1941, p. 435

Six years previously, unknown to Columbus, another anatomist had made the same discovery, though both observers
retained the Galenic idea of *spiritus*, and neither appears to have
had any true conception of the general circulation of the blood.
The unfortunate Spaniard, MICHAEL SERVETUS (1509–53), published his account of the pulmonary circulation in a theological
work, *Restitutio Christianismi*, and on that account it attracted little
attention.[1] Its main effect was to focus upon the author the
wrath of the Church. Accused by Calvin of heresy, he was condemned and burned alive at Geneva on October 27, 1553, and his
works with him.[2] Only three imperfect copies are preserved, at
Paris, Vienna, and Edinburgh. The passage in the *Restitutio* dealing with the circulation states that the blood is " transmitted from
the pulmonary artery to the pulmonary vein, by a lengthened
passage through the lungs, in the course of which it becomes of
crimson colour," and is " freed from fuliginous vapours by the
act of expiration." [3] There is, however, no suggestion in the
argument, of any systemic circulation, nor is the word " circulation " used.

At this point mention may be made of one for whom it is
claimed, though on slender grounds, that he anticipated Harvey's
discovery. ANDREA CESALPINO (1519–1603) taught anatomy at
Pisa and Rome, and was also a great botanist and mineralogist.
It is true that Cesalpino affirmed that the blood-vessels originated
from the heart, and not from the liver as Galen and his followers
had affirmed. Although he also stated that the blood passed
from the heart to all parts of the body, he believed that it coursed
through veins and arteries alike, and it appears as though he still
adhered to the old " ebb and flow " idea, rather than to any
conception of a " circulation." Much stronger evidence than
that at present available would be required to remove Harvey
from his accepted place as the great discoverer. Nevertheless
these anatomists did much to pave the way for Harvey. One
of the successors of Vesalius at Padua was FABRICIUS AB ACQUA-
PENDENTE (1533–1619). He was a distinguished anatomist and
embryologist, and among his pupils was William Harvey.
Fabricius made a special study of valves in the veins, though

[1] W. Osler, " Michael Servetus," *Johns Hopk. Hosp. Bull.*, 1910, vol. xxi. p. 1
[2] G. H. Williams, " Michael Servetus, Physician and Heretic," *Ann. Med. Hist.*,
1928, vol. x. p. 287
[3] R. Willis, *Servetus and Calvin*, 1877

these structures had been known to anatomists before him (Plate xxxvi). He believed that they served to regulate the flow of blood, but he failed to appreciate, as Harvey did, that such valves were effective only in a one-way current. Fabricius was not only an anatomist, but also a leading surgeon who devoted part of his fortune to the building of a magnificent anatomical theatre at Padua.

Fallopius and Eustachius

Many other great anatomists lived and worked during this brilliant and busy period. Casserius (1552–1616), who succeeded Fabricius at Padua, was a pioneer in comparative anatomy ; of earlier dates were Coiter (? 1534–76), of Groningen, who gave a complete account of the anatomy of the ear ; Platter (1536–1614), of Basel, who made numerous dissections out of which emerged many new facts in pathology ; and Ingrassia (1510–80), of Naples, who discovered the stapes and the tensor tympani muscle, and also differentiated measles from scarlet fever. In order to complete the picture, two men must still be mentioned, their names being household words in anatomy.[1]

GABRIEL FALLOPIUS (1523–62) succeeded Vesalius at Padua after the brief interregnum of Columbus. He took up the work of reconstruction where Vesalius had left it, and he was even more forceful than his predecessor in his criticism of the Galenic ideas. During his short life he accomplished much besides his discoveries of the " aqueduct " and " tubes " which bear his name. He held the combined professorship of anatomy, surgery, and botany at Padua, and his work in all these subjects was of outstanding merit. Withington has claimed that " in the beauty of his personal character as well as in the amount and excellence of his work, Fallopius stands first of Italian anatomists."[2]

While Vesalius was at Padua the Chair of Anatomy at Rome was held by BARTOLOMEUS EUSTACHIUS (1510–74). Although he was a follower of Galen, his anatomical discoveries were many. His fame rests chiefly upon the atlas of excellent copperplate illustrations which were completed only a few years after the publication of Vesalius's *Fabrica*. Owing to financial or other difficulties, the *Tabulae Anatomicae* did not appear in the lifetime of Eustachius. The plates were lost for 138 years. Then they

[1] C. Singer, *The Evolution of Anatomy*, 1925, p. 135
[2] E. T. Withington, *Medical History from the Earliest Times*, 1894, p. 214

were discovered in the papal library at Rome, and were published by Lancisi, the Pope's physician, in 1714. The text was never found. Professor Charles Singer is of opinion that had the plates appeared when completed, the name of Eustachius would have stood beside that of Vesalius as the joint-founder of modern anatomy. Those illustrations, though less artistic than the plates of Vesalius, are in some respects more accurate, and constitute a record of numerous discoveries. Among them may be mentioned the thoracic duct, the ciliary muscle, and details of the facial muscles, the larynx, the kidney, and other structures, while the first plate of the series is an engraving of the sympathetic nervous system. Curiously enough, the Eustachian tube is not shown in the *Tabulae*, but it is described in the *Epistola de auditus organis*, which was printed in 1563 and is probably the first complete book on the anatomy of the ear. The number of new facts elucidated by Vesalius and his associates was so enormous that it is not surprising that the practical significance of the new anatomy was only gradually appreciated.

Humane Surgery. Ambroise Paré

It was the invention of gunpowder, with all its dire consequences, rather than the application of new anatomical facts, that drew surgery into the Renaissance movement. War has ever been a great teacher of surgery, and the leading surgeons of this, as of other periods, were army surgeons. The real renaissance of surgery did not take place until the nineteenth century. During the epoch under review no such spectacular change took place. Surgery showed no sudden upheaval comparable to the revolutionary and dramatic alteration of anatomy by Vesalius, or the forceful and intolerant revolt from tradition in medicine, led by Paracelsus, to whose work reference will be made presently. Already, in mediæval times, good surgical work had been done by Guy de Chauliac, John of Arderne, and others. A steady advance had been taking place during the years which are so often regarded as sterile of ideas. The ground had been well prepared for a great surgical reformer, who by his noble personality, his courage, his humanity, and his zeal raised surgery to a higher level, and well earned for himself the title of the Father of Modern Surgery. This was AMBROISE PARÉ (1510-90), the greatest surgeon of the Renaissance, and one of the greatest surgeons of all time.[1] Essentially humanist rather than scholastic, he knew no Latin or Greek, and he trusted to observation rather than to books. Nevertheless he rose to great eminence, and became surgeon to four kings of France in succession. Withal, he was a man of shrewd judgment and of simple piety, who loved his profession, his home, and his country ; a worthy model for all modern surgeons. So let us approach him a little more closely.

Of humble parentage, he was born at Laval in Moyenne, where his father was a cabinetmaker, or, from some accounts, barber and valet to the Comte de Laval. His sister Catherine married Gaspard Martin, a barber surgeon of Paris, and his brother Jean became a barber surgeon, with a practice at Vitré in Brittany. Ambroise may have been apprenticed to this brother, who, he tells us, was clever in unmasking the tricks of street beggars. One impostor had acquired the arm of a hanged criminal, which he passed off as his own ; another, by means of coloured wax, had modelled, for his own benefit, a hideous sore on his body. At all events, the early training of the young apprentice was by no means academic. Yet he eventually reached Paris, and, freeing himself from the hair-cutting part of his work, he concentrated on surgery, and was successful in obtaining a resident appointment at the great hospital, the Hôtel-Dieu, where he remained for three years, laying a sound foundation to a brilliant career [2] (Plate XXVIII).

" Journeys in Divers Places "

During the lifetime of Paré, France was engaged in many wars : against Italy, Germany, and England, and eventually, at home, in the civil war so disastrous to the Huguenots. It was natural that so keen a surgeon should seek scope for his talents in service with the army. Ambroise Paré joined the Forces, and for the next thirty years, with a foothold in Paris in the intervals of fighting, he engaged in many campaigns. There was no organized medical corps in those days. The surgeon accompanied

[1] F. R. Packard, *The Life and Times of Ambroise Paré*, 2nd ed., 1926 ; Stephen Paget, *Ambroise Paré and his Times (1510–90)*, 1897. (The biography by Stephen Paget gives a vivid picture of the great surgeon and contains many quotations from his autobiographical *Journeys*.)

[2] D. M. Quynn, " A Medieval Picture of the Hôtel-Dieu of Paris," *Bull. Hist. Med.*, 1942, vol. xii. p. 118

the troops, attended them when required, and received such rewards as they were willing to give. Paré's first taste of active service was in the attack on Turin by the great king, Francis I, in 1537.[1] He tells the story, with his own graphic and inimitable touch, in his "Journeys in Divers Places" (*Voyages faits en divers lieux*), a most attractive journal, full of adventure and good stories, and giving a clear picture, sometimes pathetic, sometimes amusing, but always interesting, of the life of an army surgeon in the sixteenth century.

Paré was an old man when he wrote these reminiscences in reply to an attack upon him by Gourmelen, Dean of the Faculty of Physicians of Paris. There was much rivalry and wordy warfare between physicians and surgeons at that period. It was often a triangular contest, as the college of St. Côme, consisting of surgeons " of the long robe," would have nothing to do with the barber surgeons, who were regarded as altogether inferior. The physicians, thinking themselves superior to both, bitterly reproached any surgeon who dared to dabble in physic. Imagine, therefore, the rage of Dean Gourmelen against a barber surgeon who wished to publish a book which dealt, not only with surgery, but with plague and other diseases, with obstetrics, and with the folly of the physicians in employing such remedies as powdered mummy and unicorn's horn. Moreover, this upstart author had written in his mother tongue, and not in dignified Latin. We can never be too grateful to the Dean for his annoyance, as it called forth from the pen of Ambroise Paré one of the most delightful journals in literature, a book worthy to stand beside the diary of Pepys or the reminiscences of Cellini. The reply to Gourmelen is direct, and often ironical, as when he calls his accuser " mon petit maître," yet it is free from bitterness. " Dare you teach me Surgery, you who have never come out of your study ? Surgery is learned by the eye and by the hands. You, mon petit maître, know nothing else but how to chatter in a Chair." (See also Supplement, page 455.)

He proceeds to tell of his first sight of Turin, and to show how he "found a way to learn the art of surgery." " We entered pell-mell into the city . . . and in a stable where we thought to lodge our horses, found four dead soldiers, and three propped against the wall. . . . They neither saw, heard, nor spoke, and their clothes were still smouldering, burned with gunpowder. As

[1] Stephen Paget, *Ambroise Paré and his Times (1510–90)*, 1897, p. 30

PLATE XXVII VESALIUS TEACHING ANATOMY

Title-page of the *Fabrica* of Vesalius, published in 1543. This work laid the foundation of scientific anatomy (page 138)

PLATE XXVIII   SURGERY UNDER AMBROISE PARÈ

A ward in the Hôtel-Dieu of Paris about the thirteenth century. Several sisters are teaching novices how to feel the pulse. Most of the beds are occupied by two patients. The hospital had probably undergone little change before the time of Paré. From a contemporary manuscript at the Hôtel-Dieu (page 143)

(*l.*) Instruments for the removal of darts and arrowheads.   (*r.*) Type of illustration known as " Wound Man " (page 130, *cf.* Plate xxv). From *The Works of that famous chirurgeon Ambrose Parey* (English translation of 1678)

I was looking at them with pity there came an old soldier who asked me if there were any way to cure them. I said, No. Then he went up to them and cut their throats, gently and without ill will. I told him he was a villain : he answered he prayed God, when he should be in such a plight, he might find some-one to do the same for him, that he should not linger in misery."

Paré found many wounded in Turin, and he proceeded to treat them as John de Vigo had advised, " with oil of elders (sambucus) scalding hot." But his supply of oil was soon finished, and he was then forced to apply " a digestive of eggs, oil of roses, and turpentine." That night he could not sleep, fearing that he should find those patients dead in the morning. He rose early, and to his great surprise found that those who had been dressed with the " digestive " had little pain and that their wounds were not inflamed, while those to whom boiling oil had been applied were "feverish, with great pain, and swelling of their wounds." Then he discovered that gunshot wounds were not poisoned, or, as he put it, " do not partake of any venenate quality," and needed no such drastic treatment. " Then I resolved never more to burn thus cruelly poor men with gunshot wounds." In Turin he met another surgeon, who had discovered a balm for wounds which gave wonderful results. It was made by boiling together oil of lilies, young whelps, and earthworms in turpentine, " a remedy like that which I had obtained by chance. See how I learned to treat gunshot wounds, not out of books."

One day Paré heard a nobleman remark to his general, " Thou hast a surgeon young in age but old in knowledge and experience ; take good care of him." " But," adds our hero in his naïve way, " the good man did not know that I had lived three years with the patients at the Hôtel-Dieu in Paris." His next journey was to Brittany, where a landing of the English was expected, and though this never took place, there was plenty of surgical work as a result of the wrestling bouts then so popular. Paré describes in detail a particularly savage contest which ended fatally. A few years later, at Boulogne, contact was made with the English army, and Ambroise, under fire for the first time, " ducked his head low " as he felt the moved air, " though the ball was already far away." " Mon petit maître, if you had been there I should not have been afraid all alone."

" *I dressed him and God healed him* "

Germany was the seat of another campaign, and Paré tells how a soldier, attempting to gain victuals from the peasants by force, returned so mutilated that his fellows had already dug a grave for him. Here was a case to test the utmost skill of the surgeon, and the surgeon proved equal to the task. " I did him the office of physician, apothecary, surgeon, and cook. I dressed him to the end of his case, and God healed him."

" *Je le pansay ; Dieu le guarit,*" as it is written in Old French, was a favourite expression which occurs many times, with variations, in Paré's descriptions. At the end of the German war, referring to another patient, he writes : " The camp was dispersed and I returned to Paris with my gentleman whose leg I had cut off ; I dressed him, and God healed him. He said he had got off cheap, not to have been miserably burned to stop the blood, as you write in your book, mon petit maître."

The book of journeys continues, and Ambroise Paré after telling of his adventures at the siege of Metz and of his attendance on the king of Navarre, mortally wounded, relates how after the battle of St. Quentin the ground was covered with dead men and horses, and " so many blue and green flies rose from them that they hid the sun ; where they settled, there they infested the air and brought the plague with them.[1] Mon petit maître, I wish you had been there." He describes how he found that the ligature might supplant the cautery as a haemostatic in amputations, and he tells many a good story in his own intimate fashion. Early in his career as an army surgeon Paré had entered the service of the king, had married, and had acquired the house in Paris close to the Pont St. Michel, where he lived and died. He had become a barber surgeon in 1541, and thirteen years later, after numerous formalities, had been admitted to the close fraternity of the College of St. Côme, which was forced to recognize so distinguished a man, be he barber surgeon or no, and Latin or no Latin.

Ambroise Paré at Court

After 1559, his campaigning days being over, he resided permanently in Paris. It has been mentioned that Paré was surgeon to four kings of France, not counting the king of Navarre.

[1] R. H. Major, *Classic Descriptions of Disease*, 1932, p. 83

On June 29, 1559, Henry II was grievously wounded while engaged in a friendly tournament with Count Montgomery, captain of the Scottish Guard. The lance struck him above the right eye. Paré and several other surgeons attended him, and Vesalius came from Brussels by the order of Philip of Spain. They dissected the heads of four criminals, to ascertain what direction the lance may have taken, but to no purpose. The king died on the eleventh day, leaving a widow, the notorious Catherine of Medici, and three weakly and worthless sons, to carry on his work. The eldest, Francis II, husband of Mary Stuart, Queen of Scots, survived his father by only eighteen months. At the age of seventeen he died from disease of the ear, with severe headache, probably meningitis of otitic origin. Paré was suspected of having put poison in his ear by command of the Queen Mother. Despite this malicious accusation, Paré retained his Court appointment under Charles IX, who died of phthisis fourteen years later, and then under Henry III, who was assassinated a year before Paré died.

In the terrible massacre of St. Bartholomew, August 22, 1572, Ambroise Paré, who two days previously had attended Admiral Coligny, the Huguenot general, mortally wounded by an assassin, was himself in great danger, as he was believed to be a Huguenot. Charles IX, though in favour of the slaughter, sheltered Paré in his own room, as he agreed that " it was not reasonable that one who was worth a whole world of men should be thus murdered." Whether Ambroise was Huguenot or Catholic has often been argued. Certainly his two marriages were celebrated with Catholic rites, and all his nine children were baptized into the Roman Church.

His services to surgery did not merely concern gunshot wounds. He discussed in detail the treatment of fractures and dislocations, he abolished castration in herniotomy, he suggested that syphilis was a cause of aneurysm, he invented artery forceps and many another instrument, and he knew all that was to be known about sick nursing.[1] Keenly interested in all aspects of medicine, he investigated old wives' cures, and even purchased the recipes of charlatans so that they might be generally available.

Even if he did believe in evil spirits, in the power of the saints, and in the influence of the stars, his works are still

[1] E. Gurlt, *Geschichte der Chirurgie*, Berlin, 1898, Bd. ii. p. 688

well worth reading. Here are a few of his *Surgical Canons and Rules :*

He who becomes a surgeon for the sake of money will accomplish nothing.

Mere knowledge without experience does not give the surgeon self-confidence.

A remedy thoroughly tested is better than one recently invented.

It is always wise to hold out hope to the patient, even if the symptoms point to a fatal issue.

Like John Hunter, with whom he has often been compared, Ambroise Paré was one of the master surgeons of history. (See also Supplement, page 455.)

Itinerant Lithotomists

Of the many good surgeons of the Renaissance period, only a few need be mentioned to illustrate the trends of the time. It was the custom to entrust the care of cases of stone in the bladder, a very common complaint, to itinerant lithotomists. Many of them possessed great skill and experience, and some undertook other operations as well. One of the best known of this class was PIERRE FRANCO (1505–70), a native of Provence, who made his headquarters at Berne, and later at Lausanne.[1] According to Malgaigne, Franco was a surgical genius. He was the first to perform suprapubic lithotomy, removing a large stone which he had failed to extract by the perineal route, but he did not advise the routine adoption of this new method. Indeed, it was not until 1718 that John Douglas of London, brother of James Douglas the anatomist, revived the operation. Franco invented strong forceps for crushing a stone, so that the fragments might more easily pass through the wound. He did not approve the idea, then prevalent, that a stone might be dissolved by remedies given by the mouth. He wrote a treatise on hernia, and he was the first to describe the operation for strangulated hernia. Cataract was another condition for which he operated, claiming success in the great majority of his cases. That his lot was not always a happy one, despite his success, is shown by his remark, " The physicians and surgeons can defend themselves when unfortunate, but if we lithotomists have a mishap, we must run for our lives."

[1] D. Bail, " Un Chirurgien urologiste au XVIᵉ Siècle : Pierre Franco," *Bull. d'Hist. Méd.,* 1932, vol. xxvi. p. 204

PLATE XXIX SIXTEENTH-CENTURY SURGERY

Dental forceps, or "Instruments to pull out, cutt, and file Superfluous teeth."

Amputating set, or " Instruments, and Cauters actuals, for extirpation "

Both illustrations from *A Discourse of the Whole Art of Chyrurgery*, by Peter Lowe, 4th edition, 1654 (page 154)

PLATE XXX   THE BARBER-SURGEONS RECEIVE THEIR CHARTER

Painting attributed to Holbein, showing Henry VIII in 1540 handing to Thomas Vicary the Act of Union between the Barbers and the Surgeons of London. Vicary was the first Master of the new company, called the " Masters and Governors of the Mystery and Commonalty of the Barbers and Surgeons of London," which later became the Royal College of Surgeons of England (page 150)

Two later practitioners of this class were the French monks, Frère Jacques and Frère Jean.[1] FRÈRE JACQUES DE BEAULIEU (1651–1719), a native of Central France who travelled widely in order to practise his art, made it a rule only to operate in the presence of a physician or surgeon, and he charged no fees but merely took what was offered, retaining only just sufficient money for living expenses and giving the surplus to the poor. In 1697 he visited Paris, where his success aroused the jealousy of the surgeons to such an extent that he was obliged to resume his wanderings through Europe. He practised the operation of lateral lithotomy, which came into general use, and was often associated with his name.

In the following century FRÈRE JEAN DE SAINT CÔME (1703–81), a professional and ecclesiastical brother of Frère Jacques, and like him a Franciscan monk, practised lithotomy with such creditable results that he was able to maintain a private hospital in Paris.[2] Frère Côme, as he was called, invented a lithotome with a concealed knife, which ensured greater accuracy of incision. He was able to claim 90 per cent. of cures in over 1,000 cases.

Surgery in Italy and Germany

As has been mentioned, the Italian anatomists of the Renaissance were also surgeons. It is said that Vesalius met Paré in consultation at the deathbed of Henry II. Fabricius of Acquapendente had a large surgical practice, and so had GUIDO GUIDI, or Vidius, of Pisa (d. 1569), whose name is familiar to anatomists. Special mention, however, must be made of the perfecter of rhinoplasty, or restoration of loss of the nose by a plastic operation. He was GASPARE TAGLIACOZZI (1540–99) of Bologna, and his operation consisted in the transplantation of a flap of skin from the arm, the limb being bandaged in contact with the nose, until the grafted part had established itself.[3] This procedure was strongly condemned by the Church, which discountenanced any attempt to improve upon the handiwork of the Almighty, and the operation was not revived until the nineteenth century.

Reference has already been made to German surgery of the

[1] A. H. Buck, *The Growth of Medicine from the Earliest Times to About 1800*, Yale, 1917, p. 549
[2] A. Pousson and E. Desnos, ed. of *Encyclopédie Française d'Urologie*, 2 vols., 1914, vol. i. p. 166
[3] E. T. Withington, *Medical History from the Earliest Times*, 1894 p. 285

period, but one name which must be added is that of Wilhelm Fabry of Hilden, near Düsseldorf, or FABRICIUS HILDANUS (1560–1634).[1] He acquired much experience during the Thirty Years War when he introduced the tourniquet, and proved the necessity of amputating through healthy tissue in cases of gangrene. It was said that he used a red hot knife for amputation in order to check bleeding. Despite the severity of his methods he had a private hospital at Berne, and he worked hard to raise the surgeon to a position of dignity equal to that of the physician. In his *Observationes Medico-Chirurgiae* may be found many illustrations of the instruments he invented.

Another ingenious German inventor of surgical instruments was JOHANN SCULTETUS, whose *Armamentarium Chirurgium*, published in 1655, contains many interesting illustrations.

English Surgery in the Sixteenth Century

As early as the fourteenth century the barber surgeons of England were organized in groups or " gilds." Every town of importance had its gild, and it is estimated that there were twenty or thirty of them, although most of the records are lost. Of the individual members we know little beyond a few names. John of Arderne, whose work we have noted, was one of the few English surgeons who wrote on his subject and gave to posterity some idea of the prevailing practice. Yet it is not until the sixteenth century that the picture becomes more clear.[2]

The name of THOMAS VICARY (1495–1561) is memorable for two reasons. He was the author of the first textbook of anatomy to be written in English, and he was the first Master of the United Company of Barber Surgeons.[3] Originally a practitioner in Maidstone, he went to London as a barber surgeon, and rapidly rose to fame, becoming chief surgeon to the king, Henry VIII, in 1535. His work on anatomy bore the title, *A Treasure for Englishmen, containing the Anatomie of Man's Body*. It is said to have appeared in 1548, but no trace of this first edition can be found. It was reprinted in 1577, after his death, by his col-

---

[1] E. Gurlt, *Geschichte der Chirurgie*, Berlin, 1898, Bd. iii. p. 107
[2] Sir H. Rolleston, " The Early History of the Teaching of Anatomy," *Ann. Med. Hist.*, 1939, 3rd Series, vol. i. p. 203
[3] D'Arcy Power, " The Education of a Surgeon under Thomas Vicary " (Vicary Lecture), in *Selected Writings*, 1931

leagues on the staff of St. Bartholomew's Hospital, and it held its place as a textbook until the seventeenth century. The anatomy contained in it is of the mediæval type, despite the fact that the author had studied at Padua.

Vicary was instrumental in securing in 1540 the Royal Assent to a union of the gilds of barber surgeons and surgeons. The occasion is commemorated in a well-known picture by Holbein in the possession of the Royal College of Surgeons (Plate xxx). The Act of 1540 declared that surgeons should no longer be barbers, and that barbers should restrict their surgery to dentistry. The new Company was empowered to impose fines upon unlicensed practitioners in London, and was entitled to have two bodies of executed criminals each year for the study of anatomy.

One of the earliest teachers of anatomy under the new scheme was JOHN BANESTER (1533–1610), who had a great reputation both as a physician and surgeon, at Nottingham, and later in London.[1] He strove hard to reunite surgery and medicine, which union, he stated, would be to the benefit of both. In his own words, " Some of late have fondly affirmed that the chirurgeon hath not to deal in physic. Small courtesy it is to break faithful friendship . . . for the one cannot work without the other, nor the other practise without the aid of both." In the Hunterian Museum of Glasgow his anatomical figures are preserved, and also a contemporary painting showing Banester delivering the " visceral " lecture at the Barber Surgeons' Hall of London in 1581.[2] The open book beside him is the book of Columbus, who succeeded Vesalius at Padua. Thus it is evident that Banester was following the new knowledge of anatomy.

In England, as in France, war was a teacher of surgery, and there was at this time a military surgeon whose quaint writings give some interesting details of army practice. WILLIAM CLOWES (1540–1604), who became surgeon to Queen Elizabeth and to St. Bartholomew's Hospital, distinguished himself on service with the army in Flanders, and with the navy in the repulse of the Armada.[3] His works include a treatise on venereal disease (1579),[4] in which he dwells on the importance of writing in the vernacular

[1] J. F. South, *Memorials of the Craft of Surgery in England*, 1886, p. 90
[2] H. Lett, " Anatomy at the Barber Surgeons' Hall," *Brit. Jour. Surg.*, 1943–44, vol. xxxi. p. 101   [3] G. Parker, *The Early History of Surgery in Great Britain*, 1920, p. 74
[4] William Clowes, *A Short and Profitable Treatise touching the cure of the disease called Morbus Gallicus, or Lues Venerea, by unctions, etc.*

rather than in Latin, and an important work on gunshot wounds, a short book with the long title, *A profitable and necessarie book of observations, for all those that are burned with the flame of gunpowder, etc., and also for curing of wounds made with Musket and Caliver shot and other weapons of warre commonly used at this day both by Sea and Land* (1591).[1] Clowes makes many interesting observations, as he had conducted experiments on the vexed question of whether or no gunshot wounds were poisoned. He noted that when arrows were fired from a musket the feathers were not singed. Clearly, therefore, he argued, the bullet could not be purified by heat, and might well carry poison into a wound. He gives some interesting accounts of the surgical instruments then in use.

THOMAS GALE (1507–86) was another army surgeon who, in his *Treatise of Wounds with Gonneshot* (1563), proves that, contrary to the prevailing idea, " the bullet does not acquire such heat in its motion as to render the wound similar to cautery." Gale was a man of high principle, and his ethical rules for surgeons must have exercised a salutary influence at a time when the field of surgery was invaded by many charlatans.

Another of Queen Elizabeth's surgeons was JOHN WOODALL (1569–1643),[2] who had an extensive experience, both afloat and ashore, in the service of the East India Company, and on the Continent. His books, *The Surgeon's Mate* (1617) and *The Viaticum, or The Pathway to the Surgeon's Chest* (1639) give details of the necessary instruments and equipment, and describe how they are to be used. Woodall is sometimes credited with the discovery of lime or lemon juice as a cure for scurvy, long before James Lind published his treatise on the subject (1753). Woodall commends " the juice of vegetables and fruits, and where none of these can be had, oil of vitriol."

Early Scottish Physicians and Surgeons

Only scanty records exist of the practice of medicine and surgery in Scotland in early times. The name of MICHAEL SCOT (? 1175–? 1232) has been already mentioned (p. 107), and details

[1] R. H. Major, " William Clowes and his *Profitable and Necessarie Booke of Observations*," *Ann. Med. Hist.*, 1932, vol. iv. p. 1 ; F. N. L. Poynter, ed. *The Selected Writings of William Clowes*, 1948
[2] J. Aikin, *Biographical Memoirs of Medicine in Great Britain*, 1780, p. 93 (Gale), p. 238 (Woodall). (Aikin's *Memoirs*, though now rather a rare book, supplies interesting information which cannot be found elsewhere) ; S. Jenkinson, " John Woodall, Surgeon, Royal Navy, 1569–1643," *Jour. Roy. Naval Med. Service*, 1940, vol. xxvi. p. 107

of a number of Gaelic medical manuscripts dating from the twelfth century to the fourteenth century, are described in Comrie's *History of Scottish Medicine*. Comrie mentions several pioneers, including one WILLIAM SCHEVEZ (1428–97), who practised at St. Andrews, and being as well versed in theology as in medicine, became Archbishop or Primate of Scotland in 1487. Schevez was a renowned scholar who had studied at Louvain, and founded a valuable library at St. Andrews.[1] Little is known of his medical work, save that he was the best-known practitioner of Scotland in the fifteenth century and physician to King James III at a salary of £20 per annum.

Surgery in Scotland, as elsewhere, was in the hands of surgeons and barbers, and in 1505, in response to a petition from the two crafts,[2] a " Seal of Cause " was granted by the Town Council of Edinburgh and was confirmed in the following year by King James IV. This decree conferred certain rights and privileges on the new body, the Incorporation of Barber Surgeons, which became the Royal College of Surgeons of Edinburgh in 1778. This gild was to have the sole right of practising within the burgh, and of examining candidates who desired to join them. The examination was to include " the anatomy, nature, and complexion of man's body," the position of the veins so that phlebotomy might be performed, and the signs of the zodiac and facts governed by them. Every prospective surgeon must be able to read and write, or as the document has it, " baithe wryte and reid." Further, the gild was entitled to claim each year, " ane condampnit man efter he be deid to mak anatomea of quhairthrow we may haif experience " ; in other words, one executed criminal might be claimed for dissection purposes. Lastly, and most strange of all, the gild was to have the monopoly of making and selling aqua vitae (whisky) within the burgh, a privilege which apparently has been allowed to lapse ! It may be added that each candidate for admission was to pay a fee of £5, and to entertain to dinner the existing members of the craft. Unfortunately no record of the meetings was kept until 1581. At this date the business was in the capable hands of GILBERT PRIMROSE, or Prymross (1535–1616), who was, in 1581–82, and again in 1602, elected Deacon, as the President was then called.

---

[1] J. D. Comrie, *History of Scottish Medicine*, 2 vols., 1932, vol. i. p. 83
[2] C. H. Creswell, *The Royal College of Surgeons of Edinburgh* (*Historical Notes from 1505 to 1905*), Edinburgh, 1926, p. 4

Unfortunately he left no writings, and we know little of his career. He was a member of the well-known family of which Lord Rosebery is now the chief representative. Primrose appears to have compounded his own drugs. In 1904 Lord Rosebery presented to the Royal College of Surgeons of Edinburgh a replica of a mortar, bearing the name of Gilbert Primrose, which had been found in a field near Hawick. The replica is now preserved in the College Museum.

A contemporary Scottish surgeon, better known on account of his authorship, was PETER LOWE of Glasgow (1550–1612).[1] His chief work, *A Discourse of the Whole Art of Chirurgerie*, 1597, was dedicated to his friend Gilbert Primrose, and it is said to be the first textbook of surgery to be written in English (Plate XXIX). Lowe was a native of Glasgow who had spent more than twenty years in France and Flanders as a student and army surgeon, and had then returned to practise in his native city.[2] He was an apostle of medical reform who, noting the prevalence of ignorant practitioners and the lack of organization within the profession, did not rest until he had obtained from King James VI, in 1599, a charter for the Faculty of Physicians and Surgeons of Glasgow, which still exists, the prefix Royal being added in 1909. The purpose of this body was to unite all who practised medicine or surgery, and not merely the surgeons and barber surgeons, as in London and Edinburgh.

The Faculty was empowered to examine candidates, and to control practice in Glasgow and the south-west of Scotland. This authority remained in the hands of the Faculty until the Medical Register was established. It was unquestioned until early in the nineteenth century, when the University of Glasgow, although it did not then grant a surgical degree, claimed for its graduates in medicine the privilege of practising surgery, as well as medicine, within the area. The Faculty, resenting such interference with their rights, raised an action in the Court of Session in 1815 against four general practitioners of Glasgow, graduates of the four Scottish Universities, with a view to having them interdicted from the practice of surgery. The view of the Faculty was upheld, it being decided that the offenders, although all entitled to practise medicine, were not legally qualified to practise surgery in or near Glasgow until they had passed an examination by the Faculty. The University then introduced the degree of Master of Surgery, but in 1826 the Faculty raised another action with a view to interdicting those holding this degree. Again judgment was given in their favour, although only after a law suit lasting fourteen years, during which the University was obliged to meet heavy expenses on behalf of its graduates. All those polemics were soon forgotten, as the Medical Act of 1858 changed the entire outlook by transferring to the General Medical Council the responsibility of deciding who should be permitted to practise.

One of the original functions of this Faculty of Glasgow established by Peter Lowe was the provision of free treatment for the poor, or, as the Charter states, " to give counsell to puir disaisit folk gratis." This practice continued for two centuries. Then, as hospitals became available, free vaccination took the place of free treatment, and this was provided throughout the nineteenth century. Even to this day the spirit of the foundation is kept alive in word, if not actually in deed, as the minutes of each meeting conclude with the phrase, " The poor were treated gratis, and the Faculty adjourned."

[1] A. F. Fergus, *The Origin and Development of the Glasgow School of Medicine from Maister Peter Lowe to Sir William T. Gairdner*, Glasgow, 1911
[2] A. Duncan, *Memorials of the Faculty of Physicians and Surgeons of Glasgow (1599–1850)*, Glasgow, 1896, p. 21

BOOKS FOR FURTHER READING

BALL, J. M.   *Andreas Vesalius, the Reformer of Anatomy*, St. Louis, 1910
BUCK, A. H.   *The Growth of Medicine from the Earliest Times to 1800*, Yale, 1917
CRESWELL, C. H.   *The Royal College of Surgeons of Edinburgh (Historical Notes from 1505 to 1905)*, Edinburgh, 1926
FERGUS, A. F.   *The Origin and Development of the Glasgow School of Medicine from Maister Peter Lowe to Sir William Gairdner*, Glasgow, 1911
MACCURDY, E.   *The Notebooks of Leonardo da Vinci*, 2 vols., 1938
McMURRICH, J. P.   *Leonardo da Vinci the Anatomist*, Baltimore, 1930
MICHELET, LEON.   *La Vie d'Ambroise Paré*, Paris, 1930
PACKARD, F. R.   *The Life and Times of Ambroise Paré*, 2nd ed., New York, 1926
PAGET, STEPHEN.   *Ambroise Paré and his Times (1510–1590)*, 1897
PARKER, G.   *The Early History of Surgery in Great Britain*, 1920
ROTH, M.   *Andreas Vesalius Bruxellensis*. (In German.)   Berlin, 1892
SINGER, C.   *The Evolution of Anatomy*, 1925
SOUTH, J. F.   *Memorials of the Craft of Surgery in England*, 1886
SPIELMANN, M. H.   *The Iconography of Andreas Vesalius*, 1925
TAYLOR, H. O.   *Thought and Expression in the Sixteenth Century*, 1930
WILLIS, R.   *Servetus and Calvin*, 1877

CHAPTER IX

PHYSICIANS OF THE RENAISSANCE

HAVING now traced the spread of Renaissance surgery from the days of Ambroise Paré to those of Peter Lowe, let us turn back and attempt to follow the progress of Renaissance medicine. The leader in the revolt against the past and the search for new and better methods was that strange man known as Paracelsus.

The Enigma of Paracelsus

It is difficult to assess at its true value the influence of Paracelsus upon the progress of medicine.[1] He had many opponents during his lifetime, and for centuries after his death the prevailing opinion classed him as a charlatan, a mere drunken quack and disreputable braggart, while the more kindly critics said that he was of unsound mind.[2] In the nineteenth century, however, Robert Browning wrote a poem on Paracelsus, in which he discusses the greatness of a reformer who had been misunderstood. Osler designates Paracelsus " the Luther of Medicine," and Garrison calls him " the most original thinker of the sixteenth century," which is praise indeed. Withington, on the other hand, regards him as a mere trumpet blower, " vastly inferior to Vesalius or Harvey." It must be admitted that the writings of Paracelsus are by no means easy to understand. They are highly appraised by German medical historians, notably by Sudhoff,[3] but the complexity of his theories, and the fact that no complete English translation is available, places Paracelsus beyond the comprehension of the average student, and tends to perpetuate this unpopularity.[4]

Philippus Aureolus Theophrastus Bombastus von Hohenheim, better known as PARACELSUS (1493-1541),[5] was born at Einsiedeln,

[1] J. R. Russell, *History and Heroes of the Art of Medicine*, 1891, p. 157
[2] H. E. Sigerist, "Paracelsus in the Light of Four Hundred Years," in *March of Medicine*, New York, 1941
[3] K. Sudhoff, *Paracelsus : ein deutsches Lebensbild aus den Tagen der Renaissance*, Leipzig, 1936 ; *Paracelsus : Sämtliche Werke*, ed. K. Sudhoff, 12 vols., Jena, 1926-32
[4] F. Medicus, " The Scientific Significance of Paracelsus," *Bull. Hist. Med.* 1936, vol. iv. p. 353
[5] Anna M. Stoddart, *Life of Paracelsus*, 1911

PLATE XXXI MEDICINE AND MATHEMATICS

Jerome Cardan of Milan (pages 161–64)

Horoscope of Archbishop Hamilton of St. Andrews,
drawn by Cardan during his visit to Scotland in
1552 (page 162)

PLATE XXXII   CAIUS COLLEGE, CAMBRIDGE

The Gate of Honour (page 168)

near Zurich, the son of a studious and well-educated country doctor who had married the matron of the local pilgrim hospital. When the boy was nine years old, his father was appointed town physician of Villach in Carinthia. Near this place were the Fugger lead mines, where Paracelsus was first attracted to mineralogy and chemistry, assisting in the laboratory and laying the foundation of his later work. He is said to have attended the University of Basel, but we have no record of his student days. What we do know is that at the age of twenty-three he set out on the long wanderings which were to last for twelve years. " The doctor must be a traveller," he wrote, " because he must inquire of the world." Experience must be added to experiment.

He spent some time in Montpellier, and at the Italian centres of learning, Bologna and Padua. Then he travelled far and wide throughout Europe. He visited France and Spain, he saw military service in the Netherlands, he visited the tin mines of Cornwall, explored the mineral wealth of Sweden, and journeyed as far east as Turkey and Russia. During those years he was busily engaged in writing and teaching when he could, so that he became well known, and on his return to Switzerland in 1526 he was appointed, through the influence of Erasmus, town physician at Basel, and Lecturer on Medicine in the University. There, he allowed his intolerance to outweigh his discretion, and incurred the grave displeasure of the authorities by lecturing in German instead of Latin, by compounding his own medicines, and by his vehement condemnation not only of the ancient writers but of the methods of his colleagues and contemporaries. " I pleased no one," he writes, " except the sick whom I healed." He prefixed his lectures by publicly burning the works of Galen and Avicenna, holding that a complete break from the past was essential to progress. " My beard knows more than you and your writers ; my shoe-buckles are more learned than Galen or Avicenna."

Paracelsus did not favour the velvet robe of the physician, but chose simple garments, and he carried a sword, which, it is said, he was wont to brandish in the privacy of his study, and which appears in several of his portraits.[1] One is not surprised to learn that by his impetuous and forceful iconoclasm

---

[1] C. G. Cumston, " The Portrait of Parcelsus at the Museum at St. Gall, Switzerland," *Proc. Roy. Soc. Med.* 1916, vol. ix. p. 113

he made many enemies, and that within two years, the contention having culminated in a dispute regarding fees, he was obliged to leave Basel and to resume his wanderings. We find him at Colmar, at St. Gallen, at Zurich, and at other places, in each of which he practised with great success, acquiring, despite much opposition, a European reputation. Eventually in 1541 he reached Salzburg, worn out with strenuous work in the search, not for gold or rank, but for knowledge and truth. His travels were ended, and he died there on September 24, 1541.

Paracelsus as a Writer

Whatever side one takes in the controversy, which still continues, regarding the character and influence of Paracelsus, one is bound to admit that he was one of the most interesting figures in the medicine of the Renaissance.[1] He was a voluminous writer, although but little of his work was published during his lifetime. He himself predicted that he would not be understood until at least twenty years after his death, and it was so, for the first edition of his works, edited by J. Huser of Basel, did not appear until 1591.

Much that he did not write has been attributed to him. Some of it was written by the " Paracelsists," who, notably in England and Germany, carried on his teaching for a century or more. Many of those were members of that curious sect known as Rosicrucians, said to have been founded by a monk called Rosenkreuz, now known to be a fictitious person. The leading exponent in England was an alchemist, ROBERT FLUDD (1574-1637).[2]

A book entitled The Triumphal Chariot of Antimony (1604), which resulted in a vogue for that metal as a medicament, was said to have been written in the fourteenth century by a monk, Basil Valentine. His reality has never been confirmed, and some attribute the book to Thölde [3] the publisher, while others even suggest it is the work of Paracelsus.[4]

[1] K. Sudhoff, " The Literary Remains of Paracelsus," in Essays in the History of Medicine, trans. F. H. Garrison, New York, 1926, p. 275
[2] J. B. Craven, The Life and Writings of Robert Fludd, 1902 ; H. Jennings, The Rosicrucians, Their Rites and Mysteries, 1887
[3] John Read, Prelude to Chemistry, 1936
[4] A. C. Wootton, Chronicles of Pharmacy, 2 vols., 1910, vol. i. pp. 224, 376

A Chemical View of Life

It is not easy to epitomize the teaching of Paracelsus, and in any case no useful purpose would be served by discussing at length the obscure and now completely obsolete ideas that flowed from his pen. A brief outline will suffice. In his principal work, which he called the " Paramirum," he stated that man was composed of three elements—sulphur, mercury, and salt.[1] " What burns is sulphur, what smokes is mercury, the ashes are salt." Every action of the body depends upon the proportions and actions of these principles, and all disease is the result of maladjustment of the three, and may be cured by one of them or by its derivatives. Basically, therefore, there were only three diseases and three remedies.

To our modern ears all this sounds nonsensical, but at least it must be admitted that Paracelsus simplified prescribing. While there is no need to elaborate the doctrine of the three principles, reference must be made to another important foundation of Paracelsian teaching. He alleged that all medicines rested upon four pillars or columns : philosophy, astronomy, alchemy, and virtue. Philosophy was the gate of medicine ; all who entered by other ways were thieves or murderers. Astronomy was essential ; the path to true therapy was in the heavens. Alchemy was needful, to prepare the essential remedies for disease. Virtue was the most important of all, though it was given to only a few physicians to understand the ways of Providence. [2]

By the pillar of philosophy Paracelsus implied knowledge of natural phenomena, as he was a true follower of Hippocrates in his insistence upon observation as opposed to theorizing. He was fond of coining words, and he gave the name " archaeus " to " the heart of the elements," the natural renovating and reparative mechanism of the human body. He despised anatomy, and failed to see how any knowledge could be gained from the dead body, but it must be remembered that it was some years before Vesalius changed the outlook and made of anatomy a living science.

The astronomy of Paracelsus, his second pillar, was not the astrology of the time. Although he admitted that life upon this earth was influenced by the stars, he did not agree that they controlled the destiny of individuals, nor did he believe in horoscopes.

[1] D. Riesman, *The Story of Medicine in the Middle Ages*, New York, 1935, p. 338
[2] B. Telepnef, *Paracelsus, a genius amidst a troubled world*, St. Gallen, 1945

The third pillar, that of alchemy, which he practised, was not a search for the philosopher's stone, but rather an attempt to explain health and disease in terms of chemistry.[1] He stated that the aim of the alchemist was to separate poison from food, for if this was not accomplished, the poison became deposited upon the teeth, or in the organs. To this deposit he applied the name " tartar " and he held that it was the cause of gout and of stone.

As for the fourth pillar, virtue, this was the most potent healing factor of all. The physician must be a God-fearing man, for medicine was more than a collection of facts. There was a spiritual side of healing, and " just as the lily produces invisible perfume, so does the invisible body send forth its healing influence." Only faith in God, he alleged, could prevent such influence from being evil. Surely the man who could write thus was more than " a mere drunken sot," as Paracelsus is termed by one of his opponents.

It is said that he believed in the weapon salve, or " powder of sympathy," that strange practice, extolled later by Sir Kenelm Digby, of applying certains drugs to the weapon that caused a wound rather than to the wound direct. Reference has already been made to this curious mode of treatment (p. 14). It was sometimes a dangerous theory ; Van Helmont suffered imprisonment for stating that this was the reason for the cures wrought by relics of the saints.

Paracelsus also believed in the doctrine of " signatures " or " similars." For example, the plant cyclamen was used for ear diseases because the leaf resembles the human ear. The lungs of foxes were used for lung diseases, a yellow remedy was the treatment for jaundice, and so on. But those ideas played no great part in his system of treatment. Medicine is indebted to him for the introduction of iron, antimony, mineral salts, and other inorganic substances into therapeutics. He sought out the " quintessence " of his remedies, or " active principles " as we now call them. There has been much controversy regarding the " laudanum " which was one of his favourite remedies, and no definite conclusion has been reached, save that it was not the opium preparation known to us.[2] His surgery was sound as far as it went, and although to his mind lithotomy was the only

[1] H. Redgrove, *Alchemy, Ancient and Modern*, 2nd ed., 1911, p. 58
[2] A. C. Wootton, *Chronicles of Pharmacy*, 2 vols., 1910, vol. i. p. 243 ; H. E. Sigerist, " Laudanum in the Works of Paracelsus," *Bull. Hist. Med.*, 1941, vol. ix. p. 530

operation which was justified, he pointed out Nature's method of healing wounds by sealing the edges with a natural " balsam " manufactured by the body.

The Mission of Paracelsus

Whatever view one may take regarding the personal character of Paracelsus and his contribution to medical progress, one is bound to admit that he must have given a powerful stimulus to original thought, for he was nothing if not original. His motto, which is inscribed beneath many of his portraits, was the following :

> Eins andern Knecht soll niemand seyn
> Der für sich bleyben kann alleyn,

or, as translated by Mrs. Stoddart in her excellent work : [1]

> That man no other man shall own
> Who to himself belongs alone.

Paracelsus was not a Vesalius nor yet a Harvey. He may have suffered from congenital syphilis, as has been stated, and he may have been addicted to alcohol. He certainly was boastful, intolerant, and injudicious, and he exemplified the Philistine in medicine. Yet he was sincere and honest, and even pious in his own way. A mystic and an enigma, he has been misinterpreted and misunderstood ; nevertheless he will always remain one of the great figures of medical history.

Our account of Paracelsus may fitly conclude with the words, put into his mouth by Robert Browning :

> If I stoop
> Into a dark tremendous sea of cloud,
> It is but for a time ; I press God's lamp
> Close to my breast ; its splendour, soon or late,
> Will pierce the gloom : I shall emerge one day.

Astrology, Algebra, and Medicine

While Paracelsus was blowing the trumpet of criticism and brandishing the sword of reform in Switzerland, there lived in Italy a versatile scholar who, though now almost forgotten, was the most popular philosopher and the most fashionable physician of the sixteenth century.

JEROME CARDAN (Hieronymus Cardanus, 1501–76), (Plate XXXI), was born in Milan, and according to his horoscope, to

[1] Anna M. Stoddart, Life of Paracelsus, 1911

which he attached great importance, an unlucky star ruled his nativity. Astrology was only one of the many interests of this paradoxical character, whose views represent a mixture of mediæval absurdity and Renaissance wisdom. " His life," wrote Morley,[1] " was one of the most curious on record, full of extremes and contradictions, the most wonderful sense and the wildest nonsense." His unhappy childhood and youth, his struggle with poverty as a country practitioner, his gambling for a livelihood, his eventual and astonishing rise from this level to that of Professor of Medicine at Bologna and Pavia, his mathematical achievements, his fame as a physician, his broken-hearted old age, following the execution of his son as a murderer, finally his death in Rome as a pensioner of the Pope ; all these details of his eventful career are recorded in the biographies of Morley and of Waters, as well as in Cardan's autobiography, *De Vita Propria Liber*, 1575, which has been translated by Jean Stoner, and which well deserves to stand alongside the better known life story of Cardan's compatriot and contemporary, Benvenuto Cellini. It is a unique document of self-revelation.

A Consultation at Edinburgh

The most interesting episode in the tragic career of Jerome Cardan was his journey to Scotland in 1552 in order to attend Archbishop Hamilton, brother of the Earl of Arran, Regent of Scotland during the minority of Mary Stuart. The archbishop was not only Primate of Scotland, but, as his brother's adviser, was virtually the ruler, and his health was an affair of national importance.[2] It is a commentary upon the backwardness of British medicine at that time that the archbishop's personal physician, a Spaniard named Cassanate, was obliged to summon a consulting physician from Italy.

Jerome Cardan spent several months in Edinburgh and at Monimail, in Fife, conducting the treatment of this case of asthma on surprisingly modern lines, with a highly successful result. Although he survived for twenty years, the unfortunate archbishop was ultimately executed for treason (Plate xxxi).

During his journey Cardan met a number of distinguished persons : in Paris, Jean Fernel the leading physician, and Sylvius

[1] H. Morley, *The Life of Girolamo Cardano of Milan, Physician*, 2 vols., 1854; W. G. Waters, *Jerome Cardan, a Biographical Study*, 1898 ; Jerome Cardan, *The Book of My Life (De Vita Propria Liber)*, trans. Jean Stoner, 1931
[2] J. D. Comrie, *History of Scottish Medicine*, 1932, vol. i. p. 179

the anatomist ; in London, the boy king Edward VI ; and in Zurich, the great naturalist Conrad Gesner.

The Versatile Physician

Jerome was an industrious author. His collected works, published by Spon of Paris a hundred years after his death, comprise ten large closely printed folios. About one-third of the material is of medical interest.

Besides the autobiography, which was his last work, he wrote a treatise on algebra which he called *The Book of the Great Art* (1545), and in which he propounds the rule for solving cubic equations. Though this was really discovered by a rival mathematician named Tartaglia, it is still known as Cardan's rule. Cardan's chief claim to fame probably rests upon his contribution to mathematics.[1] A book of very different nature, which remained unpublished until 1658, contained an account of " metoposcopy," or the significance of lines on the forehead, a study analogous to palmistry, and surely one of the most absurd and fantastic subjects of investigation. Sir Walter Scott mentions it in his novel, *The Abbot*, chapter xxxii, thus : " His learned face stooping until a physiognomist might have practised the metoposcopial science upon it."

Cardan's most popular work was *De Subtilitate* (1551), a sort of household encyclopædia, dealing with all manner of subjects, such as the marking of household linen, the raising of sunken ships, the identification of mushrooms, the origin of mountains, the twinkling of stars, signalling by torches, and the universal joint, now known as the " Cardan shaft."

De Subtilitate was Cardan's masterpiece, although now altogether obsolete. *De Vita Propria Liber* is still worth reading, as one of the quaintest literary relics of that fruitful age, especially his observations on things supernatural, for he attached great weight to dreams and omens. The little book of precepts which he wrote for the benefit of his children, *Praeceptorum Filiis Liber*, contains sound advice, such as, " Never associate with a stranger on a public road " ; " When you talk with a bad or dishonest man, look at his hands, not at his face " ; " Do not talk to other people of yourself, your children, or your wife."

[1] D. E. Smith, " Medicine and Mathematics in the Sixteenth Century," *Ann. Med. Hist.*, 1917, vol. i. p. 125

Another small work, *De Consolatione*, was the only book by Cardan translated into English during his lifetime. The translation, by Thomas Bedingfeld, is entitled *Cardanus Comforte* (1573).

Jerome Cardan's writings have attracted the attention of many scholars. Robert Burton quotes from Cardan repeatedly in his *Anatomy of Melancholy*, and Sir Thomas Browne acknowledges his great intellectual influence.

Cardan made no great discovery in medicine, and he was an empiric physician. Nevertheless, like John Hunter, by his collection of facts and clarifying of ideas, he made the path of investigation easier for others, and he well deserves to be more fully acknowledged as a great Renaissance doctor. (See Supplement, pages 455–6, for JEAN FERNEL and ANTONIO BENIVIENI.)

The Origin of Syphilis

History is punctuated by the appearance from time to time of plagues and epidemics which, however disastrous in their effects, acted as a stimulus to the medical profession. The Black Death was one such visitation ; the Sweating Sickness, as we shall see, was another. In 1495, when Charles VIII of France laid siege to Naples, there broke out in the city a new and dreadful disease, consisting of widespread skin eruptions and ulceration, with great destruction of all the tissues, causing many deaths, and persisting for years in those who survived the initial illness. It was said to have been brought to the Spanish occupants of Naples by the sailors of Christopher Columbus, who had acquired it in the West Indies.[1] The Spaniards, in turn, passed it on to the French invaders. The French called it the Neapolitan disease, the Spaniards named it the French disease, while Fracastorius was the first to apply to it the name " syphilis," which it retains to this day.[2]

Whether syphilis was known before that date is still open to argument ; certainly there is no mention of it by the ancient writers, and if it did exist it was in a mild form. In any case, it was either reactivated or introduced at the siege of Naples, where it at once assumed epidemic proportions and a severity which has never since been equalled.

[1] K. Sudhoff, " The Origin of Syphilis," in *Essays in the History of Medicine*, trans. by F. H. Garrison, New York, 1926, p. 257
[2] J. Johnston Abraham, " The Early History of Syphilis," *Brit. Jour. Surgery*, xxxii, 1944

Syphilis in Poetry

It was in 1530 that Fracastorius published "that Divine poem," written in 1521, and entitled *Syphilis, sive morbus Gallicus*.[1] HIERONYMUS FRACASTORIUS (1483–1553) was of noble family, and being thus favoured by fortune was able to devote himself to a life of study.[2] Born at Verona, he spent most of his life at his villa there, studying mathematics, geology, and astronomy, practising medicine, and adding to those serious studies the lighter pursuits of music and poetry. He was a student at Padua along with his friend Copernicus, but while Copernicus concentrated upon astronomy, Fracastorius was attracted chiefly to medicine. The poem on syphilis was his first and best known work.[3] In elegant verse modelled upon the style of Virgil, he tells of a mythical young shepherd named Syphilus, who incurred the anger of the gods by some act of impiety and was smitten with a loathsome and contagious disease.

> He first wore Buboes dreadful to the sight.
> First felt strange pains, and sleepless passed the night.
> From him the malady received its name.
> The neighbouring shepherds catch'd the spreading Flame.

There is no story in the poem. Syphilus was merely the patient on whom the poet grafted his description of syphilis, and of the treatment by mercury and guaiacum, or Holy Wood, a remedy of American origin which had accompanied the disease to Europe.

In 1519, ULRICH VON HUTTEN of Tübingen, himself a sufferer from the disease, extolled the virtue of this drug in a treatise which was translated into English twenty years later under the title, *Of the wood called guaiacum that healeth the French pockes and also helpeth the goute in the feete.*

The First Epidemiologist

Fracastorius did much more than merely describe and name syphilis. He became keenly interested in epidemic diseases, and

[1] G. L. Henrickson, "The 'Syphilis' of Girolamo Fracastoro," *Bull. Hist. Med.*, 1934, vol. ii. p. 515
[2] D. W. Montgomery, "Hieronymus Fracastorius," *Ann. Med. Hist.*, 1930, vol. ii. p. 406 ; C. and D. Singer, "The Scientific Position of Girolamo Fracastoro (?1478–1553)" *Ann. Med. Hist.*, 1917, vol. i. p. 1
[3] R. H. Major, *Classic Descriptions of Disease*, 1932, p. 37

was among the first to recognize typhus fever.[1] In 1546 he published the great work, *De Contagione*, in which he described the three methods of infection : infection by direct contact, infection by "fomites," a word which he was the first to apply to infected clothing, utensils, etc., and infection at a distance, as in smallpox or plague. The description is wonderfully modern, and although bacteria were as yet unknown, Fracastorius presumes the existence of imperceptible particles or "seminaria, the seeds of disease which multiply rapidly and propagate their like." Centuries elapsed before any practical use was made of such enlightened views, nevertheless Fracastorius must be regarded as the founder of modern epidemiology. A more genial and friendly character than either Paracelsus or Cardan, his contribution to medicine was entirely positive. His death was much lamented, and a few years later there was erected a statue to his memory, a monument which still adorns one of the principal squares of Verona.

Early Physicians of England

The new learning, born in Italy, grew slowly. Some years elapsed before it reached England. It is doubtful whether the physicians whose names will be mentioned presently were direct products of the Renaissance. They certainly revived an interest in the classics, but they remained followers of Galen, and it was not until the Elizabethan age that men like Francis Bacon, Descartes, and Galileo pointed the way to the inductive method of reasoning, and so guided science into fruitful fields. It needed the genius of William Harvey to integrate the knowledge of the past, and to fashion, step by step, the wonderful idea of the circulation of the blood. Mention has already been made of the men who raised the level of surgery in England and in Scotland to a status worthy of royal recognition. Now we must turn to those who performed a similar service for medicine.

The Royal College of Physicians

THOMAS LINACRE (1461–1524) was born in Canterbury, and after taking his degree in Oxford went to travel in Italy.[2] At

[1] A. Terson, "Sur Fracastor, son Iconographie et les Traités de la Contagion," *Bull. Soc. de l'Hist. de Méd.*, 1932, vol. xxvi. p. 171
[2] J. Aikin, *Biographical Memoirs of Medicine in Great Britain*, 1780, p. 28

Bologna he was recognized as " an elegant Latinist " ; at Florence he was fortunate in meeting Lorenzo de' Medici, who permitted him to share a tutor with his own son. At Rome, where he studied medicine, he is said to have been the first Englishman who understood Aristotle and Galen in the original Greek. On his return to Oxford he taught Greek in the university, and he was responsible for the health and education of Prince Arthur, son of Henry VII. His appointment as court physician was continued during the three successive reigns.

Linacre's greatest achievement, apart from his translations of Greek classics, was the establishment of an authoritative body to control the practice of medicine. He had noted with concern that medicine was engaging the attention of illiterate monks, often with the connivance of their bishops, and of charlatans and empirics. He therefore obtained from the king, Henry VIII, in 1518, letters patent for a body of regular physicians, which later (1551) became the Royal College of Physicians of London. This body was empowered to decide who should practise within the city or within a radius of seven miles around it, and also to examine and license practitioners throughout the kingdom. Graduates of Oxford and Cambridge were exempted. The college also had authority to examine prescriptions and drugs in apothecaries' shops, and to inflict fines and even imprisonment upon those who broke the laws. The first President of the new college was the learned Dr. Thomas Linacre. Not only was he the leading classical scholar of his day—the original, it is said, of Browning's *Grammarian*—but his skill in practice was widely recognized, and he included Erasmus among his patients. Linacre was " a hater of fraudulent dealings, sincerely faithful to his friends, and well beloved of all ranks and degrees of men." He died of stone, and was buried in St. Paul's Cathedral. The well-known portrait by Holbein may be seen in All Souls College, Oxford, of which Linacre was a Fellow.

The sister university of Cambridge may also claim a distinguished and scholarly physician of this period.[1] JOHN CAIUS, sometimes written Kaye or Keys (1510–73), a native of Norwich, became at an early age a Fellow of Gonville Hall, Cambridge, and then studied medicine at Padua, where he lodged in the same house as Vesalius. He practised medicine for a time at Norwich,

---

[1] Sir W. Langdon-Brown, "John Caius and the Revival of Learning," *Proc. Roy. Soc. Med.* (Sect. Hist.), 1941, vol. xxxv. p. 61

and at Shrewsbury, with such success that he was called to court during the reign of Henry VIII, and he remained as court physician to Edward VI, Mary Tudor, and Elizabeth. He succeeded Linacre, for whom he had a high regard, as President of the College of Physicians, which office he held for nine years. During the reign of Mary, he obtained permission to rebuild Gonville Hall as a college (1557), and this was accomplished largely through his own benefactions. Over the gates of " Gonville and Caius " college he caused to be inscribed the words, Humility, Virtue, and Honour (Plate xxxii). The later years of his life were spent as master of the college which perpetuates his name, and in the chapel of which he was buried. His tomb bears, as he had directed, the brief epitaph, " Fui Caius." A few years before his death he was subjected to some indignity when it was found that he possessed certain vestments worn in Roman Catholic ritual, and these articles were burned in public. It is said that his life was shortened by this demonstration of religious intolerance.

Oxford v. Cambridge

Caius was a diligent author. His works include Latin versions of Galen, treatises on the pronunciation of Greek and Latin, on rare plants of Britain, *De Ephemera Britannica*, on the antiquity of Cambridge, and a quaint volume on British dogs, *De Canibus Britannicis*, which he wrote at the request of his friend Conrad Gesner of Zurich, " the German Pliny," who died of plague in 1565. The history of Cambridge was his contribution to a wordy contest with the rival University of Oxford regarding priority of foundation. When Queen Elizabeth visited Cambridge in 1564, the public orator, rather unwisely, claimed superior antiquity for Cambridge. This called forth a spirited challenge from one Thomas Caius of Oxford who stated that his Alma Mater was founded by Alfred the Great in A.D. 870. Cambridge found her champion in one John Caius (apparently no relation), who sought to prove that Cambridge had been a seat of learning since the days of a Spanish Prince named Cantaber in 394 B.C., and therefore antedated Oxford by more than a thousand years. The arguments of both sides are now regarded as completely mythical.

The Sweating Sickness

Caius' principal contribution to medical literature is the classical account of that remarkable disease, the English Sweat, or Sweating Sickness, which ravaged the country in a series of severe epidemics, one of which occurred in 1551 while Caius was practising at Shrewsbury.[1] It is greatly to his credit that he wrote *A Boke of Conseill against the Disease commonly called the Sweat or Sweating Sickness*, 1552, because other physicians, finding no mention of the disease by the Greek writers, had viewed it with singular hopelessness.[2] Caius, although he also strove to explain the illness as a corruption of the humours, wrote a direct and popular book, which is the only good contemporary account of the Sweat. He blamed the gross and unhygienic mode of life of the time, and he gave sound advice, claiming no specific remedy as his own, though mentioning China root, guaiacum, and even theriac. The outbreak observed by Caius at Shrewsbury was the fifth and last of a series of epidemics.

The Sweating Sickness originally broke out among the soldiers of Henry VII, Earl of Richmond, who, landing from France at Milford Haven, secured a great victory at the Battle of Bosworth on August 22, 1485, and was about to ascend the throne of England, thus to inaugurate the prosperous Tudor dynasty. The epidemic spread so rapidly that it was at its height in London by the middle of September, and the coronation had to be postponed. It is said that not one in a hundred escaped; the death-rate was terrifying. Two Lord Mayors and six Aldermen died within a week, for the disease spared none ; indeed it appeared to be more severe among robust young men, and to attack the higher classes more severely than the poor. Business was at a standstill. Oxford University was closed. Thousands died, many of them while walking in the streets. Within a few weeks, however, the force of the epidemic was spent ; it vanished as quickly as it came. It swept through England, but did not spread to Scotland or Ireland, nor to the Continent.

The disease began very suddenly with shivering and violent fever, headache, lethargy, abdominal pain, and profuse perspiration. It lasted only for twenty-four hours, but many died within

[1] M. B. Shaw, " A Short History of the Sweating Sickness," *Ann. Med. Hist.*, 1933, vol. v., p. 246
[2] R. H. Major, *Classic Descriptions of Disease*, 1932, p. 149

the day, and some within the first hours of the attack. There was a characteristic stench, and sometimes a vesicular rash. Creighton in his *History of Epidemics in Britain*, quotes a contemporary description of the symptoms as " a grete swetyng and stynkyng, with redness of the face and body, and a contynued thurst, with a grete hete and hedeche because of the fumes and venoms." [1]

Among the circumstances favouring the disease, according to various historians, were excess of meat in the diet, the drinking of cider, lack of fresh vegetables, excess of clothing and especially the thick cloth caps worn by men, and—probably the most potent factor —dirty personal habits and the scarcity of soap. As for treatment, it was soon found that the only hope for the patient was to take to bed at once, in order to favour the perspiration, and to avoid chill or the least exertion. He was on no account to be permitted to sleep until the twenty-four hours had elapsed. No immunity followed, and many persons suffered from two or three or even more attacks. [2]

Epidemics occurred again in 1508, 1517, 1528, and 1551, each time during the summer months. The epidemic of 1508 was not severe, and fatal cases were not numerous, but in 1517 there was again a violent outbreak which claimed many victims all over England, and which, beginning in July, lasted until the end of the year. Moreover, it was on this occasion accompanied by other epidemic diseases ; plague, measles, and diphtheria took heavy toll of those who survived the sweating sickness.

The most severe epidemic of all appeared in May 1528, and not only did it spread rapidly with a very high mortality, but contrary to its usual habit it spread to Northern Europe during 1529 with severe malignity. From Hamburg it spread through Germany to the Netherlands and to the Scandinavian countries. Once again it vanished as quickly as it came.

The final visitation, which began in Shrewsbury in April 1551, was also a severe pestilence. Nine hundred persons died in that town within a few days ; " No one thought of his daily occupations, women filled the streets with lamentations and loud prayers, and funeral bells tolled day and night." " The disease came completely without warning ; at table, on journeys, at all times of the day, and had lost none of its old malignity, so that many died within an hour or two."

[1] C. Creighton, *A History of Epidemics in Britain*, 2 vols., 1891–94
[2] J. F. K. Hecker, *The Epidemics of the Middle Ages*, trans. B. G. Babington, Sydenham Society, 1844, p. 181

This was the epidemic described by John Caius in his famous pamphlet, the last outbreak of a strange disease, the nature of which has often been discussed, but never satisfactorily explained. It was not influenza, nor was it a modified form of typhus. Had it occurred to-day, it would probably have been classed as one of the virus infections.

Long after the sweating sickness disappeared from England, there broke out in Northern France an epidemic of what was known as the Picardy Sweat, or " Suette des Picards." Appearing first in 1718, it returned almost every year for the next century. The symptoms resembled those of English Sweat, but lasted longer. A rash appeared within two days, and desquamation followed about a week later. In some respects it resembled malignant scarlet fever, but there was no sign of throat infection. It is now generally conceded that both diseases were " miliary fevers," allied to rheumatic fever.

Early English Medical Books

Our brief study of Renaissance medicine may be suitably concluded by a short account of a few contemporary works, which were among the first medical books printed in English and in England. Although none of them bears the stamp of originality, all are of interest as examples of current medical practice, and they appear to demonstrate clearly that not until the time of William Harvey did the renaissance of medicine exercise much influence in Britain. Garrison, in his well-known history,[1] remarks that the first medical work to be printed in England was a little plague tract entitled, *A Passing Gode Lityll Boke Necessarye and Behovefull Against the Pestilence* (*cf.* p. 128). It was a translation from Bishop Kanutus of Västernås, Sweden (1461), who in turn had copied it from Johannes Jacobi of Montpellier (1364). The copy in the John Rylands Library, Manchester, reproduced in facsimile in 1910, consists of ten pages. It has no titlepage, and it commences in the following manner : " Here begynneth a litil boke the whiche traytied and reherced many gode thinges necessaries for the infirmite a grete sekeness called Pestilence the whiche often times enfecteth us made by the most expert Doctour in phisike Bisshop of Arusiens in the realme of Denmark."

It is believed to have been printed in London in 1485 by

---

[1] F. H. Garrison, *History of Medicine*, 3rd ed., 1924, p. 195

Willelmus de Machlina (of Malines, in Brabant), who had set up a printing press in Holborn. Only two other copies are known ; one is in the British Museum, the other in Cambridge University Library. The work was originally written about 1461–63, just after Sweden had been devastated by plague, and the author was Knutsson, Bishop of Arusiens or Arosias, the Latin name of Västerås, near Stockholm. There is a Latin edition of the little book, dated 1494, in the Royal College of Physicians of London. The earliest original medical work to be printed in Scotland, at Edinburgh in 1568, was *Ane Breve Description of the Pest*, by Gilbert Skene, who practised in Aberdeen and then in Edinburgh. The only copy extant is in the National Library of Scotland.

In the opinion of some authorities, the first *original* English medical book to be printed was *The Breviarie of Health*, by Andrew Boorde, which appeared in 1547 (?1542) (Plate xxxiii).

ANDREW BOORDE (1490–1549), or Andreas Perforatus (bored) as he called himself, was rather an odd character. Physician, traveller, and sometime Carthusian monk, he was educated at Oxford, and led a roving life " in and through and around all Christendom," so he tells us. He studied medicine at Montpellier, which he designated " the noblest university of the world for physicians and surgeons," and he visited many other places on the continent and in Britain. It was said that during his travels he was wont to make humorous speeches at fairs and markets, and that he was the original " Merry Andrew." [1] Some regard this as a myth ; in any case, it would be a capital mistake to class Andrew Boorde as a buffoon. As one of the physicians to Henry VIII he had a good standing at court. His writings, though witty, are also wise, and show that he was a man of considerable learning. These works include, *The Introduction of Knowledge*, *The Dyetary of Health*, and *The Breviarie of Health*. The first-named is a most interesting treatise, dealing with each of the countries he visited ; also with " the naturall disposycion of the people and theyr speche." As one of the objects of the book is " to teach a man to speake parte of all maner of languages," in truly modern fashion he appends lists of phrases in many tongues, including Cornish, Welsh, Castilian, Dutch, Hebrew, and Romany Gipsy (this is the first printed example of the Gipsy language). He spent a year in

---

[1] R. C. Buist, " Andrew Boorde," *Caled. Med. Jour.*, vol. xi. p. 292 ; Douglas Guthrie, " The ' Breviarie ' and ' Dyetary ' of Andrew Boorde," *Proc. Roy. Soc. Med.* (Sect. Hist.), vol. xxxvii. Dec. 1, 1943

Scotland, at " a lityle unyuersyte named Glasco, where I study and practyse physyk for the sustentacyion off my lyvyng," but it is evident that he did not love the Scots. " Trust no Skott," he wrote, " they youse flatteryng wordes and all ys falshode."

The *Dyetary* deals not only with food and drink, in health and in sickness, but with the choice of a house, the best use of one's income, and such aspects of personal hygiene as clothing, exercise, and sleep. He counsels his readers to keep their bedroom windows closed, to sleep on the right side with the head high, and to wear " a skarlet nyght-cap."

" The Breviarie of Health "

From the medical standpoint, the *Breviarie* is Boorde's most interesting work. Brevity was the keynote in the mind of the author of this little household medical dictionary, " for," said he, " if I should write all my mynde, everie bongler would practise Phisicke uppon my booke." The writing of it was a labour of love ; Boorde " did never look for no reward, neither of Lord nor of Printer nor of no man living, nor will I never have none as long as I do live, God helping me " (Plate xxxiii).

Some idea of the contents of this quaint volume may be gathered from the following extracts. Writing on " Spleen," he proceeds thus : " Spleen is the Greek word, in Latin it is Liena. In Englysche it is named a man's splene, a spongious substance lienge under the ribbes on the left side, and it doth make a man to bee mery and to laughe, although melancholy resteth in the splene if there be impedimentes in it. If any man be splenitike let him use mery company, be joconde, and not to study upon any supernatural thynges." " Let him be bloud of a veyne named Basilica on the left side."

There is a chapter on " Lowsiness," which begins, " Pediculacio or Morbus pediculorum be the Latin wordes. In Greek it is Phthiriasis. In Englysche it is named lowsiness, and there be foure kyndes, head lyce, body lyce, crabbe lyce, and nits. This impediment doth come by unclene kepynge or lyenge with lousy persons or in a lousy bedde or the not changynge of a mannes sherte." The Breviarie also has chapters on Drunkenness, Tears, Music, Woman, Pestilence, and many another subject.

Andrew Boorde's works are still well worth reading. Several have been excellently edited for the Early English Text Society by F. J. Furnivall (1870).

Pediatrics in England

About the same time as Boorde there lived a physician named THOMAS PHAER, or Phayre (1510–60), of whom we know little, save that he was originally a lawyer in London before he took to medicine, and that he wrote *The Boke of Children*, which was published in 1545, and was the first English work on Pediatrics [1] (see page 367). Aikin, in his medical biographies,[2] states that it was a translation from the French. It shows no originality, but it is a good compilation of all that was known of the subject. Here are fragments of Phaer's advice : " To procure easy breding of teeth, annoint the gummes with the braynes of a hare mixed with capon's grece and hony." The cause of " terrible dreames and feare in the slepe " is " the arysyng of the stynking vapours out of the stomake into the fantasye and sences of the brayne," and the treatment consists in giving " honey and powdered seeds of peony," after which one must not rock or move the infant too much, for " overmuch shaking maketh the chylde to vomyte."

" The Byrth of Mankynde "

The first English printed book on midwifery was a translation of Eucharius Roesslin's *Rosgarten, Der schwangern frawen und hebammen roszgarten*, a work which enjoyed a very wide circulation and was translated into many languages.[3] Roesslin, or Rhodion, was a medical man who practised in Worms and then in Frankfort-on-Main, and his book was the first separate work on midwifery to be printed. It appeared in 1513. An improved version, entitled *De conceptu et generatione hominis*, was published in 1554 by Jacob Rueff. One of the woodcuts is reproduced in Plate xxxiv. It was from the Latin version of Roesslin's book, which had appeared in 1532 under the title *De Partu Hominis*, by E. Rhodion, that the English translation, entitled *The Byrth of Mankynde*, was prepared by THOMAS RAYNALDE in 1545. The first edition of *The Byrth of Mankynde*, of which the British Museum possesses the only copy known to exist, was the work of Richard Jonas. It is dated 1540, and marked, " Imprynted at London by T.R.,"

[1] G. F. Still, *A History of Pædiatrics*, 1931, p. 108 ; J. Foote, " Ancient Poems on Infant Hygiene," *Ann. Med. Hist.*, 1919, vol. ii. p. 216
[2] J. Aikin, *Biographical Memoirs of Medicine in Great Britain*, 1700, p 78
[3] I. S. Cutter, Historical Chapter in *Obstetrics and Gynaecology*, ed. by A. H. Carter, Philadelphia, 1933, p. 5

presumably Thomas Raynalde.[1] Subsequent editions, fourteen in number, between 1545 and 1676, according to Ballantyne,[2] who made a careful bibliographical study of the work, all bear the name of Thomas Raynalde, although it is uncertain whether there were two men of this name, one a printer, the other a physician. All the editions are now very rare. The book is illustrated by anatomical drawings from the *Fabrica* of Vesalius, by a series of " Byrth Fygures " depicting the various positions of the child in the uterus, and by a woodcut showing a birth stool (The Woman's Stoole). *The Byrth of Mankynde* maintained its place as a textbook of midwifery until the eighteenth century.

We shall have occasion to note in the next chapter that William Harvey not only solved the problem of the circulation of the blood, but also made the first original contribution to British midwifery (p. 183). It was he who really brought the Renaissance to Britain.

[1] J. L. Miller, "Renaissance Midwifery. The Evolution of Modern Obstetrics (1500–1700)," in *Mayo Foundation Lectures on the History of Medicine*, Philadelphia, 1933.
[2] J. W. Ballantyne, *The Byrth of Mankynde : Its Author, Editions, and Contents*, 1907. (Reprinted from *Journ. of Obst. and Gynaecol. of the British Empire*, 1906 and 1907.)

BOOKS FOR FURTHER READING

CARDAN, JEROME. *The Book of My Life (De Vita Propria Liber)*, trans. J. Stoner, 1931
CREIGHTON, C. *A History of Epidemics in Britain*, 2 vols., 1891–94
FURNIVALL, F. J. Ed. of *The Introduction and Dyetary of Andrew Boorde*, Early English Text Society, 1870
HECKER, J. F. K. *The Epidemics of the Middle Ages*, trans. B. G. Babington, Sydenham Society, 1844
MACMICHAEL, W. *Lives of British Physicians*, 1830
MACNALTY, Sir A. S. *The Renaissance and its Influence on English Medicine* (Thomas Vicary Lecture), 1945
MAJOR, R. H. *Classic Descriptions of Disease*, 1932
MORLEY, H. *The Life of Girolamo Cardano of Milan, Physician*, 2 vols., 1854
STILL, G. F. *A History of Pediatrics*, 1931
STODDART, ANNA M. *Life of Paracelsus*, 1911
SUDHOFF, K. *Paracelsus ; ein deutsches Lebensbild aus den Tagen der Renaissance*, Leipzig, 1936
WATERS, W. G. *Jerome Cardan, a Biographical Study*, 1898
WOOTTON, A. C. *Chronicles of Pharmacy*, 2 vols., 1910

CHAPTER X

WILLIAM HARVEY AND HIS TIMES.
XVII-CENTURY MEDICINE

THE seventeenth century was a period of intense intellectual activity in all the arts and sciences.[1] In the realm of medicine it was indeed a golden age. New ideas took root and flourished, new discoveries were made and adopted. There was a general feeling of dissatisfaction with the past, and a thirst for fresh knowledge. Nevertheless, during the period of transition old methods and concepts persisted, so that we find Sir Theodore Turquet of Mayerne, the most fashionable physician of his day, still making use of theriac and of a decoction of earthworms, the great Sir Thomas Browne still believing in witches, many distinguished practitioners still regarding the stars as potent influences in the control of health and diseases, and, as every student of Shakespeare knows, the Galenic pathology of the " humours " still holding its own.

The conservative worshippers of Galen and his school were, however, far outnumbered by the seekers after new truths, some of whom in their eagerness to find something to replace antiquated notions constructed " systems," which in turn became obsolete.

Among the unbiased investigators of the seventeenth century there stands forth the noble figure of William Harvey, who by his genius and insight revolutionized medical science. Before referring to Harvey's achievement, it may be interesting to glance at the philosophical and scientific background which existed during the early part of this great century of medical progress.

Philosophers and Scientists

The reform of philosophy was a necessary prelude to scientific discovery. Bacon and Descartes were among the reformers. Each stated his views with caution, not desiring to become a martyr for truth, yet each made a valuable contribution to the sum of human knowledge, and both were actuated by utilitarian motives.

[1] Basil Willey, *The Seventeenth-Century Background*, 1934

PLATE XXXIII "THE BREVIARIE OF HEALTH"

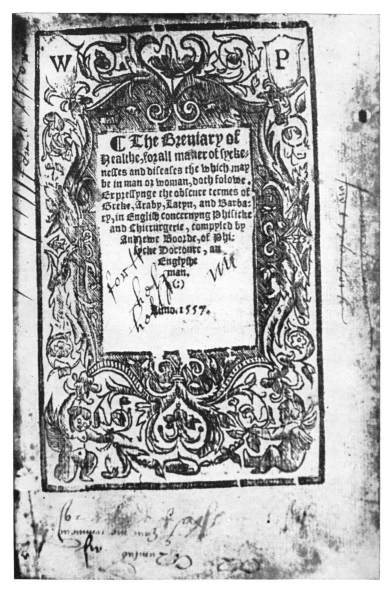

Title-page of the 1557 edition of Andrew Boorde's *Breviarie of Health.* From the copy in the Hunterian Library of Glasgow University (pages 172–73)

PLATE XXXIV BIRTH SCENE IN THE SIXTEENTH CENTURY

PRIMVS.   3

CAPVT II.

De mixtura vtriusque sexus seminis, eius q̃ substantia & forma.

Postquam autem vterus, quod genitale fœminei sexus membrum est,
viri genituram conceperit, suum quoque semen illi admiscet, ita vt ex

A 3   ambobus

Woodcut from Rueff's *De Conceptu et Generatione Hominis*, showing the patient,
seated on a birth stool, attended by three midwives. At the window in the background an astrologer is casting the horoscope of the child about to be born.
From the copy in Edinburgh University Library (page 174)

FRANCIS BACON, Lord Verulam (1561–1626),[1] philosopher and statesman, has often been compared with his greater namesake, Roger Bacon (p. 120), to whom he makes no reference in his writings. Both were antagonistic to the current methods of scholarship, both favoured experiment as opposed to argument, and both spurred men on to think for themselves, to make experiments, and to hold fast to facts. Truth, they argued, was not derived from authority but from experience. Roger was a scientist as well as a philosopher ; Francis was content to point the way and to leave scientific verification to others. The legal training of a Lord Chancellor, which admitted of no imagination, was not the best preparation for a scientist. Consequently Francis Bacon was well content merely to " ring the bell which called the wits together." Nor did he found any new school of philosophy, as Descartes did. Nevertheless he was a man of great wisdom and learning who expressed the new spirit of the age. He simply revived the Platonic method of reasoning. In his *Novum Organum* (1620) he urged men to abandon the four " idols " —accepted authority, popular opinion, legal bias, and personal prejudice—and to replace them by the " inductive " method of reasoning based upon experience.[2] Naturally, this " great secretary of nature," as Isaak Walton called him, was bound to affect the march of scientific endeavour. His immediate influence was not great ; indeed, his ideas were not generally adopted until the following century, but science and medicine must have been influenced to some extent by this philosopher, whom Pope, apparently with mixed feelings, deemed " the noblest, wisest, meanest of mankind."

Far different in personal character was the austere yet kindly French philosopher, Descartes. Greater, too, was his immediate influence, for not only did he found a new school of thought, but he wrote a remarkable work on physiology, *De Homine*, which, however, was not published until some years after his death.

RENÉ DESCARTES (1596–1650) was a brilliant student who after leaving college joined the army in order to see the world, a strange calling indeed for a philosopher.[3] The main part of his life,

---

[1] G. W. Steevens, " Medical Allusions in the Writings of Francis Bacon," *Proc. Roy. Soc. Med.* (Sect. Hist.), 1913, vol. p. 76 ; J. R. Russell, *History and Heroes of the Art of Medicine*, 1861, p. 177
[2] Sir B. W. Richardson, *Disciples of Aesculapius*, 2 vols., 1896, vol. i. p. 402 (" Francis Bacon")
[3] E. S. Haldane, *Descartes, his Life and Times*, 1905

however, was spent in Holland, where he lived in seclusion for over twenty years, devoting himself to the elaboration of his ideas. Eventually he accepted an invitation from Queen Christina of Sweden to join her court, but the rigour of the climate proved too severe for him, and he died of pneumonia within a few months.

The effect of " Cartesian " philosophy upon medical science was considerable. At the commencement of his mental pilgrimage, which Descartes so delightfully describes in his *Discours de la Méthode* (1637), he endeavoured to rid his mind of all that he had previously learned, in order that he might base his opinions on a foundation wholly his own.[1] The central idea in his philosophy was that mind and matter constituted the universe, but that there was no connection between them, although by some strange reasoning he located the soul in the pineal gland of the human brain (Plate XLI). For Descartes the body was " a machine made by the hand of God : incomparably better than any machine of human invention." Animals did not possess minds and souls ; they were, in fact, mere automata. Man, on the other hand, although he likewise was a machine, was possessed of a mind which acted upon the body. The proof of the existence of mind was conscious thought. " Except our own thoughts," wrote Descartes, " there is absolutely nothing in our power." Thought could be no illusion ; indeed, nothing else was certain. The kernel of his philosophy was his famous dictum, " I think, therefore I am." Such a conception could not fail to influence medical progress, and it was peculiarly attractive to the school of " Iatro-physicists," who regarded the human body as a mechanical contrivance. Furthermore Descartes commanded the respect of medical men by his interest in physiology and in the work of Harvey, who was " the first to teach that there are small passages at the extremity of the arteries through which the blood passes into the vein and returns to the heart."

Just as the progress of medicine was influenced by philosophy, so also was it guided by science. Astronomy, which up to the time of the Renaissance had been diverted into astrological channels, had acted as a distraction and a hindrance. Copernicus had established this science on a sound basis. Tycho Brahe and his pupil Kepler had made wonderful discoveries without the aid of any telescope. Then, in the period under discussion, there

[1] R. Descartes, *A Discourse on Method* (Everyman's Library, No. 570), 1912, p. 21

appeared a versatile Italian who by his discoveries made a valuable contribution to medicine.

GALILEO GALILEI (1564–1642) did indeed study medicine, and at this period he avoided mathematics, as he felt that the two subjects might conflict.[1] Born in Pisa and educated there, he made his first great discovery before he was twenty. In the cathedral he watched the movement of a swinging lamp, compared it with the beat of his own pulse, and realized that it might be used in the recording of time.[2] Thus he discovered the principle of the pendulum. He perfected, if he did not actually invent, the telescope, and although his instrument magnified only thirty-two diameters, he showed that the Milky Way was formed of stars, that there were mountains on the moon's surface, and that there were spots on the sun which moved as that orbit rotated.[3] Such heretical discoveries could not escape the censure of the Church, and Galileo was forced to deny them on oath, though there is a legend that after his recantation he murmured, " Nevertheless, it does move." The stress which Galileo laid upon mechanics and measurement in science accelerated the discovery of various methods of diagnosis in medicine.[4]

At the very beginning of the seventeenth century there appeared the first book on physical science to be published in England. This was *De Magnete* (1600), by WILLIAM GILBERT (1540–1603). Gilbert was born in Colchester, educated at Cambridge, and practised in London, becoming physician to Queen Elizabeth and to James I, and also President of the College of Physicians.[5] His work on magnetism entitles him to be regarded as the Father of Electrical Science ; indeed, it was he who, noticing that amber could be electrified by friction, introduced the word " electricity," derived from " elektron," the Greek name for amber.

Thus did the philosophers and scientists of the seventeenth century supplant the theorizing of the Schoolmen by the practice of observation and experiment.

[1] L. Vaccaro, " Galileo Galilei," *Ann. Med. Hist.*, 1935, vol. vii. p. 372
[2] J. J. Fahie, " The Scientific Works of Galileo (1564–1642)," article in *Studies in the History and Method of Science*, ed. by C. Singer, 1921, vol. ii. p. 206
[3] L. Olschki, " The Scientific Personality of Galileo," *Bull. Hist. Med.*, 1942, vol. xii. p. 248
[4] A. Castiglioni, " Galileo Galilei and his Influence on the Evolution of Medical Thought," *Bull. Hist. Med.*, 1942, vol. xii. p. 226
[5] Sir B. W. Richardson, *Disciples of Aesculapius*, 1896, vol. i. p. 33 (" Gilbert ")

The Genius of William Harvey

There now entered upon the scene one who was to revolutionize medical science, to change the centre of outlook, and to lay the foundation of modern practice. The facts of his life and labours are so well known through the medium of many biographies and hundreds of Harveian orations that only a brief synopsis need be given.

WILLIAM HARVEY (1578–1657) was born at Folkestone, the eldest of the seven sons of Thomas Harvey, who was Mayor of Folkestone in 1600, and his wife Joan, whose tomb may still be seen in the parish church. Five of the sons became well-known men of business in London. William received a good education at the Grammar School of Canterbury and at Caius College, Cambridge. Next he proceeded to the renowned University of Padua, then at the height of its fame as a centre of medical learning.[1] Harvey spent four years at Padua, graduating with high honours as Doctor of Medicine in 1602. Representing his nation as a " councillor," he was entitled to a " stemma," or coat of arms, in the hall of the university, and Harvey's stemma, showing a hand grasping a lighted candle around which two serpents are entwined, was discovered in 1892. Among his teachers at Padua was the successor of Vesalius, Hieronymus Fabricius, who had published a work on " the little doors of the veins," *De venarum ostiolis.* Fabricius did not grasp the true significance of the valves of the veins. He thought that they simply prevented over-distension, and it was left to Harvey to show their true significance as part of his proof of the circulation of the blood [2] (Plate XXXVI).

On his return to London Harvey engaged in practice, and within a few years he became a Fellow of the College of Physicians and physician to St. Bartholomew's Hospital.[3] Under the terms of the latter appointment he was obliged to attend the poor " one day in the week through the year," and this he did in the hall of the hospital, which was heated by a great fireplace stoked with wood from the Royal forest at Windsor.

---

[1] D'Arcy Power, *William Harvey* (Masters of Medicine Series), 1897
[2] R. B. Hervey Wyatt, *William Harvey, 1578–1657*, 1924. (Almost every phase of William Harvey's life and work has been discussed by many generations of Harveian orators)
[3] Sir W. Herringham, " The Life and Times of Dr. William Harvey," *Ann. Med. Hist.*, 1932, vol. iv. pp. 109, 249, 347, 491, 575

PLATE XXXV   THE PHYSICIAN'S VISIT

Jan Steen, who was born at Leyden in 1626, was responsible for at least twenty
paintings of varying design each entitled " The Physician's Visit."   The above,
from the Stephenson Clarke Collection, is an excellent example of his work
(pages 130, 194)

PLATE XXXVI THE VALVES OF THE VEINS

Woodcut from *De venarum ostiolis*, 1603, by Fabricius, Harvey's teacher
at Padua (page 141)

Woodcuts from *De motu cordis*, 1628, where they are used by Harvey to
support his proof of the circulation of the blood (page 180)

The appointment which brought him greatest renown, however, was that of Lumleian Lecturer on Anatomy and Surgery.[1] The lectureship was founded in 1581 by Lord Lumley and Dr. Caldwell. It provided for a series of lectures, twice a week, throughout the year. The subjects differed each year until, at the end of six years, the entire course was recommenced. Each year the lecturer was " to dissect all the body of man for five days together, as well before as after dinner ; if the bodies may last so long without annoy." The " anatomies " were open to the public, and Mr. Pepys, under the date February 27, 1662, gives a spirited account of his attendance to view a dissection by Dr. Terne, a successor of Harvey. Harvey delivered his first lecture on April 16, 1616, a week before the death of Shakespeare, and he held the appointment for the next forty years. Notes of his first course are still preserved in the British Museum. Written in the very illegible hand which is favoured by so many medical men, and in a curious mixture of Latin and English, the notes show that even then Harvey had reached a conclusion regarding the circulation of the blood. " The movement of the blood," he writes, " is constantly in a circle, and is brought about by the beat of the heart." Yet it was not until twelve years later, having meantime carefully verified each proof of his discovery, that he published the full results of his great work in the little book of seventy-two pages, *Exercitatio Anatomica De Motu Cordis et Sanguinis in Animalibus*, which was printed in Frankfort in 1628.

At the outset of his career, Harvey has been described by one who knew him as a man of short stature, of dark complexion, and with keen dark eyes and hair black and curling, rapid in speech and given to gesture, and with a habit of fingering nervously the small dagger which he wore. Although Harvey was not distinguished as a clinician, he had a good practice which, however, fell away greatly when he announced his great discovery. Patients do not favour unorthodox views in a regular practitioner, however much they may condone such views in a " quack." According to the fashion of the time Harvey made his rounds on horseback, his man following him on foot.

In 1618 he was appointed Physician Extraordinary to the king, James I, whose son Charles I made him Physician in

[1] D. F. Fraser-Harris, " William Harvey's Knowledge of Literature—Classical, Medieval, Renaissance, and Contemporary," *Proc. Roy. Soc. Med.* (Sect. Hist.), 1934, vol. xxvii. p. 1099

Ordinary. Harvey was closely associated with the Court of King Charles. He attended the Duke of Lennox on a mission to France and Spain, during which he wrote to Lord Dorchester, Secretary of State, complaining of the lack of anatomical material, for he " could scarce see a dog, cow, kite, or any other bird or thing to anatomise." Some years later he accompanied the Earl of Arundel to Germany, and it was recorded by one of the gentlemen-in-waiting that during the journey, " little Dr. Harvey would be making observations of strange trees and plants," and came so near to being lost that he incurred the ambassador's displeasure.

A much more important duty was undertaken in 1633.[1] Harvey was then in attendance on the king when His Majesty journeyed to Scotland to be crowned in the Abbey Church of Holyrood and to hold court there. During the visit to Edinburgh Harvey found time to visit the Bass Rock, and in his treatise on Development he describes the solan geese, or gannets, which congregate there in such numbers. Fortunately the king was interested in Harvey's researches, for he allowed him to make observations on the deer in the royal parks [2] (Plate xxxvii). The study of comparative anatomy was highly regarded by Harvey, as it also was by John Hunter more than a century later. Harvey observed, for example, that the movement of the heart could be observed more readily in cold-blooded animals such as frogs and fishes. He ranged the entire animal kingdom for his material, and it is unfortunate that many of his writings on comparative anatomy have been lost.

Shortly after the Scottish visit he was commanded by the king to conduct a post-mortem examination of Thomas Parr, who had died at the alleged age of 153 years. Parr was a country-man of Shropshire, who had enjoyed perfect health, had married twice, first at the age of 88, and again at 120, and who, had he not come to London as a member of the household of the Earl of Arundel, might have lived still longer. Harvey found that his death was due to pleuropneumonia, brought on by the impure London atmosphere, and the sudden adoption of a high mode of living and rich diet.[3]

A few years later King Charles was faced with the troubles of the civil war, which led to his own tragic end. Harvey was

[1] W. MacMichael, *Lives of British Physicians*, 1830, p. 41
[2] J. Aikin, *Biographical Memoirs of Medicine in Great Britain*, 1780, p. 290
[3] J. Timbs, *Doctors and Patients*, 2 vols., 1873, vol. i. p. 37 (Harvey dissects Old Parr)

present at the battle of Edgehill in 1642, and it is said that he had charge of the two young princes and was reading a book not far from the battlefield, when his studies were interrupted by a stray cannon shot, so that he was obliged to " remove his station."

After the defeat of the Royalists Harvey retired to Oxford, and there continued his studies in embryology which led to the publication of his second great work, *De Generatione Animalium*, in 1651.[1] Although the main theme of the work is indicated in its title, it may also be regarded as the first original book on midwifery to be published by an English author.[2] A contemporary obstetrician, PERCIVALL WILLUGHBY (1596–1685), of Derby and London, left a manuscript on *Observations in Midwifery* which was printed for private circulation so recently as 1863. One chapter of Harvey's book on Generation, entitled " De Partu," is devoted to obstetrics. He advanced the view that the foetus assisted its own delivery by active movement, which he compared to that of the chick emerging from the egg or the butterfly from the chrysalis. He also described a case of spurious pregnancy, ending with the remark, " All my arguments could not remove that persuasion from her, till at the last all her hopes vanished into flatulency and fatness."

Harvey was now over seventy years of age, but although he was a martyr to gout his brain was active as ever. His generosity is shown by his gift at this time of a library and museum to the College of Physicians. The honour of Presidency was offered to him ; this, however, he was obliged to decline on account of age and infirmity. He died in his eightieth year on the 3rd of June 1657, and his body, uncoffined but " lapped in lead," was buried at Hempstead in Essex, some fifty miles from London.

" De Motu Cordis et Sanguinis "

The *Anatomical Treatise on the Movement of the Heart and Blood in Animals*, to quote the English title of *De Motu Cordis*, is probably the greatest book in medical literature.[3] It is dedicated to Charles I, and Harvey compares the king to the heart, the centre

---

[1] J. Needham, *A History of Embryology*, 1934, p. 112
[2] H. R. Spencer, *History of British Midwifery*, 1927, p. 1 ; A. H. Curtis, ed. of *Obstetrics and Gynaecology*, Philadelphia, 1933, p. 9
[3] D. Flourens, *Histoire de la découverte de la circulation du sang*, Paris, 1857

of all strength and power, adding that " the knowledge of his own Heart cannot be unprofitable to a King." Before Harvey's time it was known that the blood moved, but a to-and-fro motion was envisaged.[1] The dilatation or diastole of the heart and arteries was the motive power which drew the blood along, and it was believed that blood could pass from the right to the left ventricle through pores in the septum. Furthermore, the liver was regarded as the central blood organ. It is true that Cesalpino described " a perpetual movement from the vena cava through the heart to the aorta," but he still believed in the to-and-fro movement, and alleged that " the native heat," not the blood, passed from the arteries to the veins during sleep. Servetus certainly discovered the pulmonary, or lesser, circulation, but he did not by analogy suggest that there might be a systemic circulation. Vesalius had doubted whether there were pores in the septum between the ventricles, though his view was not at once accepted.

The genius of Harvey led him far beyond his predecessors.[2] He altered the entire conception of the blood system, and proved the heart to be the central motive force. Step by step, and confirming each advance by experimental proof, he built up his great discovery, so that every objection to the new idea might be met with irrefutable argument. He showed that the heart was indeed a hollow muscle, and that the blood, impelled into the arteries, gave rise to the pulse. He compared the sequence of movements to a flint-lock ; the flint, striking the steel, ignites the powder, causes the explosion, and ejects the bullet, " all in the twinkling of an eye." Proceeding, Harvey attacks another problem. Where does all the blood come from and where does it go ? The veins are not drained, nor are the arteries ruptured, as might be expected. Harvey ligated arteries and veins at various points, and noted the effect : he calculated the amount of blood expelled at each heart-beat so as to show that the entire volume of the blood would be used up within a short time, and as a result of all this careful thought and experiment he " began to think whether there might not be a motion, as it were, in a circle." In those words Harvey first introduced a new conception of the functions of the human body, just as Vesalius had given a

[1] J. J. R. Macleod, " Harvey's Experiments on Circulation," *Ann. Med. Hist.*, 1928, vol. x. p. 338
[2] Sir H. Rolleston, " Harvey's Predecessors and Contemporaries," *Ann. Med. Hist.*, 1928, vol. x. p. 323

new view of its structure. Harvey advanced no dogmatic view as to the reason why the blood circulated. He wrote that " whether for the sake of nourishment or for the communication of heat, is not certain."

Lacteals, Lymphatics, and Capillaries

Apparently Harvey did not accept the discovery of the lacteals, which had been made by GASPARE ASELLI of Cremona (1581–1626), nor the demonstration, by JEAN PECQUET in 1647, of their connection with the blood-stream.[1] This is shown in a letter written by Harvey a year after the latter discovery, in which he attributed the presence of chyle in the lacteals to " too ample a supply of nourishment." Nevertheless these two works had added greatly to the significance of Harvey's researches. Aselli's book, De lactibus sive lacteis venis, the first anatomical work to have coloured illustrations, appeared in 1627, the year before Harvey's De Motu Cordis.[2] The author describes how he noted the whitish vessels spread over the mesentery and intestine of a dog which he was dissecting. Pecquet, while still a student, completed Aselli's discovery by tracing the entire course of the lacteals, and OLOF RUDBECK, a Swedish student at Padua, discovered the lymph vessels in 1653, and distinguished them from the lacteals. (See also Supplement, page 456.)

One is not surprised to learn that the publication of De Motu Cordis gave rise to much heated controversy. Harvey treated his critics with patience and with dignity.[3] Only to one, JEAN RIOLAN of Paris, did he reply in any detail. This he did in a small book, De Circulatione Sanguinis, published in 1649. Riolan was Professor of Anatomy in Paris, and like his friend GUY PATIN, the Professor of Medicine and author of the well-known Lettres, who also questioned Harvey's work, he was an ardent supporter of Galen.[4] Nevertheless Harvey's supporters soon outnumbered his opponents and he lived to see his views accepted and applied. His discovery of the circulation was indeed an

[1] W. Stirling, Some Apostles of Physiology, 1902, p. 13
[2] E. T. Withington, Medical History from the Earliest Times, 1894, p. 400
[3] J. Donley, " Riolan and Harvey," Ann. Med. Hist., 1923, vol. v. p. 26
[4] F. R. Packard, " Guy Patin and the Medical Profession in Paris in the Seventeenth Century," Ann. Med. Hist., 1922, vol. iv. pp. 137, 251, 357 (reprinted in book form, 1924) ; J. W. Courtney, " The Multiple Personality of Dr. Guy Patin," Ann. Med. Hist., 1924, vol. vi. p. 1

immense achievement, and the method by which the results were secured was as admirable as the work itself. It has served as a model for all research scholars since that day.

There was only one link in Harvey's remarkable chain of evidence which awaited the strengthening touch of visual confirmation. Harvey knew that there was some sort of channel between the smallest arteries and the smallest veins along which the blood must pass so as to complete the circulation. The introduction of the microscope enabled MARCELLO MALPIGHI (1628–94) of Bologna to furnish the necessary evidence. In examining a frog's lung he saw a network of tiny blood-vessels which connected the venules with the arterioles. The circulation of the blood was now completely demonstrated. Malpighi made other discoveries with his primitive microscope. He was the first to describe the layers of the skin, the lymph nodes of the spleen, and the glomeruli of the kidney.[1] Investigating the entire world of plant and animal life, he was a tireless worker who may well be honoured as the founder of microscopic anatomy. He was succeeded by his pupil ANTONIO VALSALVA (1666–1723), whose contributions to the anatomy and physiology of the ear, in *De Aure Humana* (1704) established his fame (p. 244).

Although he demonstrated so clearly and conclusively the course and mechanism of the circulation, Harvey gave no explanation of the reason *why* the blood circulated. The prevailing view was that the heart heated the blood, which then became cooled down as it coursed through the vessels. Harvey makes a brief reference to the matter in stating that he did not know whether or not the heart added " heat, spirit, or perfection " to the blood, nor whether the movement of circulation was " for the purpose of cooling or for nutrition."

The problem was solved, step by step, by the genius of four young Oxford scientists, already mentioned among the founders of the Royal Society. Each of them was responsible for a definite contribution to the physiology of respiration.

First came the Hon. ROBERT BOYLE (1627–91), son of the Earl of Cork, who devoted his wealth and talent to the service of science. Experimenting with his air pump, he showed that in a vacuum a mouse or a small bird could not live, nor would a candle burn. If, however, the supply of air was renewed in time,

[1] J. M. Hayman, " Malpighi's *Concerning the Structure of the Kidneys*," *Ann. Med. Hist.*, 1925, vol. vii. p. 242

the bird or animal would recover. Clearly, therefore, air was essential for life and for combustion.[1] (See Supplement, page 457.) Then Boyle's assistant, ROBERT HOOKE, to whose work as a miscroscopist we shall presently refer (p. 190), proved that it was the air, and not merely the movement, which sustained life. The lungs were no longer to be regarded as bellows which cooled the fiery heart. After removing the greater part of the chest wall in a dog, Hooke made some openings in the surfaces of the lungs. Then, by blowing into the windpipe, so that the air escaped through the openings, he was able to keep the animal alive. This was, in fact, the first demonstration of artificial respiration.

The interaction between the air and the blood was not yet understood. This aspect of the problem of respiration was solved by two Cornishmen, Lower and Mayow. RICHARD LOWER (1631–91) tells us in his *Tractatus de Corde* (1669) that the surface of a fresh blood clot becomes bright red when turned round and exposed to air. Did this change in colour take place also as blood circulated through the lungs? [2] Lower repeated the experiment of Hooke and found that it was indeed so. He noted that when the artificial respiration was stopped, the blood in the lungs became dark and venous, and that it became bright red again when the respiration was resumed. Further, he took some dark blood from the vena cava and " perfused " it through the lungs, noting that it then acquired the bright red hue of arterial blood. The conclusion to be drawn from those experiments was that the entrance of fresh air into the blood was essential for the maintenance of life.[3] " Were it not so, we could breathe as well in the most filthy prison as in the most delightful pastures." Lower was the first to perform blood transfusion from one animal to another. This led to attempts to transfuse blood from an animal into man as a means of resuscitation after haemorrhage. The results were not encouraging, as nothing was then known of haemolysis or of blood grouping.[4] (See Supplement, page 457.)

To Lower, also, medicine is indebted for the proof that the

[1] W. Stirling, *Some Apostles of Physiology*, 1902, p. 39
[2] E. C. Hoff and P. M. Hoff, " The Life and Times of Richard Lower, 1631–91," *Bull. Hist. Med.*, 1936, vol. iv. p. 517 ; K. J. Franklin, " Richard Lower and his De Corde," *Ann. Med. Hist.*, 1931, vol. iii. p. 599
[3] K. J. Franklin, " The Work of Richard Lower, 1631–91," *Proc. Roy. Soc. Med.* (Sect. Hist.), 1932, vol. xxv. p. 113
[4] M. W. Hollingsworth, " Blood Transfusion by Richard Lower in 1665," *Ann. Med. Hist.*, 1928, vol. x. p. 213 ; Geoffrey Keynes, *Blood Transfusion*, 1949

increased flow of nasal mucus which accompanies a cold arises from the nasal mucous membrane, and not from " purging of the brain " as was previously imagined.

The last of this brilliant school of Oxford physiologists was JOHN MAYOW (1643–79), who achieved much during his short life of thirty-six years, and whose *Tractatus Quinque* is a medical classic. Mayow was a lawyer before he turned his attention to medicine, a fact which may partly account for the precision and clarity of his writing. He reviewed the entire knowledge of respiration, adding his own contribution.[1] His description of the mechanism—the inspiratory movement accomplished by the diaphragm and the intercostal muscles, the expiratory phase a passive movement—holds good to this day. As for the object of respiration, it was obvious to Mayow that " some constitutent of the air necessary to life enters into the blood in the act of breathing." It was not the entire air, for when a small animal or a lighted candle were sealed up in the same vessel the candle went out and the animal died, although the air remained. There was something in the air which was necessary to enable the candle to burn and the animal to live. Combustion and breathing were identical. Now the substance which was attracting the attention of chemists of that day was nitre, that constituent of gunpowder which was not by itself inflammable but which burned fiercely even in a vacuum when mixed with sulphur. In the above experiment the candle, or the animal, represented the sulphur. The nitre, so argued Mayow, was supplied by the air which contained " igneo-aerial particles " or " nitro-aerial spirit." It was essential to life ; and when breathing stopped, the nitrous particles were not supplied, the heart-beat ceased, and death followed. Mayow suspected the presence in the air of the constituent we now know as oxygen, but more than a century was to pass before it was isolated by Priestley and named by Lavoisier (p. 261).[2]

The Early Microscopists

The microscope, which enabled Malpighi to complete the work of Harvey, was probably known to the ancients, although the evidence is inconclusive. In its earliest form it consisted of

[1] Sir M. Foster, *Lectures on the History of Physiology*, 1901, p. 185 (" Mayow ")
[2] T. S. Patterson, " John Mayow in Contemporary Setting," *Isis*, vol. xv, Nos. 45 and 47, 1931

PLATE XXXVII HARVEY AND THE KING

William Harvey demonstrating his researches on the deer to Charles I and the
boy Prince (page 182)
Painting in Royal College of Physicians, London, by R. Hannah

PLATE XXXVIII EARLY MICROSCOPES

Leeuwenhoek's microscope. The object to be examined, mounted on holder A, may be moved in two directions by screw adjustments so as to bring it within focus of the small lens B, which is firmly fixed between two perforated brass plates (page 189)

Robert Hooke's microscope, from his *Micrographia*, 1665. The objective is a tiny double convex lens of short focus, mounted in a cell close to a pin-hole diaphragm. A wider field might be secured by a plano-convex lens within the tube at fixed distance from the eye. Hooke often dispensed with this (page 190)

a simple biconvex lens.[1] Roger Bacon first suggested the use of lenses as spectacles, and a simple lens was used by Malpighi and also by Leeuwenhoek. It was ZACHARIAS JANSEN, a spectacle-maker of Middelburg in Holland, who, about the year 1609, accidentally discovered the principle of the telescope and micro-scope by placing two lenses together in a tube.[2] Galileo turned this invention to practical use, but the instrument remained merely a toy for some years.

One of the first to apply the microscope to the study of disease was ATHANASIUS KIRCHER (1602–80),[3] Professor of Philosophy at Würzburg, who in examining the blood of plague-stricken patients found " countless masses of small worms, invisible to the naked eye." It is generally agreed that what Kircher really saw were masses of red blood corpuscles, as he could not have seen plague bacilli with lenses of such low power. Yet his inference was correct, for he stated that contagious diseases were conveyed by minute living organisms. (See Supplement, page 457.)

Fracastorius had advanced a similar idea but had produced no evidence to support it.

One of the greatest of the early microscopists was that remark-able man ANTONY VAN LEEUWENHOEK (1632–1723), a merchant of Delft, who, blessed with leisure, was able to devote his long life of ninety years to microscopical study [4] (Plate XXXVIII). Leeuwenhoek ground his own lenses and constructed his own microscopes, more than two hundred of them, and although he used a simple lens and obtained a magnification of only 160 at most, and usually of much less, he made many valuable observations, some of which were translated and published by the Royal Society, as the writer knew no language but his own Dutch. He amplified the work of Malpighi by finding capillaries in the tail of the tadpole ; he discovered red blood corpuscles, noting that these were oval in fishes and amphibians, and round in men and mammals. He also described the striation of muscle fibres, the compound eyes of insects, and many of the animalculae so familiar to students of stagnant ponds. From the medical standpoint, the greatest achievement of this energetic amateur was that he was the first to see and describe bacteria and also protozoa. Examin-

[1] R. H. Haden, " The Origin of the Microscope," *Ann. Med. Hist.*, vol. i. No. 1, p. 30
[2] C. Singer, " Notes on the History of Early Microscopy," *Proc. Roy. Soc. Med.* (Sect. Hist.), 1914, vol. vii. p. 247
[3] R. H. Major, " Athanasius Kircher," *Ann. Med. Hist.*, 1939, vol. i. 3rd Series, p. 105
[4] Clifford Dobell, *Antony van Leeuwenhoek and his " Little Animals,"* 1932

ing the white film which collected on his teeth, he saw " little animals, more numerous than all the people in the Netherlands, and moving about in the most delightful manner." Although Leeuwenhoek never visited London, the Royal Society made him a Fellow in 1680. Another pioneer of microscopy, also a Dutchman, was JAN SWAMMERDAM (1637–80) of Amsterdam, a man of intense energy but indifferent health, who crowded into his short life a vast deal of original work. His discoveries mainly concern the structure of insects, and he made some wonderful dissections of the internal organs of bees, dragonflies, and many other types.[1] His manuscripts, illustrated by excellent drawings, were not published until years after his death, when another great Dutchman, Boerhaave, sponsored the appearance of some of them in 1738 under the title, *Bybel der Natuure*. Swammerdam's " Bible of Nature " is the greatest collection of microscopical observations ever made by a single worker.

Meanwhile, in England, other microscopists were blazing the trail. The earliest, and the most brilliant, was ROBERT HOOKE (1635–1703), who acted as Curator to the Royal Society.[2] His *Micrographia* (1665) is a classic work, the beauty of the drawings being equalled only by those of Swammerdam.[3] In describing a section of cork, " much like a honeycomb," he was the first to use the word " cell " (Plate XXXVIII).

It was not until 1839 that MATTHIAS JACOB SCHLEIDEN (1804–81) and THEODOR SCHWANN (1810–82) enunciated the cell theory, which opened a new viewpoint in biology, to be developed later by Goodsir and Virchow [4] (p. 283). Thenceforth the cell was regarded as the unit of all organic structure, and cytology, the science of the cell, took its place as an important branch of biology.

In the field of microscopic botany NEHEMIAH GREW (1641–1712) led the way. Grew was a London physician, and secretary of the Royal Society.[5] In his *Anatomy of Plants* (1682), he traced the vascular structure, showing how plants resemble animals and noting the presence of sex in plants. Many beautiful drawings adorn his work.

[1] S. G. B. Stubbs and E. W. Bligh, *Sixty Centuries of Health and Physick*, 1931
[2] W. S. Middleton, " The Medical Aspect of Robert Hooke," *Ann. Med. Hist.*, 1927, vol. ix. p. 227
[3] W. Stirling, *Some Apostles of Physiology*, 1902, pp. 34, 135
[4] E. B. Wilson, *The Cell in Development and Heredity*, 1928
[5] A. C. Wootton, *Chronicles of Pharmacy*, 2 vols., 1910, vol. i. p. 343

Societies and Journals

Mention has been made of the Royal Society, one of a group of scientific societies which arose during the seventeenth century. Italy led the movement when, in 1603, the Accademia dei Lincei was founded in Rome by an enlightened aristocrat, Duke Federigo Cesi. This academy of " lynx-eyed " scientists applied their penetrating vision to the solution of many problems, and included Galileo among their early members.

In Paris, the Académie des Sciences came into being, and was accorded royal patronage by Louis XIV in 1666, through the influence of his minister, Colbert. The society published many important scientific works.

In Germany, the Collegium Naturae Curiosorum was inaugurated at Halle in 1652.

Most renowned of all was the Royal Society, which began in a small way about 1645, when a group of scientists formed the " Invisible College," which held meetings for discussion, at first in each other's rooms, then in Gresham College, not without some risk of ecclesiastical censure. A few years later a number of scientists in Oxford, mostly physiologists, instituted meetings for the advancement of their interests.[1] They included Thomas Willis, Francis Glisson, Richard Lower, Robert Boyle, Robert Hooke, John Mayow, and Christopher Wren,[2] all great men who fulfilled the object of the Royal Society, viz. the " improvement of natural knowledge." At last a royal charter was granted by Charles II, in 1663, and the Royal Society, now well established, commenced the publication of its *Philosophical Transactions* two years later.[3] The Royal Society became responsible for many publications, including Newton's *Principia*, the greatest of all works on physical science, which appeared in 1687 when the famous Samuel Pepys was president.

It was at one time believed that the mace of the Royal Society was the identical " bauble " which had incurred Cromwell's contempt in Parliament, but this pretty story has since been disproved.

---

[1] T. Sprat, *The History of the Royal Society of London*, 3rd ed., 1722
[2] P. Musser and J. C. Krantz, " The Friendship of Robert Boyle and Christopher Wren," *Bull. Hist. Med.*, 1939, vol. vii. p. 970
[3] C. R. Weld, *A History of the Royal Society*, 2 vols., 1848 ; Sir Henry Lyons, *The Royal Society of London : 1660–1940*, Cambridge, 1944

About this time, too, museums and botanical gardens became popular. Of the latter, the best known was the Jardin des Plantes in Paris, founded in 1626 by Cardinal Richelieu ; but every medical school had its physic garden for the cultivation of medicinal plants.

The leading physicians of Edinburgh, led by Sir Robert Sibbald (p. 225), determined to establish the Royal College of Physicians of Edinburgh (1681), and also to lay out a physic garden at Holyrood, which was the first of a series of such gardens in or near the city (p. 225).

In London, Sir Hans Sloane had a garden at Chelsea, which he presented to the Apothecaries' Company in 1722,[1] and which still exists.

The nucleus of the British Museum was the collection of specimens belonging to the Royal Society. This was transferred in 1676 to Montague House, designed for the purpose by the redoubtable Robert Hooke. Later, there was added the large accumulation of plants and animals brought from the West Indies by Sir HANS SLOANE (1660–1753), a well-known physician who lived in Bloomsbury Square and later in Chelsea, who attended Queen Anne, and who gave his name to more than one London Street.[2] He succeeded Sir Isaac Newton as president of the Royal Society.

Another scientific activity of the seventeenth century was the publication of journals. The *Philosophical Transactions* of the Royal Society contained contributions from scientists of all countries, but it was preceded by the *Journal des Sçavans* (savants) (1665) which was the first scientific journal to be published in the vernacular. The first medical journal,[3] also French, was *Nouvelles Descouvertes sur toutes les Parties de la Médecine* (1679–81), edited by Nicolas de Blegny (1652–1722), surgeon to Louis XIV and his queen. It was followed by an English medical journal,[4] *Medicina Curiosa* (1684), also a short-lived periodical, of which only two numbers were issued. The rise of medical journalism will be discussed more fully in a later chapter (p. 393).

---

[1] F. D. Drewitt, *The Romance of the Apothecaries' Garden at Chelsea*, 1924
[2] J. C. Jeaffreson, *A Book about Doctors*, 1870, p. 30 (" Sir Hans Sloane ") ; B. Chance, " Sir Hans Sloane," *Ann. Med. Hist.*, 1938, vol. x. p. 390
[3] A. G. Nicholls, " Nicholas de Blegny and the First Medical Periodical," *Canad. Med. Assoc. Jour.*, 1934, vol. xxxi. p. 198
[4] P. Johnston-Saint, " The First English Medical Journal," *Med. Press and Circ.*, 1939, vol. cci. p. 117

PLATE XXXIX DECORATIVE ANATOMY

Many early anatomical illustrations were works of art, and this standard was
extended to museum specimens, reaching a high degree of excellence in the
preparations, or "cabinets," of the Dutch anatomist Frederik Ruysch (1638–
1731), as illustrated above. Skeletons, organs, calculi, and above all, blood-
vessels injected with a coloured solidifying fluid, were grouped together in an
indiscriminate and often grotesque fashion (page 194)

PLATE XL AN EARLY EXPONENT OF METABOLISM

Sanctorius, seated in his balance, determines the variations of his
" invisible perspiration." The illustration forms the frontispiece of
his work, entitled *Medicina Statica*, 1614 (page 197)

Leyden, the Medical Centre

Reference has been made to the work of two Dutch pioneers in microscopy, Swammerdam and Leeuwenhoek, neither of whom had a degree in medicine. Nevertheless the great medical school of Leyden had come into being before that time. In 1575 William of Orange desired to reward the town of Leyden for its valiant and successful defence against the Spaniards in the previous year. He asked the inhabitants to choose between a remission of taxes for ten years and the establishment of a university. They wisely chose the latter, and it was a happy choice. By this time the Reformation had lessened the popularity of the Italian and French centres of learning, and the University of Leyden, although of Protestant foundation, was to be open to all students —Protestants, Catholics, and Jews alike. By Papal decree all non-Catholics had been excluded from the Italian universities, and although Padua had evaded the edict by establishing a separate university for non-Catholics, such an action could not revive the glory of the Italian Renaissance, which was now fading fast. The educational centre of medicine which had passed from Greece to Salerno, then from Salerno to Montpellier, and eventually to Padua, was now to shift still farther north, and to become established at Leyden. To Leyden, in increasing numbers, came students from many lands : from England, Scotland, Ireland, and even from America. The first medical student to matriculate was an Englishman, John James, afterwards a distinguished London physician.[1] As Latin was the academic language, Leyden (Lugdunum Batavorum) was able to acquire an international reputation. Among the many learned medical teachers at Leyden there were well-known anatomists. There was Franz de la Boë, or SYLVIUS (1614–72), a popular teacher, discoverer of the fissure of Sylvius in the brain, to whom further reference will be made, and GOVERT BIDLOO (1649–1713), who published a magnificent atlas of anatomy which was unfortunately plagiarized by the English anatomist William Cowper.[2]

One of the most versatile professors at Leyden was PIETER

[1] R. W. Innes-Smith, *English-speaking Students of Medicine at the University of Leyden*, 1932
[2] F. Beekman, " Bidloo and Cowper, Anatomists," *Ann. Med. Hist.*, 1935, vol. vii. p. 113

PAAW (1564–1617).[1] He had studied under Fabricius at Padua and also at Paris, and on his return home had been appointed director of the Botanical Garden as well as Professor of Anatomy. He was largely responsible for the foundation of the Anatomical School of Leyden, and it is said that during his twenty-two years as occupant of the Chair he dissected sixty bodies, a remarkable achievement for that time. He was a pioneer in anthropology, describing in his treatise on osteology the cranial differences to be found in the various races of mankind. He also practised medicine, showing much zeal and courage during a plague epidemic, and he wrote an account of the disease, which was published after his death. He deserves to be remembered as one of the great figures of the Leyden School.

Another anatomist of Leyden was FREDERIK RUYSCH (1638–1731), who devised a method of preserving anatomical specimens by injecting the blood-vessels with a material which solidified on cooling.[2] Of these specimens he had a large number, mounted in fantastic style and arranged in cabinets, decorated by dried plants and corals (Plate XXXIX). The collection was eventually sold to Czar Peter the Great. Most familiar of all Dutch anatomists as the central figure in Rembrandt's painting, " The Lesson in Anatomy " was NICOLAS TULP (1593–1674) of Amsterdam, who was also a physician and the first to describe the disease beri-beri from East Indian cases. Dutch artists were fond of painting anatomical scenes,[3] and they also included among their models the less reputable practitioners, such as itinerant tooth-drawers and blood-letters and the quacks who removed fictitious stones from the heads of their victims. Jan Steen's " Dentist " is an example, as is his " Physician's Visit " (Plate xxxv).

Anatomy flourished exceedingly in other countries during this century. The names of Bartholin, Stensen, Wirsung, Brunner, Pacchioni, Peyer, Vieussens, Wharton, Meibom, and Schneider will recall to the mind of the reader who knows his anatomy a

---

[1] L. Hahn, *Dictionnaire encyclopédique des Sciences médicales*, Paris, 1884, vol. xix. p. 617
[2] N. T. Hazen, " Johnson's Life of Frederic Ruysch," *Bull. Hist. Med.*, 1939, vol. vii. p. 324 ; F. J. Cole, " The History of Anatomical Injections," in Singer's *Studies in the History and Method of Science*, 1921, vol. ii
[3] F. Regnault, " Frans Hals vu par un Médecin," *Bull. d'Hist. de Méd.*, 1929, vol. xxiii. p. 28
[4] H. Meige, " Les Médecins de Jan Steen, *Janus*, 1900, vol. v. pp. 187, 217 ; J. W. Churchman, " The Physician in the Paintings of Jan Steen," *Johns Hopk. Hosp. Bull.*, 1907, vol. xxiii. p. 480

duct, a gland, or some other anatomical structure named from the discoverer. (See also Supplement, page 457.) Dutch anatomy was well represented by REGNIER de GRAAF (1641–73), who discovered the Graafian follicles of the ovary and made observations on the secretion of saliva and bile.[1] The leading obstetrician was HENDRIK VAN DEVENTER (1657–1724), who practised at The Hague and was the first to make a study of the variations of the female pelvis and their effect upon labour.[2] The relationship of the school of Leyden to that of Edinburgh will be discussed in a later chapter.

[1] H. R. Catchpole, " Regnier de Graaf (1641–73)," *Bull. Hist. Med.*, 1940, vol. viii. p. 1261
[2] B. J. Kouwer, " Hendrik van Deventer," *Janus*, 1912, vol. xvii. pp. 425, 506

BOOKS FOR FURTHER READING

BAYON, H. P.   *William Harvey, Physician and Biologist* (Annals of Science), 1938–9
CLAY, R. S. and COURT, T. S.   *The History of the Microscope*, 1932
DOBELL, CLIFFORD.   *Antony van Leeuwenhoek and his " Little Animals,"* 1932
DREWITT, F. D.   *The Romance of the Apothecaries' Garden at Chelsea*, 1924
FULTON, J. F.   *A Bibliography of Robert Boyle*, 1932
HALDANE, E. S.   *Descartes, his Life and Times*, 1905
INNES-SMITH, R. W.   *English-speaking Students of Medicine at the University of Leyden*, 1932
MORE, L. S.   *The Life and Works of the Hon. Robert Boyle*, 1944
NEEDHAM, J.   *A History of Embryology*, 1934
PACKARD, F. R.   *Guy Patin and the Medical Profession in Paris in the Seventeenth Century*, New York, 1925
POWER, D'ARCY.   *William Harvey* (Masters of Medicine), 1897
SPRAT, T.   *History of the Royal Society of London*, 3rd ed., 1722
WILLEY, BASIL.   *The Seventeenth-Century Background*, 1934

CHAPTER XI

SCIENCE AND SUPERSTITION : THE QUEST FOR A NEW BASIS

IN addition to the wonderful work of Harvey, of the Dutch anatomists, of the pioneer microscopists, and of the young Oxford physiologists, the period under review is noteworthy for certain trends which marked an important phase of medical progress. The seventeenth century produced a series of brilliant investigators, some of whom sought to explain all the phenomena of health and disease on a materialistic basis.

About the middle of the century, a salutary corrective to such theorizings appeared in the teaching of Thomas Sydenham, who counselled a return to Hippocratic methods, and reminded physicians that medicine was not only a science but also an art. There remained also a substratum of superstition in the medicine of the time. Richard Wiseman, the leading surgeon of his time, believed in the efficacy of the Royal Touch in cases of scrofula, and even the learned Sir Thomas Browne affirmed that witches did exist. Let us now examine a little more closely each of the above movements.

The Human Body : Machine or Test-tube ?

In the early years of the seventeenth century two curious trends in medicine made their appearance.[1] There was at that time a general desire to discard the past, and to replace obsolete opinions by new and fresh ideas. Some of the ideas were far-fetched, and when pushed to extreme limits were even absurd, yet they served as stepping-stones to greater wisdom, and therefore deserve to appear in any account of the medicine of the period.

One school regarded the body as a machine, and sought to explain all its workings, whether in health or disease, as physical or mechanical in nature. This was the " iatro-physical " or " iatro-mechanical " theory. Another school preferred to view

[1] Basil Willey, *The Seventeenth Century Background,* 1934

life as a series of chemical processes or reactions, assuming that the body was a sort of test tube. This theory was designated " iatro-chemical."

As already mentioned, Descartes (p. 177) upheld the iatro-physical view of *l'homme-machine*, but Descartes was primarily a philosopher, and only incidentally a physiologist.

The first of the iatro-physicists was SANCTORIUS SANCTORIUS (1561–1636) of Padua, who applied his mechanical skill to the service of medicine by designing a number of ingenious instruments.[1] He invented the first clinical thermometer, a trocar and cannula for the performance of tracheotomy, and a pulsilogium, or pulse clock, which antedated by a century a similar invention, the watch of Sir John Floyer, which he described in his book (p. 257), " *The Physician's Pulse Watch* (1707).[2] The most famous creation of Sanctorius, however, was the weighing machine or balance in which he literally passed a great part of his life. Seated in this balance, eating and even sleeping in it, he estimated the weight of the " invisible perspiration," upon which he laid great stress (Plate XL). The results of this pioneer work in what we now call metabolism he embodied in a collection of aphorisms, published in 1614 under the title *Medicina Statica*, and which was translated into English in the following century by John Quincy. Perspiration, Sanctorius tells us, must be distinguished from sweating. " The perspiration which is beneficial is not what goes off with sweat, but that insensible steam which exhales to the quantity of about fifty ounces in the space of one day." " The Perspiration, which is insensible, is natural, and a token of health ; but Sweat is the contrary." " Insensible perspiration is greater during sleep than in waking hours, and has been found to be about forty ounces." " Imperceptible perspiration lightens the body more than all the sensible evacuations together." Although Sanctorius was obviously obsessed by his idea, his aphorisms contain much sound wisdom, and his book is one of the most interesting of medical classics.

Another Italian of the iatro-physical school is often regarded as its founder, as he went further than Sanctorius in his application of mechanical principles to the solution of problems of health and disease. GIOVANNI ALFONSO BORELLI (1608–79) was Professor

---

[1] R. H. Major, " Santorio Santorio," *Ann. Med. Hist.*, 1938, vol. x. p. 369 ; Sir M. Foster, *Lectures on the History of Physiology*, 1901, p. 145 (" Sanctorius ")
[2] H. E. Sigerist, *Great Doctors*, 1933, p. 150

of Mathematics at Pisa, and a close personal friend of Malpighi, when he undertook his researches on animal movement and wrote his great work, *De Motu Animalium*, which, however, was not published until after his death. Like Descartes, he was indebted to the patronage of Queen Christina of Sweden, who then resided in Rome. Borelli busied himself with the mechanics and statics of the body, calculating with mathematical accuracy the force expended by the muscles and the physical laws involved in animal locomotion and bird flight. He believed that all muscles increased in bulk during contraction, and that the hardening and tension were due to " inflation of the muscular substance by something from without." " Some corporeal substance," he alleged, " must be transmitted along the nerves to the muscles." For Borelli this substance was " succus nervens " which circulated through the nerves, just as the blood circulated through the arteries and veins. He also showed that the action of the heart was like that of any other muscle. All the theories of Borelli are now merely of historic interest.[1]

It soon became evident, however, that the working of the body did not strictly conform to mathematical rules. This was evident to the third member of our group of Italian iatro-physicists.

GIORGIO BAGLIVI (1668–1707) was not only a clever physicist but also a brilliant clinician and a popular teacher.[2] As Professor of Anatomy at Rome, he compared the human body to a collection of mechanical contrivances. The teeth were scissors ; the thorax, bellows ; the heart and vessels, waterworks ; the stomach, a grinding mill. But when he became Professor of Medicine, Baglivi soon discovered that all could not be explained in terms of physics. Dissatisfied with current views, he discovered that the best book of medical knowledge was the narrative of the sick man. He discarded theory, and placed the patient in the centre of the picture. " The two chief pillars of Physick," he wrote in his *De praxi medica*, are " Reason and Observation." Here was a true disciple of Hippocrates, who held that the healing art could be learned only by a study of the patient himself, and that Nature was the best physician. We are not surprised to learn that Baglivi had a large practice, and was held in high esteem, and that his early death was much deplored.

Having surveyed the human body from the standpoint of the

[1] Sir M. Foster, *Lectures on the History of Physiology*, 1901, p. 55 (" Borelli ")
[2] F. Stenn, " Giorgio Baglivi," *Ann. Med. Hist.*, 1941, 3rd Ser., vol. iii. p. 183

iatro-physicist, let us now turn to that of the iatro-chemist, who regarded life as a collection of chemical experiments, and who compared the human body to a test tube. The founder of the iatro-chemical school was JEAN BAPTISTE VAN HELMONT (1577–1644) of Brussels.[1] This follower of Paracelsus refused the M.A. degree of Louvain because he did not feel that he was Master of any Arts. In choosing a profession, he declined to take Holy Orders, because his livelihood would be derived from the sins of the people. Law he also rejected, as it was not always based on truth and justice. Medicine, the last hope, remained, and to Medicine he devoted his life.[2] He set himself to develop the views of Paracelsus, for whom he had a great regard.[3] Like Paracelsus, he believed that a life force or archaeus, which he called " Blas," dominated all the bodily processes. It produced fever, cough, etc., in an effort to get rid of harmful products, but it was often too energetic and required to be pacified by treatment.[4] " Blas " has been long since forgotten, but Van Helmont was on surer ground when he introduced the word " Gas," which he alleged was a ferment or a number of ferments, which presided over nutrition, movement, digestion, and indeed over all vital functions. He discovered that a gas, which we now know to be carbon dioxide, but which he called " gas sylvestre," was produced during the fermentation of wine, and during combustion. Van Helmont's chemistry was largely tinged with the mysticism of the alchemist, which renders his writings rather obscure.

It was a professor at Leyden who placed chemical physiology upon a sounder basis. FRANCISCUS SYLVIUS (1614–72), or Francis de la Boë, would not accept the speculations of the alchemists.[5] He showed that fermentation, with the escape of gas, was only one of the many chemical changes which took place in the body. Sylvius studied the nature of the juices of the body—saliva, pancreatic juice, bile, etc., and drew his deductions therefrom. For him, a knowledge of acids and alkalis furnished not only a key to the problems of life, but also an index of the appropriate treatment. Yet Sylvius was not merely a chemist and physio-

[1] R. O. Moon, " Van Helmont, Chemist, Physician, Philosopher, and Mystic," *Proc. Roy. Soc. Med.*, 1932, vol. xxv. p. 23 ; C. G. Cumston, *History of Medicine*, 1926, p. 279 (" Van Helmont ")
[2] A. C. Wootton, *Chronicles of Pharmacy*, 1910, vol. i. p. 257
[3] H. Redgrove, *Alchemy, Ancient and Modern*, 1922, p. 75
[4] H. E. Sigerist, *Great Doctors*, 1933, p. 157
[5] Sir M. Foster, *Lectures on the History of Physiology*, 1901, p. 147 (" Sylvius ")

logist ; he was a truly great clinician.[1] It is said that he was the first to introduce clinical instructions at Leyden, and he attracted many students by the excellence of his teaching.

Contemporary with Sylvius, there was in England another great clinician who developed the ideas of the iatro-chemical school. THOMAS WILLIS (1621–75) said that the physician, watching the fermentations of the body, ready to correct or prevent any irregularity, might be compared with a brewer or vintner. This Professor of Natural Philosophy at Oxford, a staunch Royalist during the Civil War, who afterwards became a fashionable physician in London, is perhaps best known for his researches on the nervous system.[2] His *Cerebri Anatome* (1664), one of the first descriptions of the brain, was illustrated by no less a person than Sir Christopher Wren (1632–1723), who not only designed St. Paul's Cathedral but assisted to found the Royal Society ; and although he was not a medical man, was the first to suggest intravenous medication (Plate XLI). The name of Willis is still familiar in its application to the arrangement of arteries at the base of the brain, the " circle of Willis," also to the phenomenon of hearing better in a noise, " paracusis of Willis." Willis is also credited with the discovery of the presence of sugar in diabetic urine.[3]

Clinical Medicine in England

A distinguished contemporary of Willis was FRANCIS GLISSON (1597–1677), who succeeded Harvey as Lumleian Lecturer, and became Professor of Physic at Cambridge.[4] In his *Anatomia Hepatis* (1654) he gave the first accurate description of the capsule of the liver ; his *De Rachitide* (1650) is well known as a classical account of infantile rickets, and he described the inherent " irritability " of the tissues of the body, an idea which was·later elaborated by Von Haller. Of rickets, he wrote that the affected children " do not shake and brandish their little Joynts, and are not delighted like other children, with the agitation of their bodies, being pleased only with gentle usage and quiet rest." The rickety

[1] E. T. Withington, *Medical History from the Earliest Times*, 1894, p. 303
[2] R. S. Dow, "Thomas Willis (1621–75) as a Comparative Neurologist," *Ann. Med. Hist.*, 1940, 3rd Ser., vol. ii. p. 181
[3] J. H. Barach, "Historical Facts on Diabetes," *Ann. Med. Hist.*, 1928, vol. x. p. 387
[4] Sir W. Langdon-Brown, "Francis Glisson and the Insurgent Century," *Proc. Roy. Soc. Med.*, 1942, vol. xxxvi. p. 17 ; Sir N. Moore, *The History of the Study of Medicine in the British Isles*, 1908, p. 111 (" Glisson ")

chest he compared to " the Keel of a Ship inverted, or the Breast of a Hen or Capon, for the middle riseth to a point and the sides are pressed down." Glisson was one of the three great clinical physicians of the seventeenth century, the other two being Mayerne and Sydenham. Those were the pioneers of the study of clinical medicine in England.

Sir THEODORE TURQUET OF MAYERNE, near Geneva, who is usually called, simply, Mayerne (1573–1655), studied medicine at Heidelberg and Montpellier, and practised for a time in Paris.[1] In 1611 he settled in London, where his skill as a physician soon won for him an immense reputation.[2] He became a Fellow of the Royal College of Physicians and Physician to King James I, who honoured him with knighthood. He edited the first edition (1618) of the Pharmacopoeia of the College of Physicians, and although some of his prescriptions contain such ingredients as powdered human skull, the blood of weasels, and " balsam of bats," he was responsible for the introduction of calomel and of the mercurial lotion known as " black wash." [3] That Mayerne was a careful observer is shown by his record of the medical history of James I, still preserved in the British Museum (Sloane MS.). He writes that the king, now aged fifty-seven years, " has a very steadfast brain, which was never disturbed by the sea, by drinking wine, or by driving in a coach." He is " easily affected by cold," " bolts his food owing to want of teeth," and " has the strongest antipathy to water and all watery drinks." Mayerne goes on to describe the king's former illnesses, noting everything, and producing a record which might well serve as a pattern of case-taking.[4] The king cared little about the causes of illness, but demanded relief from pain, and he must have caused a good deal of trouble to Mayerne, who writes that, " The King laughs at medicine and declares physicians to be of very little use and hardly necessary." The above quotations are from the translation by Sir Norman Moore, the original manuscript being in Latin.

[1] T. Gibson, " A Sketch of the Career of Theodore Turquet de Mayerne," *Ann. Med. Hist.*, 1933, vol. v. p. 315
[2] T. Gibson, " Letters of Dr. Theodore Turquet de Mayerne," *Ann. Med. Hist.*, 1937, vol. ix. p. 401 ; " The Iconography of Sir Theodore Turquet de Mayerne," *Ann. Med. Hist.*, 3rd Ser., vol. iii. p. 288
[3] W. Wadd, *Memorabilia*, 1827, p. 193 (" Biographical Notes ")
[4] Sir N. Moore, *The History of the Study of Medicine in the British Isles*, 1908, p. 97

The Return to Hippocrates : Thomas Sydenham

By far the greatest clinical physician of the seventeenth century was THOMAS SYDENHAM (1624–89),[1] well named " the English Hippocrates." Such a man was needed to shake medicine free from the bonds of such schools and systems as had been introduced in place of the mediæval scholasticism. " As a clinician Sydenham was unrivalled ; his word pictures are unsurpassable." That he had no patience with book-learning in medicine, and little respect for the fundamental sciences, is obvious from the well-known tales of his retorts to two of his pupils.[2] To Sir Richard Blackmore, who asked him to recommend a textbook of medicine, he replied : " Read *Don Quixote*, a very good book ; I read it myself still." His rejoinder to Sir Hans Sloane (p. 192), whose testimonial described him as " a good botanist and a skilful anatomist " was, " Anatomy, botany, nonsense ! No, young man, go to the bedside ; there alone can you learn disease," and when Sloane at a later date mooted his project of collecting plants in Jamaica, Sydenham told him that he had better drown himself in the pond in St. James's Park on his way home. Such were the opinions of the physician who, at an opportune time in the history of medicine, demonstrated that common sense was better than vague theory.

Born at Wynford Eagle in Dorset, Sydenham came of a well-to-do Puritan family, but little is known of his early life. His studies at Oxford were interrupted by the Civil War. As his father and four of his brothers were already serving in Cromwell's army, young Thomas also enlisted, and served for four years as captain of a troop of horse. In his works he makes no reference to his military experiences, which must have given him that sympathy and insight into human nature, so clearly shown in his later life.[3] Among his friends at Oxford were Robert Boyle the chemist, and John Locke, physician and philosopher.[4] It is unlikely that he ever met Harvey, who of course was on the side of the Royalists.

Graduating at Oxford, Sydenham continued his medical

---

[1] D. Riesman, " Thomas Sydenham, Clinician," *Ann. Med. Hist.*, 1925, vol. vii. p. 174
[2] Sir. B. W. Richardson, *Disciples of Aesculapius*, 1900, vol. ii. p. 656
[3] J. D. Comrie, *Selected Works of Thomas Sydenham, M.D., with a Short Biography*, 1922
[4] John Brown, " Locke and Sydenham," in *Horæ Subsecivæ*, 1st Ser., 1st ed., 1858. (One of the best of this charming collection of essays, though less famous than *Rab and his Friends* in the 2nd Ser.)

studies at Montpellier, and on his return he practised in London. Owing to his political views, he never became a Fellow of the Royal College of Physicians. It is greatly to his credit that he accomplished so much, in spite of difficulties and opposition.[1] Although he was not a Court physician, his extensive practice included many distinguished persons. His portraits reveal Sydenham as a robust man, his hair worn long, his expression grave but kindly.[2] Benevolent and modest, he disliked popularity.[3] The value of his work was not fully recognized until after his death, when his books became very popular, and it is said that Boerhaave, when lecturing at Leyden, always raised his hat on mentioning the name of Sydenham.

Yet he had many admirers in his day. One of them was his ardent pupil, THOMAS DOVER (1660–1742), ship surgeon and buccaneer,[4] the rescuer of Alexander Selkirk (Robinson Crusoe). Dover's famous powder is still in use, and his book, quaintly entitled, *The Ancient Physician's Legacy to His Country* (1732), is fascinating to read.[5] He refers to " the honest and good Dr. Sydenham, whose reason was much superior to mine," and relates how Sydenham treated him during an attack of smallpox, with no fire in the room, the windows constantly open, the bedclothes no higher than the patient's waist and " twelve bottles of Small Beer every twentyfour hours." [6]

Sydenham, who had suffered from gout since early manhood, was in later years much troubled with stone. He died at his house in Pall Mall, and was buried in St. James's Church, Piccadilly, where the College of Physicians, in 1810, erected a tablet to his memory. He was not a voluminous writer. His best-known works are *Medical Observations*, in which he discusses fevers, and *A Treatise on the Gout*. A short extract from each, in abridged form, will show how clear and concise were his descriptions. Of measles he writes : " The measles generally attack children. On the first day they have cold and shivers. On the second they have the fever in full, a white tongue, thirst and somnolence. The nose

---

[1] W. MacMichael, *Lives of British Physicians*, 1830, p. 84
[2] H. W. Jones, " The Portraits of Thomas Sydenham," *Ann. Med. Hist.*, 1940, 3rd Ser., vol. ii. p. 265
[3] W. Wadd, *Memorabilia*, 1827, p. 213 (" Sydenham ")
[4] L. Eloesser, " Pirate and Buccaneer Doctors," *Ann. Med. Hist.*, 1926, vol. viii. p. 45
[5] W. Osler, " Thomas Dover," in *An Alabama Student and Other Essays*, 1908 ; M. P. Russell, " Thomas Dover, 1660–1742," *Edin. Med. Jour.*, 1942, vol. xlvx. p. 259 ; T. H. Howell, " Dover's *Legacy*," *Edin. Med. Jour.*, 1942, vol. xlix. p. 266
[6] J. A. Nixon, " Salt-water Surgeons," *Lancet*, 1941, vol. ii. p. 774

and eyes run continually. The symptoms increase until the fourth day. Then there appear on the face and forehead small red spots like flea-bites which increase and cluster together so as to mark the face with large blotches. The spots spread to the trunk. . . . On the eighth day they disappear. On the ninth, there are none anywhere."

Of gout Sydenham could speak from intimate experience.[1] " The victim goes to bed and sleeps in good health. About two o'clock in the morning he is awakened by a severe pain in the great toe. . . . Then follow chills and shivers and a little fever. The pain becomes intense. Now it is a violent stretching and tearing of the ligaments, now it is a gnawing pain and now a pressure or tightening. . . . The night is passed in torture . . . and in vain effort by change of posture to obtain an abatement of the pain. At last the patient has a respite. . . . In the morning he finds the part swollen. . . . A few days after the other foot swells and suffers the same pains."

Sydenham was essentially a clinician; he rejected entirely the ideas of iatro-physics or iatro-chemistry.[2] His method consisted in the careful observation and recording of the phenomena of disease, and he had the greatest veneration for the Hippocratic outlook.

In treatment, he preferred simple remedies. Fevers he treated by cooling methods ; phthisis by open air exercise on horseback. Blood-letting he practised with circumspection. Sydenham was one of the first to prescribe iron for anaemia ; he popularized the use of the quinine-yielding cinchona bark, lately introduced from Peru, in the treatment of ague or malaria, so serious and so prevalent a disease in England during the seventeenth century.[3] Syphilis he treated by mercurial inunctions until free salivation occurred, and he believed that it was the salivation, rather than the mercury, which wrought the cure. One of his favourite drugs was opium, in the form of a tincture to which were added saffron, cloves, and cinnamon. " Sydenham's laudanum," as it was called, remained a popular remedy for many years. The greatest service, however, which Sydenham rendered to medicine was to divert men's minds from speculation, and to lead them back to the bedside, for there only could the art be studied.

[1] M. A. Schnitker, " A History of the Treatment of Gout," *Bull. Hist. Med.*, 1936 vol. iv. p. 89
[2] S. G. Stubbs and E. W. Bligh, *Sixty Centuries of Health and Physick*, 1931, p. 175
[3] A. C. Wootton, *Chronicles of Pharmacy*, 1910, vol. ii. p. 93

The History of Cinchona

Mention has been made of Sydenham's use of " the bark " in cases of ague. To this statement, a further note may be added. The romantic tale of the discovery of cinchona is familiar to every student of medical history. Early in the seventeenth century, the Countess of Chinchon, wife of the Viceroy of Peru, was miraculously cured of a fever by the use of a remedy suggested by a local governor, a powder (quinine) prepared from the bark of a tree, which came to be known as Countess's Powder. As a thank-offering for her recovery, she distributed large quantities to the citizens of Lima, and is said to have afterwards introduced the drug into Spain. The story was first recorded by Sebastian Bado in 1663, and was repeated by Sir Clements Markham in his *Memoir of Lady Ana de Osorino, Countess of Chinchon*, London, 1874.

Unfortunately, the pretty legend has recently received a rude shock from the researches of Mr. A. W. Haggis,[1] who, after a study of the original diary of the Count of Chinchon, has proved that the Countess died in Spain before her husband was sent to Peru ; and, further, that his second wife, who accompanied him, led a remarkably healthy life, and never returned to Spain at all, so that she was neither cured by cinchona, nor did she introduce it into Europe.

Haggis has gone further in his exposure of the errors relating to cinchona. He states that the Indian name Quina-quina (literally, bark of bark), originally applied to the tree Myroxylon which yielded Peruvian balsam, came to be used also to designate the plant Cinchona, and thus the two products or barks were often confused. Moreover, Peruvian bark was in such great demand in Europe that adequate supplies were not available ; and the cargoes were sometimes fraudulently adulterated with the more plentiful cinchona bark. The deception passed unnoticed for many years, the two barks being used indiscriminately and naturally with conflicting results. Eventually Peruvian bark, or Jesuit's bark, as it was called, fell into disuse, and was supplanted by cinchona bark, and eventually by quinine prepared from it.

[1] A. W. Haggis, " Fundamental Errors in the Early History of Cinchona," *Bull. Hist. Med.*, 1941, vol. x. p. 417

The Great Plague of London

Among the diseases described by Sydenham was plague, which he had ample opportunity of observing in London during 1665, although, as most of his patients had fled to the country, he had deemed it prudent to follow, with his family, while the epidemic was at its height. There had been previous outbreaks of plague in London, but " The Poore's Plague " of 1665 eclipsed them all in fury. It was well named, as it commenced in the slums, where the wooden houses, with little light or air, and neither water supply nor sanitation, favoured the spread of any epidemic.[1] Conditions were made worse by the enforced closure of infected houses, which, locked and guarded, were marked with a red cross and the words, " Lord have mercy on us." Samuel Pepys in his diary records how he saw several marked houses in Drury Lane, and his fear that he might be a victim, for, said he, " the season is so sickly that it is much to be feared how a man can escape, for which the Lord God bless me or make me fitted to receive it."

No one might enter or leave the sealed house, save the physician, when available, which was seldom, or the old women who performed the gruesome task of " searchers," their duty being to view the dead bodies in order to report the cause of death. The bodies often showed dark red patches, which had appeared shortly before death. and were known as " tokens " or God's marks.[2]

Almost invariably the tokens foretold a fatal issue. Notification of death was not then compulsory, and needless to say, the " Bills of Mortality," which were the only index of the extent of the plague, were by no means accurate.[3] The law was often evaded. Many escaped from infected dwellings and spread the disease. Of those who remained, few survived. Defoe, in his *Journal of the Plague Year*, though he was only six years old in that year, and can hardly be regarded as an eye-witness, tells us that " whole families, indeed whole streets of families, were swept away altogether," and that the plague " defied all medicines, the very physicians were seized with it, with their preservatives in their

---

[1] G. R. Owen, " The Poore's Plague and Mr. Pepys," *Ann. Med. Hist.*, 1926, vol. viii. p. 249

[2] R. Crawfurd, *Plague and Pestilence in Literature and Art*, 1914, p. 187

[3] Three years before the Great Plague, John Graunt, a London draper, had published his *Natural and Political Observations . . . upon the bills of mortality*, which may be regarded as the first book to deal with Vital Statistics. Registration of births and deaths did not become compulsory until 1842. (See also p. 388.)

mouths," and "men went about prescribing to others till the tokens were upon them and they dropped down dead, destroyed by the very enemy they directed others to oppose." [1] All honour to those brave physicians who remained in London to fight the pestilence, albeit with such imperfect weapons.

One of the physicians who stayed in the city to fight the plague was Dr. NATHANIEL HODGES (1629–88),[2] to whom we are indebted for the best contemporary account, entitled *Loimologia*, the Greek word "loimos" meaning pestilence. The first edition, dated 1672, is now a rare book. Describing his daily round while the plague was raging, Hodges tells us that he rose early, took a dose of antipestilential electuary and then, for two or three hours, saw "crowds of citizens, as in a hospital." Then he breakfasted, and visited the sick at their homes.[3] On the threshold of each dwelling he "immediately had burnt some proper thing upon coals," by way of fumigation. Meanwhile he sucked lozenges containing myrrh, cinnamon, and angelica root, and he took care to recover his breath and coolness before entering the sickroom. On returning home to dinner, he drank a glass of sack before and after the meal. After a further round of visits, "until eight or nine at night," he "concluded the evening at home, by drinking to cheerfulness of my old favourite liquor, which encouraged sleep and an easy breathing through the pores all night." On two occasions he felt ill and feared he might be smitten with plague, but a glass of sack proved a sure antidote.

Hodges treated his plague patients very sensibly, insisting on complete rest, with light diet, and promoting perspiration by serpentarium, or Virginian snake root, his favourite remedy. He tells us that he tried bezoar stone, unicorn's horn, and dried toad powder, but that these much vaunted cures were of no value. He quotes a number of prescriptions, including the " Plague water " of the Pharmacopoeia of the College of Physicians, which contained twenty-one ingredients, and Sir Theodore Mayerne's cordial with its twenty-nine component drugs. Recognizing that the infection was air-borne, Hodges noted the benefit of fresh air,

[1] Daniel Defoe, *A Journal of the Plague Year*, London, 1722. (Entirely a work of fiction, though based on reliable information.)
[2] G. H. Evan, " Nathaniel Hodges," *Ann. Med. Hist.*, 1940, 3rd Ser., vol. ii. p. 79 ; W. Wadd, *Memorabilia*, 1927, p. 105 (" Hodges ")
[3] Nathaniel Hodges, *Loimologia*, 3rd ed., 1772, ed. John Quincy. (English editions of this work are still occasionally obtainable. The book is of great interest as a first-hand account of the plague.)

" brisk winds which help to dissipate the poisonous miasmata," and of fumigation, not with coals, which " exhale a fetid and suffocating sulphur," but with " resinous woods, which throw out a clear and unctious smell."

A contemporary physician, GEORGE THOMSON, made a praiseworthy though futile effort to discover the cause of the disease by post-mortem examination as he records in his book entitled *Loimotomia* (Plate XLII).

It was believed that dogs carried the infection, and they were therefore slaughtered in great numbers. No war was waged against the rats, which were the real source of the trouble.

The plague raged throughout the summer of 1665, commencing in June, reaching an appalling climax in September, and then gradually abating until by November it was gone. The king and his court fled to Salisbury, and thence, when the plague reached Salisbury, to Oxford. The poor people who could not thus escape were in dreadful plight. Trade stood still ; the streets were deserted. The silence was broken only by the tolling of bells, the rumble of the dead carts, and the cry of " Bring out your dead." Funerals were forbidden, coffins became unobtainable, and churchyards were soon filled.[1] Then great pits were dug for the reception of the corpses, and even so, the air was polluted by the stench of bodies buried too near the surface in a summer which was unusually hot and sultry. The bills of mortality showed a steadily rising death rate, so that three, four, five thousand died in a week, when the entire population of London was some 500,000. In the third week of September the mortality had mounted to 8,297.[2] " The biggest Bill yet," wrote Pepys, " which is very grievous to us all. Settling my house and all things in the best order I can, lest it should please God to take me." Hodges states that during that third week of September 12,000 perished, and his estimate is probably more correct than the official figure. Thereafter, the epidemic gradually declined, fear was replaced by hope, the death rate became steadily less, and by the month of December people were flocking back to the city, shops re-opened and life resumed its normal course. Nevertheless the plague dragged on in the country during the following year, so that

[1] W. G. Bell, *The Great Plague in London in 1665*, 1924. (The most complete and reliable modern account.)
[2] Geddes Smith, *Plague On Us*, 1941. (A well-documented history of plague, with special reference to America.)

PLATE XLI THE ANATOMY OF THE BRAIN

In 1664 Thomas Willis of Oxford published his *Cerebri Anatome*, illustrated by (Sir) Christopher Wren, and the above represents the arrangement of blood-vessels known as " the circle of Willis " (page 200)

Descartes regarded the human body as a machine controlled by the soul, which was located in the pineal gland, marked H in the above figure from his book *De Homine* (page 177)

PLATE XLII THE GREAT PLAGUE OF LONDON

The Manner of Dissecting
the
PESTILENTIALL BODY.

Frontispiece from " Loimotomia, or The Pest Anatomised,"
by George Thomson, in which he gives an account of his
efforts to ascertain the cause of plague by post-mortem
examination (page 208)

Norwich, then the second city of England, had 2,500 deaths, and many other towns suffered likewise.

Meanwhile, London was purified by the Great Fire, and thus ended the plague which had killed more than a fifth of the inhabitants. Apart from slight sporadic outbreaks, Britain has never again been visited by plague.

The King's Evil and the Royal Touch

The seventeenth century was not marked by any great advance in surgery. Germany produced such men as Fabry of Hilden, whom we have mentioned, and JOHANN SCULTETUS of Ulm (1595–1645), whose *Armamentarium Chirurgium* contains illustrations of many instruments of his devising. GOTTFRIED PURMANN (1649–1711) was a German army surgeon whose writings were highly esteemed. In France, there was PIERRE DIONIS (*d*. 1718) of Paris, who gave courses of operative surgery on the cadaver, publishing a textbook with illustrations of the instruments required for each operation.

England was represented by one who accomplished for British surgery a work similar to that achieved by Thomas Sydenham for British medicine. The name of RICHARD WISEMAN (1622–76),[1] the " Father of English Surgery," is worthy to stand beside that of Sydenham, although they served on opposite sides during the Civil War, Wiseman as Cavalier, and Sydenham as Roundhead. The military career of Wiseman need not detain us long, and indeed we have scant knowledge of his adventurous life. For a time he was a surgeon in the Dutch Navy. Then he served with the army of Charles I until the final defeat by Cromwell at Worcester in 1651. Next came a period of service with the Spanish Navy. After the Restoration Wiseman returned to London, and was appointed Surgeon to Charles II, a post which he faithfully occupied until his death sixteen years later. Wiseman made excellent use of the years of experience in naval and military surgery. His book, modestly entitled *Severall Chirurgicall Treatises*, published in the year of his death, was the greatest work on surgery in England which had appeared up to that time, and it helped to raise the status of the surgeon, which had previously been altogether subservient to that of the physician.

[1] G. Parker, *The Early History of Surgery in Great Britain*, 1920, p. 113 ; Sir T. Longmore, *Richard Wiseman, a Biographical Study*, 1891

Perhaps the most interesting of the treatises is that devoted to King's Evil, the name applied to struma or scrofula, or in modern language, " surgical " tuberculosis, chiefly affecting the lymph glands of the neck. It was called King's Evil, as it was believed to be curable by the " Royal Touch." In France this divine attribute of kings dated back to Clovis the Frank (A.D. 496). Louis XIV is said to have " touched " 2,500 persons, and the practice continued in France until 1775.[1] The first English king to treat the " evil " was Edward the Confessor, and as time went on the cure was attended with great ceremony and was incorporated in the liturgy. Each patient received a gold coin, or " touchpiece," and thus, as Wadd quaintly remarks in his *Memorabilia* (1827), " some were cured of the king's evil, who never had any other evil than that of poverty, which brought more patients and more fame to those royal practitioners than they deserved." [2] The custom reached its zenith during the Stuart period, and John Browne, whose work entitled *Adenochoiradelogia, or Kings-Evil-Swellings* (1684), is the standard authority on the subject, states that Charles II " actually touched, on an average, 4,000 persons every year" (Plate XLIII). In 1660, the year of his restoration, he touched 6,725 persons, and the grand total, from then to the end of his reign, was 92,107. Even during his exile in Holland he was so besieged by sufferers seeking relief that on one occasion six persons were trampled to death. King William was sceptical of the royal power, for he touched but few, saying, " God grant you better health and more sense," but Queen Anne restored the custom, though she was the last of the royal healers.[3] One of the patients touched by her was no less a person than Dr. Samuel Johnson, he being then about two years old.

To return to Richard Wiseman, it is not surprising that he chose to write on King's Evil, which his royal master claimed to cure on so lavish a scale. Wiseman gave an excellent account of scrofula, and that he believed in the miracle performed by the king is evident from his statement, " I have myself been an eye witness of hundreds of cures performed by His Majestie's Touch alone, without any assistance of Chirurgery." Nevertheless he

[1] D. Riesman, *The Story of Medicine in the Middle Ages*, New York, 1935, p. 247
[2] W. Wadd, *Memorabilia*, 1827, p. 134
[3] Raymond Crawfurd, *The King's Evil* (Fitzpatrick Lectures), 1911. (Contains illustrations of the ceremony and of " touch-pieces.") ; Helen Farquhar, " Touch-pieces for the King's Evil," *Brit. Numismatic Jour.*, vol. xii. p. 39 ; vol. xiii. p. 101 ; vol. xiv. p. 173 ; vol. xv. p. 205. (Well documented and illustrated.)

shows what chirurgery can do when the king is not available ; in his own words, " for such as had not the opportunity of receiving the benefit of that stupendous power." Scrofula was very common at that time, so that Wiseman had ample clinical material upon which to base his description. Here are a few sentences from the treatise : " The parts usually affected are either Glandules, Muscles, Viscera, Membranes, Tendons, or Bones. I do not remember ever to have seen the Nerves or Brain affected." " Glandules are a very notorious seat of this Distemper insomuch that authors generally have confined it to them as its Subject." " Bones are frequently affected . . . and the Bone swells and the outward shell thereof appears hard, yet the inward juices are all putrid and rotten."

In another of his treatises, Wiseman gave a graphic account of gunshot wounds, and described many cases from his vast experience. He was well qualified to establish British surgery on a sound basis, and right well did he perform this task.

(For the beginnings of *pathology*, see Supplement, page 456.)

" *Religio Medici* "

This chapter, which opened with an account of some philosophers who influenced medicine, may fitly close with a reference to a medical man and philosopher who made an immortal contribution to English literature.

Sir THOMAS BROWNE of Norwich (1605–82), is better known as an author, yet he fills an important place in medical history, and his writings deserve the attention of every medical man.[1]

Born in London, he was educated at Oxford and later at the then leading medical schools of the Continent—Montpellier, Padua, and Leyden.[2] Shortly after his return from abroad, he settled in Norwich, where he lived and worked for forty-six years. He married Dorothy Mileham, who bore him ten children ; the eldest boy, Edward, wrote a notable book of travel,[3] attained eminence in medicine, and became President of the Royal College of Physicians. Thomas Browne was a Royalist, but in his works he preserved a discreet silence on politics. In Norwich he conducted a large and extensive practice, and was well known

[1] Sir Edmund Gosse, *Sir Thomas Browne* (English Men of Letters), 1905
[2] Sir H. Rolleston, " Sir Thomas Browne, M.D.," *Ann. Med. Hist.*, 1930, vol. ii. p. 1
[3] Edward Browne, *A Brief Account of some Travel in Divers Parts of Europe*, 2nd ed., 1685

as a naturalist and antiquary. King Charles II, in visiting the town in 1671, conferred on Browne the honour of knighthood.[1]

His best known work is *Religio Medici*, which he wrote at the age of thirty, just after his return from his three years of continental study (1635).[2] It was not intended for publication, but was circulated, in manuscript, among his friends. Printed by one of them without permission, a copy reached the notorious Sir Kenelm Digby, who wrote his *Observations* on it, and thus hastened the appearance of the authorized edition of 1643, which had a great reception in England and on the Continent, despite its unorthodox views. Twenty editions appeared during the author's lifetime, and there have been innumerable editions since then. *Religio Medici* was written at a time when the new thought had separated science and medicine from the Church. The very title was a paradox, as it was inconceivable that a medical man could be a religious man. Browne seeks to reconcile faith and reason, although he recognizes that " many things are true in Divinity which are neither inducible by reason nor confirmable by sense." His scientific mind would not accept a literal interpretation of the scriptures. " For the first chapters of Genesis, I must confess a great deal of obscurity," he wrote ; he " would gladly know how Moses burnt the Golden Calf, for that mystical metal consumeth not in fire ; " he could not dream " that there should be at the last day any Judicial proceeding or calling to the bar as indeed the Scripture seems to imply," as the idea of Hell was inconceivable to him. A loyal son of the Church of England, he was no slave to creed, for he had " no antipathy in dyet, humour, air, or anything," and for him " all places, all airs, make one Countrey."

His training as a physician induced him to remark upon the intricacy of human anatomy, and to marvel how health was preserved. " I that have examined the parts of a man and know upon what tender filaments that Fabrick hangs, do wonder that we are not always sick." But he found in the Fabrick " no Organ or Instrument for the rational Soul." " Thus we are men and we know not how : there is something in us that can be without us and will be after us." Whence it came he could not tell. It is

[1] Sir N. Moore, *The History of the Study of Medicine in the British Isles*, 1908, p. 69
[2] W. Osler, " Sir Thomas Browne," *The Library*, January 1906. (Reprinted in *An Alabama Student and Other Essays*.)

tempting to multiply quotations from the *Religio*, although these can convey no idea of the symphonic nature of the work.[1] Like music, it suggests more than its words express. It stimulates thought and "gives a man a sane outlook on the complex problems of life." The mystery of death ever intrigued Sir Thomas Browne, though he confessed "We are but embryon philosophers. . . . A dialogue between two infants in the womb concerning the state of this world might handsomely illustrate our ignorance of the next " (*Urn Burial*).

One is not surprised to learn that many have found in Browne a kindred spirit ; among them Coleridge, Lamb, Johnson, Lowell, and, in modern times, that illustrious and versatile physician Sir William Osler. Browne was for Osler a hero and example whose writings he was wont to recommend to students of medicine in such words as the following : " Not only does the charm of high thoughts clad in beautiful language win readers to a love of good literature, but the *Religio* is full of counsels of perfection which appeal to the mind of youth. Mastery of self, devotion to duty, deep interest in human beings : these best of all lessons may be gleaned from the writings of Sir Thomas Browne " (*An Alabama Student*, 1908).

In *Urn Burial, or Hydriotaphia* (1658), Browne discourses with great eloquence on his favourite theme, death and immortality.[2] *The Garden of Cyrus* (1658) treats of ancient gardens and of much else besides. Quaintest of all is *Pseudodoxia Epidemica, or Enquiries into Vulgar and Common Errors* (1646), which contains observations on every department of knowledge, and is a plea for the use of the Baconian principle in research. Strange indeed that Browne, so modern in his outlook, should have believed in witches, even adding his evidence in the condemnation of two old women, convicted of witchcraft. It has been widely believed that Sir Thomas Browne was responsible for the hanging of Amy Duny and Rose Cullender, who were convicted of witchcraft before Sir Matthew Hale at Bury in 1664. That this view is erroneous has been shown by Dr. W. W. Francis,[3] who drew attention to two

---

[1] Sir Thomas Browne, *Religio Medici and Other Works*, Everyman's Library, No. 92, 1906. (This is a handy edition and readily obtainable, but some of the earlier editions are very attractive. A facsimile of the first edition was published in Oxford in 1909 from a copy in the possession of Sir William Osler.)
[2] M. L. Tildesley, *Sir Thomas Browne, his Skull, Portraits, and Ancestry*, 1924
[3] W. W. Francis, " Sir Thomas Browne and the Witch-Trials : a Vindication," *Lancet*, 1912, vol. i. p. 158

articles in the *Norfolk Chronicle* of December 1911, written by Mr. Malcolm Letts after a study of the contemporary official report of the trial. Sir Thomas Browne was present in court, and at an early stage in the trial the judge asked him to state his opinion. He thereupon expressed his belief in the reality of witchcraft, a view shared by the great majority of his learned contemporaries, but he took no part in the condemnation of the accused. It is highly probable that the witches were convicted on the evidence adduced by the prosecution without reference to Sir Thomas Browne's opinion. It is indeed unfortunate that some of Browne's biographers have perpetuated a statement so damaging to the high reputation of one whose character was so gentle and saintly. Belief in the supernatural retained this mediæval flavour long after the Renaissance, and need not detract from the homage due to the Sage of Norwich.

(See Supplement, page 458, for *Witches and Witch-hunting*.)

BOOKS FOR FURTHER READING

BELL, W. G.   *The Great Plague in London in 1665*, 1924
COMRIE, J. D.   *Selected Works of Thomas Sydenham, M.D.*, 1922
CRAWFURD, RAYMOND.   *Plague and Pestilence in Literature and Art*, 1914
FOSTER, Sir M.   *Lectures on the History of Physiology*, 1901
GOSSE, Sir EDMUND.   *Sir Thomas Browne* (English Men of Letters), 1905
LONGMORE, Sir T.   *Richard Wiseman, a Biographical Study*, 1891
PARKER, G.   *The Early History of Surgery in Great Britain*, 1920
REDGROVE, H.   *Alchemy, Ancient and Modern*, 1922
RIESMAN, D.   *The Story of Medicine in the Middle Ages*, New York, 1935
STUBBS, S. G., and BLIGH, E. W.   *Sixty Centuries of Health and Physick*, 1931
LONG, ESMOND R.   *A History of Pathology*, 1928

CHAPTER XII

XVIII-CENTURY MEDICINE

MANY years elapsed before the brilliant discoveries of the new age, or Renaissance, could be applied with advantage in the daily round of medical practice. New facts had accumulated without being assimilated, and then there came a time when it was necessary to pause and take stock of the situation. A mass of new knowledge awaited arrangement and classification, if some semblance of law and order was to be achieved.

This was the condition of affairs at about the beginning of the eighteenth century, when two great scientists supplied the need of the age. To the apparent chaos Newton applied law, and Linnaeus brought order. In medicine the outstanding figure was that of Boerhaave, one of the most eminent physicians of all time.

SIR ISAAC NEWTON (1642–1727) was not directly concerned with medicine. Nevertheless his proof that certain laws governed not only the human body, not only all things on the earth, but also all the heavenly bodies, in fact the entire universe, and that there was one set of laws for all, was bound to exercise a profound effect upon all the sciences. Newton's *Principia*, published in 1687, has been called "the greatest triumph of the human mind."

At a slightly later date Carl von Linné, known as LINNAEUS (1707–78),[1] a successful physician as well as one of the greatest botanists of all time, whose garden may still be seen at Upsala, introduced the binomial method of classifying plants, each having its genus and its species, and thus gave science a means of classification which brought order and uniformity in place of confusion. The *Systema Naturae* was published in 1735, and the method, extended to animals as well as plants, included as its leading representative *Homo sapiens*.

In addition to the general principles laid down by Newton and Linnaeus, many other "systems" and theories were evolved at about this time. Most of them are now obsolete and forgotten,

[1] B. H. Larsson, "Carolus Linnæus, Physician and Botanist," *Ann. Med. Hist.*, 1938, vol. x. p. 197 ; B. D. Jackson, *Linnaeus : The Story of His Life*, 1923

but as they played an important part in the evolution of modern medicine, some reference must be made to the theories and to their sponsors, if only to emphasize the far greater importance of Boerhaave, to whose life and work we shall afterwards direct the reader's attention.

Animism and Vitalism

The action and reaction between medicine and religion throughout the ages is one of the most interesting aspects of medical history. In the age under discussion a wide gulf had formed between them, and each advanced along a separate path. Medicine, as we have noted, had become so materialistic that the functions of the human body in health and disease were simply questions of physics and chemistry. Nevertheless there were those who thought otherwise, and at this stage we encounter a medical prophet who dared to reaffirm the existence and importance of man's immortal soul. This was GEORG ERNST STAHL (1660–1734), Professor of Medicine in the newly constituted University of Halle. Stahl discarded chemistry or physics, and he even denied that anatomy was essential to the physician. Nor would he admit, like Descartes, that soul and body each went their separate ways. In Stahl's opinion soul and body were closely blended, and the source of all vital movement was the soul or " anima." [1] The soul he alleged, prevented the putrefaction which takes place after death in the soulless body. It was true that the body did eventually die, but that was only when it no longer provided a suitable habitation for the soul. Stahl's idea was not new.[2] His " anima " had been described previously as nature, archaeus, or pneuma, and in modern times as the subconscious or unconscious mind. Stahl strove to reconcile the views of physicians and theologians, but he satisfied neither party. To the physicians, animism was simply so much nonsense, devoid of proof, and it involved a policy of undue simplicity in the treatment of disease. The theologians, on the other hand, resented the apparent degradation of the soul into a kind of defender of the body against death and disease, the defence being often ineffective. Thus Stahl's views were open to question and were not very convincing. Moreover, Stahl was not gifted with an engaging

[1] E. T. Withington, *Medical History from the Earliest Times*, 1894, p. 334
[2] Richard Koch, " War Georg Ernst Stahl ein selbständiger Denker ? " *Arch. f. Gesch. Med.*, 1926, vol. xviii. p. 20

personality. He was intolerant of criticism, blunt in manner, and appears to have deserved the criticism of Boerhaave, who called him "the sour metaphysician." Nevertheless he served his generation well by provoking some degree of reaction against materialism, and by suggesting that the psychical aspect of disease should not be neglected. Had he lived to-day, he would probably have become a distinguished psychiatrist.

JOSEPH BARTHEZ of Montpellier (1734–1806), who was born in the year of Stahl's death, recognizing the difficulty of championing the claim of "soul" or of "body," introduced a dominant force which he alleged was neither the one nor the other. This he called the "vital principle." The idea made little progress, as it was obvious that this was merely another name for the life force which had eluded so many inquirers. "Vitalism" presented no advantage over animism.

Often associated with the name of Stahl in medical history is that of his fellow-professor at Halle, FRIEDRICH HOFFMANN (1660–1742). Nevertheless Stahl and Hoffmann had little in common. A man of kindly and urbane temperament, Hoffmann had all the qualities of the successful physician. Not only did he conduct a large practice, but he also gained a great reputation as a teacher. His system of medicine was based upon the belief that the universe was pervaded by a vital substance, "finer than all other matter, but not exactly spirit, soul, or mind," and that this subtle something maintained the body in a state of tonic equilibrium. In Hoffmann's view, disease resulted from excess or deficiency of "tonus." Excess of tonus, or spasm, caused acute disease, while lack of it, or atony, caused chronic disease. Treatment, therefore, consisted for the most part in the administration of sedatives for the former condition, and tonics for the latter. Even the modern patient still demands "a tonic" from his doctor.

The fact that Hoffmann employed and sold certain secret remedies need not detract from his good name, as this was a universal practice at the time. One of his preparations, Hoffmann's anodyne (Spiritus Aetheris Co)[1] still survives, although his extensive work, *Medicina rationalis systematica*, in nine volumes, 1718–40, has long since been forgotten.

[1] A. C. Wootton, *Chronicles of Pharmacy*, 2 vols., 1910

Doses, Large and Small

While Hoffmann was approaching the end of his life, there was born in Scotland a man whose views, which closely followed those of Hoffmann, became the subject of much controversy. JOHN BROWN (1735–88),[1] a child of poor parents in a Berwickshire village, was educated at the grammar school of Duns and at Edinburgh University. He devoted himself to education and to theology in turn, but achieving no success in either he turned his attention to medicine.[2] Unfortunately for himself, he was of fickle temperament and of convivial habits, while his boastful manner made him unpopular with his colleagues. He was at first befriended by Cullen (p. 221), who employed him as secretary and tutor to his family, as Brown was an excellent Latin scholar. Continuing his medical studies, Brown even ventured to give extra-academical lectures in medicine, and to publish his work entitled, *Elementa Medicinae* (1780). Success attended those activities, and the views expressed in the so-called " Brunonian System " were warmly espoused by his students.[3] Stormy debates raged in the Royal Medical Society, of which Brown was twice President, between the students of Brown and those of Cullen, the two teachers having come into open enmity. One result of the quarrel was that Brown could not hope to graduate at Edinburgh, and was obliged to proceed to St. Andrews for his M.D. degree. News of the Brunonian doctrine reached the Continent, where it gave rise to violent controversy, so violent, indeed, that at the University of Göttingen it became necessary to call out the military to quell the disturbance.[4] Yet in his own city the prophet was without honour, although popular with his students. He was at war with all his colleagues, and had even been in prison for debt. Consequently, in 1786, he determined to remove to London. There, alas, his record did not improve, and he died in poverty two years later. Such is the brief history of " the Paracelsus of Scotland."

The Brunonian system was really very simple. Life, according to Brown, depended upon continuous stimulation. The stimulants were warmth, food, muscular movement, intellectual energy,

[1] T. J. Pettigrew, *Medical Portraits*, 1838–40, vol. iv.
[2] Sir B. W. Richardson, *Disciples of Aesculapius*, 2 vols., 1896, vol. i. p. 245
[3] F. H. Garrison, *History of Medicine*, 3rd ed., 1924, p. 319
[4] E. T. Withington, *Medical History from the Earliest Times*, 1894, p. 351

emotion, etc. Disease was the result of excess of stimulation, or, much more frequently, defect of stimulation. Acting upon this assumption, Brown classified all diseases as sthenic or asthenic. No other diagnosis was required, and the treatment was obvious, consisting, as a rule, in large and even " heroic " doses of stimulating drugs. Little wonder that it has been remarked that the Brunonian methods killed more persons than the French Revolution and the Napoleonic wars taken together.

At the opposite extreme, as regards dosage, stands a contemporary of Brown, who likewise moulded medical thought in less drastic but more permanent fashion, and whose influence is still felt to-day. SAMUEL HAHNEMANN (1755–1843), who spent most of his life in Leipzig, was the originator of homoeopathy, a system of medical treatment which is usually associated in our minds with the use of drugs in infinitesimal doses.[1] The chief principle of homoeopathy, however, lies not in the absurdly small dose but in the selection of the drug. *Similia similibus curantur*, " like cures like." In other words, drugs which, when administered to healthy persons, cause certain symptoms, are to be given in illness when such symptoms are present. As a result of numerous experiments on himself and his friends, Hahnemann succeeded in classifying the drugs which served his purpose.[2] Belladonna causes symptoms resembling those of scarlet fever, therefore it was used in scarlet fever. Similar reasoning determined the use of cinchona for ague and ipecacuanha for asthma. There can be no doubt that, setting aside the value of his deductions, Hahnemann added greatly to our knowledge of the action of drugs. Another rule of his system was that only one remedy should be used at a time, and that a second dose should not be given until the first had ceased to act. The third principle of homoeopathy was that the dose should be so small that it would act only upon the disease. Hahnemann argues that the smaller the dose, the greater was the potency, and he defended his use of solution of a drug, diluted and rediluted many times, by stating that disease produced an abnormal sensitiveness to the given drug, provided that the correct remedy had been chosen. His views were embodied in a work entitled *Organon der rationellen Heilkunde*, 1810. Naturally the new idea was strenuously opposed by the apothecaries, who

[1] H. Haeser, *Geschichte der Medizin*, 1845, p. 682
[2] O. E. Guttentag, " Trends Towards Homoeopathy, Past and Present," *Bull. Hist. Med.*, 1940, vol. viii. p. 1172

were likely to be deprived of their profits. Yet homoeopathy has had many followers, and when first introduced it served a useful purpose in checking the dangerously excessive drugging which was then prevalent.

Clinical Medicine under Boerhaave

It is a relief to turn from these theorists and extremists to those who were content to make the best use of the existing knowledge, and to devise methods of teaching which would yield the best results in medical practice.

By far the greatest clinical teacher of the eighteenth century, and one of the greatest of all time, was HERMANN BOERHAAVE of Leyden (1668–1738).[1] The son of a country pastor, who was " poor in money but pure in spirit," Hermann distinguished himself as a student by the ease with which he acquired a sound knowledge of mathematics and of classical and modern languages. It may have been his attendance at lectures on anatomy, then regarded as an essential part of a liberal education, which first attracted him to medicine. Yet his father felt that so clever a youth must not be lost to the Church. Hermann would study theology ; his younger brother James would enter medicine. Eventually it was James who became the minister and Hermann the doctor, the result, it is said, of the following encounter. Young Hermann was travelling in a packet boat when a discussion arose among the passengers regarding Spinoza, who had just startled Europe by affirming that God was everywhere. One speaker was particularly severe in his condemnation of such heresy, until Boerhaave asked him whether he had ever read the works which he so hotly attacked. This silenced the critic, but he had his revenge. On reaching Leyden, Boerhaave found that there had arrived before him the rumour that he was a follower of Spinoza. It was useless to protest. Instead, the young divine determined to change his profession, and to adopt the calling to which he was already strongly attracted. Success came rapidly. As a junior

[1] F. H. Garrison, *History of Medicine*, 3rd ed., 1924, p. 320 ; W. Burton, *The Life and Writings of Hermann Boerhaave*, 2nd ed., 1746 ; H. E. Sigerist, " A Boerhaave Pilgrimage in Holland," *Bull. Hist. Med.*, 1939, vol. vii. p. 257 ; E. C. van Leersum, " How did Boerhaave Speak? " *Janus*, 1912, vol. xvii. p. 145 ; " Hermann Boerhaave," *Janus*, 1918, vol. xxiii. p. 193. (Oration on the 250th anniversary of the birth of Boerhaave) ; H. Barnes, " On Consultations with Boerhaave " (extracts from the notebook of a Carlisle physician), *Proc. Roy. Soc. Med.* (Sect. Hist.), 1917, vol. xi. p. 1

Lecturer on Medicine he attracted many students, and on his appointment to the Chair of Botany and Medicine at Leyden in 1709 his fame spread so widely that students from all over Europe, and even from America, came to attend his classes. For over twenty years he was the central figure of European medicine, lecturing extempore in well phrased Latin, and adopting any theory or system which might serve his purpose, for Boerhaave was a partisan of no special method except, perhaps, that of Hippocrates. Like Hippocrates, he placed the patient in the centre of the picture, and favoured observation rather than argument. Although only twelve beds were allotted to him, he made excellent use of this scanty material.

His enormous private practice drew patients from the entire civilized world, so that it is easy to believe the well-known tale of a letter from China, addressed to " Dr. Boerhaave, Europe," which was delivered without delay. Needless to say, he was a man of intense activity and boundless energy, possessed also, no doubt, of a sound physique, though he suffered greatly from gout in his later years. He was dignified, though kindly, in manner, and gifted with a keen memory and a wide knowledge of affairs, qualities of great value to the popular teacher and fashionable physician which he was (Plate XLIV).

His chief works are the *Institutiones Medicae*, 1708, and *Aphorismi*, 1709, both of which passed through many editions and were the subject of various commentaries. The *Index Plantarum*, 1710, is a catalogue of the Botanical Gardens of Leyden, which he classified and enlarged. Not content with his reputation as a leading physician and botanist, he accepted the Chair of Chemistry in 1718, and in 1731 he published *Elementa Chemiae*, which had engaged his attention for some years.

Beloved and honoured during his lifetime, Boerhaave is still commemorated at Leyden by an elegant statue ; by the Boerhaave Kwartier, as the Medical Buildings are called ; by his town house, once the seat of such intense activity ; by his lovely country house, a present from a grateful patient ; and by the botanical gardens which he so greatly loved.

Only second in importance to Boerhaave as an eighteenth-century teacher was WILLIAM CULLEN (1710–90).[1] Cullen was born at Hamilton, in Lanarkshire, where his father was a lawyer,

[1] J. Thomson, *Life of Dr. William Cullen*, 2 vols., 1879 ; J. D. Comrie, " An Eighteenth-Century Consultant," *Edin. Med. Jour.*, 1925, vol. xxxii. p. 17

and factor to the Duke of Hamilton. From the Grammar School of Hamilton young Cullen proceeded to Glasgow University, but as there was as yet no organized Medical Faculty he became apprenticed to a surgeon in Glasgow, and later to an apothecary in London. He also undertook a voyage to the West Indies as ship's surgeon. After this training he felt justified in setting up his plate in his native town, especially as he enjoyed the patronage of the Duke. About this time he formed a friendship with William Hunter, also a native of Lanarkshire, and the two determined to practise in partnership, each releasing the other, alternately, for further study of medicine. Next year Hunter went to London, to become engrossed in anatomical work, and by mutual and friendly consent the partnership was dissolved. Cullen, too, was ambitious, and we next find him in Glasgow conducting a large practice, and lecturing, with the approval of the authorities, not only on his favourite subject, chemistry, but also on botany, materia medica, and the practice of physic.[1] He may indeed be regarded as the founder of the Glasgow School of Medicine (Plate XLV).

In 1751, when he was forty-one years of age, he became Professor of Medicine in Glasgow, and he continued to lecture on this subject, and on chemistry, until 1755, when he obtained the Chair of Chemistry in Edinburgh.[2] His lectures were the first to be given in the vernacular instead of Latin.[3] To Edinburgh, Cullen brought the distinction which he had conferred upon Glasgow. In Edinburgh, also, his versatility was apparent. Not content with chemistry alone, he delivered lectures on clinical medicine in the Royal Infirmary. Nor was that all, for in 1766 he added the Chair of Institutes or Theory of Medicine, or Physiology as we now call it, which had become vacant by the death of Robert Whytt. At the same time he resigned from the Chair of Chemistry in favour of Joseph Black[4] (p. 261), who had been his pupil in Glasgow, and who achieved great distinction in his subject.

Finally, he arranged with JOHN GREGORY (1724–73), who had come from Aberdeen to be Professor of the Practice of Medicine, that he and Gregory should lecture on this subject alternately. When Gregory died, Cullen became sole professor. Cullen was

[1] A. F. Fergus, *The Origin and Development of the Glasgow School of Medicine*, 1911 ; A. Kent (ed.), *An Eighteenth Century Lectureship in Chemistry*, Glasgow, 1950
[2] W. MacMichael, *Lives of British Physicians*, 1830, p. 234
[3] F. H. Garrison, *History of Medicine*, 3rd ed., 1924, p. 368
[4] Sir W. Ramsay, *The Life and Letters of Joseph Black, M.D.*, 1918

now sixty-three years old. Nevertheless he continued to teach for other fifteen years, when he retired to his country seat at Kirknewton near Edinburgh, and there he died two years later. Cullen's successor was James Gregory, of " Gregory's Powder " fame, son of the Dr. John Gregory just mentioned. Both were members of the distinguished Aberdeen family which produced no fewer than sixteen professors within five generations.[1]

Although Cullen was the author of a successful textbook, *First Lines of the Practice of Physic*, 1777, and although he is credited with having drawn attention to the importance of the nervous system in disease, as well as with an attempt to classify diseases, as Linnaeus classified plants, he cannot be regarded as a discoverer. Theories he only used to illustrate his remarks, and he was no slave to systems. " There must be a tub to amuse the whale," he would say. His pupil and secretary, John Brown, who, as we have seen, took himself so seriously and pursued his "system" like a fanatic, would have been well advised to imitate the philosophic calm of his master. The fact that Cullen taught in the vernacular added interest to his lectures. His gifts of infinite patience and of unruffled temper added to his success. Taking a keen personal interest in his students, he placed at their disposal his house, his library, and even his purse. Among Cullen's admirers was the South American physician and patriot HIPOLITO UNANUE (1755–1833), who transferred to Lima in Peru the methods of Leyden and Edinburgh. His monograph, *El Clima de Lima* (1806), is a medical classic which deserves to be more widely known.

Pupils of Boerhaave

Boerhaave and Cullen were two great teachers of Clinical Medicine in the eighteenth century, the former at the beginning, the latter towards the end. We shall secure a better understanding of the medical history of the time if we survey the lives and work of a few of the colleagues and pupils of those two distinguished men. Boerhaave had attracted to Leyden so many students who subsequently became famous that it is only possible to mention a few of them. One of the most eminent was ALBRECHT VON HALLER (1708–77), a native of Berne.[2] He was a precocious

[1] J. D. Comrie, *History of Scottish Medicine*, 2 vols., 1932, vol. i. p. 383
[2] O. Klotz, " Albrecht von Haller (1708–77)," *Ann. Med. Hist.*, 1936, vol. viii. p. 10 ; Sir M. Foster, *Lectures on the History of Physiology*, 1901, p. 205 ; H. E. Sigerist, *Great Doctors*, 1933, p. 191

child, but, unlike many other infant prodigies, his achievements in adult life really did fulfil the promise of his early years. His name lives in history as a poet, as a botanist and, above all, as a great pioneer physiologist. He wrote Latin verse at the age of ten, and composed scientific lectures before he was fifteen years old. After studying at Leyden under Boerhaave, he visited Paris and London, and had commenced practice in Berne when he was called to be professor at the newly established University of Göttingen.[1] There he worked hard for seventeen years ; then he returned to his native Berne, where he continued his researches and writing until the date of his death. His poetry was of high standard, especially the poem "Die Alpen," descriptive of the Swiss mountains he loved so well. In botany his work on *The Flora of Switzerland* earned high fame.[2] Especially eminent in physiology, he has been acclaimed, with good reason, as the founder of modern physiology, for he collected and arranged all the work on that subject which had been done prior to his time, and added many facts of his own discovery. His greatest achievement was his demonstration of the irritability of muscles and of the sensibility of nerves.[3] He proved that irritability was an attribute of muscular tissue, inherent in the muscle itself, and not dependent upon the nerve supplying the muscle. Glisson had already suggested the hypothesis, but Haller proved it by a series of experiments upon excised muscle tissue. It was Haller who originated the myogenic theory of the action of the heart. His *Elementa Physiologiae*, in eight volumes, 1759–66, was an immense undertaking, and was only a fraction of his work. Medical science owes much to this brilliant scholar. He is one of the most imposing figures in medical history.

The Old Vienna School

Another of Boerhaave's pupils who achieved fame was GERHARD VAN SWIETEN (1700–72) who, after completing his studies at Leyden, acted as a lecturer there with great success. His name was even mentioned as a possible successor to Boerhaave. As he was a Roman Catholic, this post was closed to him. Fortunately, however, he had won the confidence of the Empress Maria Theresa by his skilful treatment of her sister. The Empress

[1] C. G. Cumston, *Introduction to the History of Medicine*, 1926, p. 340
[2] T. J. Pettigrew, *Medical Portraits*, 1838–40, vol. i. (" Haller ")
[3] R. H. Major, *Classic Descriptions of Disease*, 1933, p. 376

PLATE XLIII THE ROYAL GIFT OF HEALING

Charles II " touching," to cure King's Evil. Illustration from John
Browne's *Adenochoiradelogia*, 1684 (page 210)

PLATE XLIV A MEDICAL LECTURE AT LEYDEN

Hermann Boerhaave, 1668–1738, was the greatest physician and medical teacher of his time. The above title-page of one of his works represents him addressing a large audience at Leyden (pages 220–21)

persuaded Van Swieten to come to Vienna as her physician. This he did, but not content to be a mere courtier, he determined to reconstruct the medical school in Vienna, and he did so with characteristic skill and energy. The university was brought under the control of the State, and Van Swieten was appointed principal. Naturally enough, this innovation was severely criticized. Other members of the faculty resented the intrusion of a Dutchman and the limitation of their authority. Yet Van Swieten's masterly handling of the situation overcame all difficulties, and under his able administration the Medical School of Vienna [1] (the Old Vienna School) took root and flourished, and continued to do so under his successor, ANTON DE HAEN (1704–76), who was also a Dutchman. De Haen, though an austere and arrogant man, was a hard worker and an excellent clinician. Recognizing the importance of bedside observation and teaching, he inaugurated a system of careful case-taking, followed by detailed notes of progress or changes from day to day. He was the author of a treatise on therapeutics, in which he condemned the excessive drugging which was then prevalent, and supported the expectant or Hippocratic method.

Leyden and Edinburgh

Many British students found their way to Leyden while that school enjoyed world-wide fame. Among them was Sir Thomas Browne, who graduated there in 1633. The torch of learning which had been lit in Greece had passed to Salerno, then to Montpellier and Padua, then to Leyden, and early in the eighteenth century it was handed on to Edinburgh, which then became the centre of medical learning.

As early as 1660, Sir ROBERT SIBBALD (1641–1722) spent a year and a half at Leyden under Sylvius and other teachers, and then returned to Edinburgh, to become famous as the founder of the Royal College of Physicians of Edinburgh (1681), the first Professor of Medicine in the Town's College (later University) of Edinburgh, Geographer Royal for Scotland, and the author of a number of works on history and archæology.[2] He was one of a trio of professors of medicine appointed by the town (1685), the others being Dr. JAMES HALKET, another Leyden student, and

[1] M. Neuburger, *British Medicine and the Vienna School*, 1943, p. 15
[2] F. P. Hett, ed. of *The Memoirs of Sir Robert Sibbald (1641–1722)*, 1932

Dr. ARCHIBALD PITCAIRNE (1652–1713).[1] Pitcairne was only thirty-three years of age when appointed professor, and he became the most celebrated Scottish physician of his day. To his influence, and to that of ALEXANDER MONRO, may be traced the origin of the Edinburgh Medical School. Pitcairne, a member of a well-known Fifeshire family,[2] had graduated in divinity and in law before turning to medicine. He studied in Edinburgh and Paris, graduating M.D. at Rheims in 1680. Next year he became an original fellow of the Royal College of Physicians of Edinburgh, the youngest to receive this distinction. About this time he wrote an able defence of Harvey's claim to the discovery of the circulation of the blood, a claim which was then by no means universally accepted. Pitcairne adopted the views of the iatro-physical school of thought, which, as we have noted, explained all the activities of the body on a mechanical basis. His writings, published under the title *Dissertationes Medicae*, increased his reputation and led to his appointment as Professor of Medicine at Leyden in 1692. At Leyden he enhanced the reputation of the medical school although, for family reasons, he was obliged to return to Edinburgh at the end of his first year in Holland. Among his pupils in Leyden were his successor, Boerhaave, who was to become so famous, and the celebrated London physician, Dr. Richard Mead (p. 254).

Pitcairne was a man of strong personality, and when we learn that he was a Jacobite and an Episcopalian we may readily understand why he was not universally popular. Yet his is a name worthy to be revered in the annals of medicine. Pitcairne died at the age of sixty-one and was buried in Greyfriars churchyard. Among other bequests he left a " jeroboam " of wine, with instructions that it was to be drunk on the restoration of the Stuart kings. That event was not forthcoming, and in 1800 a number of medical men in Edinburgh, led by ANDREW DUNCAN (1744–1828), who had succeeded Gregory as Professor of the Institutes of Medicine, decided that the restoration of the tomb of Pitcairne might well fulfil the terms of his will. Accordingly the tomb was restored, and the memory of the deceased duly honoured with the contents of the jeroboam.[3]

[1] J. D. Comrie, *History of Scottish Medicine*, 2 vols., 1932, vol. i. p. 277
[2] Constance Pitcairn, *The History of the Fife Pitcairns*, Edinburgh, 1905
[3] R. Thin, " Archibald Pitcairne, 1652–1713," *Edin. Med. Jour.*, 1928, vol. xxxv. p. 368

Influence of the Monros

Among Pitcairne's students at Leyden was JOHN MONRO
(*d.* 1737), surgeon in the army of William of Orange, a man of
sound education and of high standing in his profession.[1] His
great ambition was to establish a Medical School in Edinburgh
on the lines of the Leyden School. Accordingly he set out to
interest the physicians and surgeons in this project. As we have
already noted, some progress had been made by the appointment
of Sibbald, Halket, and Pitcairne as Professors of Medicine, and
the subjects of botany and chemistry had been taught, while
classes in anatomy had been held by Monteith, Eliot, McGill,
and Drummond in the anatomical theatre of the New Surgeons'
Hall. In 1705 Robert Eliot had been appointed "public
dissector" in the "Town's College," as the university was then
called, at a salary of £15 per annum. The time was now ripe for
a further step, and John Monro seized the opportunity and
specially educated his son Alexander to fill the post of Professor
of Anatomy. After studying in Edinburgh, Alexander continued his studies in London under Cheselden and in Leyden
under Boerhaave. Meanwhile his father had done everything
possible to smooth his path and promote his success, and on returning to Edinburgh ALEXANDER MONRO (1697–1767), called PRIMUS,
to distinguish him from his son and grandson of the same name,
then only twenty-two years of age, was appointed Professor of
Anatomy.[2] His first course was attended by fifty-seven students,
and the number rose steadily each year. It is reported that at the
first lecture the presence of the Lord Provost and Magistrates and
the leading physicians and surgeons of Edinburgh so disconcerted
the young professor that he entirely forgot his discourse, but he
rapidly recovered his composure, and delivered an extemporane-
ous lecture with great success. According to another account he
had left his notes at home. In any case he emerged creditably from
the ordeal. At first Monro taught in the Surgeons' Hall, but in
1725, in consequence of a public demonstration against "body
snatching," he was obliged to seek sanctuary within the university.
Among other incidents, there had been a fight between the students
and the relatives of the deceased for the possession of the body of a

[1] J. A. Inglis, *The Monros of Auchinbowie*, Edinburgh, 1911
[2] S. W. Simon, "The Influence of the Monros on the Practice of Medicine," *Ann. Med. Hist.*, 1927, vol. ix. p. 244

woman criminal who had just been executed. While the fight was in progress, the " body " came to life, and lived for many years, being known as " Half-hangit Maggie Dickson." According to another account, Maggie Dickson was a native of Musselburgh, and it was on the journey thither, while the funeral procession was resting at Peffermill, that the corpse revived, to the consternation of the bearers and the delight of the mourners. This was about a century before the days of the terrible Burke and Hare murders. Monro continued to teach, with great acceptance, for thirty-eight years. He taught surgery as well as anatomy, and conducted a large practice. He was active in his attendance upon the wounded after the battle of Prestonpans in 1745. Of him Struthers wrote, " a great and good man, he well earned the title of father of the Edinburgh Medical School "[1] (Plate XLVI).

Foundation of the Edinburgh School

Stimulated by Monro's success, four leading Fellows of the College of Physicians, Drs. St. Clair, Rutherford, Plummer, and Innes, petitioned the Town Council to be appointed professors in the university, and this was done in 1726. Each of the new professors had studied in Leyden under Boerhaave, as also had the Professors of Chemistry (JAMES CRAWFORD) and of Botany (CHARLES PRESTON). ANDREW ST. CLAIR taught the Institutes of Medicine (Physiology) ; JOHN RUTHERFORD, the maternal grandfather of Sir Walter Scott, dealt with the Practice of Medicine ; while ANDREW PLUMMER and JOHN INNES shared between them the subjects of Chemistry and Materia Medica.

In the same year, 1726, another Chair was founded, that of Midwifery, and JOSEPH GIBSON, who practised in Leith, was its occupant, and indeed was the first Professor of Midwifery to hold office in any university. He died in 1739. Systematic lectures on the subject were not given, however, until THOMAS YOUNG was elected professor in 1756, and it was through the exertions of Young's successor, ALEXANDER HAMILTON (1739–1802) that a maternity hospital was established, independently of the Infirmary, in 1793. Naturally a great impetus had been given to the clinical teaching by the provision of hospital beds, at first on a small scale in a " hired house," and eventually by the opening of an infirmary in 1741. The Edinburgh Medical School was then securely founded.

[1] J. Struthers, *Historical Sketch of the Edinburgh Anatomical School*, 1867

PLATE XLV
THE FOUNDER OF THE GLASGOW SCHOOL

WILLIAM CULLEN, 1710–90 (page 221)
From an engraving by T. Sommers, in the National Portrait Gallery of
Scotland, of a painting by W. Cochrane

PLATE XLVI
THE FOUNDER OF THE EDINBURGH SCHOOL

ALEXANDER MONRO (primus), 1697–1767 (page 227)
(From an engraving by J. Basire of the painting by Allan Ramsay)

Alexander Monro was succeeded in 1758 by his son ALEXANDER MONRO, SECUNDUS (1733–1817). Monro secundus was even more brilliant than his distinguished father.[1] He had studied in London under William Hunter, in Berlin under Meckel, and in Leyden under Albinus. He was a clear and eloquent lecturer, and like his father he spoke without notes. It is estimated that during his forty years' tenure of the Chair about 40,000 students attended his classes. Among his discoveries was the foramen of Monro, familiar to every student of anatomy, and he published original observations on the " bursae mucosae " and on the lymphatics. None of his great work was published until he was fifty years of age. Besides being a famous anatomist, he was the leading physician of his time, and he was also consulted regarding surgical cases, though he did not himself operate. He certainly deserved his successes ; his father was obliged to " achieve greatness," but Monro secundus was " born great." It is often unfortunate to be the son of a distinguished father, yet Monro held his place, intellectually and socially, among the great men of his period.

Unfortunately the high standard was not maintained in the next generation. Again the Professorship of Anatomy passed from father to son, this time, in 1798, to ALEXANDER MONRO, TERTIUS (1773–1859), who was content to read to his students his grandfather's lectures, a century old, and although he had never been to Leyden, he did not even trouble to delete the remark, " When I was a student at Leyden in 1719."[2] Nevertheless he occupied the Chair for thirty-eight years. Thus anatomy was taught in Edinburgh by three generations of Monros, during a period of one hundred and twenty-six years.

During the early part of the eighteenth century surgery was taught by the professor of anatomy as a mere appendage to his subject. The surgeons of the time were general practitioners, such as ALEXANDER WOOD (1725–1807), a tall, striking figure, familiarly known as " Lang Sandy Wood," who was often accompanied on his professional rounds by a tame raven and a sheep, and he was the first person in Edinburgh to carry an umbrella.[3] Despite such eccentricities, he was recognized as the leading surgeon of Edinburgh. He added to the reputation of the Infirmary by his

[1] A. Miles, " The Dynasty of the Monros," *University of Edinburgh Jour.*, 1925–26, vol. i. p. 54
[2] J. D. Comrie, *History of Scottish Medicine*, 1932, 2 vols., vol. ii. p. 493
[3] J. Kay, *Edinburgh Portraits*, Edinburgh, 1877

skill, while by his genial and friendly manner he promoted the harmony of his profession (Plate XLVII).

The Teaching of Surgery

Of slightly later date was BENJAMIN BELL (1749–1806), who has been acclaimed as "the first of the Edinburgh scientific surgeons" (Plate XLVII). He studied in London and Paris, acquiring a knowledge of surgery such as could not then be obtained in Scotland.[1] Appointed as surgeon to the Royal Infirmary at the of age twenty-four, he soon became the first surgeon in Scotland. He wrote a *System of Surgery*, in six volumes, which was translated into French and German, and was for many years a standard authority.[2] Benjamin Bell was an ancestor of Dr. JOSEPH BELL (1837–1911), also a well-known surgeon, who became still more widely famous when his pupil, Conan Doyle, portrayed him as "Sherlock Holmes."[3] (Plate LVIII). Another eminent Edinburgh surgeon, of the same name, but no relation to Benjamin, was JOHN BELL (1763–1820). He was a clever surgeon and had a large practice, although as a result of a malicious attack by the irritable Professor James Gregory, to which he replied with dignity, he found himself excluded from the Royal Infirmary.[4] His younger brother was Sir Charles Bell, to whom we shall refer later (p. 266).

Home, Whytt, and Gregory

Meanwhile the teaching of other subjects was passing on from the original occupants of the Chairs to capable successors. Another pupil of Boerhaave, CHARLES ALSTON, succeeded to the Chair of Botany, to which was added Materia Medica, in 1738. Materia Medica was made a separate Chair in 1768, when FRANCIS HOME (1719–1813) became its first occupant.[5] Home, while serving with the army in Flanders, had ordered his dragoons to drink only boiled water, and doubtless he had thus saved many lives (Plate XLVII). While on the Continent he had taken the oppor-

[1] Sir B. W. Richardson, *Disciples of Aesculapius*, 2 vols., 1896, vol. ii. p. 482
[2] J. D. Comrie, *History of Scottish Medicine*, 2 vols., 1932, vol. i. p. 311
[3] Sir A. S. MacNalty, "Conan Doyle," *Ann. Med. Hist.*, 1935, vol. vii. p. 532
[4] A. Miles, *The Edinburgh School of Surgery before Lister*, 1918, p. 60
[5] E. E. Hume, "Francis Home, M.D., 1719–1813, the Scottish Military Surgeon Who First Described Diphtheria as a Clinical Entity," *Bull. Hist. Med.*, 1942, vol. xi. p. 48

tunity to attend Boerhaave's lectures ; still another Leyden student to become an Edinburgh professor. The stamp of Leyden, and especially the tradition of Boerhaave, served Edinburgh well in those early days.

Another great professor was ROBERT WHYTT (1714–66). He taught both the theory and the practice of medicine, and made extensive research on the possibility of dissolving stones in the bladder by the injection of lime-water and soap. He was the first to localize the seat of reflex action in the spinal cord, and to show that it was independent of the brain. His work on diseases of the nervous system was of high standard, and his original descriptions of tuberculous meningitis and of diphtheria are medical classics.[1] One of the most brilliant of the early Edinburgh professors, Whytt was succeeded in the Chair of Practice of Medicine by John Gregory, and in that of the Institutes of Medicine by William Cullen, of whose work some account has been given.

JAMES GREGORY (1753–1821), who followed Cullen, had studied at Leyden, although by that time the death of Boerhaave had deprived that school of its chief ornament. As has been already mentioned, Gregory was a member of a famous family.[2] He achieved great success in practice and as a teacher, and his textbook, *Conspectus Medicinae*, had a large circulation. It was regarded as " a model of exactness and classical elegance."[3] His powder containing magnesia, rhubarb, and ginger is still well known.[4] Unfortunately he was rather contentious, and became involved not only in an altercation with the surgeon John Bell, as already mentioned, but also in a violent quarrel with a colleague of similar temperament to his own, JAMES HAMILTON (*d.* 1839), who had succeeded his father, Alexander Hamilton (p. 228), as Professor of Midwifery.[5] The difference of opinion led to blows and ended in court, where Hamilton was awarded £100 of damages. Gregory is said to have remarked that the pleasure of beating Hamilton was worth the money. Such were the polemics of eighteenth-century Edinburgh. It is interesting to note that Professor James Hamilton was the last person in Edinburgh to visit his patients in a sedan chair, which conveyance he used as late as 1830.

[1] J. D. Comrie, " An Eighteenth-century Neurologist," *Edin. Med. Jour.*, 1925 vol. xxxii. p. 755
[2] J. D. Comrie, *History of Scottish Medicine*, 2 vols., 1932, vol. i. p. 383
[3] *Life of Robert Christison*, ed. by his sons, 2 vols., 1885, vol. i. p. 80
[4] A. C. Wootton, *Chronicles of Pharmacy*, 1910, 2 vols., vol. ii. p. 137
[5] J. D. Comrie, *loc. cit.*, vol. ii. p. 485

Medicine in the Army and Navy

As a conclusion to this sketch of the rise of the Edinburgh Medical School, it is fitting to pay a brief tribute to two Edinburgh graduates who distinguished themselves by their services to the army and navy respectively.

Sir JOHN PRINGLE (1707–82) was the son of Sir John Pringle, Bart., of Stitchel, Roxburghshire.[1] After a brilliant undergraduate career at St. Andrews, Edinburgh, and Leyden, he became M.D. of the last-mentioned university in 1730, and returned to settle in Edinburgh. There he was appointed Professor of Moral Philosophy. He combined the duties of this Chair with the practice of medicine, and attained eminence in both fields. In 1742 he was appointed physician to the Earl of Stair, then in command of the British Army on the Continent. At the battle of Dettingen (1743), it was on Pringle's suggestion that arrangements were made with the French commander that military hospitals on both sides should be considered as sanctuaries and be mutually protected. This arrangement, which was rigidly observed, led eventually to the development of the " Red Cross " organization in modern warfare.[2] Actually it was the publication by the Swiss banker, Jean Henry Dunant, of his impressions of the horrors of the battlefield, in a little book entitled *Un Souvenir de Solferino*, 1862, which prepared the way for the Geneva Convention of October 1863, at which international agreement was reached regarding the protection of the sick and wounded and of those who attended them. In the following year the Convention reassembled and resolved that neutral status should be accorded to all persons in attendance on the wounded, and the emblem of the Red Cross (in Moslem countries, the Red Crescent) was adopted as their distinguishing mark. (See Supplement, p. 458.)

To complete our story of Pringle, when he returned to England he served, under the Duke of Cumberland, in the army sent to quell the Jacobite Rebellion of 1745, and he was present at the battle of Culloden. There he encountered, among 270 wounded men, a new type of wound, " cuts with the broadsword, which bled much at first, but easily healed."

The Chief Medical Officer to the army of Prince Charles

[1] W. MacMichael, *Lives of British Physicians*, 1830, p. 172.
[2] R. H. Major, *War and Disease*, 1944, p. 92 ; Dermot Morrah, *The British Red Cross*, 1944, p. 16

Edward Stuart was another baronet, Sir STUART THREIPLAND, a graduate of Edinburgh University and an ardent Jacobite, who afterwards settled in Edinburgh and became President of the Royal College of Physicians. In 1752 Pringle published *Observations on the Diseases of the Army*, a famous work which passed through many editions, and which was translated into French, German, and Italian. In it he made suggestions for the better ventilation of barracks, jails, and hospitals, and certain other recommendations which contributed to the comfort and health of the troops. Often it was said of him that " few physicians have rendered more definite services to humanity." Among his other works was a series of short papers on *Experiments upon Septic and Antiseptic Substances*, read before the Royal Society (1750–52), in which the word " antiseptic " is used for the first time. Those papers are included as an Appendix to the *Observations* mentioned above. Pringle became a Fellow of the Royal College of Physicians, Physician to King George III, and President of the Royal Society. He married a daughter of Dr. Oliver of Bath, the physician whose name strangely survives in a biscuit.[1]

About the same period there lived a surgeon who rendered to the navy a service similar to that which Sir John Pringle had given to the army. JAMES LIND (1716–94), born and educated in Edinburgh, entered the navy at the age of twenty-three and served for nine years, most of the time in tropical seas. Retiring from the sea in 1748, he practised in Edinburgh for ten years, and was then appointed physician to Haslar Hospital, a post which he held for twenty-five years. When he joined the navy he found the conditions most unfavourable to health.[2] The cabins were " cold, damp, and unwholesome," the diet consisted of " putrid beef, rancid pork, mouldy biscuit, and bad water," so that scurvy was rampant on every voyage. " In such a situation, the ignorant sailor and the learned physician will equally long, with the most craving anxiety, for green vegetables and the fresh fruits of the earth, from whose healing virtues relief only can be had." So wrote James Lind in his book, *A Treatise of the Scurvy*, 1753, one of the most interesting and important works in medical literature[3].

[1] E. B. Krumbhaar, " Bath Olivers—Doctor and Biscuit," *Ann. Med. Hist.*, 1929, vol. i. p. 253

[2] Sir H. Rolleston, " James Lind, Pioneer of Naval Hygiene," *Jour. Roy. Nav. Med. Service*, 1915, vol. i. p. 181

[3] R. Stockman, " James Lind and Scurvy," *Edin. Med. Jour.*, 1926, vol. xxxvii. p. 329

John Knyveton, another naval surgeon of this time, writes in his diary of the " scores of poor wights lying helpless with swollen discoloured limbs and bleeding mouths." [1] Lord Anson had lost seventy-five per cent. of his ship's company from scurvy during his voyage round the world (1740–44). It was the scourge of the navy, and Lind often had three to four hundred cases in his wards at Haslar. He knew nothing of vitamins, but he recommended the use of lemon juice, and made other suggestions to improve the health of seamen. Thanks to his efforts, scurvy disappeared as if by magic, though he did not live to see the full result of his efforts.

Lind was not the first, and did not claim to be the first, to suggest the use of lime juice or lemon juice for scurvy. John Woodall mentioned it in *The Surgeon's Mate* a century earlier (p. 152), and JOHN HUXHAM (1692–1768), a well-known physician of Plymouth, who wrote a *Treatise on Fever*, in 1750, and papers on malignant sore throat and on Devonshire colic, recommended the use of cider and vegetable diet as a means of preventing scurvy.[2] The Devonshire colic studied by Huxham was proved by Sir GEORGE BAKER (1722–1809) to be lead poisoning arising from the lead pipes of cider presses.[3]

(For *Medical Teaching in Aberdeen* see Supplement, page 459.)

[1] E. Gray, *Surgeon's Mate : The Diary of John Knyveton, Surgeon in the British Fleet During the Seven Years' War, 1756–1762*, 1942
[2] F. H. Garrison, *History of Medicine*, 3rd ed., 1924, p. 373
[3] R. H. Major, *Classic Descriptions of Disease*, 1932, p. 285

BOOKS FOR FURTHER READING

CHRISTISON. *Life of Sir Robert Christison by His Sons*, 2 vols., 1885
COMRIE, J. D. *History of Scottish Medicine*, 2 vols., 1932
HETT, F. P. Ed. of *The Memoirs of Sir Robert Sibbald (1641–1722)*, 1932
JACKSON, B. D. *Linnaeus : The Story of his Life*, 1923
MILES, A. *The Edinburgh School of Surgery before Lister*, 1918
PETTIGREW, T. J. *Medical Portraits*, 2 vols., 1838–40
PITCAIRNE, C. *The History of the Fife Pitcairns*, Edinburgh, 1905
STRUTHERS, J. *Historical Sketch of the Edinburgh Anatomical School*, 1867
THOMSON, J. *Life of Dr. William Cullen*, 2 vols., 1879
WOOTTON, A. C. *Chronicles of Pharmacy*, 2 vols., 1910

CHAPTER XIII

XVIII-CENTURY MEDICINE (*Continued*)

IN the medical world of London early in this eventful century surgery was in the capable hands of Cheselden and Pott, and, above all, of John Hunter. In medicine the leaders were Radcliffe and Mead, Fothergill and Lettsom, Withering, Baillie, and Heberden, and many others. The third great branch of medical science, obstetrics, was now to be established on a scientific basis.

The Man-Midwife. Smellie and Hunter

Prior to this time the practice of obstetrics had remained for the most part in the hands of midwives. A change was now imminent, and there came on the scene a new type of specialist who was appropriately called the "man-midwife." [1] He was unpopular with some of his colleagues, who held that the assistance of a surgeon was demanded only in exceptional obstetric cases, and for obvious reasons he was even more unpopular with the midwives.

A number of distinguished men had already specialized in obstetrics. We have noted that William Harvey was the first Englishman to write on the subject (1651), and since then Sir RICHARD MANNINGHAM,[2] the first to institute " lying-in " wards (1739),[3] WILLIAM GIFFARD, the first, after the Chamberlens, to use the forceps or " extractor " (1726), EDMUND CHAPMAN, the first to illustrate and describe the forceps (1733), and other " man-midwives " had contributed to the knowledge of obstetrics ; while in Ireland Sir FIELDING OULD (*b.* 1710) helped to found the famous Dublin School of Midwifery.[4]

The master of British midwifery was WILLIAM SMELLIE (1697–1763). Born at Lanark, he studied medicine in Glasgow, and

[1] W. F. Menjer, " The Origin of the Male Midwife," *Ann. Med. Hist.*, 1932, vol. iv. p. 453
[2] It was Sir Richard Manningham who, in 1726, was sent to Godalming in Surrey by King George I to investigate the strange case of Mary Toft, who claimed to have given birth to seventeen rabbits. " The Rabbit Woman " provided the sensation of London for a season, until the hoax was exposed.
[3] A. H. Curtis, ed. of *Obstetrics and Gynaecology*, Philadelphia, 1933, vol. i. p. 16
[4] H. R. Spencer, *History of British Midwifery*, 1927, p. 30

practised in his native town for sixteen years.[1] Then after a short stay in Paris he settled in London in 1739. He soon became the leading obstetrician, and as a teacher he was also very successful. During his twenty years in London 900 students attended his classes, and along with these pupils he attended 1,150 cases of labour. He lived in Pall Mall, and later in Wardour Street. On his retirement in 1759 he returned to Lanark, where he had acquired the small estate of Smyllum, now an orphanage, and there he died. His library, which he bequeathed to the town of Lanark, is still preserved there, and his portrait, said to have been painted by himself, is in the Royal College of Surgeons of Edinburgh (Plate XLIX). Smellie's well-known *Treatise on Midwifery* appeared in 1752. In it he gave a clear account of the mechanism of labour, and he also corrected many errors and laid down sensible rules for obstetrical practice. (See Supplement, page 459.)

He was not, as is sometimes stated, the inventor of the forceps, though he was one of the first to use this instrument. Nevertheless he made it a rule to employ forceps as seldom as possible. So great was the prejudice against forceps on the part of patients and midwives that it was customary to apply them without the knowledge of either. Smellie at first employed wooden forceps in order to avoid the clinking noise of the metal blades, and at a later stage in his practice he had the blades covered with leather (Plate XLIX). He modified the shape of the forceps, improved the lock, and added the pelvic curves. The "axis traction" handles were a later invention by Tarnier (1828–97). The history of obstetric forceps has been a subject of much discussion, but it is now agreed that the inventor was PETER CHAMBERLEN (the elder) (1560–1631), a Hugenot refugee, and that the invention was held as a secret by the Chamberlen family for one hundred and twenty-five years.[2] This Peter Chamberlen, the first of his dynasty, had the honour of being called to attend Henrietta Maria, wife of Charles I, in 1628, after the midwife in charge had "swooned with fear" on entering the queen's chamber.

In four generations of Chamberlens there were seven medical men (including three Peters and two Hughs), each of whom doubtless inherited the secret of the forceps, of which, it now

---

[1] J. Glaister, *Dr. William Smellie and His Contemporaries*, Glasgow, 1894
[2] J. H. Aveling, *The Chamberlens and the Midwifery Forceps*, 1882 ; K. Das, *Obstetric Forceps : Its History and Evolution*, Calcutta, 1929. (An excellent and comprehensive account, with 878 illustrations.)

PLATE XLVII EDINBURGH DOCTORS OF THE EIGHTEENTH CENTURY

ALEXANDER WOOD (page 229)

FRANCIS HOME (page 230)

BENJAMIN BELL (page 230)

JOHN SHIELDS

John Shields, a typical general practitioner of the time, made his rounds on horseback, as was the custom. He kept an apothecary's shop in Nicolson Street, and although he charged only a shilling per visit he amassed a considerable fortune. (From Kay's *Edinburgh Portraits*)

PLATE XLVIII ARTISTIC OSTEOLOGY

Illustration from Cheselden's *Osteographia*, 1733, showing skeleton of child grasping an adult humerus (page 239)

appears certain, Peter the Elder was the inventor. In 1818, several pairs of forceps were found at Woodham Mortimer Hall, near Maldon, Essex, a house which had once belonged to Dr. Peter Chamberlen (1601–83), nephew of the inventor and the most distinguished member of the family. When Dr. Hugh Chamberlen died in 1728, he left no son to carry on the tradition. The secret instrument gradually became known, and many other patterns of forceps were introduced (Plate L).

For example, JEAN PALFYN (1650–1730), a surgeon of Ghent, demonstrated in Paris a form of forceps or tire-tête, consisting of two steel spoons, and known as Mains de Palfyn. The inventor published no description of his instrument.[1]

The writer is indebted to Professor Miles Phillips, whose interest in the subject is well known, for the following notes on the " lock " and the " pelvic curve " : " Chapman did not invent the ' English lock,' as still used, though some authors think so : he certainly did away with the screw (a French idea) and used a simple groove on each blade. It was Smellie who, in 1744–45, added flanges to the grooves and so contrived the ' English ' lock, and he is usually credited with this invention. The ' pelvic curve ' seems to have been independently introduced by Pugh, who writes in 1754 of ' the forceps I invented upwards of fourteen years ago,' by Levret who, in 1747, exhibited to the Paris Academy his forceps with ' la nouvelle courboure,' and by Smellie who, with characteristic honesty, wrote in 1753 of his long forceps with double curve, ' they were contrived some years ago by myself as well as other practitioners.' "

William Smellie had been in London for three years when he was joined by a young fellow-countryman who was destined to become famous as an anatomist and obstetrician, though his fame was eclipsed by that of his younger brother, who followed him to the metropolis a few years later. WILLIAM HUNTER (1718–83), like his brother John, was born at the farm of Long Calderwood, East Kilbride, seven miles from Glasgow.[2] As already noted (p. 222), he practised for a short time in the town of Hamilton, along with Dr. William Cullen. Soon after his arrival in London William Hunter accepted the invitation of Dr. James Douglas, the anatomist, to reside with him and to act as tutor to his son. After the death of this patron Hunter commenced to teach

[1] A. H. Curtis, *Obstetrics and Gynaecology*, Philadelphia, 1933, vol. i. p. 56
[2] G. R. Mather, *Two Great Scotsmen : The Brothers William and John Hunter*, 1893

anatomy, and a few years later, along with young Dr. Douglas, he visited Leyden, and saw the work of the great anatomist Albinus, then at the height of his fame. William Hunter founded the Windmill Street School of Anatomy, the centre of anatomical learning in London during many years.[1] He accumulated a collection of anatomical and other specimens which, along with Dr. John Fothergill's collection, now forms the Hunterian Museum of Glasgow, and he became the leading obstetrician of London. This honour he shared at first with Smellie, but his career was longer than that of Smellie. Moreover, Hunter was elegant in dress and refined in manner, in contrast to Smellie who was somewhat uncouth. He led an austere life, never married, and worked hard to the end, although his later years were clouded by an unfortunate controversy with his brother. His greatest work was an atlas of *The Anatomy of the Human Gravid Uterus* (1774). In his obstetrical practice he was conservative, his rule being to leave the case to Nature whenever possible. Forceps he seldom used ; in fact, he was wont to exhibit his own rusty pair as proof of this fact.

Eighteenth-Century Surgery

The two leading surgeons of the early years of the eighteenth century were William Cheselden and Percivall Pott, both of them able and distinguished men, although their work was perhaps overshadowed by that of their brilliant pupil, John Hunter.

WILLIAM CHESELDEN (1688–1752), a student under William Cowper the, anatomist, became surgeon to St. Thomas's Hospital, famous. as a lithotomist, and one of the best known men of his time.[2] He attended Sir Isaac Newton and Alexander Pope. The latter referred to his medical attendants in the couplet :

> I'll do what Mead and Cheselden advise,
> To keep those limbs and to preserve those eyes.

Cheselden was one of the first to perform iridotomy, restoring sight to a blind boy by constructing an artificial pupil. In operations for stone (lithotomy) he excelled.[3] Incredible though

[1] S. C. Thomson, " The Great Windmill Street School," *Bull. Med. Hist.*, 1942, vol. xii. p. 377
[2] F. R. Packard, " William Cheselden," *Ann. Med. Hist.*, 1927, vol. x. p. 533 ; F. G. Parsons, *The History of St. Thomas's Hospital*, 3 vols., 1932
[3] Sir B. W. Richardson, *Disciples of Aesculapius*, 2 vols., 1896, vol. i. p. 128

it may seem, he frequently completed the operation in one minute, and it was said that his record time was fifty-four seconds. He improved the technique of the operation, at first adopting the suprapubic route, which had been advised by John Douglas, but later abandoning this in favour of the perineal route. Lateral lithotomy had been already preferred to median lithotomy by Frère Jacques, as it was safer and easier. Cheselden modified this operation and reduced the mortality to seventeen per cent., a surprising figure in pre-anaesthetic days. His chief literary work was a beautifully illustrated monograph on the bones of man and animals, entitled *Osteographia* (1733). Some of the illustrations are as amusing as they are elaborate (Plate XLVIII).

Like many other anatomists and surgeons, Cheselden was a good draughtsman. Fulham Bridge, a wooden structure spanning the Thames, was built to his design in 1729.

PERCIVALL POTT (1714–88), another well-known London surgeon, gave classical descriptions of the tuberculous disease of the spine, and of the fracture just above the ankle, still known respectively as Pott's disease and Pott's fracture. Pott was surgeon to St. Bartholomew's Hospital until his death at the age of seventy-four, as there was no retiring age in those days. From his house in Bow Lane he conducted a large surgical practice, attending such distinguished patients as Samuel Johnson and David Garrick. A lively and sociable man, he was popular with all ranks of society.[1]

It is said that every surgeon ought to experience operation or injury in his own person. Pott acquired experience of this personal nature in 1756 when, riding down the Old Kent Road, he was thrown from his horse and sustained a compound fracture of the tibia. His injury was not, as is sometimes stated, a " Pott's fracture," but something much more serious. As he lay on the ground he realized just how serious it was, and how it might be aggravated by movement. Accordingly he sent for a door and two chair poles, to make a stretcher, and on this he was carried home. Fortunately his old " chief," Edward Nourse, was able to save the limb, no small achievement at a time when amputation was the treatment for almost every compound fracture. Naturally the recovery was slow, but Pott improved the time by writing a treatise on hernia, which was

---

[1] G. M. Lloyd, " The Life and Works of Percivall Pott, 1714–88 " (Wix Prize Essay), *St. Barth's Hosp. Repts.*, 1933, vol. lxvi. p. 291

his best work.[1] Although less great than his pupil, John Hunter, Pott did much to place surgery on a rational basis and to bring it into line with the new thought in physiology and medicine.

Why Think? Why not Try the Experiment?

In 1748, JOHN HUNTER (1728–93), youngest of the family of eleven children, set out on horseback from his home at Long Calderwood, near Glasgow, to join his brother William in London, and reached his destination in about a fortnight.[2] John had no inclination for scholarship but had an insatiable curiosity regarding "birds and bees and grasses" and all the works of Nature. William, ten years his senior, set him to dissect the upper limb, and the excellence of his work as an anatomist was immediately apparent. John also commenced the study of surgery under the two great surgeons, Cheselden and Pott. The life story of John Hunter has been so often narrated by numerous "Hunterian Orators" that it need only be briefly sketched.[3] Threatened by tuberculosis, he was advised to seek rest in a warmer climate, and this advice he followed by enlisting in the army and serving as a staff surgeon in Belle Isle and Portugal for four years.[4] During John's absence on military service, his brother William was assisted by WILLIAM HEWSON (1739–74), a brilliant young man who demonstrated the existence and function of the lymph vessels in animals, and established the fact that the coagulation of the blood was due, not to a solidification of the corpuscles, but to a substance in the plasma which he called "coagulable lymph," later known as "fibrinogen." Hewson died from septicaemia following a dissection wound at the age of thirty-five.[5] (See also Supplement, p. 459.)

When John Hunter returned from Portugal he commenced those vast researches in comparative anatomy and physiology to which the remainder of his life was to be devoted. He taught anatomy, although he was never a good lecturer, and on one occasion he asked the porter to bring in the skeleton so that he

[1] Sir J. Earle, *The Chirurgical Works of Percivall Pott ; With a Short Life of the Author*, 3 vols., 1790
[2] G. C. Peachey, *A Memoir of William and John Hunter*, 1924 ; G. R. Mather, *Two Great Scotsmen : The Brothers William and John Hunter*, Glasgow, 1893
[3] Stephen Paget, *John Hunter, Man of Science and Surgeon, 1728–93*, 1897
[4] G. E. Gask, " John Hunter in Portugal," *Brit. Jour. Surg.*, 1936–37, vol. xxiv. p. 640
[5] G. H. Bailey, " William Hewson, F.R.S., 1739–74, His Life and Work," *Ann. Med. Hist.*, 1923, p. 209

PLATE XLIX   THE MASTER OF BRITISH MIDWIFERY

Wm Smellie

1697–1763

Smellie's long forceps, the
blades bound with leather
strips (page 236)

PLATE L EARLY PATTERNS OF OBSTETRIC FORCEPS

1 Forceps invented by Peter Chamberlen (the elder) about 1630, and
retained as a family secret for many years (page 236)

2 Palfyn's forceps (Mains de Palfyn, 1720) ; two spoons, with handles
clamped together (page 237)

3 Smellie's short wooden forceps, 1745, with the " English " lock
(see page 235 and Plate XLIX)

4 Dusée's forceps, 1733 ; the first attempt to articulate Palfyn's
instrument by means of the " French " lock

5 Chapman's forceps, 1733 ; the blades united by a simple groove,
easily detachable (page 235)

6 Burton's forceps, 1751 ; slender blades controlled by screw handle.
Burton, of York, was the original Dr. Slop of *Tristram Shandy*

(All figures are ⅛ natural size)

might preface his remarks with the word " Gentlemen." Later in his career he lectured on " the whole circle of the sciences around surgery," and he certainly raised surgery from the level of a technical accomplishment to that of a definite science. John Hunter was the founder of surgical pathology.[1]

Among his pupils were Abernethy and Astley Cooper of London, Physick of Pennsylvania, and Edward Jenner, the country doctor whose great invention saved innumerable lives. The letters written by John Hunter to Jenner have fortunately been preserved, and one of them contains the oft-quoted advice, " Why think ? Why not try the experiment ? " The experiment related to the temperature of hibernating hedgehogs, one of many problems investigated by Hunter and Jenner. They also studied the plumage of nestlings, the habits of the cuckoo, the life history of eels, and many other interesting matters. Vaccination did not fully engage the attention of Jenner until after Hunter's death.

As John Hunter prospered in surgical practice he removed from Golden Square to his brother's house in Jermyn Street, and then to a large establishment in Leicester Square. This was his home, and here also were his consulting rooms, his lecture rooms, and his museum. For many years he worked incessantly to study and collect the 13,600 specimens which the museum eventually contained (Plate LI). Many tales are told of his quest for material and of his dissections ranging from bees to whales.[2] The skeleton of Byrne, the Irish giant, which Hunter long coveted during the lifetime of its owner, and at last secured for £500, was one of the treasures of the museum, and the feet appear in the famous portrait of John Hunter by Sir Joshua Reynolds.

In addition to this town establishment Hunter had a country house and grounds at Earl's Court. There he kept all kinds of

---

[1] Sir E. Home, *Life of John Hunter*, 1794 ; Jesse Foot, *The Life of John Hunter*, 1794 ; J. Adams, *The Life and Doctrines of the the Late John Hunter*, 1817 ; J. F. Palmer, ed. of *The Works of John Hunter, F.R.S. ; With a Life by Drewry Ottley*, 4 vols., 1835 ; Sir W. Jardine, " Memoir of John Hunter," vol. x. of *Naturalists' Library*, 1843

[2] G. T. Bettany, *Eminent Doctors*, 2 vols., 1885, vol. i. p. 133 ; Sir B. W. Richardson, *Disciples of Aesculapius*, 2 vols., 1896, vol. ii. p. 501 ; T. J. Pettigrew, *Medical Portraits*, 1838–40, vol. ii

There are many shorter biographical notices of John Hunter, as well as numerous Hunterian Orations including those by Sir James Paget (1877), Sir William MacCormack (1899), and Mr. Wilfred Trotter (1932), which are especially noteworthy. G. Mather and G. A. Peachey have each added to the attraction of these works by including both the Hunter brothers. Perhaps the best of the earlier biographies is the work of Drewry Ottley, and among the more recent accounts that of Stephen Paget holds a high place.

animals, birds, and fishes, and there he conducted many experiments and dissections. In 1773 there occurred the first attack of angina pectoris, from which disease John Hunter died twenty years later. There can be no doubt that he also suffered from cerebral syphilis, contracted as the result of a foolhardy inoculation of himself in order to ascertain whether syphilis and gonorrhœa were the same disease.[1] He died suddenly at a meeting of the governors of St. George's Hospital, to which institution he had been surgeon for some years. His body rested in St. Martin's Church until 1859, when it was re-interred in Westminster Abbey at the instance of Frank Buckland.[2]

John Hunter made no great discovery, yet in a sense he was the originator of many discoveries. His writings are full of fresh observations which pointed the way for other pioneers.[3] His great collection in the Royal College of Surgeons' Museum was destroyed by enemy action in World War II, but the name of John Hunter will always remain one of the greatest in the history of surgery.

Pupils and Contemporaries of John Hunter

John Hunter had many pupils who achieved fame ; among them were the distinguished London surgeons, Abernethy and Astley Cooper, and the first great American surgeon, Philip Syng Physick.

JOHN ABERNETHY (1764–1831),[4] who was born in London of Scots-Irish parentage, succeeded Pott as surgeon to St. Bartholomew's Hospital, and fell heir to much of the practice of his teacher, John Hunter. He was a clear and dramatic lecturer, very popular with his students. In practice, he adopted a brusque and even rough manner with his patients, and many stories are told to illustrate this peculiarity.

" Live on sixpence a day, and earn it," was his advice to a luxurious alderman. Another patient, a hypochondriac, he sent to consult a fictitious Dr. Robertson of Inverness. Fear of the unknown verdict on the northward journey, combined with anger against Abernethy as he returned, made the patient forget his ills and completed the cure.

[1] D'Arcy Power, " John Hunter, a Martyr to Science," in *Selected Writings*, 1931
[2] Frank Buckland, *Curiosities of Natural History*, 4 vols., 1866, vol. iv. p. 159
[3] Morley Roberts, " John Hunter and Evolution," *Med. Press and Circ.*, 1929, May 29 and June 5 and 12
[4] Sir B. W. Richardson, *Disciples of Aesculapius*, 2 vols., 1896, vol. ii. p. 786

Abernethy alleged that all diseases which were not surgical and external were due to digestive disturbance, and his favourite remedies were calomel and blue pill. Nevertheless he was a bold and skilful surgeon, being the first to ligate the external iliac artery for aneurysm.

Sir ASTLEY PASTON COOPER (1768–1841) was the son of a Norfolk clergyman and a descendant of the family of Paston made famous by *The Paston Letters*, which give so intimate a picture of domestic life in the fifteenth century.[1] Astley Cooper was a man of strong personality. Handsome and dignified in appearance, courteous and agreeable in manner, he inspired the confidence of his patients and the admiration of his students. He was a brilliant and careful operator, and he soon acquired an enormous practice. For some years his annual income was never less than £15,000. His servant " Charles " was said to make £600 a year by showing in patients out of their turn.[2] Astley Cooper's boldest operation was ligation of the aorta in a case of aneurysm. He was also the first to amputate at the hip joint. His most famous operation was the removal of a sebaceous cyst from the head of King George IV, a successful achievement rewarded by a baronetcy.[3] Among his many contributions to surgical literature were his treatises on hernia, on fractures and dislocations, and on diseases of the breast.

Another of John Hunter's pupils was PHILIP SYNG PHYSICK (1768–1837), who has been called the Father of American Surgery.[4] Hunter pressed him to remain in London as his assistant, but he preferred to return to America. No sooner had he settled in practice than a violent epidemic of yellow fever broke out. Physick gave faithful service to many patients until he was himself attacked by the fever. Fortunately he recovered, although he never regained his original vigour.[5] Nevertheless he soon became noted for his excellence as a surgeon, and was appointed surgeon to the Pennsylvania Hospital, and Professor of Surgery

[1] Bransby B. Cooper, *Life of Sir Astley Cooper*, 2 vols., 1843 ; R. C. Brock, *The Life and Work of Astley Cooper*, 1952   [2] J. C. Jeaffreson, *A Book about Doctors*, 1870, p. 111
[3] G. T. Bettany, *Eminent Doctors*, 2 vols., 1885, vol. i. p. 202 ; Sir D'Arcy Power, " The Removal of a Sebaceous Cyst from King George IV," *Brit. Jour. Surg.*, 1933, vol. xx. p. 361
[4] W. S. Middleton, " Philip Syng Physick, Father of American Surgery," *Ann. Med. Hist.*, 1921, vol. i. p. 562
[5] S. D. Gross, ed. of *Lives of Eminent American Physicians and Surgeons*, Philadelphia, 1861, p. 351 (" Life of Physick," by J. Bell)

A HISTORY OF MEDICINE

at the University. Like his master, John Hunter, he was a conservative surgeon, and his operative work was for the most part limited to lithotomy and the extraction of cataract.[1] He modified and improved the treatment of fractures. A hard worker, a good lecturer, and a man of sterling character, he was in every respect a worthy leader of the many great Americans who have advanced the profession of surgery since then.[2] (See also Supplement, page 459.)

On the Continent there were a number of distinguished surgeons. Italy was represented by ANTONIO SCARPA of Pavia (1752–1832), whose name survives in various anatomical descriptions, but who was also famous as a surgeon and ophthalmologist. A contemporary Italian was DOMENICO COTUGNO of Naples (1736–1822), who investigated the cerebro-spinal and labyrinthine fluids, enunciated a theory of hearing, and wrote a famous monograph on sciatica.[3] Another name familiar to every otologist is that of ANTONIO VALSALVA of Bologna (1666–1723), (p. 186) who published his *Tractatus De Aure Humana* in 1704. The leading German surgeon was LORENZ HEISTER (1683–1758), whose *Chirurgie,* published in 1718, was an interesting and well-illustrated treatise which became very popular as a textbook.[4]

In France the best-known surgeon was JEAN LOUIS PETIT (1674–1750) of Paris, inventor of the screw tourniquet, and the first to perform a successful operation for mastoiditis. He used a trephine, and " had scarcely got through the outer table when there escaped a quantity of foul-smelling exudation." [5] The patient made a rapid recovery. Petit's description of the procedure was not published until after his death ; it therefore attracted little attention. About a century later the mastoid operation was established on a sound basis by Schwartze (p. 379).

Other Parisian surgeons of the time were FRANÇOIS CHOPART (1743–95), who improved the technique of amputations, and PIERRE-JOSEPH DESAULT (1744–95), who devised better methods of treating fractures.

[1] G. Edwards, " Philip Syng Physick, 1768–1837," *Proc. Roy. Soc. Med.*, 1940, vol. xxxiii. p. 145
[2] A. Randall, " Philip Syng Physick's Last Major Operation," *Ann. Med. Hist.*, 1937, vol. ix. p. 133
[3] A. Livinson, " Domenico Cotugno," *Ann. Med. Hist.*, 1936, vol. viii. p. 1 ; H. R. Viets, " Domenico Cotugno : His Description of the Cerebro-spinal Fluid," *Bull. Hist. Med.*, 1935, vol. iii. p. 701
[4] T. Meyer-Steineg and K. Sudhoff, *Geschichte der Medizin*, 1921, p. 379
[5] Sir C. Ballance, *The Surgery of the Temporal Bone*, 2 vols., 1919, vol. i. p. 35

Applied Pathology

During the eighteenth century there appeared the pioneers who demonstrated the importance of morbid anatomy, and who showed how important to the physician was a knowledge of pathology. The leader of the movement was GIOVANNI BATTISTA MORGAGNI (1682–1771), whom Castiglioni refers to as " a master in the best sense of the word and a tireless investigator." [1] He studied under Valsalva at Bologna and then returned to practise in his native town of Forli. An ardent student of the classics, a poet and archaeologist, and already an anatomist of repute, his fame spread, so that at the age of twenty-nine he was called to be Professor of Anatomy at Padua, a position which he held with distinction for fifty-six years. His great achievement was the union which he effected between anatomy and pathology on the one hand, and clinical medicine on the other. Post-mortem findings became correlated with clinical symptoms. Morgagni was, in fact, the founder of pathological anatomy. Throughout his long life he strenuously pursued his search for the causes of disease, and for the changes which are found on post-mortem examination. He did not publish his results until he had reached the age of seventy-nine. [2] The masterpiece which he then wrote gives details of case histories and pathological appearances in no less than seven hundred cases. Many were the discoveries he described, including cirrhosis of the liver, pneumonic consolidation of the lung, and many forms of tumour. He was the first to show that cerebral abscess was a result rather than a cause of suppurative otitis. This great work, *De sedibus et causis morborum* (On the sites and causes of diseases), in five volumes, appeared in 1761.

During the later years of the century pathological anatomy was enriched by the work of another gifted observer, MARIE FRANÇOIS XAVIER BICHAT (1771–1802), the pupil and assistant of Desault in Paris. [3] He it was who founded the science of histology, the study of tissues or " membranes," by directing attention to the pathological changes in cellular, nervous, osseous, fibrous, muscular, and other tissues, twenty-one in all. His views were the

[1] A. Castiglioni, *A History of Medicine*, trans. by E. B. Krumbhaar, New York, 1941, p. 602 ; E. R. Long, *A History of Pathology*, 1928 ; H. E. Sigerist, *Great Doctors*, 1933, p. 229
[2] Sir B. W. Richardson, *Disciples of Aesculapius*, 2 vols., 1896, vol. i. p. 283
[3] T. J. Pettigrew, *Medical Portraits*, 1838–40, vol. i ; E. T. Withington, *Medical History from the Earliest Times*, 1894, p. 358

subject of his *Traité des Membranes*, published in 1800. Pathological changes, according to Bichat, affected tissues rather than organs. This view marked a great advance, which held its own until the further discoveries of Virchow transferred the seat of disease to the cells of which tissues and organs are composed. Although Bichat died at the age of thirty-one, his is one of the great names of medical history.

A third famous pathologist was our own MATTHEW BAILLIE (1761–1823), the nephew of the Hunters and son of the Professor of Divinity at Glasgow.[1] Educated at Balliol College, Oxford, he settled in London, where he taught anatomy for twenty years and eventually acquired a large fortune as a physician. He was physician to St. George's Hospital and physician to King George III, whom he attended during his last illness. His greatest achievement, however, was the publication of his *Morbid Anatomy* in 1793. This complete work, the first of the kind, was illustrated by a series of excellent engravings, and it is interesting to note that the figure illustrating emphysema of the lung depicts the lung of Dr. Samuel Johnson.[2]

Inoculation and Vaccination

Smallpox, now a comparatively rare disease, was very prevalent during the eighteenth century. The mortality was high, and among the survivors there were many pock-marked faces and cases of blindness. Any relief from such a plague was welcome, and when Lady Mary Wortley Montagu, wife of the British Ambassador in Turkey, introduced " inoculation " into England in 1717, it was eagerly welcomed and widely practised. After the method had been tried successfully upon six condemned criminals, several members of the Royal House were inoculated. Inoculation had been popularized in Europe early in the eighteenth century by Emmanuel Timoni, who was one of the first to describe the practice in writing.

It had been long in use in the East. In China, it consisted in blowing or sniffing into the nose the powdered dried crusts from a case of smallpox. The method employed in England was to make a superficial incision in the arm, and to draw through it a

[1] W. MacMichael, *The Gold-headed Cane*, 1827 (chap. v, " Baillie "). See p. 253-4.
[2] R. H. Major, *Classic Descriptions of Disease*, 1932, p. 546

thread soaked in the fluid from a smallpox pustule. By those means there was produced a mild form of the disease, and the patient was safe-guarded from future infection.[1] Medical practitioners throughout the country became specialists in inoculation, and maintained isolation hospitals or " inoculation houses " for the purpose.

One of the most successful virus inoculators was THOMAS DIMSDALE (1712–1800), a Quaker physician who practised at Hertford.[2] News of his fame reached the Empress Catherine of Russia, who forthwith sent for him to inoculate herself and her son. It was a perilous mission. Dimsdale's journey to St. Petersburg, his arrangements to escape should any disaster attend his efforts, his complete success, and his great reward of £10,000, a pension of £500, and the rank of Baron, form one of the most romantic episodes in the history of medicine.[3] What relief Dimsdale must have felt as he wrote in his journal, " She has had the smallpox in the most desirable manner ; which now, thank God, is over ! " He inoculated almost two hundred other persons in St. Petersburg and in Moscow, and all did well. His method was to use a minute incision or a mere scratch, and he frequently inoculated children while they were asleep. None the less, inoculation, though beneficial to individuals, did not check the spread of the disease nor reduce the mortality.

The Career of Edward Jenner

Such was the state of affairs when there came upon the scene a country practitioner named EDWARD JENNER (1749–1823), one of the greatest benefactors to mankind.[4] We have already mentioned this pupil of the " dear man," as his intimates affectionately termed John Hunter, and reference has been made to the researches in physiology and natural history which Jenner carried out in collaboration with his great teacher. That he was a lover of Nature and a keen observer is shown by his verses, " Address to a Robin," and " Signs of Rain," which appear in

[1] E. M. Crookshank, History and Pathology of Vaccination, 2 vols., 1889
[2] W. J. Bishop, " Thomas Dimsdale, M.D., F.R.S., 1712–1800, and the Inoculation of Catherine the Great of Russia," Ann. Med. Hist., 1932, vol. iv. p. 321
[3] R. Hingston Fox, Dr. John Fothergill and His Friends, 1919 (" Baron Dimsdale," chap. ix.)
[4] J. Baron, The Life of Edward Jenner, 2 vols., 1838

every biography of Jenner.[1] The son of the vicar of Berkeley, in Gloucestershire, Rev. Stephen Jenner, he practised in his birthplace, and there he made his great discovery. City life never appealed to him ; nor indeed did fortune, for when, at the height of his fame, he was urged to come to London, and was assured of an income of £10,000 a year, he declined this prospect and wrote to a friend, " My fortune is sufficient to gratify my wishes. And what is Fame ? A gilded butt, for ever pierced with the arrows of malignancy." So in Berkeley he lived and died.

The idea of vaccination was conveyed to Jenner by the chance remark of a dairymaid, " I can't take smallpox, for I have already had cowpox." Now cowpox was a relatively mild disease, transmitted from the udder of the cow to the hands of the milker, and consisting of a pustular eruption, accompanied by transient general malaise. It was generally known in Gloucestershire that the dairymaid's statement was true. Jenner felt that such knowledge might be put to practical use. For more than twenty years he considered the problem, and even bored his medical friends with his views to such an extent that he was threatened with expulsion from the Convivio-Medical Club, as the local medical society was called.

At last, on 14th May 1796, he summoned sufficient courage to try the crucial experiment. He " vaccinated " James Phipps, a boy of eight years, with pus from the hand of a dairymaid, Sarah Nelmes, who had become infected with cowpox. Eight weeks later Jenner inoculated the boy with smallpox, and no disease appeared. The proof was now complete, and Jenner recorded his views and observations in a little book of seventy-five pages, with the long title, *An Inquiry into the Causes and Effects of the Variolae Vaccinae, a Disease discovered in some of the Western Counties of England, particularly Gloucestershire, and known by the name of " The Cow Pox."*

The advantage of vaccination was everywhere confirmed, at home and abroad. Honours and congratulations showered upon Jenner. Had he been selfish enough to keep his method secret he would have made a large fortune. With true scientific generosity he had freely proclaimed his discovery. He had even suffered financial loss, and it was only fair that the Government should recompense a discoverer who had conferred so great a benefit

[1] W. MacMichael, *Lives of British Physicians*, 1830, p. 252

upon humanity. Accordingly in 1802 he was voted £10,000, and a further sum of £20,000 was added in 1807.[1] For a short time he practised in London, but soon returned to be the village doctor of Berkeley. There, he used to vaccinate the poor in an arbour of his garden.[2] Meantime the incidence and mortality of smallpox fell steadily. The value of vaccination had been proved, and a principle had been established which was eventually to lead to the immunization of man against typhoid, cholera, and other diseases. Later, Dr. Monckton Copeman described in his *Milroy Lectures* (1898) how the extraneous bacteria in vaccine lymph could be destroyed by glycerine.

Quaker and American Physicians

" Let us preserve the memory of the deserving ; perhaps it may prompt others likewise to deserve." So wrote Dr. John Fothergill in 1769, and none is more deserving of remembrance than he. The Society of Friends, ever noted for its wide sympathies and love of justice, was well represented in medicine during the eighteenth century by such versatile and great-hearted practitioners as Fothergill and Lettsom, as well as by WILLIAM TUKE, who at his mental hospital, The Retreat, at York (1792),[3] inaugurated a humane treatment of the insane, who before that time had been imprisoned and chained in a merciless fashion, or even, as at Bedlam, exhibited like menagerie animals (p. 372).

JOHN FOTHERGILL (1712–80)[4] was born at Wensleydale, Yorkshire, and during his career as a student in Edinburgh he assisted Monro in his work on osteology, and distinguished himself in other subjects. Settling in London, he soon acquired a large practice by " climbing on the backs of the poor to the pockets of the rich." His *Account of the Sore Throat*, 1748, the result of his observations during a violent epidemic of what was probably a malignant form of scarlatina, brought him fame.

As his status and wealth increased he became greatly interested in botany, and in the introduction of new plants into England. To this end, in 1762, he planted a large botanical garden of five

[1] G. T. Bettany, *Eminent Doctors*, 2 vols., 1885, vol. i. p. 169
[2] T. J. Pettigrew, *Medical Portraits*, 1838–40, vol. ii
[3] S. G. Stubbs and E. W. Bligh, *Sixty Centuries of Health and Physick*, 1931, p. 338
[4] R. Hingston Fox, *Dr. John Fothergill and His Friends*, 1919

acres at Upton in Essex (later the birthplace of another famous Quaker, Joseph Lister), and there, in hothouses and in the open, he accumulated many thousands of exotic plants which were collected for him by friends, by sea captains, and by collectors whom he employed. His garden, now incorporated in the West Ham public park, ranked next to Kew in importance.

An authority on materia medica, he extended the use of cinchona bark, and he even grew a cinchona tree in his garden.[1] He advised hemlock (conium) for neuralgia, introduced the astringent gum known as kino, and revived the use of antimony. He popularized the use of coffee, and promoted the cultivation of the plant in the West Indies. In the garden at Upton there was a coffee shrub fifteen feet in height.

One of the most interesting of his papers deals with the " History and Use of Coffee." Another noteworthy work was his account of " Weather and Disease," consisting of monthly records during a period of four years, from 1751 to 1754. His " Observations on recovering a man dead in appearance, by distending the lungs with air," 1744, is a forecast of artificial respiration. He wrote on epilepsy, hydrophobia, angina pectoris, sick headache, and other subjects, and his style is always precise and readable. Fothergill's efforts were further directed towards the abolition of slavery, the registration of births and deaths (although this did not become compulsory until 1837), the widening of certain London streets, the use of maize or potato to augment the supply of wheaten flour, and the supply of cheaper fish for the poor.

He collaborated with his friend, JOHN HOWARD (1726–90), in promoting a scheme for prison reform. Most important of all, though unsuccessful, were his untiring efforts in 1774, along with his close friend, BENJAMIN FRANKLIN (1706–90), that great philosopher and statesman, to prevent rupture between England and her American colonies.

One of the effects of the War of the Revolution was to bring into prominence a number of American physicians and surgeons who, while giving good service to the army, turned their attention to hospital organization and medical education. Foremost among them were Morgan and Shippen ; before them was Cadwalader and after them came Rush. THOMAS CADWALADER

[1] Sir H. Rolleston, " The History of Cinchona and its Therapeutics," *Ann. Med. Hist.*, 1931, vol. iii. p. 261. (See also page 205)

(1708–99) was a colonial pioneer who had studied medicine in London. He was the first to teach anatomy in Philadelphia, and he helped to found the hospital and library. His best-known work was an *Essay on the West-India Dry-Gripes* (lead poisoning) which was printed by Benjamin Franklin in 1745.

The founder of the School of Medicine in the University of Pennsylvania, originally the Pennsylvania College, and indeed the pioneer of all medical education in America, was JOHN MORGAN (1735–89), a native of Philadelphia, and an Edinburgh graduate.[1] While in Edinburgh he had studied under Monro ; he had also visited Morgagni at Padua, spending altogether five years in Europe. Appointed to the Chair of Medicine in his native city, the first American to confine his practice to medicine, he was called to be Director-General to the army medical department on the outbreak of war. Political squabbles led to his unjust dismissal in 1777, when WILLIAM SHIPPEN (1736–1808), another American who had studied at Edinburgh, was appointed to succeed him. Morgan was afterwards acquitted and restored to favour, but he never recovered from the blow. Shippen was the first teacher of obstetrics in America, although his professional Chair was that of anatomy and surgery. There is little doubt that Fothergill, who had befriended Morgan and Shippen during their studies in Europe, exerted his influence with William Penn on their behalf, and thus indirectly assisted to found this new medical school.

Another student from Philadelphia, who came to London with an introduction to Fothergill, and who proceeded to graduate M.D. at Edinburgh in 1768, was BENJAMIN RUSH (1745–1813), a famous Quaker physician who succeeded Morgan as Professor of Medicine in Philadelphia.[2] There, he taught medicine for forty-four years, and acquired a great reputation as " the Sydenham of America," although his active opposition to war, slavery, alcohol, and the death penalty led to some decline in his practice. His name is perpetuated in Rush Medical College.

When John Fothergill died of a prostatic tumour at the age of sixty-eight, he was succeeded by another Quaker physician, Lettsom, whose name is even more familiar than that of Fothergill.

---

[1] W. S. Middleton, " John Morgan, Father of Medical Education in North America," *Ann. Med. Hist.*, 1927, vol. ix. p. 13
[2] S. Jackson, " Life of Benjamin Rush," in *Lives of Eminent American Physicians, etc.*, ed. by S. D. Gross, 1861, p. 17

JOHN COAKLEY LETTSOM (1744–1815), the son of a cotton planter in the West Indies, was one of the seventh set of twins, and the only pair to survive. He was sent to England to be educated, and after attending school in Lancashire, was apprenticed to a surgeon-apothecary at Settle in Yorkshire. As soon as he came of age, he returned to his birthplace to claim his heritage. Meanwhile his father had died and his mother had married again, so that the only property accruing to young Lettsom consisted of a number of Negro slaves. Although this was his sole patrimony, he promptly set them all free, and thus " began the world without fortune, without a friend, without person and without address." [1] Nothing daunted, he commenced practice in the island of Tortola, and soon saved sufficient money to enable him to return to Europe. After a period of study at Edinburgh, Paris, and Leyden, he commenced practice in London, as had ever been his ambition. Aided by Fothergill, who had moved farther west, he soon prospered, and indeed his success was phenomenal. For many years he enjoyed an annual income of £5,000. It is said to have risen as high as £12,000, and that in 1795 he actually attended 82,000 patients. It is also said that on his long rounds he wore out three pairs of horses a day. Lettsom's house in Lanebrook Court, close to the Guildhall, has long since gone. In time he built for himself and his wife a country residence at Camberwell, then a village four miles from the city. Grove Hill, as he named the house, stood in pleasant grounds, with an apiary of sixty-four hives and a well-stocked garden, for like his predecessor Fothergill, he was an ardent botanist. It was he who introduced the mangold wurzel into England. Lettsom was a tall spare man, his face yellow and lined since his residence in the West Indies ; his dress was the Quaker attire, " but not with strictness " ; he was good-tempered and genial in manner and moderate in all his habits. His great popularity arose from his genuine kindness and liberality. He championed the cause of vaccination, defending Jenner against his critics when the fight was most fierce. One of his earliest benefactions, in 1773, was the foundation of the Medical Society of London, which still flourishes.[2] The membership at first was limited to thirty physicians, thirty surgeons, and thirty apothe-

[1] J. J. Abraham, Lettsom : His Life, Times, Friends, and Descendants, 1933. (One of the most delightful of medical biographies.)
[2] Sir St. Clair Thomson, John Coakley Lettsom and the Medical Society of London (Presidential Address to the Society), 1917

caries. During the early days Lettsom contributed many papers when no material was forthcoming ; he worked hard to ensure the success of the society, and even presented to it a good house as a meeting-place (Plate LII).

Another society to which Lettsom gave ardent support, and which he assisted to establish in 1774, was the Royal Humane Society ; he thus followed up the work of Fothergill in his advocacy of artificial respiration.

Still another institution owing its inception to Lettsom was, and still is, the Royal Sea-bathing Hospital at Margate, established in 1796, although the original reason for its existence, the provision of sea-bathing facilities for weakly and tuberculous children, is no longer its principal object. It was a forerunner of modern open-air sanatoria. Lettsom visited this hospital once a year, driving down from London during the night by coach, a practice he was wont to follow in visiting patients in the country. He also inaugurated in London a system of dispensaries which enabled poor patients to be treated as out-patients, and even to be attended in their own homes by physicians of high rank. This was before the days of hospital " out-patient departments," and the system was adopted in many towns throughout the country.

This tireless and energetic physician is commemorated in the following lines, of which many versions exist, well known to many who know naught else of Lettsom, and said to have been written by himself :

> When any sick to me apply,
> I physicks, bleeds, and sweats 'em ;
> If after that they choose to die,
> What's that to me, I. Lettsom.

The Gold-headed Cane

The fashionable doctor of the eighteenth century was somewhat of a dandy, with his buckskin breeches and top boots, or stockings and buckled shoes, his velvet or satin coat with gilt buttons, his wig and three-cornered hat, his gloves, and even his muff. Another essential part of the physician's equipment was a cane, with a gold or silver top, perforated and hollow so as to contain some aromatic compound which was believed to prevent infection.

Such a cane, having a gold-mounted cross-piece as handle

instead of the usual knob, was carried by John Radcliffe, to whom reference will presently be made. It was handed by him to his successor in practice, Richard Mead, and was then passed down to various successive physicians until it came to Matthew Baillie (p. 246). Baillie's widow presented it to Sir Henry Halford, President of the Royal College of Physicians, and when the new college building in Pall Mall East was opened in 1825, Halford deposited the cane in the college. There it remains to this day, preserved in a glass case in the library.

An account of some of the physicians who carried the cane is contained in a charming volume, purporting to be the reminiscences of the relic itself. It is entitled *The Gold-headed Cane*, and was first published in 1827, the work of WILLIAM MACMICHAEL (1784–1839), a distinguished Fellow of the college and physician to the king. A second and enlarged edition appeared in 1828, and a third, edited by William Munk, in 1884. The earlier editions contain quaint illustrations. The first two bearers of the cane, Radcliffe and Mead, present a striking analogy to Fothergill and Lettsom, although they flourished during a slightly earlier period.

JOHN RADCLIFFE (1650–1714),[1] who practised in Oxford, where he had been educated, and later in London, was a physician who owed his great success more to his natural sagacity and sound common sense than to scholarship. Indeed, when asked where his library was, he pointed to a corner of the room where lay a herbal, a skeleton, and a few bottles of drugs. Yet he built up such a large and remunerative practice that he left funds sufficient to endow in Oxford the institutions which still bear his name, the Radcliffe Infirmary, the Radcliffe Observatory, and the Radcliffe Library. He attended King William, whom he offended by his curtness, and in her last illness Mary his queen, who died of smallpox. It was Radcliffe who first made the remark, since attributed to others, that " as a young practitioner he possessed twenty remedies for every disease, and at the close of his career he found twenty diseases for which he had not one remedy."

To his successor, the learned and courtly RICHARD MEAD (1673–1754), he gave the following advice : " I love you, Mead, and I'll give you an infallible recipe for success in practice ; use

<hr>

[1] J. C. Jeaffreson, *A Book about Doctors*, 1870, p. 69 ; W. MacMichael, *Lives of British Physicians*, 1830, p. 112 ; C. R. Hone, *The Life of Dr. John Radcliff*, 1950

all mankind ill." Dictatorial methods may be of use at times in medical practice, but Radcliffe had carried them too far, and Mead resolved to adopt gentler tactics. His name has been already mentioned as a student at Leyden under Pitcairne, and as the physician of Alexander Pope. When he moved into Radcliffe's house in Bloomsbury Square he achieved success which eclipsed that of his predecessor. In the placid days of Queen Anne, his principal patient, life moved in a slow and leisurely fashion, and there was time to cultivate the arts and sciences.[1] Mead was well known, not only as a physician but as a scholar and collector. He possessed one of the best libraries in the country, besides a magnificent museum which became a Mecca for every distinguished visitor to London. His services were greatly sought by the apothecaries, who came to him with their problems, which he sought to solve without seeing the patients. For this kind of practice, which occupied part of his day at Tom's Coffee House in Covent Garden, his fee was half a guinea. Mead was not a voluminous writer. In *A Mechanical Account of Poisons* he records some original observations on snake venom. Still more interesting is *A Treatise concerning the Influence of the Sun and Moon on Human Bodies*, as it indicates that even at that date astrology still held a place in medical practice.

Among his many friends was JOHN FREIND (1675–1728),[2] who was imprisoned for some months for his advocacy of the Stuart cause, and who during his incarceration in the Tower wrote a *History of Physick* (1726), which must still be regarded as authoritative (p. 412). Tradition has it that when Freind was released, Mead paid him several thousand pounds, which he had received from patients during his absence. It was of Dr. Richard Mead that Samuel Johnson remarked that he " lived more in the broad sunshine of life than almost any other man."

From Mead the gold-headed cane passed to Askew, to David Pitcairn, and then to Baillie, after whose death " it ceased to be considered any longer as a necessary appendage of the profession."[3]

Of the many other distinguished physicians of the eighteenth century it may suffice to mention two, each of whom holds an honoured place in medical history.

[1] T. J. Pettigrew, *Medical Portraits*, 1838–40, vol. i.
[2] Sir B. W. Richardson, *Disciples of Aesculapius*, 2 vols., 1896, vol. i. p. 362
[3] W. MacMichael, *The Gold-headed Cane*, 1827

Heberden and Withering

WILLIAM HEBERDEN the Elder (1710–1801) was a man who well upheld the dignity and honour of medicine, and who added considerably to our knowledge.[1] A graduate of Cambridge, he conducted a large practice in London for many years and was physician to King George III. Dr. Samuel Johnson was another of his patients. He made careful notes of all his cases, and at the age of seventy-two he wrote, for the benefit of his son, his single volume of *Commentaries* which, according to his wishes, was not published until the year after his death.[2] It is a remarkable book, which may still be read with profit, as it contains many excellent descriptions of disease, as, for example, angina pectoris, though he was not the first to describe this disease. Heberden writes : " There is a disorder of the heart marked with strong and peculiar symptoms, considerable for the danger belonging to it, and not extremely rare. The seat of it, and the sense of strangling and anxiety with which it is attended, may make it not improperly be called Angina Pectoris. The termination is remarkable. The patients all suddenly fall down, and perish almost immediately."[3]

The first mention of such a tragic end was not recorded by a medical man. It occurs in the *Life of Edward, Earl of Clarendon* (1609–74), by his son, who thus describes the death of his father : " The pain in his arm seizing upon him, he fell down dead, without the least motion of any limb."

Another important service to medicine was rendered by Heberden when he published early in his career his *Essay on Mithridatium and Theriaka*, which gave the death-blow to these fantastic antidotes, and led to their expulsion from the Pharmacopoeia. Heberden lived to the age of ninety-one, retaining his mental faculties to the last. Dr. Johnson called him " the last of the Romans." (See Supplement, page 460.)

WILLIAM WITHERING (1741–79) was the son of a country doctor in Shropshire.[1] He graduated at Edinburgh in 1766,

---

[1] T. J. Pettigrew, *Medical Portraits*, 1838–40, vol. iii ; P. B. Davidson, " William Heberden, M.D., F.R.S.," *Ann. Med. Hist.*, 1922, vol. iv. p. 336
[2] Sir H. Rolleston, " The two Heberdens : William Heberden the Elder, 1710–1801 ; William Heberden the Younger, 1767–1845," *Ann. Med. Hist.*, 1933, vol. v.
[3] R. H. Major, *Classic Descriptions of Disease*, 1932, p. 389
[4] R. Musser and J. C. Krantz, " The Friendship of William Withering and Erasmus Darwin," *Bull. Hist. Med.*, 1940, vol. viii. ; T. W. Peck and K. Wilkinson, *William Withering of Birmingham*, 1950

PLATE LI THE WORK OF JOHN HUNTER

Spur growing on cockscomb after transplantation. Hunter
carried out many experiments in tissue transplantation
(page 241)

Dissection by John Hunter of the Olfactory Nerves (page 241)

PLATE LII THE MEDICAL SOCIETY OF LONDON

John Coakley Lettsom addressing the Medical Society of London, which he founded in 1773. Membership was at first limited to thirty physicians, thirty surgeons, and thirty apothecaries. The figure standing in the background fifth from left is Edward Jenner (pages 252–253). From a painting by Samuel Medley in the Society's house practised for a time at Stafford, and then, at the suggestion of Dr. Erasmus Darwin (grandfather of Charles Darwin), he settled in Birmingham.[1] A good botanist, he published a British Flora which became very popular, and he was a member of the Lunar Society of Birmingham, which held its meetings at full moon.[2] Like Jenner, he was a provincial practitioner ; like Jenner, too, the inspiration for his great discovery came from folk medicine. Withering was aware that the country folk of Shropshire used a decoction of foxglove leaves (foxglove tea) as a cure for dropsy. He showed that the dropsy might be due to cardiac disease, and that digitalis, if carefully used and stopped if any nausea was caused, was an excellent remedy.[3] His views were stated in An Account of the Foxglove, 1785, a medical classic now very rare and valuable. The new drug was mentioned in a contemporary rhyme :

> The Foxglove leaves, with caution given,
> Another proof of favouring Heaven
>   Will happily display.
> The rapid pulse it can abate,
> The hectic flush can moderate
> And, blest by Him Whose will is fate,
>   May give a lengthened day.

Percussion and Auscultation

There were few aids to physical diagnosis before the eighteenth century. The physician, since the earliest days of his existence, had felt the pulse, but it was not accurately timed until Sir JOHN FLOYER of Lichfield (1649–1734) introduced his Physician's Pulse-watch, and wrote his book with this title in 1707[4] (p. 197). A special watch, which ran for one minute, had to be invented, as watches did not then record seconds on their dials.

The clinical thermometer was hardly used until the end of the century, when JAMES CURRIE (1756–1805), a Scot who practised

[1] H. Pearson, Doctor Darwin, 1930, p. 107
[2] A. R. Cushny, " William Withering," Proc. Roy. Soc. Med. (Sect. Hist.), 1915, vol. viii. p. 95 ; C. J. Moorman, " William Withering ; His Work, His Health, His Friends," Bull. Hist. Med., 1942, vol. xii. p. 355
[3] L. H. Roddis, " William Withering and the Introduction of Digitalis into Medical Practice " Ann. Med. Hist., 1936, vol. viii. pp. 93 and 185 ; M. S. Jacobs, " The History of Digitalis Therapy," Ann. Med. Hist., 1936 vol. viii. p. 492
[4] J. Rosenbloom " The History of Pulse Timing," Ann. Med. Hist. 1922 vol. iv. p. 97 ; J. A. Gunn, " Sir John Floyer (1649–1734)," Med. Press and Circ., 1934, vol. 189, p. 297

in Liverpool, took up the idea inaugurated by Sanctorius, and while treating typhoid fever with cold baths, checked his results by thermometry.

Meanwhile, in Vienna, there had been published a monograph of ninety-five pages which contained the first account of percussion as an aid to diagnosis, and bore the lengthy title, *Inventum Novum ex percussione thoracis humani ut signo abstrusos interni pectoris morbos detegendi*, 1761. LEOPOLD AUENBRUGGER (1722–1809) was the son of an innkeeper of Graz, and he had often used percussion to ascertain the level of wine in his father's casks. This principle he applied to the human chest when he became physician to the Military Hospital of Vienna. The *Inventum Novum* commences with the words, " I here present the reader with a new sign which I have discovered for detecting disease of the chest. It consists in percussion of the human thorax, whereby . . . an opinion is formed of the internal state of that cavity." [1] The work attracted little notice for twenty years. Then, JEAN NICHOLAS CORVISART (1755–1821) of Paris,[2] personal physician and friend of Napoleon Bonaparte, translated it into French a year before Auenbrugger died, popularizing the method, and according full credit to the discoverer. It is interesting to note that Auenbrugger was musical, and that he had composed, at the request of Maria Theresa, an opera entitled *The Chimney-sweep*.

Although he really belongs to the following century, it is convenient to mention here the discoverer of the stethoscope, RENÉ THÉOPHILE HYACINTHE LAËNNEC (1781–1826). Born at Quimper, in Brittany, where his statue may still be seen, he commenced his medical career by assisting his uncle, a physician at Nantes.[3] Next, he proceeded to Paris where he studied under Corvisart and Dupuytren, acquitting himself with great distinction, although unfortunately to the detriment of his health, for he was attacked by tuberculosis which eventually caused his death at the age of forty-five years. Shortly after his appointment as physician to the Necker Hospital in 1816, he had occasion to examine a patient whose stoutness made it difficult for the phy-

---

[1] J. Forbes, " On Percussion of the Chest ; A Translation of Auenbrugger's Original Treatise," *Bull. Hist. Med.*, 1936, vol. iv. p. 373
[2] B. B. Beeson, " Corvisart, His Life and Works," *Ann. Med. Hist.*, 1930, vol. ii. p. 297 ; A. L. McDonald, " The Aphorisms of Corvisart," *Ann. Med. Hist.*, 1939, vol. i. pp. 243, 374, 471, 546 ; and 1940, vol. ii. p. 64
[3] H. Saintignon, *Laënnec, sa vie et son œuvre*, Paris, 1904 ; G. B. Webb, " René Théophile Hyacinthe Laënnec," *Ann. Med. Hist.*, 1937, vol. xi. p. 27

sician to hear the heart sounds. Inspired, it is said, by having noticed two children playing with a log of wood, one tapping or scraping it while the other listened by holding his ear against the sawn end, Laënnec rolled a quire of paper into a cylinder, and, placing one end on the patient's chest and the other to his own ear, discovered that he could hear the heart's action, " in a manner more clear and distinct than I had ever been able to do by the immediate application of the ear." [1] Auscultation by the direct application of the ear to the chest of the patient had been long known in medicine, and even Hippocrates had described the " creaking, as of leather," which is audible in pleurisy. But, as Laënnec stated, " the older method was not only ineffective but inconvenient, indelicate, and, in hospitals, even disgusting." The stethoscope described by Laënnec in his book, *Traité de l'Auscultation médiate* (1819), was " a cylinder of wood an inch and a half in diameter and a foot long, perforated by a bore three lines wide and hollowed out into funnel shape at one of its extremities " (Plate LVI). The labour necessary to perfect his discovery and to compose his treatise was nearly fatal to the author, and he was obliged to retire to Brittany to recuperate.

The work created a sensation in Paris, and was well received in other countries, as Laënnec not only described the sounds heard by the stethoscope, coining new terms such as pectoriloquy, aegophony, crepitations, rhonchi, but in the second edition he added a detailed account of the diseases of the chest as then known, making his book of permanent value. He liberally acknowledges the labours of others, mentioning, for example, that " the employment of the new method must not make us forget that of Auenbrugger." In 1822 he had sufficiently recovered to accept the Chair of Medicine in the College of France, but the strain was too great for him, and by the irony of fate he died four years later of the disease, pulmonary tuberculosis,which he had done so much to elucidate.

Public Health and Hygiene

The eighteenth century witnessed an awakening of interest in matters pertaining to the health of communities, and the prevention of disease by various hygienic measures.

[1] Sir W. Hale-White, *Laënnec : Translation of Selected Passages from " De l'Auscultation médiate,"* with a Biography, 1923

In 1700 BERNARDINO RAMAZZINI (1633–1714), professor at Modena and Padua, published the first comprehensive work on diseases of occupation, bearing the rather clumsy title, in the English translation, *On the Diseases of Artificers, which by their particular Callings they are most liable to.* Ramazzini describes the lung diseases of miners and stonemasons, the eye diseases of blacksmiths, gilders, and " cleansers of the jakes," the lead poisoning of printers and potters, mercurial poisoning of surgeons who treat patients by inunction, and the diseases of midwives, bearers of corpses, vintners, tanners, tobacconists, fishermen, washerwomen, and even learned men. One feels that the unemployed are at least healthy. Ramazzini's work is one of the most interesting books in the medical literature of his period.[1]

It was not until the end of the century that JOHANN PETER FRANK (1745–1821) evolved his great scheme for public health legislation. Frank was a poor boy who by his own efforts climbed the ladder of fame, becoming professor at Pavia, and later at Vienna. He made it his mission in life to awaken a hygienic conscience, not only in the people but in their rulers.[2] The rulers, he said, must be taught to keep their subjects healthy. His views are embodied in an extensive work, *System einer vollständigen medizinischen Polizey* in nine volumes (1779–1827).[3] This complete system of medical policy, or medical police as it was sometimes called, included water supplies, sewage disposal, and even school hygiene, but his main contention was that the government of a country should be responsible for the public health. J. P. Frank must be regarded as a great pioneer of sanitary legislation.

The importance of good ventilation for houses and for public buildings was beginning to attract attention. One of its early advocates was Rev. STEPHEN HALES of Teddington, Middlesex (1677–1761), a versatile clergyman who had been the first to demonstrate and measure blood pressure by inserting a glass tube into the artery of a horse.[4] He it was who designed a

---

[1] J. M. McDonald, " Ramazzini's Dissertation on Rinderpest," *Bull. Hist. Med.*, 1942, vol. xii. p. 529

[2] H. E. Sigerist, " The People's Misery : Mother of Diseases. An Address by J. P. Frank," *Bull. Hist. Med.*, 1941, vol. ix. p. 81

[3] L. Baumgarten and E. M. Ramsey, " Johann Peter Frank and his *System*," *Ann. Med. Hist.*, 1933, vol. v., p. 525 ; 1934, vol. vi. p. 69

[4] R. H. Major, " The History of Taking the Blood-pressure," *Ann. Med. Hist.*, 1930, vol. ii. p. 47 ; A. E. Clark-Kennedy, *Stephen Hales, D.D., F.R.S. An Eighteenth Century Biography*, Cambridge, 1929

PLATE LIII EIGHTEENTH-CENTURY PHYSICIANS
AND QUACKS

Hogarth's cartoon entitled, "The Arms of the Honourable Company of Undertakers," represents some of the physicians of the day, most of whom are sniffing
the vinaigrettes in the heads of their canes. Two of them are inspecting urine
in a flask, and one is about to taste it with his finger.
The three figures in the upper part of the picture are, from left to right, Chevalier
Taylor, Mrs. Mapp, and Spot Ward (pages 263-64)

PLATE LIV   A STUDENT'S CLASS CARDS, EARLY
NINETEENTH CENTURY

Cards of admission to medical classes and (top centre) to library of Edinburgh University. Each of the teachers is mentioned in the present work. They are Monro, Barclay, Gregory, Hamilton, Thomson, and Duncan. The fact that the earliest card is dated 1809, and the latest 1823, suggests that Mr. John McLaren spent fourteen years in completing his course of study.

ventilator on the windmill principle, and this was fitted to the roof of Newgate prison, one of the first large-scale experiments in ventilation, which reduced the death rate from gaol fever considerably. The need for fresh air was recognized all the more when the part played by oxygen was demonstrated by Lavoisier. Before mentioning his work, reference must be made to two other chemists who sought to solve the problem of respiration.

JOSEPH BLACK (1728–99),[1] already mentioned as Cullen's pupil and successor in the Chair of Chemistry at Glasgow and later at Edinburgh (p. 222), showed that when mild lime was burned into quick lime, or when it was treated with an acid, it lost in weight by yielding up a gas. Previously it had been imagined that the lime gained in weight, acquiring the mysterious substance " phlogiston." Black disproved this idea, noting also that the gas which he had discovered was a product of combustion and of fermentation, and that it was present in expired air. He named it " fixed air." Van Helmont had called it " gas sylvestre." It is familiar to us as carbon dioxide.

The next step was taken by JOSEPH PRIESTLEY (1733–1804), a Nonconformist minister whose life was a long struggle with ill-health, poverty, and disappointment.[2] Born near Leeds, he served as a minister there, and subsequently at Warrington and Birmingham. Towards the end of his life he became involved in religious controversy, and was accused of sympathy with the French Republicans. His house and chapel were burned, and he was obliged to flee to America, where he died. That Priestley was able to carry out his great chemical researches in the face of so much distraction is indeed surprising. He showed that growing plants were able to " restore " air which had been vitiated by the products of combustion or of respiration, and he actually prepared oxygen which he called " dephlogistigated air " (1775). Yet he did not completely solve the problem, for apparently he could not rid himself of the mythical " phlogiston " idea.

It was ANTOINE LAURENT LAVOISIER (1743–94) who really discovered the nature of oxygen and its importance in respiration, and who proved that inspired air contained oxygen, while expired air contained carbon dioxide.[3] Lavoisier was a great chemist,

[1] Sir W. Ramsay, *Life of Joseph Black*, Glasgow, 1904
[2] T. E. Thorpe, *Joseph Priestley* (English Men of Science), 1906
[3] Sir M. Foster, *Lectures on the History of Physiology*, 1901, p. 244 (" Lavoisier ")

who not only replaced the phlogiston theory by definite facts but also inaugurated schemes for street lighting, introduced improvements in agriculture, and investigated the value of different kinds of food. Most of his life was spent in Paris, and it ended tragically. His views were not acceptable to the revolutionaries, his great scientific services were forgotten, and he perished by the guillotine. So passed Lavoisier, the greatest reformer of chemistry since the days of Paracelsus.[1] Although not a physician, he was a pioneer of hygiene, the first to demonstrate the chemical changes occurring during respiration and to show the necessity in inhabited buildings for a definite air space for each individual.

Mesmerism, Phrenology, and Quackery

The credulity of mankind appears to have been especially well developed during the eighteenth century. Quacks and cults flourished as never before or since. Some of those unorthodox methods of healing were sponsored by medical men.

FRANZ ANTON MESMER (1734–1815), for example, had studied medicine in Vienna.[2] As has been mentioned, the cure of scrofula by the " royal touch " had been very popular during the previous century, when Valentine Greatrakes, an Irishman, had taken upon himself the royal prerogative, and had achieved a great reputation for casting out evil spirits by the laying on of hands. So now Mesmer claimed that he, too, could cure by touching. He appears to have practised hypnotism by this means, asserting that the secret of the success lay in " animal magnetism." To give Mesmer his due, he did attempt to establish his ideas upon a scientific basis, and he must be looked upon as one of the earliest exponents of psychotherapy. Originally his treatment consisted in the application of magnets, until he found that he could achieve similar results by the use of his hands. He achieved great notoriety, especially in Paris, where he was consulted by many eminent persons. (See Supplement, page 460.)

As there was as yet no legal control of medical practice, golden opportunities were afforded to charlatans who chose to make capital out of the misfortunes and ills of mankind.

[1] P. Lemay, " Iconographie française de Lavoisier," Bull. d'Hist. de Méd., 1934, vol. xxviii, p. 146, and " Les Habitations de Lavoisier," loc. cit., p. 156 ; E. Ashworth Underwood, " Lavoisier and the History of Respiration," Proc. Roy. Soc. Med. (Sect. Hist.), vol. xxxvii, No. 2, April 1944
[2] G. Zilboorg and G. W. Henry, History of Medical Psychology, New York, 1941, p. 342

There was JAMES GRAHAM, of Edinburgh, who established a
" Temple of Health " in Pall Mall, London, in 1780.[1] It was a
house sumptuously furnished, fitted with immense mirrors, globes
of glass, dragons breathing flames, and electrical apparatus, for
about this time the scientific work of Galvani and of Volta was
attracting attention, and the charlatan Graham was quick to
exploit this interest to serve his own ends. In the " Temple " he
lectured, with the assistance of Emma Lyon, who later became
Lady Hamilton and Lord Nelson's friend, charging his hearers two
guineas per lecture, with consulting fees in proportion. Although
he made a fortune, he soon lost it, and it is said that he became
insane and died in poverty.

In America, ELISHA PERKINS of Connecticut deluded the public
by his " metallic tractors," which sold for five guineas a pair, and
when applied to the skin with a stroking movement were said to
" draw out " any disease.

Another famous charlatan was JOSHUA WARD, known as Spot
Ward from the birthmark on his face.[2] His " drops " and " pills "
were sold in enormous quantities, and he was even asked to prescribe for the king, receiving as part of his reward the privilege
of driving his carriage through St. James' Park.

> Of late, without the least pretence to skill,
> Ward's grown a famed physician by a pill.

Perhaps most notorious of all was Mrs. MAPP, Crazy Sally
Mapp, the bonesetter who was actually paid by the town of
Epsom to reside there. From Epsom she drove twice a week
to London in a magnificent coach and four, with liveried attendants, to consult at the Grecian Coffee house. For a time she
achieved great success, until gradually she lost favour and died in
obscurity.

A specialist of like quality was the CHEVALIER TAYLOR, as
he styled himself. He travelled about the country, lecturing on
the eye, and practising as " Ophthalmiater Pontifical, Imperial,
and Royal." He duped many, but not Dr. Johnson, who called
him " the most ignorant man I ever knew."

Chevalier Taylor, Spot Ward, and Mrs. Mapp are depicted by

---

[1] J. D. Comrie, *History of Scottish Medicine*, 1932, vol. i. p. 336
[2] F. H. Garrison, *History of Medicine*, 3rd ed., 1924, p. 401 ; H. S. Bennet, " Joshua
Ward, 1685–1761," *Proc. Roy. Soc. Med.*, 1916, vol. ix. Pt. i. p. 100

Hogarth in his famous cartoon, entitled, " The Arms of the Honourable Company of Undertakers " [1] (Plate LIII).

Queen Anne's ophthalmologist was WILLIAM READ, a tailor, who took to treating eye diseases with such good effect that he was knighted by his royal patroness, though so uneducated that he was unable to read or write.

In quite a different category from those irregular and even fraudulent practitioners was F. J. GALL (1758–1828), the founder of the pseudo-science of phrenology. [2] Gall, who had been a student under Van Swieten in Vienna, maintained that certain areas in the brain presided over the various mental characteristics of the individual, and that those areas cause prominences on the surface of the skull. According to his theory, it was possible to ascertain the mental and moral peculiarities of any person by the inspection or palpation of his head. [3] Unfortunately phrenology, originally a subject of serious study, was exploited by quacks and fell into disrepute.

Gall travelled through Europe with his pupil, J. C. SPURZHEIM, who later went to America. Although Gall was no impostor, his new science became a subject of lively controversy. An essay on Phrenology, read before the Royal Medical Society of Edinburgh in 1823, was followed by a discussion lasting until four o'clock the next morning. The essayist was ANDREW COMBE (1797–1847), a leading Edinburgh physician, who with his brother George Combe, a Writer to the Signet, did much to promote popular interest in healthy living as well as in phrenology.

Since that time various attempts have been made to re-establish phrenology among the accredited sciences, and to prove the close relationship between the size and shape of the head and the mental attainments and proclivities of the individual. Phrenology cannot be said to have realized the ambitions of Gall and Spurzheim. Nevertheless, however absurd this pseudo-science may appear to us to-day, due credit must be given to its founders, who were at least genuine in their beliefs, and were

[1] J. C. Jeaffreson, *A Book about Doctors*, 1870 (" Ward," p. 113 ; " Map," p. 187; "Taylor," p. 191)

[2] B. Hollander, *The Unknown Life and Works of Dr. Francis Joseph Gall*, 1909

[3] G. Elliot Smith, *The Old Phrenology and the New* (Henderson Trust Lecture, Edinburgh), 1923 ; Sir J. Crichton-Browne, *The Story of the Brain* (Henderson Trust Lecture, Edinburgh), 1924

the first to draw attention to the localization of cerebral function, although many years elapsed ere the subject was placed on a more rational and scientific basis.[1]

[1] B. Hollander, *Scientific Phrenology*, 1902

BOOKS FOR FURTHER READING

ABRAHAM, J. J. *Lettsom : His Life, Times, Friends and Descendants*, 1933
AVELING, J. H. *The Chamberlens and the Midwifery Forceps*, 1882
BARON, J. *The Life of Edward Jenner*, 2 vols., 1838
COOPER, B. BRANSBY. *Life of Sir Astley Cooper*, 1843
COPE, Sir ZACHARY. *William Cheselden, 1688–1752*, 1953
FOX, R. HINGSTON. *Dr. John Fothergill and His Friends*, 1919
GLAISTER, J. *William Smellie and His Contemporaries*, Glasgow, 1894
JEAFFRESON, J. C. *A Book about Doctors*, 1870
MACMICHAEL, W. *The Gold-headed Cane*, 1827
MATHER, G. R. *Two Great Scotsmen : the Brothers William and John Hunter*, 1893
PAGET, STEPHEN. *John Hunter, Man of Science and Surgeon, 1728–93*, 1897
PEACHEY, G. C. *A Memoir of William and John Hunter*, 1924
RADCLIFFE, W. *The Secret Instrument*, 1947 (a history of the Chamberlens and forceps)
RICHARDSON, B. W. *Disciples of Aesculapius*, 2 vols., 1896
SAINTIGNON, H. *Laënnec, sa vie et son œuvre*, Paris, 1904
SPENCER, H. R. *History of British Midwifery*, 1927
THORPE, T. *Joseph Priestley* (English Men of Science), 1906

CHAPTER XIV

THE DAWN OF SCIENTIFIC MEDICINE IN THE XIX CENTURY

PARADOXICAL as it may seem, the portrayal of medical history becomes more difficult as one approaches modern times. The facts are available, to be sure ; indeed, they are available in such profusion of detail that a selection must be made if one's work is to be contained within a single volume.

There has been a tendency in recent histories of medicine to lay stress on the modern period. In Garrison's well-known history this period occupies half the book ; in Castiglioni's history about one-third.

The modern history of medicine is a matter of common knowledge, and the literature dealing with it is already very considerable in bulk.

There is, however, another reason why it is not easy to write modern medical history. We find ourselves constantly comparing the present-day condition of medicine and surgery with that of fifty or a hundred years ago. The history of more remote periods challenges no such comparison, and the facts have been studied so fully and so frequently that they have settled down to an accepted place and value in the light of the present day. Consequently, instead of trying to evaluate recent discoveries, and to set forth the facts in their true perspective, it is advisable at this stage to abandon the analytic in favour of the synthetic method, to set down the main facts briefly and concisely, and to leave criticism to subsequent generations.

This survey of medical history will accordingly be completed by glancing at some of the great medical advances of the nineteenth century, and at the lives of a few of the distinguished medical men of that time.

Sir Charles Bell and His Work

At the gate of the century stands Sir CHARLES BELL (1774–1842), the greatest medical discoverer since Harvey, and one " whose name must be placed in the front rank among those who have contributed to the progress of science and to the relief of human suffering." His father, Rev. Wm. Bell of Doune, Perthshire, and later of Edinburgh, was an Episcopalian clergyman with an income of £25 a year. Nevertheless he contrived to give a good education to three of his sons, who all became eminent men : John, the surgeon (see p. 230) ; Robert, a Writer to the Signet and Professor of Conveyancing ; and George Joseph, Professor of Scots Law, and writer of a well-known textbook. The youngest son, Charles, was only five years old when his father died, and finances became more straitened than ever. " My education," he wrote, " was the example set me by my brothers, and, by imitation, I obtained it. My mother was my only teacher." While still a boy he assisted his brother John in his class of anatomy, employing with advantage the great artistic skill with which he was endowed, and which added so largely to the success of his later work.[1] Nevertheless the association was not altogether happy, as brother John was deeply involved in medical polemics, and the prejudice against him was extended to Charles, who saw little prospect of success under such circumstances. Accordingly, in 1804, he decided to remove to London, taking with him the manuscript of his first great work, *Essays on the Anatomy of Expression*, a book for artists, which was published in 1806, and which at once established his reputation, although it did not secure for him the Anatomical Chair in the Royal Academy. Like many others before and since, he had a hard struggle to achieve success in London.[2] In 1807 he acquired a " large ruinous house " in Leicester Square. There he lived and practised and taught anatomy. That he was confident of his own success during those early days is shown by his letters to his brother George, the Edinburgh Professor of Law, to whom he was deeply attached. A few years later Charles Bell married Marion Shaw of Ayr, the younger sister of George's wife, and it was she who edited the *Letters of Sir Charles Bell*, which give so intimate an account of his life.[3] In 1812 he acquired the Windmill Street School of Anatomy, which the Hunters had made famous, and which remained a private school until it was closed in 1826. There Bell dissected and taught and pondered on the functions

[1] Sir J. Struthers, *History of the Edinburgh Anatomical School*, 1867, p. 44
[2] G. T. Bettany, *Eminent Doctors*, 1885, vol. i. p. 242
[3] Lady Bell, ed. of *Letters of Sir Charles Bell*, 1870. (Selected from his correspondence with his brother, George Joseph Bell.)

of the nerves, his masterpiece still in embryo (Plate LV). He visited Haslar Hospital to see the wounded arrive from Corunna, and to lend his assistance. In 1815 the Battle of Waterloo gave him a further opportunity for treating gunshot wounds. Without hesitation he left for Brussels, where his sensitive nature was deeply affected by the picture of human misery. He operated each day for a week, until his " clothes were stiff with blood," and his arms " powerless with the exertion of using the knife," although at first he was " almost outmanned " for such a duty. At the field of Waterloo he wrote in his diary, " Already silence dwells here, nothing but a few wretched old men gathering cannon balls . . . but there are marks of struggle, and of horses' hoofs in all directions. Letters, caps, pack-saddles, etc., cover the whole ground."

That same year he was appointed surgeon to Middlesex Hospital, an institution to which he brought a high reputation. He had now married and lived at 34 Soho Square, but he was too deeply devoted to science to acquire a large practice, and probably he was badly in need of the £3,000 paid to him by the Royal College of Surgeons of Edinburgh for his museum, which is still their property. Among its interesting contents are the oil paintings of gunshot wounds which he made after Waterloo. In 1824 he was appointed Professor of Anatomy and Surgery by the Royal College of Surgeons of England, and his lectures, carefully prepared and well-delivered, excited much interest.

His researches on the nerves culminated in his great discovery that there were two kinds of nerve, sensory and motor, each subserving its own function. In 1807 he wrote to his brother George of his new ideas of the anatomy of the brain, and in 1810 he described how he opened the spine of an animal and " pricked the posterior filaments of the nerves," noting that no motion followed. Then he " touched the anterior filaments, when immediately the parts were convulsed." Thus was the function of the spinal nerve roots demonstrated, although Charles Bell, who disliked animal experimentation, left it to Magendie of Bordeaux to confirm his results. To Magendie, as Olmsted has shown, is due the credit of the complete demonstration (p. 279). " Now you know," he wrote to George in 1814, " what I hope to prove is, that there are two great classes of nerves." This he did indeed prove, and discovered many other facts regarding nerves, as every student knows when he dissects the long thoracic or external

PLATE LV   CERTIFICATE OF SIR CHARLES BELL'S CLASS

Theatre of Anatomy
Great Windmill Street

*Hertify that Mr Andrew Dunlop
hath attended my Lectures on Surgery during
two Courses with Great Diligence*

Charles Bell

*London Soho Square
July 1825*

Sir Charles Bell displayed great skill not only as a surgeon and anatomist, but also as an artist, as is shown in the above certificate designed by him.   Original in Royal College of Surgeons of Edinburgh (pages 266–269)

PLATE LVI LAËNNEC'S STETHOSCOPE

Fig 1.ʳᵉ   Fig. 2.   Fig. 3.   Fig. 4.

Fig. 5.

Fig. 6.

Laënnec's wooden stethoscope was designed as a more permanent substitute for his original roll of paper. The cylinder (Fig. 1) was made in two pieces, screwed together (Fig. 5), with a detachable funnel fitted into one end (Fig. 4). Figs. 2 and 3 show sections of the instrument with and without the funnel, while the end view (Fig. 6, natural size), illustrates the relative size of the bore (page 259) respiratory nerve of Bell, which supplies the serratus magnus, a muscle which raises the ribs in inspiration, or when he meets with a case of Bell's paralysis, which was a common result of surgical interference until Bell proved that division of the facial nerve would not cure neuralgia. All those discoveries, together with careful notes of forty clinical cases and a number of beautiful drawings by the author, are set forth in his volume on *The Nervous System of the Human Body*, a classic of medicine, and the first text-book of modern neurology. It appeared in 1830, and in the following year Bell received the honour of knighthood. But long ere this his merit had been recognized, especially on the Continent, where he ranked even greater than Harvey. When he visited Paris, Professor Roux dismissed his class with the words " C'est assez, Messieurs, vous avez vu Charles Bell."

In 1835 the Chair of Surgery at Edinburgh became vacant, and it was offered to Sir Charles Bell. He accepted it, as he considered that " London was a good place to live in but not to die in." Nevertheless, so violent a dislocation at the age of sixty-two could not fail to have its repercussions. Naturally, he found many changes in Edinburgh ; he " seemed to walk in a city of tombs." Yet he filled the Chair with acceptance, published a book on surgery, and busied himself with the revision of his former work on the nervous system, and his Bridgewater treatise on *The Hand, Its Mechanism and Vital Endowments as Evincing Design*, which had a great vogue and passed through many editions.[1] He acquired considerable practice among the nobility of Scotland, and was thus enabled, and even encouraged, to pursue his favourite sport of fly fishing. Sketching was another passion which had attracted him since boyhood. In 1840 he spent two months in Italy, sketching and studying art. But he was already in failing health, and he died two years later whilst visiting a friend at Hallow, near Worcester.

When Charles Bell left Edinburgh in 1804, his brother John continued to practise surgery, but the leading teacher of anatomy was JOHN BARCLAY (1758–1826).[2]

Barclay, who had been educated for the Church, began at the age of thirty-eight to teach anatomy on his own account, after assisting John Bell for a time. He was the first anatomist who did

---

[1] B. Spector, " Sir Charles Bell and the Bridgewater Treatises," *Bull. Hist. Med.*, 1942, vol. xii. p. 314
[2] G. Ballingall, *Life of John Barclay*, 1827

not also practise medicine or surgery, and he greatly advanced the subject of comparative anatomy. Alexander Monro (tertius) gave no opposition to such an energetic teacher, and Barclay was obliged to lecture twice a day in order to accommodate his many students.[1] So intent was he on his subject that he would sometimes continue to lecture to empty benches after the dismissal bell had sounded.

The Tragedy of Robert Knox

In 1824 Barclay was succeeded by ROBERT KNOX (1791–1862), who was regarded as the most popular anatomist of Edinburgh. He was a born orator and an inspiring teacher.[2] Within a few years his class numbered five hundred, and included not only medical students, but also noblemen, lawyers, artists, and men of letters. During five years as a military surgeon, Knox had tended the wounded at Waterloo, and had spent three years in South Africa. He had taken full advantage of his residence at the Cape by pursuing studies in anthropology and in natural history. His papers on those researches, communicated to various learned societies in Edinburgh, obtained for him the post of Conservator to the Museum of the Royal College of Surgeons. Knox had already played a leading part in securing for this museum the collection of Sir Charles Bell.

When Robert Knox was at the height of his fame as a teacher of anatomy, his career suffered a rude shock from the repercussions of the " Burke and Hare " murders.[3] Since the early days of the eighteenth century there had been a traffic in dead bodies for dissection, and the increasing demand for subjects, especially in Edinburgh, had stimulated the nefarious activities of the "Resurrectionists," who robbed recent graves, not only in Edinburgh and neighbourhood, but in Glasgow, and even as far afield as Dublin and London, in order to sell their gruesome spoils to the anatomists.[4] In 1827 there died in William Hare's lodging-house in the West Port of Edinburgh an old man who had failed to pay his bill. Assisted by William Burke, another of his lodgers who, like himself, was an Irishman, Hare conceived the idea of clearing

[1] Sir J. Struthers, *Historical Sketch of the Edinburgh Anatomical School*, 1867, p. 56
[2] H. Lonsdale, *The Life of Dr. Robert Knox*, 1870
[3] A. S. Currie, " Robert Knox, Anatomist, Scientist, and Martyr," *Proc. Roy. Soc. Med.* (Sect. Hist.), 1933, vol. xxvi. p. 39
[4] J. M. Ball, *The " Sack-em-up " Men*, 1926

the debt by the sale of the debtor's body to Dr. Knox for £7, 10s.[1] Encouraged by this success, the two ruffians embarked upon a series of murders, luring their victims into the house, plying them with drink and then suffocating them, so that the body showed no trace of violence. At least sixteen persons were done to death, and their bodies sold for dissection, before the miscreants were brought to justice, and, as the last of the bodies were found in Dr. Knox's rooms, there was strong feeling against him, although, as Lord Cockburn tells us in *Memorials of His Time*, " our anatomists were spotlessly correct, and Knox the most correct of them all." [2] In the trying circumstances, and in the face of considerable personal danger, Dr. Knox conducted himself with bravery and dignity, and eventually when he could no longer remain silent, replied to his accusers in restrained terms, and supported his contentions by publishing the report of the committee which had been set up by his friends to make impartial inquiry into the matter. He weathered the storm, and continued his work as a teacher of anatomy. He wrote papers for the Royal Society on whales, ever a topic of interest to anatomists. By this time his pupil, JOHN GOODSIR (1814–67) [3] had succeeded Monro (tertius) as Professor of Anatomy, and had revived the prestige of the chair, which had been so feebly held by his predecessor. Whatever the reason, Knox gradually lost power and position, finally dying in obscurity in London.[4] It is, however, both unfortunate and unfair that Robert Knox should be remembered mainly in relation to the Burke and Hare murders, for he was an eminent anatomist and a great teacher.

Anatomy under Henle and Hyrtl

We have already noted the rise of anatomical teaching in America under such pioneers as Rush and Morgan and Shippen. Meanwhile, on the Continent, a number of great anatomists had appeared.

JACOB HENLE (1809–85), whose discoveries in microscopic anatomy entitle him to a high place in medical history, held professorships of anatomy successively at Zurich, Heidelberg, and

[1] G. MacGregor, *The History of Burke and Hare*, 1884 ; W. Roughead, *The Trial of Burke and Hare*, 1921
[2] H. Cockburn, *Memorials of His Time*, Edinburgh, 1872, p. 395
[3] W. Turner, *The Anatomical Memoirs of John Goodsir, F.R.S.*, 3 vols., Edinburgh, 1868
[4] *Life of Sir Robert Christison*, ed. by one of his sons, 1885, vol. i. p. 311

Göttingen.[1] When he was a student he had come under the spell of Johannes Müller, to whose encouragement he owed much. Bichat had laid the foundation of histology. Henle proceeded to build the edifice. The simile is appropriate, as Henle, in his excellent *Handbook of Systematic Anatomy* (3 vols., 1866-71), viewed the human body from an architectural standpoint. This handbook describes the macroscopic and microscopic structure of the entire body, with lovely illustrations by himself. Henle discovered the tubules of the kidney, and first described the epithelial coverings and linings of the surfaces of the body, the muscular coat of the arteries, the minute anatomy of the eye, and various structures in the brain. Yet he did not confine his attention to histology. He states his conviction that infectious and contagious diseases are caused by living organisms, thus prophesying the dawn of bacteriology. Amid all this activity he found time to play his violin : he was an accomplished musician, and in later years learned the 'cello and viola. Garrison regards Henle as one of the greatest anatomists of all time, whose histological discoveries rank alongside the anatomical discoveries of Vesalius.

Another eminent anatomist, whose ability lay in teaching rather than research, was JOSEPH HYRTL (1810–94).[2] The son of a Hungarian musician employed by Haydn, he occupied for thirty years the first Chair of Anatomy at Vienna. A popular and interesting lecturer, he attracted students from all faculties, and captivated his hearers by embellishing his subject with all manner of other information. His friendliness and generosity endeared him to generations of students. His textbook, clearly and simply written, passed through twenty editions in forty years. He was devoted to osteology, and possessed a wonderful collection of skeletons, both animal and human. He also developed the technique of making " corrosion preparations," the blood-vessels of an organ or part being injected, and then the other tissues dissolved away by acid, so that all the vessels remained clearly revealed.

Every student of anatomy is familiar with the name of HENRY GRAY (1827–61), lecturer on anatomy at St. George's Hospital, whose early death from smallpox was a great loss to medical science. *Gray's Anatomy, Descriptive and Applied* (1858) still has an immense popularity.

---

[1] G. Rosen, " Some Aspects of Jacob Henle's Medical Thought," *Bull. Hist. Med.*, 1937, vol. v. p. 509 ; H. E. Sigerist, *Great Doctors*, 1933, p. 347
[2] F. H. Garrison, *History of Medicine*, 3rd ed., 1924, p. 490

Embryology at this time received its chief stimulus from CARL ERNST VON BAER (1792–1876) of Königsberg, and later of St. Petersburg.[1] His discovery of the mammalian ovum in 1827 was only one of his numerous contributions to our knowledge of growth in its earliest germinal stages.

Anthropology owed much to PAUL BROCA (1824–80), the Parisian surgeon who discovered the motor speech centre, and who thus inaugurated the localization of cerebral functions. Broca discovered methods of measuring and delineating the skull, and he contributed to the knowledge of prehistoric trephining (p. 6).

Physiology and Physics

It was in the early part of the nineteenth century that physiology became established as a distinct science. One of its first and greatest exponents was JOHANNES MÜLLER (1801–58), who from a humble origin, for his father was a shoemaker of Coblenz, rose to be a great pioneer of physiology. Like John Hunter, he was keenly interested in comparative anatomy, but his greatest achievement was the publication of his *Handbuch der Physiologie des Menschen* (1833–40), which is full of original observations, and which established physiology as a separate science. Müller commenced his academic career as a teacher of anatomy and physiology at Bonn, where he was assisted by Jacob Henle. In 1833 he was appointed professor of anatomy and physiology at Berlin, a post which he held until his sudden death at the age of fifty-seven. A tireless and energetic worker, he contributed numerous papers to the *Archiv für Anatomie und Physiologie*, which he edited for many years. He made discoveries in embryology (Müllerian ducts) ; he confirmed the findings of Sir Charles Bell regarding the spinal nerve roots and their position ; he enunciated the law of specific nerve energies ; he investigated the production of sound by the vocal cords ; and he was one of the first to classify tumours according to their microscopic appearances.[2] In his handbook of physiology he included the subject which we now call psychology, and he quoted freely from the aphorisms of Spinoza. His masterly account of the nature of mind may still

[1] A. W. Meyer, " A Summary of Von Baer's Commentar," *Bull. Hist. Med.*, 1938, vol. vi. p. 1031

[2] R. Röss le, " Die Pathologische Anatomie des Johannes Müller," *Arch. f. Gesch. d. Med.*, 1929, vol. xxii. p. 24

be read with profit. An impressive figure and an inspiring teacher, he was worshipped by his students and assistants, as it was ever one of his chief traits to encourage his juniors and to assist them by every means in his power. Among his disciples were many who became famous : Henle, Schwann, Virchow, Helmholtz, and others. Henle (p. 271) and Schwann (p. 190) have already been mentioned. Virchow, the pathologist, belongs to a later period (p. 282). Perhaps the greatest of all Müller's pupils was Helmholtz, that master of physics and physiology to whom the world owes so great a debt. (For Purkinje, see Supplement, p. 461.)

HERMANN VON HELMHOLTZ (1821–94) was born in Potsdam.[1] On his mother's side he was a descendant of William Penn, the founder of Pennsylvania. His father, a teacher of philosophy, sought to interest his son in classical learning, but Hermann was much more devoted to physics and chemistry. Little or no livelihood was to be gained from science at that time, therefore the boy was sent to study medicine, and in due course he became a surgeon in the army. All his spare time was devoted to science. His paper, " On the Conservation of Energy," published in Müller's *Archiv*, brought him into prominence, and in 1849 he was appointed Professor of Physiology at Königsberg University. This gave him the opportunity to indulge his passion for original research. He established, by electrical means, the rate of transmission of nerve impulses. Next, at the very outset of the investigations which led to the publication of his great work on *Physiological Optics* (1856–67), he invented the ophthalmoscope, and " had the great joy of being the first to see a living human retina." Although this instrument has proved its immense value in medical diagnosis, it was at first regarded as a toy, and even Helmholtz himself regarded the discovery as a mere incident in the course of his researches. Those researches concerned the mechanism of accommodation and the problem of colour vision. In 1801, THOMAS YOUNG (1773–1829), a pioneer British ophthalmologist practising in London, had written a treatise, *On the Mechanics of the Eye* (see p. 374). Helmholtz confirmed and elaborated Young's conclusion ; hence arose the well-known Young-Helmholtz theory of colour vision. In 1856 Helmholtz made his first visit to England, attending the British Association at Hull, where, as he wrote, " some papers were

[1] J. G. McKendrick, *Hermann von Helmholtz* (Masters of Medicine), 1899 ; L. Koenigsberger, *Hermann von Helmholtz*, 1906. (A complete and interesting biography, trans. by F. R. Welby.)

important scientific contributions, and some the tomfoolery of crackbrained persons." Two years later he visited Scotland at the invitation of Sir William Thomson, afterwards Lord Kelvin. The two eminent men remained the closest friends until death separated them, forty years later.

Having completed his researches on the physiology of the eye, which resulted in a mass of new facts and ideas, Helmholtz turned his attention to the sense of hearing. This subject had a peculiar attraction for one so keenly devoted to music. On account of the delicate health of his wife, he had accepted a Chair of Anatomy and Physiology at Bonn; but finding the teaching of anatomy irksome, he was glad to be transferred, three years later, to Heidelberg, where he could concentrate once more upon physiology. In physiological acoustics he opened up a new field, in which he made many discoveries as admirable as those he had already made in physiological optics. He showed that mathematics and music, which appear so different, " are yet interrelated and mutually helpful." His brilliant work on *Sensations of Tone*, written in clear and simple language, appeals to lovers of music as well as to scientists, and remains a classic, bridging the gap between the science of acoustics and the art of music. Amid many other discoveries, he elaborated the Resonance Theory of Hearing, which still meets with general acceptance.

In 1871 Helmholtz was appointed Professor of Physics in Berlin, where he spent the rest of his life. He now turned his attention to electro-dynamics, and was assisted by HEINRICH HERTZ, a brilliant scientist who died young, and whose discovery of " Hertzian waves " made modern wireless transmission possible. Helmholtz resigned his chair in 1885 in order to become President of the great Physico-Technical Institute which had been set up by the Government. His output of scientific work was undiminished despite his seventy years. He fulfilled a cherished ambition in 1893 when he visited America, but he was already in failing health and he died soon after his return.

We have dealt at some length upon the achievements of Helmholtz, not only because he was one of the greatest scientists of all time, but also because his work showed how one science can assist another, and how physiology was enriched from physics.

A close friend of Helmholtz, also a pupil of Müller, was EMIL DU BOIS REYMOND (1818–96), who made numerous experiments with muscle-nerve preparations, discovering many new facts and founding the science of electro-physiology.

His contemporaries in the same field of work were, in England, AUGUSTUS WALLER (1816–70), who showed that degenerative changes occur in the distal portion of a severed nerve ; and in America, HENRY BOWDITCH (1840–1911),[1] whose experiments in nerve blocking were the foundation of one method of producing local anæsthesia, later perfected by G. Crile.

Another contemporary of Helmholtz, whose name is known to every medical student as an inventor of various forms of apparatus, was CARL LUDWIG (1816–95).[2] While he was Professor of Physiology successively at Zurich, Vienna, and Leipzig, he did much to advance our knowledge of blood pressure and of the function of the kidney. He attracted many pupils of all nationalities, and when he found a keen student he would give him a problem to work out, often working along with him, and always assigning to him the credit for any successful result. Much work which was really his own was then published in the name of one of his assistants or pupils. By many he was regarded as " the greatest teacher of physiology who ever lived."

About this time another branch of physiology, that of physiological chemistry, was founded by JUSTUS VON LIEBIG (1803–73) of Giessen. He made numerous contributions to organic chemistry, although he went too far when he denied that fermentation and putrefaction were due to vital agency. A meat extract still bears his name, but his claim to fame rests upon his writings, and especially his conception of metabolism.

Pioneer British Physiologists

Among British physiologists MARSHALL HALL (1790–1857) exemplifies the trend of physiology in the early part of the nineteenth century.[3] A versatile and energetic man, he contrived to conduct an extensive medical practice while making the important investigations in physiology which brought him lasting fame. After qualifying at Edinburgh and continuing his studies at Paris

---

[1] A. A. Walking, "Henry Ingersoll Bowditch," *Ann. Med. Hist.*, 1932, vol. v. p. 428
[2] G. Rosen, " Carl Ludwig and his American Students," *Bull. Hist. Med.*, 1936, vol. iv. p. 609 ; W. Stirling, *Some Apostles of Physiology*, 1902, p. 107
[3] Charlotte Hall, *Life of Marshall Hall*, 1861 ; T. J. Pettigrew, *Medical Portraits*, 1838–40, vol. iv.

PLATE LVII THE CONQUEST OF RABIES

The lad Jupille, Pasteur's second patient, grappling with the mad dog. Statue in courtyard of Institut Pasteur of Paris (page 284)

PLATE LVIII PATIENT AND DOCTOR IN THE
NINETEENTH CENTURY

The Rahere Ward of St. Bartholomew's Hospital in 1832. A contemporary
sketch in possession of the hospital

Dr. Joseph Bell of Edinburgh in his " victoria " (page 230)

and Göttingen, he commenced practice in his native city of Nottingham, making many long journeys on horseback, as was the custom. He found time, however, to write a book on *The Diagnosis of Diseases* (1817), which was commended by Dr. Matthew Baillie, and had a wide circulation. He also denounced the prevalent practice of blood-letting, regarding the lancet as " a minute instrument of mighty mischief." His reputation was increased by his appointment as physician to Nottingham Hospital, so that in 1826 he removed to London, and actually earned £800 in fees during his first year there. At his house in Manchester Square he kept a regular menagerie of animals for his experiments. Like John Hunter, he studied hibernation, but his greatest achievement was his discovery of reflex action, which originated from the observation that a headless newt moved when the skin was pricked. The integrity of the sensory and motor nerves and of the segment of the spinal cord from which they originated was noted by him to be essential. Marshall Hall showed how " reflex action " explained the act of coughing, the involuntary closure of the eyes when threatened, the first breath of a new-born child, and many other acts. This important discovery was attacked, and even stigmatized as an absurd theory, and the Royal Society refused to publish the work, although on the Continent it was accepted, and highly praised. Marshall Hall never became embittered by these reverses. He continued his researches, and eventually had the satisfaction of finding his views universally accepted. Although he lectured at St. Thomas's Hospital on nervous diseases, he never held a hospital appointment in London. His philanthropy is shown in his successful campaign to stop the practice of flogging in the army, and in his visit to the United States in order to study conditions of slave labour. Two years before his death he introduced the method of artificial respiration which bears his name. Though now superseded by other methods, it has been the means of saving many lives. Probably the work of Marshall Hall has not received full recognition even yet. He was certainly one of the greatest men of his time. " In beauty of character he resembled Sir Charles Bell, of whom he was the true successor."

The first physiologist in Britain to devote his entire attention to the subject was WILLIAM SHARPEY (1802–80)[1] He, too, was

[1] J. C. Brougher, " William Sharpey, 1802–1880," *Ann. Med. Hist.*, 1927, vol. ix. p. 124

an Edinburgh graduate who afterwards studied in Paris, where, at the clinic of the famous Dupuytren, he formed a lifelong friendship with James Syme. For a short time he joined his stepfather, Dr. Arrott, in practice at Arbroath, but science attracted him more strongly, and he resolved to devote himself to physiology. During the next three years he visited Germany, France, and Italy, travelling on foot and learning much. Returning to Edinburgh, he assisted Allen Thomson by lecturing extra-murally on anatomy, and he pursued the research which resulted in his discovery of ciliary activity. This he described in a paper, *On a Peculiar Motion excited in Fluids by the Surfaces of Certain Animals.*[1] In 1836 he was appointed Professor of Physiology at University College, London. At the same time RICHARD QUAIN was appointed Professor of Anatomy, the two subjects having been previously taught together by Quain's brother. Sharpey occupied this Chair with great acceptance for thirty-eight years. He collaborated with Quain by writing the sections on microscopic anatomy for the well-known *Elements of Anatomy,* which is still used as a work of reference. A man of kindly nature and ready wit, Sharpey was an inspiring teacher who held the same position in Britain as Müller did in Germany. Physiology had been a mere appendage of anatomy and of physics until Sharpey gave it a place among the sciences. He also rendered valuable service as secretary to the Royal Society for almost twenty years. Among his pupils were Burdon Sanderson, Michael Foster, and others, who did much to advance physiology during the latter part of the century.

An early pioneer of the subject in Edinburgh was JOHN HUGHES BENNETT (1812–75), who succeeded Allen Thomson as professor of " the Institutes of Medicine," as physiology was called. The holder of the chair was a physician in the Royal Infirmary, an arrangement which had the advantage of linking physiology with clinical medicine.[2] Hughes Bennett inaugurated the practical study of histology, he endorsed the medicinal value of cod liver oil, long used as a folk remedy, and he described the blood disease known as leucocythemia(1845).[3]

---

[1] W. Sharpey, " On a Peculiar Motion, etc.," *Edin. Med. and Surg. Jour.*, 1830, vol. xxxiv. ; W. Stirling, *Some Apostles of Physiology*, 1902, p. 120
[2] G. T. Bettany, *Eminent Doctors*, 1885, vol. ii. p. 209
[3] J. D. Comrie, *History of Scottish Medicine*, 1932, vol. ii. p. 608 ; R. H. Major, *Classic Descriptions of Disease*, 1932, p. 465

The Genius of Claude Bernard

Another name which cannot be omitted from any account of nineteenth-century physiology is that of the great French scientist, CLAUDE BERNARD (1813–78). He was of humble parentage, as his father was a vine grower at St. Julien, in the province of Beaujolais, not far from Lyons. As a youth he was apprenticed to a local pharmacist, but the work did not attract him. All his spare time was devoted to the writing of poetry and drama, until at the age of twenty-one he determined to seek his fortune in Paris. The dramatic critic to whom he submitted his work, and who was kind enough to read it, recognized that it had merit, but he wisely advised the author to study medicine, which, he said, will " much more surely gain you a livelihood." [1]

After completing his student training, Bernard began his brilliant career by assisting Magendie,[2] the leading physiologist of France and an ardent apostle of physiological experiment. Magendie seemed, however, to substitute experiment for thought, thrusting his knife here and there to see what would come of it, and prodding in all directions in the hope of finding some new truth. Claude Bernard had the good sense to recognize the defects of his master's method, and he devoted himself to research with a definite object in view.

His first work related to digestion. By a series of carefully planned experiments, he showed that digestion was not completed in the stomach, as had been believed, but that gastric digestion was only a preparatory act. Digestion was continued in the intestine, through the action of the pancreatic juice. It was during this series of experiments that one of his dogs, having a cannula fixed in its pancreatic duct, escaped from the laboratory, and was brought back by the irate owner, an inspector of police. Bernard did not know how the animal had been obtained for the laboratory, but he soon pacified the owner and restored the dog to health, the incident ending happily for all concerned.

The next important discovery, that of glycogen, was also the outcome of systematic and planned experiments. Bernard proved that the liver did not merely secrete bile ; it also produced sugar,

[1] Sir M. Foster, *Claude Bernard* (Masters of Medicine), 1899 ; J. M. D. Olmsted, *Claude Bernard, Physiologist*, New York, 1938, and " Claude Bernard as a Dramatist," *Ann. Med. Hist.*, 1935, vol. vii., p. 253
[2] J. M. D. Olmsted, *François Magendie*, New York, 1944, p. 93

and this function was independent of sugar in the diet. There was, in fact, an " internal environment," or *milieu intérieur*, and in giving it this name Bernard paved the way for the discovery of the numerous " hormones " which we now recognize. Moreover, the production of sugar by the liver showed that the animal body could build up substances as well as destroy them. At the time his discovery had a far-reaching effect, as it showed, furthermore, that the body was not simply a bundle of organs, each having its separate function. Claude Bernard pursued his discovery of the glycogen function of the liver to its logical conclusion, and he left little to be added by subsequent investigators (p. 365).

A third discovery was that of the vasomotor mechanism. Bernard was working at the subject of animal heat when he noted that division of the cervical sympathetic nerve in a rabbit raised the temperature on that side of the head and neck. With characteristic insight he saw the significance of this side issue, and turned aside from his main quest to ascertain how the nerve could influence temperature. While investigating the function of the submandibular gland, he showed that the sympathetic nerve was the constrictor of the blood vessels ; the chorda tympani was the dilator. Thus were the fundamental facts of vasomotor physiology made known.

The merit of Claude Bernard's work was recognized in 1854, when a special Chair of Physiology was created for him at the Sorbonne. Success did not spoil him, nor did he relax his efforts to improve his subject. He never repeated a routine course of lectures, but made every lecture a new exposition rather than a repetition.

Towards the end of his life he made what is perhaps his most noteworthy contribution to the advance of medicine.[1] He described the principles upon which research should be conducted. His *Introduction to the Study of Experimental Medicine*, which appeared in 1865, is one of the greatest of medical classics which ought to be read by everyone who undertakes medical research.[2]

It is significant that two great Frenchmen, Descartes and Bernard, stepped aside from the path of scientific research in order

[1] H. Bergson, " The Philosophy of Claude Bernard," *Bull. Hist. Med.*, 1936, vol. iv. p. 15
[2] Claude Bernard, *An Introduction to the Study of Experimental Medicine*, 1865, trans. by H. C. Greene, New York, 1927

to survey the principles upon which research should be conducted. Claude Bernard stated that there was no place in experimental medicine (the name he gave to physiology) for " doctrines " or " systems." " Systems," he wrote, " do not exist in Nature but only in men's minds." He also stated that " what we know may interfere with our learning what we do not know " ; in other words, he disliked accepted formulæ, and accordingly he set out to establish a good experimental standard. The true scientist, Bernard explained, had no fixed starting-point. He studied Nature, he observed facts, and from those facts he framed a hypothesis. Then, by experiment, he tested the accuracy or fallacy of the hypothesis. Imagination, though essential before and after experiment, had no place in the experiment itself. One must shed one's imagination, like one's overcoat, on entering the laboratory, and put it on again on leaving. Such was the philosophy of Claude Bernard. Perhaps the poet in him helped him to frame his hypotheses, and to plan his experiments with such success. He also possessed great technical skill. " A head without a hand," he affirmed, " is an impotent nothing." To Bernard, in marked degree, belonged that attribute mentioned in the last sentence of his treatise, " the independence and freedom of mind so essential to the progress of humanity."

Pathology and Bacteriology

The discovery of a bacterial cause in many forms of disease changed the whole face of pathology. That change did not take place until the latter part of the nineteenth century. The two greatest exponents of pathology in the nineteenth century were Rokitansky and Virchow, the latter being often regarded as the leading pathologist of all time.

CARL ROKITANSKY (1804–78) was a Czech who was Professor of Pathology at Vienna for thirty years.[1] It is said that he performed many thousands of post-mortem examinations, and from this huge material he wrote those descriptions of disease which are models of clear and logical writing, well worthy to rank alongside those of his predecessors in this work, Morgagni and Matthew Baillie.[2] He regarded pathology as the foundation of clinical

[1] F. R. Menne, " Carl Rokitansky the Pathologist," *Ann. Med. Hist.*, 1925, vol. vii. p. 379
[2] H. E. Sigerist, *Great Doctors*, 1936, p. 291 ; M. Neuburger, *British Medicine and the Vienna School*, 1943, p. 40 ; L. Schonbauer, *Medizinische Wien*, 1947, p. 209

knowledge. Among the subjects of his researches were diseases of the arteries, on which he wrote a large treatise ; defects of the heart, which was the subject of another work ; acute yellow atrophy, which he named thus, and many other diseases. A genial and kindly man, he remarked of his sons, two of whom were physicians and two musicians, that they were of two classes, the healers and the howlers : "Die Einen heilen, die Anderen heulen."[1] His handbook of pathological anatomy had a wide circulation.

By far the most distinguished pathologist, and one of the most famous medical men of the century under review, was RUDOLF VIRCHOW (1821–1902).[2] He was one of those exceptional individuals who have encompassed several careers within a lifetime, adding lustre to each of them. Virchow was eminent as anthropologist, pathologist, and politician.[3]

In the first of those wide fields he conducted a vast investigation into the physical anthropology of German children, and he investigated lake dwellings, tattooing, and allied subjects. He accompanied Dr. Schliemann to Troy in 1879, and wrote an account of the wonderful discoveries there. His political career was no less noteworthy.[4] For many years he was by far the most influential medical man in Germany. An apostle of democracy and freedom, he was strongly opposed to the policy of Bismarck.[5] From 1880–93 he was a member of the Reichstag, and it was largely owing to his efforts that the drainage system and the water supply of Berlin were reconstructed on modern lines.

It is, however, as pathologist that Virchow is known in medical history. While still in his twenties, he was sent to investigate an epidemic of typhus in Silesia. His report revealed such deplorable social conditions, and his recommendations were so revolutionary, that the responsible authorities banished him from Berlin.

Fortunately he was appointed Professor of Pathology at Würzburg, and a few years later he was recalled to a similar post in Berlin. Early in his career he had founded the journal *Archiv für pathologische Anatomie*, which came to be known as Virchow's *Archiv*. Numerous were his contributions to pathology. He was

[1] F. H. Garrison, *Introduction to the History of Medicine*, 3rd ed., 1924, p. 454
[2] R. Virchow, *Briefe an seine Eltern, 1839–64*, Leipzig, 1906
[3] W. Bartlett, " A Sketch of Virchow's Life and Time," in *Lectures on the History of Medicine* (Mayo Foundation), Philadelphia, 1933
[4] H. G. Schlumberger, " Rudolf Virchow and the Franco-Prussian War," *Ann. Med. Hist.*, 1942, vol. iv., 3rd Ser., p. 253
[5] H. G. Schlumberger, " Rudolf Virchow—Revolutionist," *ibid.*, p. 147

one of the first to record leukaemia (described about the same time by Hughes Bennet), and to enlarge the knowledge of trichinosis, leontiasis ossea, and many other diseases. His greatest achievement was his conception of the cell as the centre of pathological changes. For him there were no specific cells in diseased tissue. Every morbid structure consisted of cells derived from pre-existent cells. The motto, " Omnis cellula e cellula " was the foundation of his work on *Cellular Pathology*, which appeared in 1858, and which destroyed at a blow the old-fashioned " humoral " pathology. He dedicated the book to Professor John Goodsir of Edinburgh (p. 271), to whom he was indebted for the idea of cell domination. Since Virchow's day it has been necessary to modify his views considerably, but at the time they marked a great advance. Virchow led a life of intense activity. In the Virchow Institute he collected and mounted 23,000 specimens.

He was the recipient of many honours, and his many years of hard work in the interests of social reform and public hygiene were suitably rewarded when his eightieth birthday was celebrated as a national holiday, and when a magnificent new municipal hospital was named after him.

The Birth of a New Science

Contemporary with Virchow was a Frenchman who, though not a medical graduate, was one of the outstanding figures of medical history. The details of the life of LOUIS PASTEUR (1822–95) are so well known that they need only be recalled briefly.[1] He was born at Dôle, a little town in the Jura, where his father, a soldier of Napoleon's army, had returned to ply his trade as a tanner. Young Pasteur showed some aptitude for drawing portraits, but his scientific ability did not become apparent until his student days in Paris. Then commenced that systematic and strenuous life, devoted to the solution of one problem after another, with results which have proved of immense value to mankind. Diseases of wine, of insects, of domestic animals, and of man were in turn investigated and elucidated. Pasteur was Professor of Chemistry at Strassburg, at Lille, and eventually for over twenty years in Paris. The last six years of his life were spent in the Institût Pasteur, which had been built in his honour in 1888, and where

[1] R. Vallery-Radot, *The Life of Pasteur*, 2 vols., 1902 ; L. Descour, *Pasteur and his Work*, 1922 ; P. Compton, *The Genius of Louis Pasteur*, 1932

he worked in almost monastic simplicity, assisted by his devoted wife, who was ever his best collaborator.

His first researches concerned crystallography, and as he noted how fermentation occurred in his solutions he was led to that vast study of the causes of putrefaction and fermentation which was to engage his attention for many years. He showed that fermentation was not merely a chemical reaction, but that it was due to micro-organisms. His appointment at Lille placed him in a wine-growing district. There, he discovered that it was the action of organisms which caused wine and milk to become sour, and that this could be prevented by the application of heat, or "pasteurization," as it was called. He next set out to ascertain whether the micro-organisms which caused the fermentation were spontaneously generated, or were present in the air. It was Pasteur's proof of the existence of atmospheric germs that led Lister to apply the principle to surgery, with amazing results (p. 323).

Pasteur was still engaged in this investigation when he was asked to go to the south of France to study the silkworm disease which threatened to wreck the industry. After three years' work he discovered two distinct diseases, and he recommended measures for their prevention which saved the prosperity of the silk industry.

At this point of his career (1868) he was stricken with cerebral hæmorrhage, although he fortunately recovered from the paralysis after a long and tedious illness. By this time he was no longer a chemist, but rather a bacteriologist. His revived energy was now devoted to the prevention of anthrax, or splenic fever, which had assumed epidemic form in France, and which threatened to wipe out the sheep and cattle. Following the lines laid down by Jenner, Pasteur prepared a weak form of virus, an old culture of low virulence, which, when injected into an animal, caused a mild attack and conferred immunity. A similar means was devised for the prevention of chicken cholera, a disease which had also caused heavy losses. Pasteur's most famous discovery, however, was made on July 6, 1885, when he treated an Alsatian boy, Joseph Meister, who had been bitten by a mad dog. A few months later Pasteur had a second successful case, when he inoculated a shepherd lad from the Jura named Jupille, who had been bitten severely by a rabid dog while he grappled with it in an effort to protect his comrades. Jupille's brave action is commemorated by a statue in the grounds of the Institût Pasteur of Paris (Plate LVII). After many experiments Pasteur had reached

PLATE LIX   BRIGHT AND BRIGHT'S DISEASE

RICHARD BRIGHT, 1789–1858

The kidneys of John King, a sailor who died of nephritis in Guy's
Hospital.   It was the study of this and other cases which led Bright
to associate dropsy with disease of the kidney.   The illustration is
from Bright's *Reports of Medical Cases*, 1827 (page 291)

PLATE LX AMERICAN PIONEERS

DANIEL DRAKE (1785–1852) (page 299)

EPHRAIM McDOWELL (1771–1830) (page 300)

the conclusion that the virus which causes rabies in animals and hydrophobia in man had its seat in the nerve centres. From the spinal marrow he produced an attenuated virus for inoculation, and the success of his bold experiments led to the establishment of Pasteur Institutes in many parts of the world, and to the reduction of the mortality to less than 1 per cent.

Thus agriculture, industry, medicine, and humanity in general are eternally indebted to this illustrious and devoted scientist. Addressing Pasteur at the great and enthusiastic gathering in Paris on his seventieth birthday, Lord Lister said, " Truly there does not exist in the wide world an individual to whom medical science owes more than to you." Pasteur, who entered leaning on the arm of President Carnot, expressed in his reply the joy he felt from the presence of foreign delegates, believing as he did that " science and peace must triumph over ignorance and war, that nations will unite not to destroy but to instruct one another, and that the future will belong to those who have done most for suffering humanity. I refer to you, my dear Lister. . . ." Then Pasteur and Lister met and embraced each other amid shouts of " Vive Pasteur."

It was this historic meeting which marked the beginning of a new era in medicine and surgery. Among the pupils of Pasteur were many famous men. One of the most eminent was ÉLIE METCHNIKOFF (1845–1916), the Russian scientist to whom the Nobel Prize was awarded in 1908. Of humble parentage, he was born near Kharkoff, and as a boy, like John Hunter, he was eager to know everything, showing that keen curiosity which eventually led him to discover so much. For a time he taught zoology at Odessa, then he pursued researches in Sicily, and it was while working at the marine laboratory of Messina that his investigations of digestive processes in larval starfish and planarian worms led him to formulate the doctrine of phagocytosis, the destruction of bacteria by white blood corpuscles.[1] Metchnikoff cared nothing for position or fortune, and in 1888 he gave up his post in Russia in order to work under Pasteur in Paris. The story of Pasteur's kindness to him, and of the researches which led him to fame, is well told in a biography by his wife, Olga Metchnikoff, who, as a trained scientist, assisted him in his work.[2] In later life Metchnikoff devoted much attention to the question of intestinal

[1] W. Bulloch, *The History of Bacteriology*, 1938, p. 259
[2] Olga Metchnikoff, *Life of Élie Metchnikoff, 1845–1916*, 1921

sepsis, and to the possibility of prolonging life by the ingestion of lactic acid bacilli.

Pasteur was succeeded by his assistant ÉMILE ROUX (1853–1933), who ranks next to him as the greatest French bacteriologist. Roux made many remarkable discoveries. He perfected the preparation of anti-diphtheritic serum, and he showed that monkeys could be inoculated with syphilis. His term of office as director of the Pasteur Institute was marked by many important discoveries.

Another well-known bacteriologist of Paris was FERNAND WIDAL (1862–1929), who first applied, in 1896, the sero-diagnostic test for typhoid fever which bears his name.[1]

The great German pioneer, who must share with Pasteur the title of the founder of bacteriology, was ROBERT KOCH (1843–1910).[2] Koch, who had studied at Göttingen under Henle and had served in the Franco-German war, was a country practitioner at a village in Wollstein when he commenced his important researches. He showed that anthrax, then so prevalent in animals and man, was due to the large bacillus which had been discovered by Pollender in 1849, and was not the result of such vague causes as "miasmata" or "contagia." He published his results in 1876. This study of anthrax suggested that this very infectious disease might be caused by its special micro-organism.[3]

In Koch's opinion proof of the specificity of an organism could be accepted only when certain facts, known as Koch's postulates, were established (1881). The germ must be invariably present, must be capable of cultivation outside the body, and must, if injected into a healthy animal, reproduce the disease. Koch discovered the vibrio of cholera (1884), and showed how it was transmitted by drinking-water. He travelled to South Africa to study rinderpest, to India to investigate plague, and to Java to examine the cause of malaria.[4]

One disease which specially interested Koch was tuberculosis. In 1882 he announced the discovery of the tubercle bacillus, and in 1890 he suggested a new remedy, consisting of a glycerine extract

---

[1] The actual discovery was made by Herbert Edward Durham (1866–1945) of Guy's Hospital, although Widal was the first to apply it in clinical practice

[2] G. B. Webb, "Robert Koch—1843–1910," *Ann. Med. Hist.*, 1932, vol. iv. p. 509 ; L. Brown, "Robert Koch (1843–1910)," *Ann. Med. Hist.*, 1935, vol. vii. pp. 99, 292, 385 ; H. E. Sigerist, *Great Doctors*, 1936, p. 366

[3] G. F. Petrie, "Robert Koch : Founder of Modern Bacteriology," *Nature*, 1943, vol. clii. p. 684

[4] B. Heymann, *Robert Koch*, Leipzig, 1932

of tubercle bacilli, which he called tuberculin, but which did not fulfil his expectations. He was the recipient of many honours, including the Nobel Prize in 1905. An Institute for Infectious Diseases was built for him in Berlin in 1891. There he continued his work even after he retired in 1904 ; there his ashes were laid after his death six years later, at the close of a laborious and fruitful life, so rich in its results, and so beneficial to humanity.

A few of the distinguished bacteriologists who were trained by Koch may now be briefly mentioned.

EMIL VON BEHRING (1854–1917) spent some years in Koch's Institute, then became professor, first at Halle and later at Marburg.[1] His great achievement was his discovery, in 1890, of the principle of serum treatment, and of diphtheria antitoxin, which caused a spectacular fall in the death rate. The first patient to be treated by the new method was a child in Von Bergmann's clinic in Berlin, on Christmas night, 1891. Collaborating with von Behring was SHIBASABURO KITASATO (1852–1931), who worked under Koch for six years and then returned to his native Japan where he founded the Institute for Infectious Diseases, of which he became director in 1891. He discovered the bacillus of plague in 1894, a discovery which was also made independently at Hong Kong by the Swiss bacteriologist ALEXANDRE YERSIN (b. 1863). Von Behring and Kitasato together discovered another antitoxin which yielded remarkable results, that of tetanus. Ehrlich (p. 384) still further elaborated the antitoxin idea, and worked out a system for standardizing the dosage.

GEORG GAFFKY (1850–1918) was appointed successor to Koch, whom he had accompanied to Egypt and India on the German Cholera Commission. Gaffky was highly esteemed as a man and as a scientist. He made many contributions to bacteriology.

The successor of Gaffky was FRIEDRICH LOËFFLER (1852–1915), one of the greatest of bacteriologists and an excellent writer and teacher. Among his discoveries were the bacilli of diphtheria and of glanders ; he also devised new methods of staining and cultivating bacteria. Yet another of Koch's disciples was RICHARD PFEIFFER (1858–1945), professor at Breslau from 1909 to 1926. His discoveries were of great importance, including the influenza bacillus and micrococcus catarrhalis. It was another physician of Breslau ALBERT NEISSER (1855–1916), a dermatologist as well

[1] W. Bulloch, *The History of Bacteriology*, 1938, p. 261

as a bacteriologist, who discovered the gonococcus. The leprosy bacillus was first identified in Norway, where the disease was endemic, by ARMAUER HANSEN of Bergen (1841–1912), the leading authority on leprosy of his time.

The pneumococcus was the discovery of ALBERT FRAENKEL (1848–1916), a physician of Berlin who specialized in diseases of the chest.

Thus, in rapid succession, the causal organisms of many infectious diseases were discovered, and in many cases effective methods of treatment were devised.

In Britain, the new science of bacteriology was studied with energy and enthusiasm. Sir Almroth Wright, the pioneer of vaccine therapy and of anti-typhoid inoculation, and Sir William Boog Leishman, will be mentioned in the chapter on military medicine (Chapter XVIII).

Sir GERMAN SIMS WOODHEAD (1855–1921), Professor of Pathology at Cambridge, made many contributions to bacteriology, and was the founder and editor of the *Journal of Pathology and Bacteriology*.

Sir ALEXANDER OGSTON (1844–1929), while working at Aberdeen on the bacteriology of suppuration in 1882, first identified and named the staphylococcus, and differentiated it from the streptococcus.[1] Ogston became Professor of Surgery in the University of Aberdeen, and Senior Surgeon to Aberdeen Royal Infirmary. His considerable experience of military surgery is evident from his *Reminiscences of Three Campaigns*, 1919.

Many other British bacteriologists whose original work is familiar to every student are happily still with us.

In America one of the most eminent bacteriologists was THEOBALD SMITH (1859–1934), to whom we shall again refer in a later chapter (p. 391). He was noted especially for his work on Texas fever of cattle, anaphylaxis, and the differentiation of human from bovine tuberculosis.

WILLIAM HENRY WELCH (1850–1934) was another distinguished American bacteriologist, who studied for a time in Germany, and who occupied the Chair of Pathology at Johns Hopkins University, Baltimore, for thirty-four years, his colleague in the Chair of Medicine being William Osler.[2] In

[1] J. D. Comrie, *History of Scottish Medicine*, 2 vols., 1932, vol. ii. p. 555
[2] S. and J. F. Flexner, *William Henry Welch and the Heroic Age of American Medicine*, New York, 1941

1892 Welch discovered the bacillus of gas gangrene, *bacillus aerogenes capsulatus*, sometimes named *bacillus Welchii*. He was a man of wide culture, and an outstanding success as a teacher, his influence being felt throughout the United States. His keen interest in the history of medicine led him in later life to relinquish his work in Pathology and Public Health in order to accept the post of Professor of Medical History. The William H. Welch Library and Institute of Medical History at Baltimore is a fitting memorial of this great teacher and scholar (p. 403).

Others who enriched the science of bacteriology might be mentioned ; it may suffice to name two who were victims of the diseases they studied. HOWARD TAYLOR RICKETTS (1871–1910), who died of typhus fever in Mexico City, had shown that this disease was caused by minute organisms which were neither bacilli nor protozoa.[1] This group, now known as Rickettsia infections, include trench fever (conveyed by the louse), Japan river fever (by the harvest mite), and Rocky Mountain fever (by a tick). DANIEL CARRION (1850–85) died at Lima after self-inoculation with verruga peruana.[2]

Some of the other workers who devoted their lives to the conquest of tropical diseases will be mentioned in Chapter XVIII.

[1] H. Zinsser, *Rats, Lice, and History*, 1935, p. 224
[2] A. A. Moll, *Aesculapius in Latin America*, Philadelphia, 1944, p. 443

BOOKS FOR FURTHER READING

BALLINGALL, G. *Life of John Barclay*, 1827
BELL, Lady. Editor of *Letters of Sir Charles Bell*, 1870
BERNARD, CLAUDE. *An Introduction to the Study of Experimental Medicine*, 1865. English translation by H. C. Greene, New York, 1927
BULLOCH, W. *The History of Bacteriology*, 1938
FLEXNER, S. and J. F. *William Henry Welch and the Heroic Age of American Medicine*, New York, 1941
FOSTER, Sir M. *Claude Bernard*, 1899
HALL, CHARLOTTE. *Life of Marshall Hall*, 1861
KOENIGSBERGER, L. *Hermann von Helmholtz*. English translation by F. R. Welby, 1906
LONSDALE, H. *The Life of Dr. Robert Knox*, 1870
METCHNIKOFF, OLGA. *Life of Elie Metchnikoff, 1845–1916*, 1921
ROUGHEAD, W. *The Trial of Burke and Hare*, 1921
STIRLING, W. *Some Apostles of Physiology*, 1902
VALLERY-RADOT, R. *The Life of Pasteur*, 2 vols. 1902
ZINSSER, H. *Rats, Lice, and History*, 1935

CHAPTER XV

XIX-CENTURY CLINICIANS

HAVING noted the advances in the scientific basis of medicine and surgery during the nineteenth century, let us now turn to the more purely clinical aspect, and study the trend of medical thought and practice as exemplified in the lives and work of some of the great leaders.

It is difficult to choose from the galaxy of masters of that time a select few in whose lives the history may be unfolded. Many worthy names are omitted in order that this outline may fulfil its mission as a history of medicine, rather than a mere collection of medical biographies.

London and Edinburgh Physicians

Early in the century there appeared a number of physicians whose names became attached to various diseases and symptoms, names therefore still familiar. One of the best known for that reason, and certainly the most renowned physician of his time, was RICHARD BRIGHT (1789–1858).[1] The son of a wealthy banker of Bristol, he received his medical education at Edinburgh, graduating M.D. in 1813. While still a student he and his friend Holland, afterwards Sir Henry Holland, accompanied Sir George Mackenzie on an expedition to Iceland.[2] Bright drew the illustrations for Mackenzie's *Travels in Iceland*. He also contributed the notes on Botany and Zoology. On his return he studied for a time at Guy's Hospital before completing the medical course in Edinburgh. After graduation he spent some months on the Continent, a journey which led to the publication of his *Travels through Lower Hungary*, a well-written and beautifully illustrated work, which contains much information and some original observations on geology. Bright settled in London, practising in Bloomsbury Square, and becoming Assistant Physician to Guy's

[1] W. S. Thayer, " Richard Bright," *Guy's Hospital Reports*, 1927, vol. lxxvii. p. 253 ; B. Chance, " Dr. Richard Bright," *Ann. Med. Hist.*, 1927, vol. ix. p. 332
[2] B. Chance, " Richard Bright, Traveller and Artist," *Bull. Hist. Med.*, 1940, vol. viii. p. 909 ; Sir H. Holland, *Recollections of Past Life*, 1872

Hospital in 1820, and Physician four years later.[1] He applied himself to the work with great energy, regularly spending six hours a day at the hospital during many years.

Bright was the first to point out that dropsy, with albuminous urine, was the result of kidney disease. His observations appeared in the first volume of his well-known *Reports of Medical Cases Selected with a View of Illustrating the Symptoms and Cure of Disease by a Reference to Morbid Anatomy* (1827). Twenty-three cases of renal disease, with dropsy and albuminuria, are described in detail, together with post-mortem reports of all the fatal cases.[2] The reports are illustrated by many coloured plates of high artistic merit. He was an able writer, his aim being " to connect accurate and faithful observation after death with symptoms displayed during life " (Plate LIX). A second volume of *Reports* (1831) dealt mainly with nervous diseases. In 1842 two wards were set aside for his renal cases in Guy's Hospital, so that an intensive investigation might be made over a six months' period. By this means Bright's original observations were confirmed and new facts were revealed. He was not content to study only one disease. Other papers from his pen related to abdominal tumours, to jaundice, and to glycosuria, and he collaborated with Addison in lecturing on materia medica and in producing a work on *The Elements of the Practice of Medicine* (Vol. I, 1839), which unfortunately was never completed. Bright was an amiable and kindly man and was in high repute as a consultant. He died at the age of sixty-nine, not from " his own disease," as is sometimes stated, but from aortic valvular disease of the heart.

A distinguished contemporary of Richard Bright was his colleague on the staff of Guy's Hospital, Thomas Addison (1793–1860), who also gave his name to a disease.[3] Although Addison was born near Newcastle-on-Tyne, he was wont to consider himself a Cumberland man, as his family had long been associated with Lanercost, near Carlisle, and his father still owned Banks House, near the fine old Priory of Lanercost. Addison spent many a holiday at Lanercost, and there he lies buried in the parish churchyard. He graduated M.D. at Edinburgh in 1815, and shortly afterwards commenced practice in Hatton Garden, London,

[1] Sir W. Hale-White, *Great Doctors of the Nineteenth Century*, 1935, p. 63
[2] R. H. Major, *Classic Descriptions of Disease*, 1932, p. 493
[3] Sir W. Hale-White, " Thomas Addison, M.D.," *Guy's Hosp. Rep.*, 1926, vol. lxxvi. p. 253

a bold step for an unknown doctor from the North. Details of his early life are scanty, but his ability was soon recognized, and in 1824 he became Assistant Physician at Guy's Hospital, and in due course Physician.[1] For about forty years he was the leading teacher at Guy's, where he was revered by the students despite his rather haughty and reserved manner. His language was well chosen, his delivery eloquent and dogmatic. Owing to his retiring nature, however, he was hardly known in his day outside his own circle. The textbook of medicine which he wrote along with Bright contained a good clinical account of " Inflammation of the Appendix Vermiformis," many years before appendicitis became a household word.

Addison devoted much attention to diseases of the chest. He greatly admired the work of Laënnec, although he differed from him in certain matters. In his paper, *On the Pathology of Phthisis* (1845), he expressed the opinion that most of the changes seen in the tuberculous lung were the result of pneumonic inflammation. While it is now admitted that this statement is not entirely correct, the conception of two processes at work was in itself a great advance.

In 1849 Addison gave the first description of " a remarkable form of anaemia." In the fatal cases he found a diseased condition of the suprarenal capsules. Continuing his researches, he collected cases, and eventually, in 1855, published his little quarto of forty pages, *On the Constitutional and Local Effects of Disease of the Suprarenal Capsules.* He distinguished two separate maladies : one, the anaemia which became generally known as " pernicious," in which no organic lesion could be discovered ; the other, an anaemia associated with bronzed skin and with diseased suprarenal capsules. The latter has since been called Addison's Disease.

Addison did not acquire a large practice, and his fame was mainly posthumous. Yet he was one of the greatest physicians of the early part of last century.

In the latter part of the century, the leading London physician was Sir WILLIAM WITHEY GULL (1816–90).[2] He exemplified all that was best in clinical medicine, combining a strong personality with sound wisdom. Born near Colchester, he was only ten years

---

[1] S. Wilks and G. T. Bettany, *A Biographical History of Guy's Hospital*, 1892, p. 221
[2] T. D. Acland, *Memoir and Writings of Sir William Gull*, Sydenham Society, 1896 ; Sir W. Hale-White, *Great Doctors of the Nineteenth Century*, 1935, p. 208

old when his father died of cholera, leaving a widow and six children of whom William was the youngest. In later life Sir William Gull attributed his success to the training given to him by his mother, who instilled into her children habits of industry and perseverance. Young Gull showed ability at school, taught himself Greek and was then encouraged by the schoolmaster to teach others, for, said he, " Directly you begin to teach you will begin to learn." For a time William cherished a desire to go to sea, but at the age of thirteen he fortunately met Mr. Harrison, Treasurer of Guy's Hospital, who had already befriended Addison and Bright, and who was visiting his nephew, the rector of the parish in which the Gulls lived. Mr. Harrison invited William Gull to come to Guy's Hospital as an apprentice, offering him accommodation and a small salary. " I can help you if you will help yourself," was his wise remark. William acted upon the advice and took his M.B. degree with honours a few years later (1841).[1] He was now appointed medical tutor, and he taught materia medica and natural philosophy, for there was as yet no strict specialization. He continued to live at Guy's until his marriage in 1848. That year he joined the hospital staff, acting first as Assistant Physician, then as Physician until his retirement twenty years later. Gull soon acquired an enormous practice, and although money-making was not one of his ambitions, he left a large fortune. A baronetcy was conferred on him after his attendance on the Prince of Wales (King Edward VII), who was seriously ill from typhoid fever at Sandringham in 1871. One who knew Sir William Gull has described " his striking presence, his minute examination of every case, and the few slowly uttered words in which he delivered his judgment, often with encouragement and never without sympathy. His manner was the same in a hospital ward as in a palace." Nothing which concerned the well-being of the patient was too minute for his attention. The patient was never a case or a disease to him. " Not a typhoid fever but a typhoid man." Of a hysterical lady, he said " There is nothing really wrong ; Mrs. X. is herself multiplied by four."

Among his other aphorisms were the following : " *Cannot* is a word for the idle and self-satisfied ; it is inadmissible in science." " The young, the aged, and the sick must always be helped."

[1] S. Wilks and G. T. Bettany, *A Biographical History of Guy's Hospital*, 1892, p. 261

" However clever you are, you are sure to overlook phthisis, syphilis, and itch."

Sir William Gull used few drugs, and often none at all. One of his papers dealt with *Acute Rheumatism treated by Mint Water*, that is to say, the disease had been allowed to run a natural course. In reality his treatment was most thorough and his directions explicit. His prescriptions were always simple, and he distrusted polypharmacy. He took a deep interest in the training of nurses. " Nursing," he said, " sometimes a trade, sometimes a profession, ought to be a religion." (See Supplement, page 461.)

Although Gull wrote little, he made many original observations, noting that locomotor ataxia was a lesion of posterior spinal columns, describing myxoedema, differentiating varieties of Bright's disease, and advising male fern in the treatment of tapeworm. He was a good linguist, a lover of poetry, and a keen observer of Nature. Even the habits of the London sparrows attracted the attention of this great-hearted man.

Closely associated with Sir William Gull was Sir SAMUEL WILKS (1824–1911), a charming and kindly man and an excellent writer,[1] while his chief rival was his friend Sir WILLIAM JENNER (1815–98), who also made a fortune by practice, and whose fame lies chiefly in his contribution to the knowledge of fevers.

Among the great clinicians of more recent times were Sir WILLIAM OSLER, whose work is described in a later chapter (p. 408), Sir CLIFFORD ALLBUTT (p. 407), and many others who elected to specialize in one of the many branches of clinical medicine which were beginning to appear.

In Edinburgh, clinical medicine was upheld by ANDREW DUNCAN, whose work has been already noted (p. 226) and by JOHN HUGHES BENNETT (p. 278). There was also that eminent man, Sir ROBERT CHRISTISON (1797–1882), the son of the Professor of Latin, who, after graduating in Edinburgh, studied toxicology under Orfila of Paris, and on his return was appointed Professor of Medical Jurisprudence (1822).[2] His famous *Treatise on Poisons* enhanced his reputation, and he excelled as an expert witness, being called by the Crown on many occasions. He made valuable contributions to pharmacology, and for many years he was the leading consulting physician in Scotland.

[1] Sir S. Wilks, *Biographical Reminiscences*, 1911
[2] *Life of Sir Robert Christison*, ed. by one of his sons, 2 vols., Edinburgh, 1885

Clinical Medicine in Dublin, Paris, and Vienna

The two most eminent physicians of the Irish Medical School were Robert Graves and William Stokes. Both were the sons of Dublin professors, and both graduated in medicine at Edinburgh.[1]

ROBERT GRAVES (1796–1853), whose father was Professor of Divinity at Trinity College, Dublin, spent several years in post-graduate study on the Continent. In Italy he enjoyed the friend-ship of J. M. W. Turner, the famous painter ; and in Austria he had the unpleasant experience of being imprisoned as a German spy, so complete was his mastery of that language. On returning to Dublin he was elected Physician to Meath Hospital, where he introduced the system of clinical instruction which had impressed him on the Continent, namely, that of assigning patients to the charge of senior students, who were responsible to the physician, and who reaped the benefit of his criticism and advice. Graves was subsequently appointed Professor of the Institutes of Medicine (Physiology). He contributed a number of papers to the *Dublin Journal of Medical Science*, of which he was editor, but his chief literary work was his *Clinical Lectures on the Practice of Medicine* (1843). The book had a deservedly high reputation. It was translated into French, with an introduction by Trousseau, who regarded Graves as a " perfect clinical teacher." The name of Graves is sometimes associated with exophthalmic goitre, which he so clearly described. One of his reforms was the elimination of starvation, purgation, and bleeding from the treatment of fevers. Instead, Graves advised that plenty of good food be given : he even suggested as an epitaph for himself the words, " He fed fevers." " Nothing," writes Sir William Hale-White, " has done more to improve the treatment of disease than Graves's *Clinical Lectures*."

Graves's colleague on the staff of Meath Hospital and his life-long friend was WILLIAM STOKES (1804–78).[2] He was the son of Whitley Stokes, Professor of Medicine at Trinity College, and a well-known member of Dublin society. William took his degree in Edinburgh in 1825, and that year, whilst still only twenty-one years old, he published a small treatise on the stethoscope, in-

[1] G. T. Bettany, *Eminent Doctors*, 2 vols., 1885, vol. ii. p. 202
[2] Sir W. Stokes (his son), *William Stokes, his Life and Work* (Masters of Medicine), 1898 ; T. G. Moorhead, " William Stokes, 1804–78," *Med. Press and Circ.*, 1935, vol. 191, p. 130

spired by a study of Laënnec's book, which had appeared six years earlier. He succeeded his father as Physician to Meath Hospital, and he closely collaborated with Graves in the new system of clinical instruction, which brought fame to the school and supplanted the old fetish of " walking the hospital."

Stokes, like Graves, was a great teacher and a hard worker. He had a large practice, and he rendered valuable service during the epidemics of cholera and typhus which devastated Ireland at the time. His book on *The Diagnosis and Treatment of Diseases of the Chest* appeared in 1837, and added greatly to his reputation as a clinician. A companion volume on *Diseases of the Heart and Aorta* appeared some years later. In 1845 he was appointed Regius Professor of Medicine in Dublin University, a post which he held up to the time of his death. Stokes noted, as his experience increased, that too much stress was laid upon physical signs, especially in valvular disease of the heart, and that the condition of the heart muscle was of more importance than the state of the valves, a fact emphasized by Sir James Mackenzie fifty years later. Along with JOHN CHEYNE, a Scotsman practising in Dublin, Stokes described the type of breathing known as " Cheyne-Stokes respiration," and noted its serious import. He also recorded, along with ROBERT ADAMS, a number of cases of slow pulse, accompanied by syncopial attacks—the " Stokes-Adams syndrome." [1]

Stokes was a man of wide learning and of many interests. He inaugurated the first British Diploma in Public Health, and he greatly improved the status of the medical profession in Ireland. A lover of art and letters, he had many friends, and his house was a Mecca for distinguished visitors to Dublin.

Another eminent Irish physician of slightly later date was Sir DOMINIC CORRIGAN (1802–80).[2] After graduating in Edinburgh, Corrigan settled in his native Dublin, and soon acquired a leading position and a large practice. He is chiefly remembered for his work on aortic disease, which, he claimed, was the cause of angina pectoris. Trousseau, indeed, spoke of it as the " maladie de Corrigan." [3]

On the Continent Paris led the way in medicine during the first half of the century; then German medicine became prominent.

[1] R. H. Major, *Classic Descriptions of Disease*, 1932, p. 301 (" Stokes-Adams ")
[2] R. T. Williamson, " Sir Dominic Corrigan," *Ann. Med. Hist.*, 1925, vol. vii. p. 354
[3] R. H. Major, *Classic Descriptions of Disease*, 1932, p. 323 (" Corrigan ")

Reference has already been made to the immortal work of Laënnec (p. 258). Another Breton physician of the time who practised in Paris, though a man of much less account in medical history than Laënnec, was FRANÇOIS JOSEPH VICTOR BROUSSAIS (1772–1838).[1] Broussais, who had been a sergeant and then a surgeon in Napoleon's army, appears to have adopted military tactics in his civilian medical practice, as he was a sort of Paracelsus of France, vigorous and dictatorial, who affirmed that there were no diseases, only symptoms, that gastro-enteritis caused most of the troubles of humanity, that the healing power of Nature did not exist, and that starvation and the application of leeches would cure every ill.[2] He caused a boom in the leech industry ; it is said that forty million leeches were imported into France in 1833. Broussais has been called " the most sanguinary physician in history."

A much sounder clinician was PIERRE CHARLES ALEXANDRE LOUIS (1787–1872), well known for his observation of phthisis, based upon a study of about two thousand cases and many post-mortems.[3] He noted the predilection of the disease for the apex of the lung. He made a similar extensive study of typhoid fever, and he proved the value of statistics in medical work. As a teacher, Louis was held in high esteem, especially by his numerous American pupils.[4]

Another distinguished French clinician was PIERRE BRETON-NEAU (1778–1862) of Tours, who described diphtheria, and was the first to use that name.[5] He also introduced tracheotomy for laryngeal diphtheria (1825).

One of Bretonneau's pupils was ARMAND TROUSSEAU (1801–67), who became an eminent physician of Paris, where he was the first to aspirate the pleural cavity.[6] The procedure was improved by his pupil, GEORGES DIEULAFOY (1839–1911), an excellent physician and a gifted teacher, affectionately known as " le beau

---

[1] J. D. Rolleston, "F. J. V. Broussais, 1772–1838 : His Life and Doctrines," *Proc. Roy. Soc. Med.*, 1939, vol. xxxii. p. 405
[2] F. H. Garrison, *History of Medicine*, 3rd ed., 1924, p. 426
[3] W. R. Steiner, " Dr. Pierre-Charles-Alexandre Louis," *Ann. Med. Hist.*, 1940, 3rd Ser., vol. ii. p. 451
[4] W. Osler, " The Influence of Louis on American Medicine," *Johns Hopk. Hosp. Bull.*, 1897, Nos. 77 and 78
[5] J. D. Rolleston, "Bretonneau : His Life and Work," *Proc. Roy. Soc. Med.* (Sect. Hist.), 1925, vol. xviii. p. 1
[6] A. H. Buck, *The Dawn of Modern Medicine*, 1920, p. 265 ; F. H. Garrison, " Armand Trousseau," *Internat. Clinics*, 1916, p. 284

Dieulafoy." Dieulafoy perfected the aspirator which Trousseau had invented.

The leading exponent of clinical medicine in Vienna was JOSEPH SKODA (1805–81).[1] The son of a blacksmith of Pilsen, Bohemia, his genius was recognized by the wife of a wealthy manufacturer, who offered to assist him if he came to study medicine in Vienna. Skoda accepted the offer, walked all the way to Vienna, a six days' journey, and proved in every way worthy of the confidence of his benefactress. After graduation he devoted his attention to diseases of the chest, and wrote an important work on auscultation and percussion, attempting to assign to each of the sounds its musical pitch. He did much to lay the foundations of modern physical diagnosis, although he made no contribution to therapeutics.[2] He was the first to lecture in German in the Vienna School.

In Germany one of the soundest clinicians was CARL WUNDERLICH (1815–77), to whom we are indebted for the temperature chart which has been in regular use since his day.[3] Clinical thermometers were at that time almost a foot in length, and took twenty minutes to register the temperature. It was said of Wunderlich, then Professor of Medicine at Leipzig, that " he found fever a disease and left it a symptom."[4]

FRIEDRICH THEODOR VON FRERICHS (1819–85) was perhaps the leading exponent of clinical medicine in Germany in the latter part of the nineteenth century. An excellent lecturer and a sound diagnostician, he was professor at Breslau, and then at Berlin, where for many years he conducted a large practice. His chief interest was the biochemical aspect of medicine, to which he contributed original observations dealing with digestion, diseases of the liver, and diabetes. It was he who discovered leucin and tyrosin in the urine, and acute yellow atrophy of the liver.

Frerichs was succeeded at Berlin by ERNST VON LEYDEN (1832–1910), who carried on the high tradition as a clinical teacher in the Charité hospital. He also rendered useful public service by his advocacy of sanatorium treatment in tuberculosis.

Two other German clinicians of this fertile period, each with

[1] M. Neuburger, *British Medicine and the Vienna School*, 1943, p. 38
[2] R. H. Major, *Classic Descriptions of Disease*, 1932, p. 38
[3] H. E. Sigerist, *Great Doctors*, 1936, p. 520
[4] H. A. McGuigan, " Medical Thermometry," *Ann. Med. Hist.*, 1937, vol. ix. p. 148

an interest in neurology, although that branch of medicine had not then become differentiated, were Kussmaul and Nothnagel, both men of high culture and wide knowledge.

ADOLF KUSSMAUL (1822–1902), who eventually occupied the Chair at Strassburg, was the first to describe progressive bulbar paralysis and also diabetic coma. He contributed to our knowledge of disorders of speech, and made pioneer attempts in oesophagoscopy and gastroscopy.

HERMANN NOTHNAGEL (1841–1905), the leader of clinical medicine in Vienna, was highly respected by his colleagues and students as one of the most popular figures of the time. Like Von Leyden, whom he assisted for a time, he was interested in neurology, and contributed to the subject. His chief title to fame, from the literary standpoint, was his editorship of the comprehensive *Handbuch der speziellen Pathologie und Therapie*, in twenty-four volumes, which was completed in the year of his death and was translated into English.

Nothnagel died of angina pectoris, leaving a written record of his own painful sensations up to the very hour of his death.[1]

The trend towards specialism in clinical medicine, which became manifest about this time, will be noted in Chapter XIX.

Medical Pioneers in America

The foundation of the Medical School of Philadelphia in the eighteenth century has already been noted (p. 251). Among the graduates of that famous school were a number of men who did much to advance medicine. One of the greatest was DANIEL DRAKE (1785–1852),[2] who has been called " the most picturesque figure in American medicine " (Plate LX). Born in poverty, he rose by his own industry and ability to a position of eminence, although he never visited Europe. He led a roving life, practising in seven different localities, and thus showing how even the peripatetic physician can collect wisdom. The story of his early life is described in his *Pioneer Life in Kentucky*. He founded medical schools at Ohio and Cincinnati, and he edited the *Western Journal of Medical Science*.[3]

His most notable book dealt with *Principal Diseases of the*

[1] M. Neuburger, *Hermann Nothnagel*, Vienna, 1822, p. 352
[2] S. D. Gross, " Life of Daniel Drake," in *Lives of Eminent American Physicians and Surgeons of the Nineteenth Century*, Philadelphia, 1861, p. 614
[3] O. Juettner, *Daniel Drake and his Followers*, Cincinnati, 1909

Interior Valley of North America (1850–54), and was the result of thirty years of observation and travel. It is one of the greatest studies of the geography of disease. The conditions of life in the Mississippi Valley are described under the headings of climate, flora and fauna, diet, occupations, housing, etc. The second volume did not appear until after the author's death. It deals with the fevers and other prevalent diseases, arranged according to geographical distribution. Drake was a tall, handsome man, gentle and dignified in manner, and deservedly popular with his colleagues.

Exactly contemporary with Drake lived WILLIAM BEAUMONT (1785–1853),[1] an army surgeon who treated the Canadian Alexis St. Martin for gunshot wound of the stomach. The patient recovered with a large gastric fistula, which Beaumont recognized as providing a unique opportunity for the study of digestion. At considerable personal inconvenience and expense he followed his patient in order to complete his investigations on the rate of digestion of various foods and on the composition of the gastric juice.[2] His *Experiments and Observations on Gastric Juice and the Physiology of Digestion* (1833) recorded a fine piece of research in the face of unusual difficulties.

A Bold Ovariotomist

Another brilliant pioneer, this time in surgery, was EPHRAIM McDOWELL (1771–1830), a native of Virginia, who had studied under John Bell in Edinburgh, and who practised in the remote town of Danville, Kentucky [3] (Plate LX). In December 1809 he performed ovariotomy, a bold venture indeed under primitive conditions and before the days of antiseptics or anaesthetics. The patient was the wife of a farmer, Mrs. Jane Todd Crawford, and McDowell took her to his home at Danville, sixty miles journey on horseback from her log cabin for the operation. She made her own bed on the fifth day, returning home on the twenty-fifth day, and living for other thirty-two years. McDowell

[1] W. Osler, " A Backwoods Physiologist," in *An Alabama Student, and Other Essays*, 1908, p. 159 ; Jesse S. Meyer, *Life and Letters of Dr. William Beaumont*, St. Louis, 1912
[2] W. S. Miller, " William Beaumont, M.D. (1785–1853)," *Ann. Med. Hist.*, 1933, vol. v. p. 28 ; A. B. Luckhardt, " The Dr. William Beaumont Collection of the University of Chicago," *Bull. Hist. Med.*, 1939, vol. vii. p. 535
[3] S. D. Gross, " Life of Ephraim McDowell," in *Lives of Eminent American Physicians and Surgeons*, 1861, p. 207 ; A. Schachner, *Ephraim McDowell, " Father of Ovariotomy " and Founder of Abdominal Surgery*, Philadelphia, 1921

reported the case, with two others, in 1817. During his career he performed thirteen ovariotomies ; eight of the patients recovered. Although his celebrated operation on Mrs. Crawford was the first ovariotomy to be performed in America, and he deserves all praise for this and for his subsequent successes, priority of a century is often accorded to Robert Houston of Glasgow who, in 1701, undertook the removal of an enormous ovarian cyst, and dressed the abdominal wound with " a large napkin dipped in warm French brandy." The patient, Margaret Millar, survived in good health for thirteen years.[1] According to some authorities Houston's operation was not an ovariotomy, but the incision and drainage of a cyst. Nevertheless it was a bold procedure, worthy of record, and in no way detracting from the later work of McDowell.

In the latter part of the century JAMES MARION SIMS (1813–83) [2] did original work in gynaecology and acquired a high reputation, in Europe as well as in America, for his successful operative treatment of vesico-vaginal fistula.[3] Many women who would otherwise have been invalids were by this procedure restored to health.

America has produced many an eminent surgeon, but few more distinguished than VALENTINE MOTT (1785–1865), a pupil of Sir Astley Cooper, who excelled in arterial surgery.[4] He was the first to ligate the innominate artery for aneurysm, and he performed many other operations which were then considered to be daring feats of skill. To him the New York Medical School owes its foundation.

Of later date was SAMUEL DAVID GROSS (1805–84) of Philadelphia, a scholarly and versatile man and an able surgeon, who wrote on pathology, on surgery, and on the history of American medicine.[5]

The History of Anaesthesia

An account of early medical work in America inevitably leads one to recall the story of general anaesthesia, and the controversy which continued for years regarding the priority of its discovery.

---

[1] A. Duncan, *Memorials of the Faculty of Physicians and Surgeons of Glasgow*, Glasgow, 1896, p. 114
[2] J. Marion Sims, *The Story of My Life*, New York, 1889
[3] Chassar Moir, " J. Marion Sims and the Vesico-vaginal Fistula : Then and Now," *Brit. Med. Jour.*, 1940, vol. ii. p. 773
[4] Samuel D. Gross, *Memoir of Valentine Mott, M.D., LL.D.*, Philadelphia, 1868
[5] Samuel D. Gross, *Autobiography*, 1887

Various drugs, such as opium, mandragora, and cannabis indica, had been used to relieve pain since very early times, and various attempts had been made to render patients unconscious during surgical operations (p. 116). Mesmerism and hypnotism had been employed by Mesmer (p. 262) and his followers with uncertain results, as also had the production of syncope by compression of the carotid arteries, which is said to date from Assyrian times.

Sir HUMPHRY DAVY, in 1799, observed the intoxicating effect of nitrous oxide, or " laughing gas," as it came to be called, and he wrote that it " seemed capable of destroying pain and might probably be used with advantage in surgical operations." MICHAEL FARADAY, in 1815, noted that ether had a similar effect, and within a few years " ether frolics " became quite a popular amusement. In 1824 Dr. HENRY HICKMAN of Ludlow, Shropshire, published the results of some experiments on animals, alleging that unconsciousness and insensibility to pain could be produced by the inhalation of carbon dioxide gas, and he suggested that this might prove useful in surgery. No-one would listen to Hickman. He was regarded as a crank, and he died broken-hearted, it is said, at the age of twenty-nine.

The scene now shifts to America, where in 1842 a country practitioner named CRAWFORD LONG (1815–78) [1] of Jefferson, Georgia, had participated in " ether frolics," and had noted that bruises or minor injuries sustained at the time were unaccompanied by pain. He therefore administered ether to a boy, James Venable, and painlessly excised a tumour of the neck. Long used ether in other cases, but whether from lack of enterprise or failure to grasp its importance he did not publish his discovery until 1849.

Meanwhile, other pioneers had been at work, and their doings form an interesting if also an intricate story. It began at Hartford (Conn.) in 1844, during the visit of GARDNER COLTON, a lecturer on chemistry. Among his experiments was one with " laughing gas." HORACE WELLS (1815–48), [2] a local dentist, noticed that the victim who inhaled the gas injured his leg in his excitement, but felt no pain. Next day Wells requested

[1] H. H. Young, " Crawford W. Long, the Pioneer in Ether Anaesthesia," *Bull. Hist. Med.*, 1942, vol. xii. p. 191 (22 illustrations) ; F. L. Taylor, " Crawford Williamson Long," *Ann. Med. Hist.*, 1925, vol. vii. pp. 267, 394
[2] M. E. Soifer, " Historical Notes on Horace Wells," *Bull. Hist. Med.*, 1941, vol. ix. p. 101

Colton to administer the gas, while his friend Dr. Riggs extracted a molar tooth. As Wells regained consciousness he exclaimed, " A new era in tooth-pulling." After a further successful trial of nitrous oxide in his practice, Wells gave a public demonstration. Unfortunately this was not so satisfactory, and the failure not only discredited the drug, but ruined its discoverer, who eventually abandoned dentistry and became a picture dealer. He never recovered from his disappointment and eventually he took his own life.

It was not until 1869 that Colton re-introduced nitrous oxide as a dental anaesthetic. The following year, in London, Joseph Clover recommended it as a preliminary to ether anaesthesia.

To return to events in America, Horace Wells had a dental partner, WILLIAM THOMAS MORTON (1819–68) with whom he discussed the use of nitrous oxide. When the partnership was dissolved Morton removed to Boston, where he continued his experiments. Like Wells, he found nitrous oxide a capricious drug, and he next tried ether on the suggestion of Dr. CHARLES JACKSON. Being satisfied, by experiments on himself and then on a dental patient, Eben Frost, of the suitability of the drug, Morton persuaded a surgeon, JOHN COLLINS WARREN, to allow him to demonstrate the method to a number of medical men at Massachusetts General Hospital, on October 16, 1846. The operation appears to have involved an incision in the neck of a young man, Gilbert Abbott, and as it was painlessly made, Warren announced, " Gentlemen, this is no humbug." But there was trouble in store for Morton. He kept the nature of the drug secret, he coloured it and disguised the odour so as to elude discovery ; he even patented it, along with Jackson, under the name " Letheon." Morton was not a medical man, and he probably saw no harm in exploiting his discovery for the sake of gain. Such conduct, however, naturally aroused the antipathy of the medical profession, and the true nature of ether was soon revealed.

Now there arose " the great ether controversy." Ether was universally lauded ; the discoverer of " anaesthesia," the name proposed by Oliver Wendell Holmes, was regarded as worthy of the highest praise. But who was he ? Long, Morton, Jackson, and the relatives of Wells, now deceased, were all claimants for the 100,000 dollars offered to the inventor by U.S. Congress, who recollected that Jenner had been voted £30,000 by the British Government (p. 249). The argument continued for years, and the award was never made. In the public gardens of Boston there is a monument to commemorate " the discovery that the inhaling of ether causes insensibility to pain," but the name of the discoverer is not mentioned. Some writers have constructed a strong case in favour of Morton,[1] but it is now acknowledged that the strongest claim to the title is that of Crawford Long.

News of the discovery of anaesthesia now reached Europe. In Britain, the first major operation under ether was performed at University College Hospital, London, on December 21, 1846, by Robert Liston (p. 307), Peter Squire administering the anaesthetic.[2] Joseph Lister, then a student, was one of those who witnessed the operation—an amputation through the thigh. The patient was Frederick Churchill, a butler, aged thirty-six (Plate LXI).

Meantime the Professor of Midwifery in Edinburgh, JAMES YOUNG SIMPSON (1811–70), had been experimenting upon himself and his friends with a view to discovering a general anaesthetic.[3] He had tried ether, but had decided that it was unsuitable for use in midwifery. One evening the coterie of investigators tried chloroform, a substance which had been discovered by Guthrie, a New York chemist,[4] in 1831, also independently by Soubeiran[5] and by Liebig[6] at about the same time, and more recently described, prepared, and first named " chloroform " by J.-B. Dumas of Paris in 1835. Truly there is no lack of claimants for priority where anaesthetics are concerned, but none of those chemists dreamed that the substance would be of practical use. David Waldie, a chemist of Liverpool, had suggested the trial of chloroform to Professor Simpson,[7] and Messrs. Duncan, Flockhart and Co. of Edinburgh prepared a supply for him. On the evening in question the new drug rapidly took effect, and as Simpson recovered consciousness and saw his colleagues lying helpless under the table, he decided, " This is far stronger than

[1] H. J. Bigelow, *Surgical Anaesthesia, Addresses and other Papers*, Boston, 1900
[2] F. W. Cock, " The First Major Operation under Ether in England," *Amer. Jour. Surg.*, vol. xxix. July 1915, p. 98
[3] J. Duns, *Memoir of Sir James Y. Simpson, Bart.*, Edinburgh, 1873
[4] S. Guthrie, " New Mode of Preparing a Spirituous Solution of Chloric Ether," *Amer. Jour. Sci. and Arts*, New Haven, 1831–32, vol. xxi. p. 64, and vol. xxii. p. 105
[5] E. Soubeiran, " Recherches sur quelques combinaisons du chlore," *Ann. de Chimie*, 1831, vol. xlviii. p. 113
[6] J. von Liebig, " Uber die Verbindungen welche durch die Einwirkung des Chlors auf Alkohol, Aether, olbildenes Gas und Essiggeist entstehen," *Ann. d. Pharm.*, Heidelberg, 1832, Bd. i. p. 182
[7] A. J. O'Leary, " Who Was the Person Who Discovered Chloroform for Anaesthesia ; Was it Simpson or Waldie? " *Brit. Journ. of Anaesth.*, 1935, vol. xii. p. 41

PLATE LXI   THE FIRST USE OF ETHER ANAESTHESIA IN BRITAIN

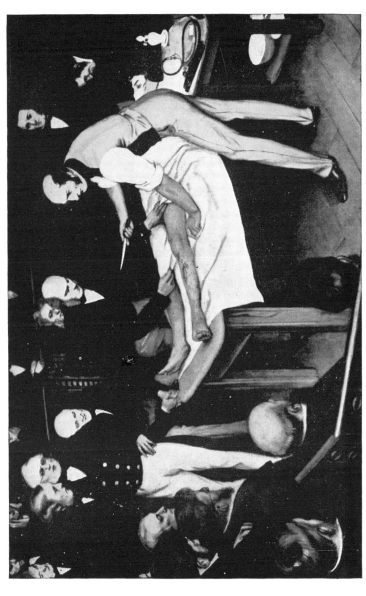

Peter Squire administering ether to a patient at University College Hospital in 1846, while Robert Liston performs an amputation. Young Joseph Lister, seen at left in profile, stands facing Liston (page 304)

PLATE LXII   A LECTURE ON SURGERY

James Syme lecturing on surgery, sketched by Alexander Peddie, one of his students, a lifelong friend of Dr. John Brown, author of *Rab and his Friends*. (From a sketch in the museum of the Royal College of Surgeons of Edinburgh (page 310)

ether." Simpson communicated his *Account of a New Anaesthetic Agent* to the Edinburgh Medico-Chirurgical Society on November 10, 1847, and five days later, at the Royal Infirmary, he administered chloroform to a "Highland boy who spoke only Gaelic," while Professor James Miller removed part of the radius for osteomyelitis. For the next fifty years chloroform was the anaesthetic of choice in Britain, and credit is due to Dr. JOHN SNOW (1813–58) for his researches on the best method of use, as described in his book, *On Chloroform and Other Anaesthetics*, 1858, now a very rare work.[1] Snow administered chloroform to Queen Victoria on two occasions. He was the first British anaesthetist, and during the last ten years of his short life he administered over four hundred anaesthetics each year. The ether inhaler he devised is surprisingly modern in design.[2] Snow was also a pioneer of preventive medicine (p. 388).

Another London anaesthetic specialist was JOSEPH CLOVER (1825–82), who advised the use of nitrous oxide and ether in sequence.

To return to our account of Sir J. Y. Simpson, he was not only the discoverer of chloroform anaesthesia. He was the most eminent obstetrician of his day, and, despite his enormous practice, found time to distinguish himself as an archaeologist, writing, among other works, papers on "Leper Hospitals in Scotland," and "Was the Roman Army provided with Medical Officers?"[3] The son of a baker in Bathgate, eighteen miles west of Edinburgh, he so distinguished himself that at the age of twenty-nine he was appointed to the Chair of Midwifery, which he held for thirty years. He was obliged to defend chloroform against its antagonists who opposed it, not on medical but on moral grounds, alleging that it would "rob God of the deep earnest cries" of women in labour. Simpson's energies were also directed to a method of haemostasis by the use of long needles, known as "acupressure," which incurred the displeasure of his surgical colleague, Syme, upon whose domain he had thus encroached. Simpson was created a baronet in 1866. He had a kindly manner and magnetic personality, which endeared him to his patients, and although he appeared to love

[1] Sir B. W. Richardson, *Disciples of Aesculapius*, vol. i. p. 227 ("Dr. John Snow")
[2] A. D. Marston, "The Centenary of the First Anaesthetic Use of Ether," *Proc. Roy. Soc. Med.*, 1941, vol. xxxv. p. 279
[3] J. Y. Simpson, *Archaeological Essays*, 2 vols., 1872, vol. ii. p. 197.

controversy, he usually proved that his was the correct view. The life-story of this versatile and forceful man is one of the most dramatic in medical history.

Although Simpson was among those who attacked the Listerian system of antisepsis, in many other respects he showed himself to be ahead of his time. He made notable advances in the technique of ovariotomy and in the use of obstetric forceps, which he improved, and he even prophesied the discovery of X-rays when he said that the day would come when "by electrical and other lights we may render the body sufficiently diaphanous for the inspection of the practised eye of the physician or surgeon." When he died, his family declined the offer of a grave in Westminster Abbey. A bust of him stands there, but his chief monument is the Simpson Maternity Hospital, now incorporated as part of the Edinburgh Royal Infirmary.

Care of the Unborn Child

JOHN WILLIAM BALLANTYNE (1861–1923), an Edinburgh obstetrician, later on the staff of the above-mentioned institution, in 1889 presented a thesis for the degree of M.D., "Some Anatomical and Pathological Conditions of the New-born Infant in their relation to Obstetrics," and was thus a pioneer in ante-natal pathology. He expanded the theme in his *Manual of Antenatal Pathology and Hygiene* (2 vols., 1902–1904). Ballantyne was the first to establish a clinic for the care of the expectant mother and unborn child. The need for such ante-natal supervision is now universally recognized.

BOOKS FOR FURTHER READING

ACTLAND, T. C. *Memoirs and writings of Sir William Gull*, 1896
DUNS, J. *Memoirs of Sir James Y. Simpson, Bart.*, Edinburgh, 1873
GORDON, H. J. *Sir James Young Simpson*, 1897
GROSS S. D. *Lives of Eminent American Physicians and Surgeons of the Nineteenth Century*, Philadelphia, 1861 ; *Autobiography*, 2 vols., Philadelphia, 1887
HOLLAND, Sir H. *Recollections of Past Life*, 1872
MAJOR, R. H. *Classic Descriptions of Disease*, 1932
PAWLING J. R. *Dr. Samuel Guthrie, Discoverer of Chloroform*, New York, 1947
SIMS, J. MARION. *The Story of My Life*, New York, 1889
STOKES, Sir W. *William Stokes : His Life and Work*, 1898
WILKS, S. *Biographical Reminiscences*, 1911
WILKS, S., and BETTANY, G. T. *A Biographical History of Guy's Hospital*, 1892

Chapter XVI

EARLY XIX-CENTURY SURGERY

EVERY other medical discovery of the nineteenth century is overshadowed by that of Lister, who by his introduction of the antiseptic method completely revolutionized the practice of surgery. By a fortunate coincidence Lister's discovery was made only a few years after the discovery of anaesthesia, and the benefit to humanity which followed the introduction of those two methods has been truly incalculable.

In order to throw into relief the vast change wrought by the antiseptic system, let us examine the methods of a few of the surgeons who immediately preceded the time of Lister. These were the days in which hospital gangrene assumed epidemic proportions, and sepsis was an inevitable sequence of operations. Compound fractures were treated by amputation, with a mortality of at least twenty-five per cent., while the surgeon wore an old blood-stained coat with a bunch of silk ligatures threaded through one of the buttonholes, ready for use. During the slow process of healing, a zinc tray contained the " laudable " pus, which dripped from the wound. The stench of the surgical wards, perhaps the least of the evils, may be readily imagined.

Small wonder, then, that a considerable degree of heroism was demanded from the unfortunate patient who, having endured the tortures of operation without anaesthesia, was still obliged to face the pains and dangers of a septic wound. As for the surgeon, he required not only " the eye of an eagle, the strength of a giant, and the hand of a lady," but also a degree of dexterity and agility with which few men are favoured.

ROBERT LISTON (1794–1847) [1] had all the attributes of a great surgeon. He was a tall, powerful man, with a commanding presence, an uncertain temper, a gift of satire, and kind to his patients, rich and poor, and his heart was in his work. His dexterity as an operator has probably never been surpassed. We have already noted (p. 304) that he was the first in Britain to employ ether anaesthesia, when at University College Hospital, London. He told the spectators that " this Yankee dodge beats mesmerism hollow."

[1] A. Miles, *The Edinburgh School of Surgery before Lister*, 1918, p. 146

Liston spent his early years in Edinburgh. His father, a country minister in West Lothian, dissuaded him from the sea-faring career which was his first fancy, and bestowed great care upon his education. As assistant to John Barclay (p. 269) the anatomist, he laid a sound foundation for his surgical career.[1] Various tales are told of his escapades as a " resurrectionist " in those days when anatomical material was scarce. He might well have been the original " Dr. Macfarlane " of R. L. Stevenson's *The Body Snatcher*. A quarrel with Barclay led him in 1818 to undertake the teaching of anatomy for himself, assisted by James Syme, his junior by only a few years. When Liston devoted his attention entirely to surgery five years later, Syme took charge of the class which had been so successful. Close friendship and co-operation then existed between Liston and Syme.[2] They assisted each other in teaching and in operating for some years. Then relations became strained and eventually there was a complete rupture. The co-operation in teaching and in practice came to an end. In 1833 the quarrel grew more bitter, and the friends of each surgeon joined in the polemics when both applied for the Professorship of Clinical Surgery, to which Syme was appointed. A reconciliation eventually took place, and Liston, shortly before his death, visited Syme in Edinburgh.

In the early years of his surgical practice Liston performed many operations in the homes of his patients. His list included the ligation of large vessels, amputations, lithotomy—which " should not occupy more than two or three minutes at most "— and the removal of a tumour of the scrotum, weighing forty-four pounds, a feat which added greatly to Liston's reputation. He treated and cured many cases which had been discharged from the Royal Infirmary as incurable, and he was even accused of diverting Infirmary patients into his own clientele. This alleged conduct led the managers, in 1822, to pass a resolution pro-hibiting Liston from entering the Infirmary " at any time, and on any pretence whatever." Although he completely exonerated himself in an open letter to the Lord Provost, the unfortunate incident delayed his appointment to the staff for other five years, during which he steadily worked and overcame the opposition of his contemporaries.

At last, in 1827, a vacancy occurred to which he was duly

[1] G. T. Bettany, *Eminent Doctors*, 2 vols., 1885, vol. ii. p. 24
[2] J. D. Comrie, *History of Scottish Medicine*, 2 vols., 1932, vol. ii. p. 593

appointed. Liston's genius lay in his operative skill rather than in any literary ability, although he published a number of papers and a textbook of surgery. Liston remained a surgeon to the Royal Infirmary after Syme had been appointed professor, but he was a disappointed man. It was natural, therefore, that he should accept the Chair of Surgery at University College, London, when it was unexpectedly offered to him in 1835. In London he was well received, soon acquired a large practice, and became eminent as a teacher. Nevertheless, he found time to indulge his favourite sports of yachting and hunting. He died suddenly at the age of fifty-three of aortic aneurysm, which was ruptured, it is said, by a blow from the boom of his yacht.

Even more distinguished in the world of surgery was JAMES SYME (1799-1870).[1] On the death of Liston in London Syme was appointed to his chair at University College, but finding the conditions unsatisfactory he resigned and returned to Edinburgh within six months, where he was reinstated in his former position, which had not been filled. Apart from this brief and unsuccessful venture in London, Syme remained in Edinburgh throughout his strenuous career, and the facts that he was born in Princes Street, that his father was a Writer to the Signet, and that he attended the High School, made him " essentially an Edinburgh type of man." [2] As a boy he was not a sportsman like Liston, but loved to spend his spare time in studying botany and chemistry. Indeed at the age of sixteen he discovered a method of waterproofing cloth, which was subsequently adopted and patented by a Glasgow manufacturer named Macintosh. As a medical student Syme was a disciple of Barclay and a close associate of Liston, commencing his career, as we have noted (p. 308), by teaching anatomy and practising surgery along with Liston. While waiting for practice he visited the Continent on two occasions in order to study surgery at the leading hospitals of France and Germany. Miles tells us that, while in Paris with his friend Sharpey (p. 277) Syme presented Dupuytren (p. 316) with a pair of " Liston's " bone-cutting forceps, that indispensible instrument which is still in daily use in many hospitals. Syme had a clear and concise literary style. Dr. John Brown said of him that " he never wasted

[1] A. Miles, *The Edinburgh School of Surgery before Lister*, 1918, p. 174; C. H. Creswell, *The Royal College of Surgeons of Edinburgh, 1505-1905*, Edinburgh, 1926, p. 250
[2] R. Paterson, *A Memorial of the Life of James Syme*, Edinburgh, 1874

a word, or a drop of ink, or a drop of blood." [1] His treatise, *On the Excision of Diseased Joints* was a plea for the conservative treatment of tuberculous joints at a time when the routine remedy was amputation. The textbook which he entitled *Principles of Surgery* (1831) was very popular and passed through five editions. Like Liston, Syme was accustomed to operate in private houses, as he had as yet no hospital appointment. With Liston's aid, he successfully performed amputation at the hip joint, an operation never before attempted in Scotland. He also removed, with success, an enormous sarcoma of the lower jaw, fifteen inches in circumference, which several other surgeons had regarded as inoperable. In 1829, being then thirty years of age, he applied for a vacancy on the surgical staff of the Royal Infirmary. Liston had been appointed in 1827, and the managers, viewing with disapproval the feud between the two surgeons, declined to appoint Syme. Further, the opposition of the Liston faction accounted for Syme's failure to secure the Chair of Surgery, to which his less eminent colleague, JOHN LIZARS (1794–1860), was appointed.

James Syme, however, was undaunted by his failure. He knew that he had ability, and his services were greatly in demand. All that he required was a hospital, and having knocked in vain at the door of the Royal Infirmary, he determined to establish a hospital of his own. He secured a large house and refitted it at his own expense, assisted to some extent by public contributions and the fees of students. There he continued to teach, to practise, and to develop those improvements in surgery with which the name of Syme is still associated. Minto House was opened on May 8, 1829. One of the most famous operations performed there by Syme was that of removal of the breast, immortalized by Dr. John Brown, Syme's clinical clerk, in that poignant sketch, " Rab and his Friends." [2]

Four years later Professor Russell, the veteran occupant of the Chair of Clinical Surgery, decided to retire, having reached the age of eighty-one. He stipulated, however, that his successor should pay him an annuity of £300. Liston declined to consider such a bargain. Syme, after open and honourable negotiation, agreed to it, and was appointed. The appointment was a great success, and during the next forty odd years Syme was one of

[1] J. Brown, *Horae Subsecivae*, 3 vols., 1882, vol. i. p. 360
[2] *Ibid.*, vol. ii. p. 363

the foremost surgeons of Europe. Despite his unfortunate tendency towards controversy, he must be regarded as one of the chief architects of surgery. He died in 1870 at his lovely house of Millbank, now part of the Astley Ainslie Institution, where his glass-houses and some of his fruit trees may still be seen, although the house has been replaced by a modern structure. The brilliant work of his famous son-in-law was just beginning to yield the first results. " The passing of Syme," writes Mr. Miles, " marked the close of a brilliant period in the history of surgery ; the advent of Joseph Lister opened one still more splendid." [1]

Three Great London Surgeons

Another Scottish surgeon may now be mentioned because his work illustrates the trend of the surgery of the time towards conservatism, and also because he forms a link between the Edinburgh School and that of London. Sir WILLIAM FERGUSSON (1808–77), born at Prestonpans and educated at Edinburgh, was appointed Professor of Surgery at King's College Hospital at the age of thirty-two, and became the most eminent surgeon in London.[2] As demonstrator to Dr. Knox, he had been an enthusiastic anatomist. In 1839 he succeeded Liston as surgeon to the Royal Infirmary, and in the following year he accepted the Chair in London, which had been offered to him at the suggestion of Sir Astley Cooper. Fergusson strongly supported Syme in his advocacy of excision of joints as opposed to amputation. He would take endless trouble to save a limb, and deemed it " a grand thing when even the tip of a thumb could be saved." He originated an operation for hare-lip which met with great success in his hands. Although he excelled in lithotomy, he preferred to crush the stone, devising his own lithotrite for the purpose, and various other instruments which are still employed in surgery. A tall handsome man, he was quiet and unassuming, kindly, and generous. These qualities naturally increased his popularity, while his skill and dexterity as an operator contributed to his success in practice. He was appointed surgeon to the Queen and to the Prince Consort, a baronetcy was conferred on him in 1866, and he became President of the Royal College of Surgeons

[1] A. Miles, *The Edinburgh School of Surgery before Lister*, 1918, p. 211
[2] G. T. Bettany, *Eminent Doctors*, 2 vols., 1885, vol. ii. p. 71

of England in 1870. His chief literary work was his *System of Practical Surgery* (1842). One of his contemporaries, Sir James Paget, called Fergusson " the greatest practical surgeon of our time."

To Paget now let us turn, and to yet another great surgeon of slightly earlier date, Sir Benjamin Brodie. Those eminent men —Fergusson, Paget, and Brodie—represent all that was best in London surgery just before the time of Lister.

Sir BENJAMIN COLLINS BRODIE (1783–1862) stands first in the chronological order.[1] From the brief autobiography of this eminent surgeon we learn that his grandfather came to London from Banffshire as a Jacobite refugee ; that his father, who was rector of Winterslow, Wilts., impressed upon him and his brothers " that he would do his utmost to give us a good education, but that he could do nothing more." All three sons did well, but Benjamin surpassed the others. He tells us how he came to London, thirteen hours by coach from Salisbury, how he attended Abernethy's lectures, how he was apprenticed to an apothecary whose stock-in-trade consisted of five large bottles of " Misturae," how he was befriended by Dr. Baillie and Sir Joseph Banks, how he assisted and eventually succeeded Sir Everard Home as surgeon to St. George's Hospital, and how he fell heir to much of the surgical practice of Sir Astley Cooper. Brodie led a very strenuous life, and his versatility expressed itself in four directions—as physiologist, as surgeon, as philosopher, and as administrator. In his younger days he distinguished himself as an experimental physiologist when he published papers on animal heat, on the nervous control of the heart's action, and on vegetable poisons. His surgical work showed the tendency towards conservatism which was at that time manifest. One can easily understand how a surgeon whose tastes were aesthetic shrank from the mutilating operations and from the septic horrors which followed. Brodie's chief surgical work was, *On the Diseases of the Joints* (1819), which was a valuable contribution to a difficult subject. That he had an enormous practice is obvious from the fact that for some years it yielded him £10,000 a year, and mainly from guinea fees. For years he took no holiday, and he paid his first visit to the Continent at the age of fifty-four. No doubt he regretted the delay, but it arose from his industrious habits and his devotion to duty rather than from any desire to make money. " Let it never be

[1] Timothy Holmes, *Sir Benjamin Collins Brodie* (Masters of Medicine), 1898

forgotten," he writes, " that it [money] forms but a part, and a small part, of professional success."

His contribution to philosophy, undertaken in later years, was as noteworthy as his physiological and surgical work. The *Psychological Inquiries* are not intended to supply a complete system of philosophy, but to show, first, that man's problem cannot be solved " by reference to only one department of knowledge," and secondly, " how to a great extent we can improve our present faculties." The facts he discusses are now matters of common knowledge, but Brodie's work must have attracted many readers when it appeared in 1854. Sir Benjamin Brodie received many honours. He was surgeon to George IV, to William IV, and to Queen Victoria ; he became President of the Royal College of Surgeons and of the Royal Society. A baronetcy was conferred on him in 1834. Perhaps his greatest honour came in 1858, when he was chosen to preside over the newly formed General Medical Council. His eminence in his profession, his administrative ability, and his charm of manner entitled him to the position, and no better choice could have been made. The passage of the Medical Act of 1858 was a most important event in the history of British medicine. At last, after many years of wrangling and of ineffective local laws, the right to practise within the British Isles had become limited to those medical men whose names were enrolled in the Medical Register. It was natural that so versatile a man as Benjamin Brodie should have been the first president of the council empowered to control medical practice.

Brodie was thirty-one years of age when another great surgeon was born, probably, with the exception of Lister, the " greatest " of the century, if we apply that overwrought word in its widest sense. Sir JAMES PAGET (1814–99) is one of the most inspiring figures in medical history. Fortunately he wrote an autobiography. Autobiographies of medical men are all too rare. Nevertheless, we have a few excellent examples such as Cardan's *De Vita Propria* (p. 163), Ambrose Paré's *Journeys in Divers Places*, the *Autobiography of Samuel D. Gross* (p. 301), and *Memoirs and Letters of Sir James Paget*.[1] The last-mentioned, perhaps, holds first place, and should be read and re-read by every medical man, especially at the beginning of his career.

[1] Stephen Paget (one of his sons), ed. of *Memoirs and Letters of Sir James Paget*, 1901

James Paget was the youngest of nine surviving children in a family of fifteen. His father, a brewer and shipowner of Yarmouth, had acquired wealth and position, although in later life he suffered much financial loss. James then paid off all the debts, even to creditors who did not press their claims, and at a time when he could least afford to do so. Early in life James Paget served for five years as apprentice to a local practitioner, Charles Costerton, and the practical experience thus gained added greatly to the interest of his subsequent studies. The apprenticeship system might be revived to-day with advantage. At this period he collaborated with his brother Charles in publishing a *Natural History of Yarmouth*, which sold at half a crown and attracted a good deal of notice. Paget was devoted to botany and sketching, noting in his memoirs, " I cannot estimate too highly the influence of botany upon the course of my life. The knowledge was useless ; the discipline of acquiring it was beyond price." In his twentieth year he entered St. Bartholomew's Hospital, which was to be the main centre of his life work. The extent of his early struggles can only be appreciated by a perusal of his *Memoirs*. As a first-year student he discovered *Trichina spiralis* in human muscle. The " little specks " were familiar to all in the dissecting rooms, but Paget revealed that each was a little worm in its capsule. After qualification he decided to settle in London. He earned about £50 a year from hack journalism, writing the medical articles for the *Penny Encyclopaedia*, and acting as curator of the hospital museum, an appointment which brought him £40 more. He also rewrote the catalogue of the Royal College of Surgeons museum, continuing the work of John Hunter's assistant, William Clift, a task which occupied part of almost every day for seven years. He wrote reviews and reported lectures for the medical press, and he taught himself German in order to translate medical work.

In 1843 he was appointed students' warden, and for the next seven years he resided in the hospital. At the same time he was appointed Lecturer on Physiology. To this work he applied himself with great energy and industry, devoting much time and care to the preparation of every lecture. Among his students was one named William Senhouse Kirkes, " one of my best pupils," and the materials of Paget's lectures formed the basis of Kirkes' *Handbook of Physiology*, which later became " Halliburton's," and is now in its 38th edition (1944).

Meantime, Paget was in practice as a surgeon, but his income from this source, beginning at £5, 1s. for the year 1836, had risen only to £15, 4s. in 1842, and he had been sixteen years in practice before he made £100 a year in fees. Eventually he had the most lucrative practice in London, when he earned £10,000 a year for some years, though he scorned a reputation which could be measured only by money, as that " might be obtained by the most ignorant through self-assertion, self-advertisement, or mere impudence." Although he was made Assistant Surgeon to St. Bartholomew's Hospital in 1847, and full Surgeon in 1861, he never shone as an operator. Diagnosis was his speciality, and it was said that one should " go to Paget to find out what was the matter, and then to Fergusson to have it cut out."

Paget was intolerant of those who separated the art from the science of medicine. He held that " the roughest country practice might be made a way of science," and that " every man ought to try to do some good bit of original work." His passion for clear observation and careful classification is shown in his writings, which are still admirable to read, and he was an eloquent orator. *Lectures on Surgical Pathology* (1853) was at once recognized as a masterly work, and was followed by *Clinical Lectures and Essays* in 1875. His name is associated with at least two diseases which he described. In an essay on *What Becomes of Medical Students*, he dealt with the careers of a thousand of his old pupils at St. Bartholomew's.

Sir James and Lady Paget had a very happy home life. He did not retire to his study to work, but in the evenings after a busy day he would sit writing letters and preparing papers, with his family around him, while they talked and played and sang apparently without disturbing him. Among his friends were many eminent persons—Browning, Tennyson, Gladstone, Darwin, Ruskin, Pasteur and Virchow.

In 1871 Paget was made a baronet, and during the same year he nearly lost his life from septicaemia contracted at a post-mortem examination. He used to say that he was the only person who had recovered after being attended by ten doctors. Sir James Paget worked hard right to the end of his long life. " There is no true success without work," he said, and his own success was the fruit of incessant toil. His life was a noble record of achievement, a worthy pattern for all surgeons.

Dupuytren, A Born Teacher

On the Continent, in the period just before Lister, there were many excellent surgeons : Dieffenbach of Königsberg, Langenbeck of Berlin, Middeldorpf of Breslau, Malgaigne, Nélaton, and Velpeau, all of Paris, and their colleague, Dupuytren, perhaps the greatest of them all. He may well represent Continental surgery early in the nineteenth century.

GUILLAUME DUPUYTREN (1777–1835),[1] in his time the most illustrious surgeon of France and a great clinical teacher, was born of humble parents in an obscure village. Although in manhood he was austere and reserved, he must have been an attractive child, since at the age of four he was carried off by a rich lady who was attracted to him. On this occasion he was rescued by his parents, but again at the age of twelve he was coveted by a cavalry officer, who offered to take him to Paris for his education. The offer was accepted, and thus commenced the career of one who greatly furthered the progress of surgery by inventing many new instruments and operations, and by making the scene of his activity, the Hôtel-Dieu, a centre of surgical teaching of wider repute than any other hospital of Paris. Dupuytren wrote little, yet he exercised a vast influence through his clinical lectures, which were very popular. His personal qualities did not attract, for he was cynical, intolerant, and " on occasions more intolerably brutal than even the cunning Abernethy." He was " a man whom all admired, few loved, and none understood." Perhaps he has been misjudged, as Sir Robert Christison (p. 294), who saw him perform lithotomy on a child, wrote that " nothing could surpass the humanity and kindliness of the reputedly rough and ill-natured-looking man." [2] An eccentricity in dress accentuated his defects, for he wore a dirty white apron, a threadbare coat, a green cloth cap, and carpet slippers. Nevertheless he had a large practice and, like Larrey (page 338), he became a Baron. He left a fortune, part of which was applied to the endowment of a museum, the Musée Dupuytren, which still exists.

Among the many distinguished pupils of Dupuytren was ANTOINE LEMBERT (1802–51), who noted that the solution to the problem of intestinal suture lay in securing union of the serous surfaces, the well-known Lembert suture.

[1] L. Delhoume, *Dupuytren*, Limoges, 1935
[2] *Life of Sir Robert Christison*, edited by his sons, 1885, vol. i. p. 229

Of slightly later date than Dupuytren was ALFRED ARMAND LOUIS MARIE VELPEAU (1795–1867), the son of a blacksmith, who became Professor of Clinical Surgery in the Paris Faculty, and who wrote a comprehensive work on operative surgery.[1]

Antecedents of the Antiseptic System

It is difficult to do full justice to the achievement of Lister. Fortunately the facts of his life and work are already so well known that the events which led to his discovery need only be briefly outlined.

We have already described the dangers of surgery before the coming of Lister, and we have recalled some of the giants of surgery who faced heavy odds. There had indeed been some groping towards the antiseptic principle before Lister's day, just as there were glimmerings of a " circulation " idea before the advent of Harvey. Even the name " antiseptic " had been used if not actually coined by Sir John Pringle in the eighteenth century.

The story really begins another century earlier with Leeuwenhoek and his " little animals," to which we have already referred (p. 189). He and Kircher were really the first bacteriologists, though they could not explain what they saw through their primitive microscopes. About the same time, FRANCESCO REDI (1626–98), the Italian poet and parasitologist, was making important observations.[2] The fruit of his observations is contained in his book of *Osservazioni intorno agli animali viventi che si trovano negli animali viventi* (Observations on living animals which are to be found within other living animals) (1684), the pioneer work on animal parasites. In the course of his researches he noted that maggots do not appear spontaneously in putrefying material, and that if meat is left covered to keep out the flies no maggots are seen. From this crude experiment, which no one had thought of trying before, Redi agreed that the widely held doctrine of "spontaneous generation" was incorrect. Life alone produces life, he said. Everything must have a parent. *Omne vivum ex ovo.*

A century later, the argument was transferred from maggots to microbes by another Italian, LAZARO SPALLANZANI (1729–99).

[1] A. Corlieu, *Centenaire de la Faculté de Médecine de Paris (1794–1894)*, Paris, 1896, p. 417
[2] R. Solla, " Francesco Redi (1626–98), der Naturforscher," *Arch. f. Gesch. d. Med.*, 1938, vol. xxx. p. 352 ; R. Cole, " Francesco Redi, Physician, Naturalist, Poet," *Ann. Med. Hist.*, 1926, vol. viii. p. 347

A tireless and ardent scientist, he proved that micro-organisms do not develop in fluids contained in flasks which have been exposed to heat and sealed.[1] Numerous experiments were necessary to enable him to answer his chief critic, an English Catholic priest named Needham, who continued to uphold " spontaneous generation " until Spallanzani finally disposed of the idea.

The next notable worker in this field was none other than the famous Pasteur, from whom Lister derived his chief inspiration, in the manner already described (p. 284).

The Tragedy of Puerperal Fever

While scientists were gradually moving nearer a solution of the cause of septic infections, surgeons and obstetricians were discovering a means of avoiding sepsis, though they could not fully explain the reason for their success. The ghastly nature of puerperal fever stimulated every thinking obstetrician to devise means for its prevention, but tradition died hard and progress was slow.[2]

In 1773 CHARLES WHITE (1728–1813),[3] an enlightened surgeon and man-midwife of Manchester, wrote *A Treatise on the Management of Pregnant and Lying-in Women*, in which he recommended the use of " emollient and antiseptic injections into the uterus in cases when the lochia have become foetid." He also insisted on strict cleanliness and adequate ventilation of the lying-in chamber. Although he has never received sufficient notice from medical historians, he was certainly a surgeon who practised methods far ahead of his time.

Another whose work is almost forgotten was ALEXANDER GORDON (1752–99) of Aberdeen, who in 1795 published a *Treatise on the Epidemic Puerperal Fever of Aberdeen*, in which he advised that the " nurses and the physicians who have attended patients affected with puerperal fever ought carefully to wash themselves and to get their apparel properly fumigated." [4]

[1] A. Castiglioni, *History of Medicine*, trans. E. Krumbhaar, 1941, p. 612
[2] C. H. Peckham, " A Brief History of Puerperal Infection," *Bull. Hist. Med.*, 1935, vol. iii. p. 187
[3] J. G. Adami, " Charles White of Manchester (1728–1813) and the Arrest of Puerperal Fever " (Lloyd Roberts Lecture, 1921), *Jour. Obst. and Gynaec. of Brit. Emp.*, 1922, vol. xxix. p. 1 ; C. J. Cullingworth, " Charles White, F.R.S. : A Great Provincial Surgeon of the Eighteenth Century," *Lancet*, 1903, vol. ii. p. 1071
[4] I. S. Cutter, historical chapter in *Obstetrics and Gynaecology*, ed. A. H. Curtis, Philadelphia, 1933

OLIVER WENDELL HOLMES (1809–94), better known in literary than in medical circles, raised a storm of hostile argument by a paper, *On the Contagiousness of Puerperal Fever*, which he read in 1843 to the Boston Society of Medical Improvement.[1] The improvement on this occasion was regarded as an insult by certain old-fashioned practitioners. Holmes regarded the dissecting room as a source of infection, and he advised washing the hands and changing the clothes before attending a confinement. The simple suggestion met with nothing but opposition and abuse. Holmes answered his critics with dignity, observing that " medical logic does not appear to be taught or practised in our schools." He was probably more proud of this medical work than of any of his better-known publications of the " Breakfast Table " series. Forty years later he wrote of it, " Others had cried out against the terrible evil before I did, but I think I shrieked my warning louder and longer than any of them . . . before the little army of microbes was marched up to support my position." [2]

Four years later the tragic Semmelweiss of Vienna made his contribution to the problem. As First Assistant in the Maternity Hospital, IGNAZ PHILIPP SEMMELWEISS (1818–65) observed that there was a much higher mortality in the wards open to students than in the wards to which only midwives were admitted.[3] The patients also noticed this and pleaded to be treated by the midwives. While Semmelweiss sought to explain this disparity in death rates, his friend Kolletschka, Professor of Medical Jurisprudence, fell ill and died of a dissection wound. Semmelweiss noted that the symptoms, as well as the lesions found on postmortem examination, closely resembled those of puerperal fever. " Puerperal fever," he wrote in 1847, " is caused by conveyance to the pregnant woman of putrid particles derived from living organisms, through the agency of the examining fingers." He insisted that students coming from the dissecting rooms or postmortem theatre should wash their hands in a solution of chloride of lime. Immediately the mortality in the wards under his care fell from eighteen per cent. to three per cent., and then to one

[1] J. H. M. Knox, " The Medical Life of Oliver Wendell Holmes," *Bull. Johns Hopk. Hosp.*, 1907, vol. xviii. p. 45
[2] J. T. Morse, *Life and Letters of Oliver Wendell Holmes*, 2 vols., 1896
[3] E. R. Wiese, " Semmelweiss," *Ann. Med. Hist.*, 1930, vol. ii. p. 80 ; I. T. Edgar, " Ignaz Phillip Semmelweiss," *Ann. Med. Hist.*, 1939, vol. i. p. 74 ; M. Neuburger, *British Medicine and the Vienna School*, 1943, p. 74

per cent. His arguments and even his results did not convince the conservative obstetricians of Vienna, and the persecution he endured led him to resign from his position and remove to Budapest.[1] There, in 1861, he published his great work, *On the Cause and Prevention of Puerperal Fever*, but he never convinced his critics. Eventually, he became insane, and died from a septic wound on the finger, the victim of the very disease he had done so much to prevent.

There were surgeons in the pre-Listerian era who insisted on strict cleanliness of the hands, the instruments, and the field of operation, although they could not clearly explain the reason for such precautions. One of the most successful was Sir THOMAS SPENCER WELLS (1818–97),[2] an eminent surgeon and gynaecologist of London, who commenced his career by seven years of service as a surgeon in the navy. He afterwards settled in practice in London, and became attached to the Royal Samaritan Hospital, which was then merely a dispensary. Wells was particularly successful in ovariotomy, an operation which he conducted with simple technique, but with great care and strict attention to cleanliness. Complete silence during the operation was the rule in his theatre. During thirty years of active practice Spencer Wells operated upon a thousand cases of ovarian tumour with an astonishingly low mortality, and he was in high repute as a " safe " surgeon. His success lay in his insistence upon " the most scrupulous cleanliness." Yet he could not explain why cleanliness was so important, and he did not possess that genius for detached investigation which led Lister to the summit of success.

[1] M. Neuburger, *British Medicine and the Vienna School*, 1943, p. 74
[2] G. T. Bettany, *Eminent Doctors*, 2 vols., 1885, vol. ii. p. 105

BOOKS FOR FURTHER READING

BETTANY, G. T. *Eminent Doctors*, 2 vols., 1885
BROWN, JOHN. *Horae Subsecivae*, 3 vols., 1882
CRESSWELL, C. H. *The Royal College of Surgeons of Edinburgh, 1505–1905*, Edinburgh, 1926
HOLMES, TIMOTHY. *Sir Benjamin Collins Brodie* (Masters of Medicine), 1898
MORSE, J. T. *Life and Letters of Oliver Wendell Holmes*, 2 vols., 1896
NEUBURGER, M. *British Medicine and the Vienna School*, 1943
PAGET, STEPHEN. *Memoirs and Letters of Sir James Paget*, 1901
PATERSON, R. *A Memorial of the Life of James Syme*, Edinburgh, 1874

PLATE LXIII LISTER AND HIS FELLOW HOUSE-SURGEONS 1854

Jn Beddoe

John Kirk

George Hogarth Pringle

Lister

Patrick Heron Watson

David Christison

Alexander Struthers

PLATE LXIV   LISTER'S EXPERIMENT

249

air but the solids which cause the decomposition. Take any fermenting liquid, say wine, and place it in a flask with an extended neck so that the heat may be carried up to 212°, and then apply a spirit lamp below the flask so as to expell the air and destroy anything that may be alive in it. Take away the spirit lamp and the air will reenter, but any germs which may happen to pass up the tube will be killed by the heat. What will be the result? You have let the air reenter but this air has been deprived of its germs and the wine in the flask will remain for any length of time, 20 years or more perfectly sweet because the air that is now in the flask deprived of its power of decomposition by being heated in a way calculated to kill anything that may be alive in it.

Facsimile page from lecture notes taken by William Stirling Anderson, one of Lister's students in Glasgow. Lister describes his experiment in support of the antiseptic principle (page 325)

Chapter XVII

LISTER AND HIS DISCIPLES

It is customary and logical to divide the history of surgery into two epochs, before Lister and after Lister. The dramatic change wrought by Lister is now universally acknowledged. Surgery had been rendered painless by the introduction of anaesthesia, but the terrible scourge of sepsis remained. The patient on the operating table "faced danger equal to that of the battlefield." So said Sir James Y. Simpson when he advised that old hospitals should be pulled down and replaced by groups of small pavilions. Lister attacked sepsis by a more direct method. With infinite patience he sought to perfect his system of preventing the entrance of germs into a wound, and of destroying them when already present. His technique was misunderstood and mis-applied, and it has since been largely superseded by " asepsis," which is simply another name, another means of achieving the same end, but those facts in no way detract from Lister's discoveries.

Joseph Lister (1827–1912),[1] who became Lord Lister, the first medical peer, was born at Upton House, near Plaistow in Essex. The district is now absorbed into the great East End of London and the house is St. Peter's Vicarage, overlooking West Ham Public Park. In Lister's day Upton was a country village. The park was the property of Samuel Gurney, a leading Quaker, and during the previous century it had been the country estate of Dr. John Fothergill, another famous Quaker to whom we have referred (p. 249). The Listers, too, were Quakers, and Joseph inherited that simplicity and placidity which characterized the Society of Friends. His father, Joseph Jackson Lister, was a prosperous wine-merchant, who devoted his spare time to science, and who had achieved a wide reputation for his improvements in microscopic technique, which also earned for him the Fellowship of the Royal Society.

Lister took the B.A. degree of London before entering University College Hospital as a student. In his early student days

<hr>

[1] Sir Rickman Godlee, *Lord Lister*, 1918 (an excellent biography by his nephew) ; G. T. Wrench, *Lord Lister : His Life and Work*, 1913 ; Cuthbert Dukes, *Lord Lister*, 1924 ; Douglas Guthrie, *Lord Lister, his Life and Doctrine*, 1949

he witnessed the first operation under ether in this country, performed by Liston (p. 307), an experience which doubtless deeply impressed him, though he did not refer to it in his letters. He graduated M.B. in 1852 and also became a Fellow of the Royal College of Surgeons. At this time he was keenly interested in physiology.[1] His paper, " On the Contractile Tissue of the Iris," confirmed and extended the observations of Professor Kölliker of Wurzburg, who praised Lister's work. A second paper by Lister, also published in the *Quarterly Journal of Microscopical Science* (1853), dealt with the muscular tissue of the skin, the pilomotor fibres which cause " goose skin."

Nevertheless he regarded physiology as the introduction to a career of surgery, on which he had set his heart. " Physiology," he wrote, " is even more important to the surgeon than to the physician."

Early Life in Edinburgh and Glasgow

His Professor of Physiology, William Sharpey (p. 277) suggested that he could not do better than continue his surgical studies in Edinburgh, and he supplied a letter of introduction to Professor James Syme (p. 309), then the leading surgeon of Europe. So Lister went to spend a month in Edinburgh ; he actually stayed for seven years. In 1853 he became Syme's house surgeon, with twelve dressers under him who affectionately regarded him as " The Chief," a name which he retained throughout his career (Plate LXIII). " I must not expect to be a Liston or a Syme," he wrote to his father, " still I shall get on. Certain it is that I love surgery more and more and . . . I am honest and a lover of truth, which is as important as anything."

A year later R. J. Mackenzie, a brilliant young Edinburgh surgeon, died of cholera while on service in the Crimea.[2] Lister was appointed to succeed him as Assistant Surgeon to the Royal Infirmary and as Lecturer on Surgery in the Extra-Mural School. He now established himself in practice in Rutland Street, and on April 23, 1856, he married Syme's eldest daughter Agnes, although in doing so he was obliged to sever his connection with the Quaker community. During the next thirty-nine years, Lister owed much to the devotion and assistance of his wife. She acted as his secretary, writing to his dictation for many hours at a stretch. She

[1] *The Collected Papers of Joseph, Baron Lister*, 2 vols., 1919
[2] J. D. Comrie, *History of Scottish Medicine*, 2 vols., 1932, vol. ii. p. 599

attended to his instruments and assisted in his experiments, and she tried to cure his unfortunate habit of unpunctuality, a defect which implied no lack of diligence, but rather the reverse, for he became so deeply absorbed in his work that he was prone to forget his next appointment. Agnes Syme deserves the highest praise for the part she played in advancing the success of her famous husband.

At this period in his career, the scientific side of surgery engaged his attention, and he investigated, in the foot of a frog captured at Duddingston Loch, " The Early Stages of Inflammation," communicating the results in a paper to the Royal Society in 1857. Next year he wrote a paper on " The Coagulation of the Blood." Practice, however, was slow to appear, as we gather from the fact that Mrs. Lister used to speak of " Poor Joseph and his one patient." Lister's election to the Chair of Surgery in Glasgow was therefore opportune. It offered a wide field for surgery and a freedom to develop his own ideas without the supervision of his father-in-law, valuable as that had been in the early years. So in 1860 Lister removed to Glasgow, which was to become the scene of his epoch-making discovery.

His wards in the Glasgow Royal Infirmary, built upon the site of an old burial ground crammed with the coffins of the victims of the cholera epidemic of 1849, were " some of the most unhealthy in the kingdom." Sir John Erichsen in London and Sir J. Y. Simpson in Edinburgh had each attributed the sources of the hospital gangrene, erysipelas, and pyaemia which then decimated surgical wards to what was called " hospitalism," an evil then much greater in hospitals than in private houses, and greatest of all in the largest hospitals.

The Antiseptic System

His researches on inflammation had led Lister to suspect that decomposition, or putrefaction, as it was sometimes called, was the cause of suppuration and infection of wounds, and that the cause was not merely the gases of the air, but something carried by the air. It was the professor of chemistry in Glasgow, Thomas Anderson, who drew Lister's attention to the work of Pasteur. Pasteur, as we have already noted (p. 284) had shown that putrefaction was a fermentation, caused by microscopic organisms which could be transmitted by air. To Lister, Pasteur's discoveries came as a revelation, and he repeatedly, in speech and in writing, acknowledged his debt to Pasteur. From a study of Pasteur's work he deduced that infection in wounds must be analogous to putrefaction in wine. Lister therefore sought for a means of destroying the organisms, and for this purpose he selected carbolic acid, which had been prepared by a Manchester chemist named Calvert, and had been used to deodorize and to disinfect sewage at Carlisle. Carbolic acid had also been employed as an antiseptic by a Parisian chemist, Jules Lemaire, although Lister was unaware of this work until two years after his own preliminary trials, which were made in 1865. If Lister had applied the word " aseptic " to his method of treatment he might have obviated the misunderstanding of those who imagined that he had merely discovered an antiseptic. Lister never claimed to have discovered carbolic acid or any other antiseptic. What he did discover was the principle involving the prevention and cure of sepsis in wounds. At first he used crude carbolic acid, and various forms of putty or plaster, such as the " lac plaster," containing carbolic acid ; later, he found that weaker applications, such as 1 in 20 or 1 in 40 lotion, would answer the purpose. To minimize the irritant action he used a " protective," such as tinfoil or oiled silk. Not content with a mere application to the wound, he insisted that everything which touched the wound, whether dressings, instruments, or fingers should be treated with the antiseptic. He even produced an antiseptic atmosphere by means of a spray of carbolic lotion. The spray, at first worked by hand, then by a pump, the " donkey engine," and finally by a steam apparatus, remained for over twenty years an essential part of the antiseptic equipment (Plate LXV). The spray was abandoned by Lister in the eighties ; by this time he had modified his views and was using a yellow gauze impregnated with carbolic acid. At a later stage he tried various salts of mercury, at first corrosive sublimate and then cyanides. Eventually he favoured " double cyanide gauze," which contained the cyanides of mercury and zinc, and was dyed a heliotrope colour for identification.

The antiseptic system was first used by Lister in March 1865 in a case of compound fracture of the leg. Such a case was peculiarly suitable for a trial of the new method, as the condition could hardly be made worse, and if the treatment was successful the limb would be saved. In 1867 Lister published his first results in *The Lancet* under the title, " On a New Method of Treat-

PLATE LXV   AN OPERATION AT ABERDEEN IN
LISTER'S DAY

The figure fourth from left is (Sir) Alexander Ogston.   An assistant attends to
the carbolic spray as used by Lister, which stands on a small plush-covered table.
The era of gowns, caps, masks, and gloves had not dawned (pages 288 and 324)

PLATE LXVI THE MAYO CLINIC

The clinic founded by William and Charles Mayo, world-famous as a centre of surgical progress. The present building, illustrated above, was opened in 1928 (page 332)

ing Compound Fracture." He described eleven cases, with nine recoveries of life and limb, one amputation, and one death. He stated that by the use of his method blood clotted instead of liquefying and becoming putrid, remained intact, and ultimately became organized. A year later he wrote in the *British Medical Journal*, " On the Antiseptic System of Treatment in Surgery," declaring his preference for carbolic acid and describing his methods.

Lister Returns to Edinburgh

In 1869 Professor Syme was smitten with paralysis, from which he died a year later, and Lister succeeded him in the Chair of Surgery at Edinburgh. While in Edinburgh Lister continued his investigations, and it was at this time that he introduced the spray. He confirmed Pasteur's findings by keeping boiled urine in flasks, open to the air but with necks drawn out and twisted, so that dust could not enter, and noting that the fluid remained clear (Plate LXIV). These famous flasks were used to illustrate his lectures, being conveyed to various medical meetings in London and elsewhere by Lister and his wife, nursed carefully on their knees in cabs and railway carriages. From Edinburgh Lister corresponded with Pasteur, and thus commenced a life-long friendship between two scientists, each of whom had a high personal regard for the other.

Lister's scrupulous attention to detail is exemplified by his recommendation of black safety pins for securing bandages, as they are more easily seen, and he further notes that they should be inserted parallel to the line of strain. The sinus forceps and the probe-pointed scissors which he invented are still used in every hospital. No detail of treatment escaped his supervision. Two of his favourite aphorisms were : " Success depends upon attention to detail," and " There is only one rule of practice : put yourself in the patient's place."

In addition to his work on antiseptics, Lister introduced the catgut ligature, and showed how it might be rendered safe by storing it in carbolized oil. He also popularized the rubber drainage tube, which had been introduced by Chassaignac a few years earlier. The first occasion on which he used it was in 1871. The case was one of abscess of the axilla, and the patient was Queen Victoria. Lister went to Balmoral to open the abscess, while Sir William Jenner, who was also in attendance, worked the bellows of the spray. A few years later Lister was placed in an awkward position when the queen asked him to make a public statement opposing " vivisection," which was then the subject of a Royal Commission. In a tactful reply he explained why he could not do so ; nevertheless this incident, it is said, delayed his honour of a baronetcy by several years.

The second Edinburgh period was probably the happiest part of Lister's life. He was now at the summit of his fame, and very popular with his students, while his clinic attracted many distinguished foreign visitors. In 1875 he visited Germany, and was received with enthusiasm in a country which was then eager to adopt new ideas. An equally warm welcome awaited him in America, when he attended an international congress at Philadelphia in September 1876.

His Work and Later Years in London

In 1877, the year of Lister's fiftieth birthday, Sir William Fergusson died, and Lister was invited to fill the vacant Chair of Clinical Surgery at King's College, London. When the Edinburgh students heard of this, seven hundred of them signed a petition imploring him to remain. Lister, however, was a man with a mission. His antiseptic doctrine, accepted in almost every part of the world, had made little headway in London. So to London he went, taking with him as his assistants Watson Cheyne and John Stewart. The reception was somewhat chilly. Students were apathetic, nurses even hostile, colleagues critical or disinterested. Surgeons were even horrified when he opened the knee joint to wire a fractured patella, yet they could not but admire his results. Gradually the critics were disarmed, and Lister's system was adopted.

He took a keen interest in the foundation of a British Pasteur Institute for the treatment of hydrophobia, opened in 1897. The Jenner Institute, as it was called at first, had a much wider scope than that of a Pasteur Institute, embracing as it did the study and treatment of all infective diseases. In 1903 it became the Lister Institute of Preventive Medicine. Lister's friendship with Pasteur has been mentioned, and also the famous meeting at the Sorbonne on Pasteur's seventieth birthday (p. 285). That year, 1892, Lister reached the retiring age, and resigned his chair and hospital appointment.

In 1893 Lady Lister died while they were on holiday in Italy. Lister did not allow his great grief to interfere with the public duties which now engaged his attention. He succeeded Lord Kelvin as President of the Royal Society in 1895, he was President of the British Association in 1896, and when he became a peer in 1897 he rendered good service by his support of the Vaccination Bill in the House of Lords. In 1902 he became one of the original members of the Order of Merit, instituted at the coronation of King Edward VII.

Lister's health now began to fail, and he gradually withdrew from public life, although he came strongly into prominence on the occasion of his eightieth birthday (1907), which was celebrated with enthusiasm throughout the world. By this time he had retreated to Walmer in Kent, owing to increasing infirmity. There he died on February 10, 1912, at the age of eighty-five. Many were the eulogies which appeared at the time of his death, but none more aptly worded than that which appeared in the Royal College of Surgeons' report : " His gentle nature, imperturbable temper, resolute will, indifference to ridicule, and tolerance of hostile criticism, combined to make him one of the noblest of men. His work will last for all time ; humanity will bless him evermore and his fame will be immortal."

Disciples of Lister

Immense advances have been made in surgery and all its branches during the short period since Lister's day. As so frequently happens, his views were accepted and their value was recognized abroad sooner than at home.

JUST LUCAS-CHAMPIONNIÈRE (1843–1913), who had studied under Lister in Glasgow, was the first to introduce " Listerism " into France, by his practice and by writing a short work entitled *Chirurgie antiseptique* (1876). Lucas-Championnière is also remembered for his advocacy of early massage and movement in the treatment of fractures.

In more recent times French surgery has been well represented by JULES PÉAN (1830–98), a leading gynaecologist of Paris and admirer of Lister, and the first in France to perform ovariotomy (1864) ; by PAUL RECLUS (1847–1914), a pioneer of local anaesthesia ; by MARIN THÉODORE TUFFIER (1857–1929), who was one of the first to employ spinal anaesthesia, and who rendered important services in many branches of surgery and in the treatment of wounds during the Great War ; and by many others whose names are familiar.

MATHIAS HIERONYMUS SAXTORPH (1822–1900), Professor of Clinical Surgery at Copenhagen, was one of the first to adopt antiseptic surgery on the Continent. He described, in a letter to Lister in 1870, how he had banished pyaemia from his hospital.

In Germany Lister had many disciples. There was KARL THIERSCH (1822–95) of Leipzig, who devised the method of skin-grafting named after him ; RICHARD VOLKMANN (1830–89) of Halle, ever associated in the minds of students with fascial contractures ; and JOHANN VON NUSSBAUM (1829–90) of Munich, an able surgeon and a prolific writer. Several of Nussbaum's letters to Lister have been preserved. " Our results," he wrote, " become better and better, the time of healing shorter, and pyaemia and erysipelas completely disappeared."

Stromeyer of Hanover, whose work is mentioned on p. 343, crystallized his opinion of Lister in light verse, and even supplied the English translation :

> Mankind looks grateful now on thee
> For what thou did'st in Surgery
> And Death must often go amiss,
> By smelling antiseptic bliss.

Abdominal Surgery Established

One of the most brilliant German surgeons of Lister's time was THEODORE BILLROTH (1829–1894), who taught at Vienna and there introduced many new operations, especially in the surgery of the abdomen, of which he is regarded sometimes as the founder.[1] Billroth was the first to excise cancer of the stomach, and the first to perform laryngectomy, feats which had been rendered possible by his early adoption of Lister's methods. In Breslau, JOHANN VON MIKULICZ-RADECKI (1850–1905), a Polish pupil of Billroth, still further extended the field of abdominal surgery. Another of Billroth's pupils, a famous teacher of surgery in the Vienna School, was ANTON VON EISELSBERG (1860–1939).

ERNST VON BERGMANN (1836–1907), professor at Berlin, was

[1] E. R. Wiese, " Theodore Billroth, Scholar, Musician, and Master Surgeon," *Ann. Med. Hist.*, 1928, vol. x. p. 278 ; M. Neuburger, *British Medicine and the Vienna School*, 1943, p. 113

another follower of Lister.[1] He introduced what he called the " aseptic " method, which was simply another means of applying the principles so clearly stated by Lister. It was Von Bergmann who introduced sterilization by steam and improved the design of operating theatres. He was succeeded in the Chair of Surgery by AUGUST BIER (1861–1949) so well known for his treatment of inflammatory lesions by " passive congestion."

Another Berlin surgeon bearing a name familiar in surgery was FRIEDRICH TRENDELENBURG (1844–1924), who pointed out the advantage of elevating the pelvis in certain operations. PAUL KRASKE (1851–1930), chief of the surgical clinic at Freiburg for thirty-six years, wrote, while he was still a junior assistant, a monograph on his method of excision of the rectum for carcinoma.

The foremost Swiss surgeon of his time was THEODORE KOCHER (1841–1917) who in his clinic at Berne revolutionized the surgery of the thyroid gland, and performed two thousand thyroidectomies with a mortality rate of five per cent. He made important contributions to other branches of surgery, achieving world-wide fame.

As a representative of the Italian surgery of modern times, the name of EDOARDO BASSINI (1844–1924) may be selected for mention. In his clinic at Rome, Bassini evolved the technique of the operation for inguinal hernia associated with his name, and he was the leading surgeon of Italy in his day.

In Russia we find an important link in the chain of modern surgery in the person of IVAN PETROVICH PAVLOV (1849–1936). Although not a practising surgeon, he was perhaps the greatest experimental surgeon of modern times. His researches on the psychic factor in the secretion of digestive juices, and his elaboration of " conditioned reflexes " have had an important bearing upon many problems of surgery and medicine.

To return to British surgery, there may be mentioned at this stage in our story the name of one of Lister's contemporaries who deserves to be honoured. Sir JONATHAN HUTCHINSON (1828–1913), surgeon to the London Hospital, was a man of encyclopaedic knowledge and of wide experience. He had an outlook similar to that of John Hunter, with whom he has often been compared. His researches on syphilis and leprosy are well

---

[1] C. L. Schleich, *Besonnte Vergangenheit*, Berlin, 1920. English trans. entitled, " Those Were Good Days," trans. by B. Miall. (Recollections of a surgeon whose name is associated with local anaesthesia.)

known, and his *Archives of Surgery* (1889–99) was a mine of surgical information.

At this period gynaecological surgery was represented by Sir Spencer Wells (p. 320) who achieved wonderful results in ovariotomy, and by ROBERT LAWSON TAIT (1845–99), a pupil of Simpson in Edinburgh who built up a large practice in Birmingham.[1] Lawson Tait was strongly opposed to Lister's views, and he denied the bacterial nature of sepsis. Nevertheless, he always insisted on absolute cleanliness, on asepsis, in fact, and this was no doubt the cause of the remarkable success of his operations.

The leading gynaecological surgeon of America was HOWARD KELLY of Baltimore (1858–1943), who introduced many new operative procedures, and who was an authority on the use of radium.

Appendicitis Defined

Sir FREDERICK TREVES (1853–1923), who operated upon King Edward VII for appendicitis in 1902, was a leader of abdominal surgery, in which great advances were being made.

The pathologist who established appendicitis as a definite lesion was REGINALD HEBER FITZ (1843–1913) of Boston.[2] His *Perforating Inflammation of the Vermiform Appendix, with Special Reference to its Early Diagnosis and Treatment*, focused attention upon the disease and upon its relation to peritonitis, which had previously been ill understood. He was the first to apply the name " appendicitis."

Among American surgeons who added to the knowledge of appendicitis were CHARLES McBURNEY of New York (1845–1913), who devised the so-called gridiron incision, and JOHN BLAIR DEAVER (1855–1931), Professor of Surgery at Philadelphia, a brilliant surgeon who wrote a monograph on appendicitis (1896), in addition to other important work.[3] Another early exponent of abdominal surgery was a Swiss, NICHOLAS SENN (1844–1908), who had come to Chicago at an early age. Senn performed intestinal anastomosis by means of bone plates, which fulfilled the same function as did " Murphy's button " a few years later.

---

[1] Stewart McKay, *Lawson Tait: His Life and Work*, 1922
[2] Sir D'Arcy Power, " Treves' First Appendix Operation," *Brit. Jour. Surg.*, 1935, vol. xxiii. p. 1 ; W. R. Bett, ed. of *A Short History of Some Common Diseases*, 1934, p. 168
[3] R. A. Leonardo, *History of Surgery*, 1943, pp. 318, 323

JOHN BENJAMIN MURPHY (1857-1916), also of Chicago, was unrivalled as a surgical teacher. He achieved success and fame in the face of much opposition. Details of his interesting career have been set forth in a biography entitled *Surgeon Extraordinary*.[1]

An eminent British exponent of abdominal surgery was BERKELEY GEORGE ANDREW MOYNIHAN (LORD MOYNIHAN) (1865-1936), Professor of Surgery at Leeds.[2] Facile alike as operator and as author, he made many contributions to the knowledge of gall stones and of duodenal ulcer. For his services during the Great War he was created a Baron.

Sir ARBUTHNOT LANE [3] (1856-1943) introduced an operative technique of " plating " fractures by uniting the bones with metal plates, a procedure which the method of Lister, who used to unite the fractured patella by wire, had rendered possible. Lane had his own views on chronic intestinal stasis, for which he advised a method of short-circuiting the bowel.

A more recent worker in the field of abdominal surgery was Sir DAVID PERCIVAL DALBRECK WILKIE (1882-1939), Professor of Surgery in the University of Edinburgh, who achieved distinction for his work on the surgery of the gall bladder.

Surgery in America

General surgery in the United States was considerably advanced by the labours of GEORGE WASHINGTON CRILE of Cleveland (1864-1943). His researches were chiefly concerned with the causes of surgical shock and the best means of avoiding shock, especially in operations for toxic goitre. WILLIAM STEWART HALSTED (1852-1922) [4] was the surgical member of the great team, " the big four," engaged in the teaching of medicine at the Johns Hopkins University, Baltimore, from its inception in 1889. The others were Welch (pathology), Osler (medicine), and Kelly (gynaecology). Halsted was a worthy disciple of Lister, and one of those who endeavoured to secure a sterile field in operating. To this end he introduced the use of rubber gloves, which marked a great surgical advance, and he perfected operations for hernia and for removal of the breast.

[1] Loyal Davis, *Surgeon Extraordinary : The Life of J. B. Murphy*, 1938
[2] Donald Bateman, *Berkeley Moynihan, Surgeon*, 1940
[3] W. E. Tanner, *Arbuthnot Lane : His Life and Work*, 1946
[4] W. G. MacCallum, *William Stewart Halsted*, 1930

A crowning triumph of American surgery was the foundation, by the brothers Mayo, of the clinic at Rochester, Minnesota, which bears their name (Plate LXVI). The fascinating story of the two brothers, "Dr. Will and Dr. Charlie," as they were familiarly called, is well told in the recent biography by Helen Clapesattle.[1] WILLIAM JAMES MAYO (1861–1939) and CHARLES HORACE MAYO (1865–1939) achieved their rise to fame almost as one man. "My brother and I" was the phrase used constantly by each of them. The Mayo Clinic soon became the surgical focus of the United States and a centre of study for surgeons the world over; and the Mayo Foundation, to advance the teaching of surgery, was another ideal successfully attained by the brothers. Will turned his attention largely to abdominal surgery. Charlie was an authority on thyroid surgery. Both were inspiring teachers, who were content with nothing but the best in their immense undertaking. "They were born at the right time, neither too early to ride the wave of advance that followed upon the work of Pasteur and Lister, nor too late to reap the advantages of the old school at its soundest and best." Every surgeon admired and respected the Mayos, and a more subtle criterion of their greatness was shown in the affectionate regard of the town folk of Rochester.

Specialism in Surgery

The trend of surgery towards specialism was already evident towards the end of the nineteenth century. The rise of specialism in the fields of medical science will form the theme of a subsequent chapter. Meanwhile a few words may be said regarding the rise and progress of various branches of surgery. Reference has already been made to the rapid growth of abdominal surgery. Even more spectacular was the surgery of the central nervous system.

Neurological Surgery, which has now reached such a high degree of perfection, had its beginnings in London, when Lister's nephew and biographer, SIR RICKMAN GODLEE (1859–1925), was the first to remove successfully a tumour of the brain. This was in 1884, and in commemorating the operation fifty years later, Mr. Wilfred Trotter, who regretted that in such great events of medical history the name of the patient is so seldom mentioned, placed it on

---

[1] H. Clapesattle, *The Doctors Mayo*, University of Minnesota, 1941

PLATE LXVII NAPOLEON'S CHIEF SURGEON

Baron Larrey, 1766–1842

Larrey's " Flying Ambulance " (page 338)

PLATE LXVIII A DIRECTOR-GENERAL OF MEDICAL
SERVICES

Sir James McGrigor, whose *Reports on Sickness, Mortality, and Invaliding among
the Troops* did so much to improve the health of the army and the efficiency
of the medical services (page 341)

record that " this young man's name was Henderson, and that he was a native of Dumfries." [1]

ARTHUR BARKER (1850–1916) was the first in this country to drain successfully an otitic brain abscess in 1886, and he was closely followed by Sir WILLIAM MACEWEN (1848–1924) of Glasgow,[2] whose series of early successes in the treatment of brain abscess (twenty-four operations, twenty-three recoveries) remains unequalled. His *Pyogenic Diseases of the Brain and Spinal Cord* (Glasgow, 1893) is a medical classic.

Sir VICTOR HORSLEY (1857–1916), who, like Godlee, was surgeon to University College Hospital, was the first, in 1887, to operate successfully for the removal of an accurately localized tumour of the spinal cord. Horsley died of sunstroke while on military service in Mesopotamia during the Great War.[3]

In America the pioneer was WILLIAM WILLIAMS KEEN (1837–1932) of Philadelphia, who made notable contributions to surgical literature, and who successfully removed a brain tumour in 1888. The greatest neurological surgeon of America was HARVEY CUSHING (1869–1939), a highly skilled neurologist and pathologist, who evolved a technique of his own, and who published classic monographs on the pituitary body (1912), and on tumours of the nervus acusticus (1917). His *Life* of his friend Sir William Osler (1926) is a gem of medical biography. He served in France during the Great War, and wrote an account of his experiences.[4] His *Bio-bibliography of Andreas Vesalius* was not published until 1943.

Early workers in the field of neuro-surgery in Europe include FRANCESCO DURANTE (1844–1934) of Rome, who introduced the osteoplastic flap in brain surgery, and PAUL BROCA (1824–80) of Paris, whose achievements as an anthropologist (p. 6) are equalled by his skill as a surgeon and anatomist. He was one of the first to apply his knowledge of cerebral localization to the diagnosis of brain tumours, and by some authorities he is regarded as the founder of modern neuro-surgery.

Another highly specialized field which at this time became differentiated from general surgery, was the surgery of the genitourinary system, briefly called *Urology*. A great impetus was given

[1] Wilfred Trotter, " A Landmark in Modern Neurology," *Lancet*, 1934, vol. ii. p. 1207
[2] A. K. Bowman, *Sir William Macewen : A Chapter in the History of Surgery*, 1942
[3] Stephen Paget, *Life of Sir Victor Horsley*, 1919
[4] Harvey Cushing, *From a Surgeon's Journal, 1915–18*, 1936

to this study by the invention of the cystoscope in 1877 by MAX NITZE (1848–1906) of Berlin.[1] At a later date he perfected the operating cystoscope. Together with FELIX GUYON (1831–1920) of the Necker Hospital, Paris, a pioneer in prostatectomy and in cystoscopy, Nitze can claim to have founded modern urology.[2] In Britain this branch of surgery was advanced by Sir HENRY THOMPSON (1820–1904) and by Sir JOHN THOMSON-WALKER (1870–1937), whose book became the standard work. A prominent urologist of America is HUGH HAMPTON YOUNG (1870–1945), who devised a technique of prostatectomy and made numerous contributions to the subject.

Among earlier surgeons who enriched this special field was HENRY JACOB BIGELOW (1818–90), who perfected the technique of crushing stone in the bladder (lithotrity). A brilliant surgeon and teacher, he was Professor at Harvard for thirty-three years.

Orthopaedic Surgery was widely practised long before it became recognized as a separate branch. It received a considerable impetus during the Great War, but if any one man must be selected as the father of modern orthopaedics, that man must be HUGH OWEN THOMAS (1834–91) of Liverpool.[3] To the craft of " bone-setting," which had been practised by his ancestors for seven generations, he added a sound knowledge of surgery. The greater part of his professional life was spent as a " club doctor " in the dock district of Liverpool ; consequently he had a hard fight to secure acceptance of his views by those who had entered surgery through the usual hospital channel. He was convinced of the importance of complete and prolonged rest in the treatment of fractures, and he devised various forms of apparatus for the correction of deformities and the treatment of injuries.[4] Thomas's splint has saved many limbs, the death rate from compound fractures of the femur falling from eighty to twenty per cent., largely as a result of its use.

The work so well begun by Thomas was continued by his successor, Sir ROBERT JONES (1858–1933), who greatly raised the status of orthopaedics by his skill and organizing ability during the Great War. " To him and his practical teaching and influence we owe it that our streets to-day show relatively so few war

[1] Brandsford Lewis, ed. of *History of Urology*, 2 vols., Baltimore, 1933, vol. i. p. 160
[2] A. Pousson and E. Desnos, ed. of *Encylopédie française d'Urologie*, Paris, 1914, p. 274
[3] D. McCrae Aitken, *Hugh Owen Thomas : His Principles and Practice*, 1935
[4] Sir D'Arcy Power, ed. of *British Masters of Medicine*, 1936, p. 159

cripples." [1] William Mayo said that he was " one of the greatest surgeons that it has been my good fortune to meet " ; and *The Times* referred to him in the following words : " The shining lustre of his name is an abiding glory of British surgery."

No account of the beginnings of orthopaedic surgery is complete without a reference to that medical classic entitled *Rest and Pain,* which appeared in 1862 from the pen of John Hilton. [2]

JOHN HILTON (1804–78) was fifty-five years of age when he delivered those lectures at the Royal College of Surgeons. Apart from the fact that he was a native of Essex, nothing is known of his early life. For twenty years he acted as Demonstrator in Anatomy and Physiology at Guy's Hospital, to which institution he was appointed Surgeon and Lecturer in Anatomy at the age of thirty-eight.

The therapeutic importance of rest and the diagnostic value of pain were the themes of his great work. He showed how Nature treats an inflamed joint by retaining it, by muscular action, in a fixed and flexed position. It was the surgeon's duty to assist the muscles and to relieve the tension by removing sources of irritation, and by ensuring rest for the affected part. Pain was provided by Nature to guide the surgeon to the seat of the disease, and in order that this guide might be correctly interpreted, an accurate knowledge of the distribution of nerves was essential.

That Hilton's teaching is no longer wholly accepted does not detract from its value. Much may still be learned from his book ; indeed, as Sir Arthur Keith remarks, [3] " never again shall anyone preach the gospel of rest so freshly, so practically, and so persuasively as John Hilton."

[1] F. Watson, *The Life of Sir Robert Jones,* 1934
[2] John Hilton, *Rest and Pain,* 1862 (2nd ed. 1876, 3rd ed. 1880)
[3] Sir A. Keith, *Menders of the Maimed,* 1919, p. 18

BOOKS FOR FURTHER READING

AITKEN, D. McCRAE. *Hugh Owen Thomas : His Principles and Practice,* 1935
BABKIN, B. P. *Pavlov, a biography,* 1951
BATEMAN, DONALD. *Berkeley Moynihan, Surgeon,* 1940
BETT, W. R. Ed. of *The History of Some Common Diseases,* 1934
BOWMAN, A. K. *Sir William Macewen : A Chapter in the History of Surgery,* 1942
CHEYNE, W. WATSON. *Lister and his Achievement,* 1925
CLAPESATTLE, HELEN. *The Doctors Mayo,* University of Minnesota, 1941

CRILE, GRACE (ed.). *George Crile, an Autobiography*, 1947
CUSHING, HARVEY. *From a Surgeon's Journal, 1915–18*, 1936
DAVIS, LOYAL. *Surgeon Extraordinary : The Life of J. B. Murphy*, 1938
FLACK, HENRY. *Lawson Tait, 1845–99*, 1949
FULTON, J. F. *Harvey Cushing*, 1946
GODLEE, Sir RICKMAN. *Lord Lister*, 1918
HUTCHINSON, H. *Jonathan Hutchinson*, 1946
LAYTON, T. B. *Sir William Arbuthnot Lane, Bt.*, 1956
LEONARDO, R. A. *History of Surgery*, 1943
LISTER, Baron. *The Collected Papers of Joseph, Baron Lister*, 2 vols., 1919
MACCALLUM, W. G. *William Stewart Halstead*, 1930
MCKAY, STEWART. *Lawson Tait : His Life and Work*, 1922
PAGET, STEPHEN. *Life of Sir Victor Horsley*, 1919
SCHLEICH, C. L. *Besonnte Vergangenheit*, Berlin, 1920
WATSON, F. *The Life of Sir Robert Jones*, 1934
WRENCH, G. T. *Lord Lister : His Life and Work*, 1913

CHAPTER XVIII

MILITARY AND NAVAL SURGERY ; CONQUEST OF TROPICAL DISEASES

WAR, which brings sorrow and suffering, becoming more and more dreadful on each occasion, is nevertheless not without its compensations. The battlefield has always been a training ground for surgeons, and in recent years war has provided opportunities for vast experiments in public hygiene and national health which could not have been carried out during the years of peace.[1]

Military Surgeons of Early Times

The first surgeons in history were doubtless military surgeons, detailed to tend the casualties resulting from single combat or from tribal fighting.

Homer sang of the bold surgeons Machaon and Podalarius, the Roman Army appears to have had its medical officers, the Knights Hospitallers treated wounded Crusaders, and so it went on until the time of Ambroise Paré, when the invention of gunpowder added so greatly to the problems confronting the military surgeon.

Paré's prototype and contemporary, Thomas Gale, was the first English surgeon to publish *An Excellent Treatise of Wounds made with Gonneshot*, 1563, although the German surgeon Hieronymus Brunschwig had given the first account of gunshot wounds in his illustrated work, *Cirurgia Hantwirckung der Wundartzny*, 1497 (p. 126).

Gale was closely followed by another Elizabethan surgeon, William Clowes, who saw service in the navy as well as in the army, and whose investigations, as we have noted (p. 151), were concerned with the burns produced by gunpowder. The great surgeon of the Civil War was Richard Wiseman, whose career has been noted (p. 209), and in that war we find a still greater campaigner in the person of William Harvey, who so closely followed

---

[1] Maj.-Gen. R. M. Downes, " What Medicine Owes to War and War Owes to Medicine," *Jour. R.A.M.C.*, 1936, vol. lxvii. p. 381 ; Surg.-Capt. H. E. R. Stephens, " The Influence of Wars on the Craft of Surgery," *Jour. R.A.M.C.*, 1934, vol. lxii. p. 40

the fortunes of his tragic royal master. Mention has also been made of the pioneer work of Sir John Pringle in the interests of military hygiene, and of certain distinguished surgeons, such as John Hunter and Charles Bell, who added to their civilian experience by a period of military service or by a visit to some centre of warfare.

Baron Larrey and the Practice of Military Surgery

The war which marked the opening years of the nineteenth century acted as a strong stimulus to surgical advance. The surgery of the battlefield had made little progress since the time of Ambroise Paré. Now another great French military surgeon appeared on the scene and achieved immortal fame. This was Baron Larrey, who took part in all Napoleon's campaigns, acted as chief surgeon to the army, and won the emperor's admiration and friendship.

DOMINIQUE JEAN LARREY (1766–1842) was a native of Baudean in the Pyrenees. When he was a boy his father died and he was brought up by an uncle, an army surgeon in charge of the hospital at Toulouse. There Larrey engaged in the study of medicine, and then, entering the navy as surgeon to a frigate *Vigilante*, he narrowly escaped shipwreck off the stormy coast of Newfoundland. The voyage lasted seven months, and afforded the young surgeon the opportunity of studying mal de mer and scurvy, as well as the scenery, the climate, the birds and animals, and the native customs of this part of the New World. On his return to France he studied in Paris at the Hôtel-Dieu.[1] Among his patients were some of the victims of the Revolution, of which he was an eye-witness.

In 1792 war broke out, and Larrey at once entered the army, and commenced the work for which he was so admirably fitted.[2] It was at this early stage of his career, when he was with the army of the Rhine, that he introduced his " ambulances volantes." These were light, two-wheeled, well sprung vehicles, each drawn by two horses (Plate LXVII). They could readily be rushed up to the front line, where no heavy ambulance could be taken, and it was thus possible to collect and deal with the wounded rapidly.[3]

[1] F. C. Stewart, *The Hospitals and Surgeons of Paris*, 1843, p. 309
[2] P. E. Bechet, " Dominique Jean Larrey," *Ann. Med. Hist.*, 1937, vol. ix. p. 428
[3] E. R. Wiese, " Larrey, Napoleon's Chief Surgeon," *Ann. Med. Hist.*, 1939, vol. i. p. 435

Larrey's flying ambulances brought him into prominence, but this was by no means his only achievement. Details of his adventurous life with the army of Napoleon are given in his *Mémoires de Chirurgie militaire et Campagnes*, 1812.[1]

Larrey showed a devotion to duty which was almost fanatical. Among the troops he was enormously popular, although on one occasion, it is said, he incurred the displeasure of his fellow officers by slaughtering some of their horses in order to make bouillon for his wounded men at a time when provisions were scarce. Hearing of this, Napoleon affected displeasure and sent for Larrey. " Have you dared to kill officers' horses in order to feed your wounded ? " he asked. " Yes," said Larrey simply. "Well," retorted Napoleon, " I will make you Baron of the Empire." This he did. Larrey treated Napoleon for an injury to the foot caused by the kick of a horse, the only wound which he ever received. Larrey himself was wounded on two occasions, in Egypt and at Waterloo. He was present at many battles. At Aboukir there were 1,900 wounded, and " many amputations were performed in the field of battle amid a shower of bullets." For his valour he received from the hands of his general a valuable sword of honour, afterwards inscribed, by order of the emperor, " Aboukir et Larrey." At the battle of Borodino he performed two hundred amputations. One of his patients during the Russian campaign was General Zayochek, whose leg was removed " under the enemy's fire and amid thickly falling snow." The general lived for fourteen years more, and was Viceroy of Poland when he died.

Larrey was a strong advocate of prompt amputation by the circular method when the limb could not be saved, and in those days amputation was the rule for compound fractures or severe injuries. Larrey became Medical Inspector-General in 1805. He was present during the fateful retreat from Moscow, when " the cold was more deadly than the enemy." His campaigning days ending at Waterloo, Larrey was compelled to face the poverty and trials which were the lot of Napoleon's followers. Yet he was not idle. He wrote his great work on military surgery. He visited England in 1826, and was well received by Sir Astley Cooper and other surgeons. He had never lost the high esteem of his countrymen, and in 1830 he was appointed Surgeon-in-Chief at the Hôtel des Invalides. Ten years later, on December

[1] Baron Larrey, *Mémoires de Chirurgie militaire et Campagnes*, 4 vols., Paris, 1812–17

15, 1840, he attended the funeral of his emperor. " Never," he wrote, " has my heart been more distressed by my memories." Napoleon bequeathed the sum of 100,000 francs " to Baron Larrey, the most virtuous man I have ever known."

Napoleon was indeed fortunate in retaining in his service a surgeon so efficient as Baron Larrey. Another man of sterling quality was Napoleon's chief physician. NICOLAS RENÉ DUFRICHE DESGENETTES (1762–1837) entered the army after completing his studies at Montpellier, and by his ability and devotion to duty rapidly rose to eminence.[1] That he possessed courage is shown by the fact that during a plague epidemic in Egypt, when the soldiers were terror-stricken by the spread of the disease, Desgenettes deliberately inoculated himself in their presence with pus from a bubonic abscess. Fortunately the foolhardy yet heroic experiment had no ill effects. He followed all Napoleon's campaigns, and carried out such measures as were available in his day for the promotion of the health and well-being of the troops. Desgenettes was the recipient of many honours, and like Larrey became a Baron of France.[2]

Among others who influenced the trend of French military surgery during the early part of the century, two men were preeminent, although neither adopted the army as a career.

JOSEPH FRANÇOIS MALGAIGNE (1806–1865), surgeon to the Hôpital Saint-Louis of Paris, was distinguished, not only as a surgeon, but also as a clear writer and as a medical historian.[3] All his writing was of high quality. He published an excellent edition of the works of Ambroise Paré (1840), and made valuable contributions of his own to surgical literature, including a treatise on fractures and dislocations in which he advised fixation of the fractured patella by " Malgaigne's hooks."

His colleague at the Hôpital Saint-Louis was AUGUSTE NÉLATON (1807–73), a modest and kindly man who declined to involve himself in controversy. He was a careful operator and a popular teacher of surgery.[4]

It is interesting, as a sign of the times, to recall that the name of Nélaton was associated with his invention of a porcelain-tipped

[1] E. Pariset, *Histoire des membres de l'Académie royale de Médecine*, 2 vols., Paris, 1845, vol. ii. p. 192
[2] L. Gazel, *Le Baron Desgenettes, 1762–1837*, Paris, 1912
[3] A. Corlieu, *Centenaire de la Faculté de Médecine de Paris (1794–1894)*, Paris, 1896, p. 344
[4] J. Becclard, " Notice historique sur la vie et les travaux d'Auguste Nélaton," in *Notices et Portraits*, Paris, 1878, p. 289

probe, which was used to locate bullets, the porcelain becoming marked when it rubbed against the leaden bullet. The first patient whose wound was probed with this instrument was Garibaldi.

British Military Surgery

While the medical services of Napoleon's army were under the able leadership of Larrey, the British army was likewise very fortunate. The Director General of Medical Services at the time was Sir JAMES McGRIGOR (1771–1858), an Inverness-shire man who studied at Aberdeen and Edinburgh, and who founded the Aberdeen Medical Society, which was largely responsible for the development of the medical school in that city [1] (Plate LXVIII). McGrigor's reports, and especially those which deal with the health of the troops in India and Egypt, are full of interesting information. No one did more than he to raise the standard of the medical department of the army so that it might attract the best class of surgeon.[2] He inaugurated at Chatham a museum and a library for army medical officers, and he originated a fund for their widows and orphans.

Among the officers who served under Sir James McGrigor was one who was his great friend, whose fame became even greater than that of his chief, and who fully earned his title of " The British Larrey." This was GEORGE JAMES GUTHRIE (1785–1856), who may be regarded as the most distinguished British army surgeon in history. Born in London of Scottish ancestry, he began his medical career as apprentice to Dr. Phillips, a surgeon in Pall Mall. While still a youth of sixteen years he entered the army as " hospital mate " at York Hospital, Chelsea.[3] Hardly had he commenced work there when an order was issued obliging all hospital mates to obtain a medical qualification. Guthrie at once submitted his name, and passed the M.R.C.S. examination with ease. There now commenced for him a long period of military service, at first five years in Canada, then in the " Peninsula " for six years, after which, although he had been placed on half pay and had commenced practice in London, he resumed military duties in order to assist in treating the wounded at

[1] E. H. B. Rodger, *Aberdeen Doctors*, 1893, p. 125 ; *Autobiography of Sir James McGrigor*, 1861
[2] T. J. Pettigrew, *Medical Portrait Gallery*, 1838–40, vol. iv. (" McGrigor ")
[3] *Ibid.*, vol. iv. (" Guthrie ")

Brussels, after Waterloo.[1] At the age of twenty-six he had three
thousand wounded under his care after the Battle of Albuera,
where he won the admiration of Wellington for his skill and
devotion to duty. He was present at many engagements, was twice
wounded, and even distinguished himself by capturing a French
gun single-handed, a feat which " greatly amused " his general.
His monograph on *Gunshot Wounds* (1815) is still worth reading.
Like Larrey, he advised that when amputation was essential it
should be performed as soon as possible after the injury, certainly
within twenty-four hours, and he preferred the circular method
in most cases. The rule appears to have been, " When in doubt,
amputate." The mortality was about fifty per cent. In 1816,
having declined the honour of knighthood, he founded an infirmary for diseases of the eye, now Royal Westminster Ophthalmic
Hospital. Guthrie served on the staff of this institution, and he
was also appointed surgeon to Westminster Hospital.[2] He was
as successful in civil surgery as he had been in military surgery.
Yet he did not forget the army. He organized courses of instruction
for medical officers of the navy and army, and his services were so
appreciated that the students presented him with a silver cup.
In his treatise on *The Operative Surgery of the Eye* (1823) he advocated the extraction, as opposed to the " couching " of cataract.
In 1830 Guthrie published an important work on *Diseases and
Injuries of Arteries*, and in 1853 there appeared his *Commentaries on
the Surgery of War*. On three occasions he was President of the
Royal College of Surgeons, in 1833, 1841, and 1854. He was a
small, active man, with a brusque military manner which concealed his kindly nature. His services to military surgery were
great, and he was one of the first to lay stress on the need for
medical representation in Parliament.

Military Surgery in Germany and Russia

Other nations besides Great Britain and France possessed
their military surgeons. Germany set a high standard in this
respect at the opening of the nineteenth century.

There was KARL FERDINAND VON GRAEFE (1787–1840), Professor of Surgery in Berlin, whom Garrison has designated " the

[1] H. A. L. Howell, " George James Guthrie, F.R.S., F.R.C.S.," *Jour. R.A.M.C.*,
1910, vol. xiv. p. 577
[2] H. Grimsdale, " George James Guthrie, 1785–1856, Founder of the Royal Westminster Ophthalmic Hospital," *Brit. Jour. Ophthalm.*, 1919, vol. iii. p. 145

founder of modern plastic surgery." He was in close touch with the army throughout his career. On his death he was succeeded in the Chair by another eminent pioneer of plastic surgery, JOHANN FRIEDRICH DIEFFENBACH (1792–1847), who had seen active military service as a combatant and also as a surgeon.

Dieffenbach was in turn succeeded at Berlin in 1847 by BERNHARD VON LANGENBECK (1810–87) who, though not specifically a military surgeon, may be mentioned at this stage as the most famous operator and teacher of his time in Germany. He devised many new operations, and he founded the German Society of Surgery as well as the influential surgical journal, *Archiv für klinische Chirurgie*.

The founder of modern military surgery in Germany, however, was GEORG FRIEDRICH LOUIS STROMEYER (1804–76). In addition to his prowess as a strictly military surgeon he was a pioneer of orthopaedic surgery, applying the operation of subcutaneous tenotomy to the relief of various deformities of the limbs.[1]

Towards the end of the century the most outstanding military surgeon was FRIEDRICH VON ESMARCH (1823–1908), who introduced the first field dressing during the Franco-Prussian War, and who advised the Esmarch elastic bandage for securing haemostasis. He was a strong advocate of "first aid," in civil as in military life. For forty-two years he held the Chair of Surgery at Kiel.

In Russia there was no organized medical profession until well on in the nineteenth century. Doctors from other lands went to seek their fortunes in Russia. Notice has been taken (p. 247) of Thomas Dimsdale of Hertford, England, who was summoned to inoculate Catherine the Great against smallpox. One of the adventurers who sought practice in Russia was an Aberdeen graduate, Sir JAMES WYLIE (1768–1854).[2] Young Wylie went to Russia at the age of twenty-two. His rise to fame was rapid. The story of his successful treatment of a courtier for an abscess of the throat reached the ears of the Tsar, who promptly raised him to the office of court physician, a post which he retained throughout the reigns of the two succeeding Tsars.

Wylie travelled far in the royal service, and took part in every Russian campaign of the time. He was said to be a good surgeon,

[1] G. F. L. Stromeyer, *Erinnerungen eines deutschen Arztes*, 2 vols., Hanover, 1874
[2] Sir R. Hutchison, "A Medical Adventurer. Biographical Note on Sir James Wylie, Bart., M.D., 1758–1854," *Proc. Roy. Soc. Med.* (Sect. Hist.), 1928, vol. xxi., Pt. 2, p. 1406. (Date of birth should have been 1768)

and he certainly was a capable administrator, who did much to found and to organize medical schools, both civil and military. When he accompanied Tsar Alexander to England in 1814 he was made a baronet by the Prince Regent, and he was the recipient of many other honours. A military hospital to his memory was opened in 1873 in the city now known as Leningrad.

The greatest of Russian military surgeons was NIKOLAI PIROGOFF (1810–81), who saw much active military service, taking part in many campaigns, and serving for over a year in the Crimea, where on the Russian side he acted as Florence Nightingale did on the British side, introducing female nursing and insisting upon a more adequate supply of medical comforts.[1] Pirogoff adopted ether anaesthesia as early as 1847, and his name is associated with a method of amputating the foot. Educated at Berlin and Göttingen, he came to the conclusion that anatomy as then taught was insufficient for surgical needs ; accordingly he published an *Atlas of Anatomy* (1852–59), with over 200 plates depicting the numerous frozen sections which he had prepared. At the age of thirty he became Professor of Surgery at St. Petersburg, a chair which he held for forty-one years. His *Treatise on Military Surgery* appeared in 1864.

The Teaching of Military Surgery

Early in the nineteenth century there arose a vogue for the teaching of military surgery as a special subject. At Edinburgh, then the centre of British medical learning, a Chair was established in 1806.[2] The first incumbent was JOHN THOMSON (1765–1846), the son of a Paisley weaver. He had studied at Glasgow, Edinburgh, and London, and was already Professor of Surgery at the Royal College of Surgeons and surgeon to the Royal Infirmary when the military Chair was instituted. This appointment he held for sixteen years, although he lent no great distinction to the Chair. He certainly endeavoured to atone for his lack of military experience by visiting the field of Waterloo and attending the wounded, thereby raising his prestige considerably. Thomson resigned from the Chair of Military Surgery in order to apply for the Chair of Medicine, rendered vacant by the death of James Gregory (p. 231). His application was unsuccessful,

[1] F. H. Garrison, *An Introduction to the History of Medicine*, 3rd ed., 1924, p. 532
[2] A. Miles, *The Edinburgh School of Surgery Before Lister*, 1918, p. 108

but ten years later he became the first professor to occupy the Chair of Pathology, which had been founded at his suggestion. It is not surprising that Dr. Robert Knox referred to Thomson, who had inaugurated and occupied Chairs in three different subjects, as " the old chair maker."

In 1813 Thomson published a book which had a wide circulation. It was entitled *Lectures on Inflammations, Exhibiting a View of the Doctrines of Medical Surgery.* It is obvious from his career that he was no advocate of specialism and that he even viewed with disfavour the separation of medicine from surgery. He therefore approached the subject of inflammation from the medical as well as the surgical point of view.

Thomson was succeeded in the Chair of Military Surgery by one whose military experience at home and in the East well fitted him for his new duties. Sir GEORGE BALLINGALL (1780–1855) was a good teacher, popular with his students, and highly esteemed by his colleagues.[1] His *Outlines of Military Surgery* (1832), which went through five editions, gives a clear picture of the state of the subject prior to the time of Lister. That extreme degree of wound infection, known as hospital gangrene, was very prevalent, and in Ballingall's opinion was best treated by the cautery. The usual dressing for wounds was the cold water compress. Tetanus was common, especially in Egypt and India, and was believed to be the result of injury to a nerve, although occasionally seen even after slight wounds. In gunshot wounds, especially wounds of joints, Ballingall had " a very high opinion of the beneficial effects of large and repeated leeching," and he advised that an ample supply of leeches should be available in military hospitals.

Of fractures he writes, " The practice of swinging or suspending fractured legs in a sort of cradle, as I have seen practised in many Continental hospitals, might well be extended. It would greatly add to the comfort of the soldier, compelled to travel with a broken leg." He gives an illustration of the apparatus, surprisingly modern in design.

He also writes of a method of treatment of compound fracture which has been recently re-discovered, and named the " closed plaster " method. First, he recalls that Larrey, in Egypt, treated compound fractures with cushions or compresses of straw, which

---

[1] A. Miles, *The Edinburgh School of Surgery Before Lister*, 1918, p. 115; J. D. Comrie, *A History of Scottish Medicine*, 2 vols., 1932, vol. ii. p. 506

were left undisturbed until cure was complete. Then he relates how " a small boy was brought to my tent in India, having sustained a compound fracture of the leg. I was preparing to amputate the limb when the parents came and carried him away to a potter who enveloped the limb in clay and finally cured the patient."

In the chapter on the selection of recruits the author expresses the opinion that " the most eligible time for enlistment is from twenty to twenty-five years of age. Boys only fill the hospitals, and not the ranks." This interesting volume concludes with an account of diseases of troops on foreign stations, namely, fever, dysentery, beri-beri, and guinea-worm.

Sir George Ballingall died suddenly in 1855, and Professor Syme wrote to the Secretary of State for War expressing the opinion that the duties of a military or naval surgeon could only be taught by actual demonstration, and that a Chair of Military Surgery was " a useless encumbrance." It was therefore abolished in 1856.

The Royal Army Medical Corps

In spite of this burst of enthusiasm for the teaching of military surgery, there was comparatively little scope for the development of the subject during the peaceful years of the nineteenth century.

Nevertheless, vigorous efforts to raise the status of medical service in the British Army were made by such men as ROBERT JACKSON (1750–1827), an indomitable Scot who, having literally fought with a Surgeon-General who was opposed to any reform, suffered a term of imprisonment for his rashness, but later rose in prestige in spite of it. Indeed his *Systematic View of the Formation, Discipline, and Economy of Armies* (1804) became a military classic.[1] Besides Sir James McGrigor, to whose work reference has been made, there were other administrators who saw the need for improvement in the medical department of the army. Nevertheless, when the Crimean War broke out in 1854, there was no organized medical corps. Each medical officer wore the uniform of the regiment to which he was attached. Some purchased their commissions ; some also purchased combatant commissions, and drew pay from both appointments. A few were posted for duty in general hospitals, but they remained subsidiary to the fighting

[1] H. H. Scott, *A History of Tropical Medicine*, 2 vols., 1939, vol. i. p. 43 ; J. D. Comrie, *History of Scottish Medicine*, 2 vols., 1932, vol. ii. p. 746

ranks, and even the Director-General could exercise little authority. There were also " Apothecaries to the Forces," who had been chemists in civil life, in charge of medical stores and equipment. In the Crimea, the need for reform became more clamant. The hospitals were still civil organizations. There were no army nurses; most of the orderlies were pensioners employed for this duty.

The first attempt to improve matters consisted in recruiting strong men for the work in place of the feeble old pensioners, many of whom were unfit to bear a stretcher. The orderlies were formed into what was called the " Medical Staff Corps." They were, however, men of scant education, they had received no special training, and had no officers of their own. The scheme was therefore doomed to failure from the first.

It was at this stage that FLORENCE NIGHTINGALE (1820–1910) took the law into her own hands and introduced women nurses into the hospital at Scutari.[1] All the world is familiar with the story of " The Lady with the Lamp," of her victorious return to England, and of the fund raised in her honour to endow a school for nurses at St. Thomas's Hospital. This was opened in 1860, and it was followed by many other similar schools.[2] Although Florence Nightingale did her great work before the antiseptic era, she revolutionized nursing, and her little handbook, *Notes on Nursing*, is still well worth reading. (See Supplement, page 461.)

To return to the main theme, it was not until after the Crimean War in 1857 that there came into being an " Army Hospital Corps " of specially trained n.c.o.'s and men, with officers, who were not, however, medical men, but who had been detailed for this duty from various regiments.

In 1873 this regimental system was abolished, and the corps became consolidated under its own officers. A further step, in 1884, was the important decision that the corps should be commanded by medical officers, the former name of " Medical Staff Corps " being revived. Eventually, in 1898, came the red-letter day, when a royal warrant of Queen Victoria inaugurated the " Royal Army Medical Corps," having all the usual army ranks and titles, and its own uniform, with the badge bearing the motto, " In arduis fidelis." [3]

[1] Sir E. T. Cook, *The Life of Florence Nightingale*, 2 vols., 1913
[2] L. R. Seymer, *A General History of Nursing*, 1932 ; M. A. Nutting and L. E. Dock, *History of Nursing*, 4 vols., New York, 1907–12 ; Victor Robinson, *White Caps, the Story of Nursing*, Philadelphia, 1946
[3] Col. Fred Smith, *A Short History of the Royal Army Medical Corps*, Aldershot, 1929

The Royal Army Medical College, for the special instruction of officers of the corps, was opened in 1902, and in the same year the auxiliary medical services were included in the corps.

When the Great War broke out in 1914, the strength of the R.A.M.C. in all ranks was 9,000. Then, for the first time in history, the entire medical profession of the country was placed at the disposal of the army, so that by the end of the war in 1918 the total strength of the corps had increased to 133,000. No less than 743 officers and 6,130 other ranks of the R.A.M.C. gave their lives in the Great War.[1] In that war, as never before, the supreme importance of a fully trained and efficient medical service was proved on many occasions.

Preventive Medicine in the Army

It has been truly said that in war the prevention of disease is infinitely more important than the actual treatment of the sick and wounded. In 1817 the mortality rate in the British Army in India was as high as eighty-seven per thousand, and there was little or no reduction of this figure during the greater part of the nineteenth century.[2] Nevertheless, the five-year period 1907–11 showed an average mortality rate of only six per thousand. Much was accomplished by improved hygiene, and by increased knowledge of the causes of disease.

During the South African War of 1899–1902 typhoid fever was a more formidable foe than the enemy, and accounted for twice as many deaths as his weapons. In the Great War typhoid fever was relatively rare, and even in the most unhealthy centre, that of Gallipoli, the incidence was very small and the enormous improvement was almost entirely due to the success of anti-typhoid inoculation. This happy result may be traced to the efforts of Sir ALMROTH WRIGHT (1861–1947), a leading pioneer in bacteriology and the discoverer of preventive inoculation. Along with his pupils and co-workers he devised a system of inoculation against typhoid, and eventually there was prepared a vaccine from a triple source, potent against the organisms of typhoid, para-typhoid A and para-typhoid B, which proved highly satisfactory in the Great War, preventing any serious epidemic and saving many lives.

[1] Lt.-Col. F. S. Brereton, *The Great War and the R.A.M.C.*, 1919
[2] Arnold Chaplin, " The Rate of Mortality in the British Army a Hundred Years Ago," *Proc. Roy. Soc. Med.* (Sect. Hist.), 1916, vol. ix., Pt. 2, p. 89

Wright's successor as Professor of Pathology in the Army Medical College at Netley was Sir WILLIAM BOOG LEISHMAN [1] (1865–1926), a medical graduate of Glasgow. Early in his career he had devised a simple method of staining the malarial parasite, and he also made original observations into the cause of kala-azar or dum-dum fever, now known as Leishmaniasis, which was associated with a heavy death-rate. Leishman became Director-General two years before his untimely death at the age of sixty-one.

The Surgery of Modern Warfare

It is interesting to read the accounts of various campaigns which have been written by military surgeons who took part in them. The graphic descriptions by Ambroise Paré show clearly the nature of gun-shot wounds in his day. The writings of Larrey, of Guthrie, and of Ballingall show clearly how dreadful must have been the terror of the battlefield in those early days. The introduction of antiseptics and anaesthetics, together with the earlier treatment afforded by " field hospitals " in the South African war, and by " casualty clearing stations " in the Great War, considerably lessened the suffering of the wounded. Wholesale amputation was no longer practised.

Three contemporary accounts of this new era in military surgery may now be mentioned, as they are well worth reading.

The American Civil War produced a historian in the person of GEORGE ALEXANDER OTIS (1830–81), who saw much active service. In 1870 he published the first volume of his *Medical and Surgical History of the War of the Rebellion*. A second volume appeared in 1876, and a third after the death of the writer.

Sir THOMAS LONGMORE (1816–95), a Deputy Director-General, wrote an excellent work on *Gun-shot Injuries* in 1877. It is interesting to note that a large part of the volume is devoted to a description of various instruments for the location and removal of bullets.

Even during the South African War the rifle remained the chief lethal weapon.[2] Sir GEORGE MAKINS (1853–1934), surgeon to St. Thomas's Hospital, London, related his surgical experiences in South Africa, his book being " mainly a clinical study of the nature and effects of injuries produced by bullets of small calibre."[3]

On the outbreak of the Great War, however, the Army

[1] H. H. Scott, *A History of Tropical Medicine*, 2 vols., 1939, vol. ii., p. 1058
[2] Col. W. F. Stevenson, *Wounds in War*, 1897
[3] Sir G. Makins, *Surgical Experiences in South Africa*, 1901

Medical Department was faced with new and difficult problems occasioned by new weapons and new methods of warfare. Deaths from wounds now exceeded those from sickness, and the injuries produced by shell-fire were much more dreadful than those caused by bullets. New modes of treatment were devised to meet the demand. New antiseptics, such as flavine and various dyes, were tried, and continuous irrigation of wounds with sodium hypochlorite solution by the Carrel-Dakin technique was introduced, as also was the procedure of excising wounds or removing the bruised and torn edges by " débridement." Team work and specialism, which had proved of value in civilian practice, were now adopted in military hospitals. The issue of steel helmets reduced the proportion of head injuries, and the menace of tetanus and gas gangrene was met by preventive inoculation, while a similar procedure reduced to a minimum the danger of typhoid fever. The new type of " trench warfare " in France brought its own peculiar afflictions, such as trench nephritis, trench fever, and trench foot, although the last-mentioned had been previously described by Larrey. The end of the Great War in 1918 was marked by a world-wide epidemic of influenza, which caused many thousands of deaths, and taxed to the utmost the resources of the medical profession.

During the period " between the wars," medicine and surgery continued to advance, but other new methods of destroying human life were also invented, so that at the commencement of the greatest conflict in history mankind was confronted with a form of warfare not only highly mechanized, but also " total," in the sense that every man, woman, and child was potentially in the front line of battle. The possibility that noxious gases might be used led to a study of suitable defensive measures. New and more deadly explosives in aerial bombs gave rise to " blast " injuries of a nature previously unknown, while vast developments in aviation created new problems relating to the health and efficiency of Air Force personnel. Facilities for blood transfusion were organized on a large scale. The sulphonamide treatment of septic infections, medical and surgical, the closed plaster method of treating compound fractures, the application of psychological tests in the assessment of fitness for service, the discovery of penicillin ; these are only a few of the advances in medical science which have appeared in time of war, and which have become adapted to the needs of peace.

Medicine and Surgery in the Navy

Much of what has been said regarding the evolution of military medicine and surgery may be applied to the navy, as the two services, together with the more modern Air Force, are now so closely associated that many medical problems of to-day apply to all three services.

In the days of sailing ships the navy was confronted with difficulties of its own, and the voice of the medical reformer was that of one " crying in the wilderness." Attention has already been drawn (p. 233) to the trying conditions under which seafaring men lived and worked in those early days. One need only read the vivid descriptions of life in the navy in the pages of *Roderick Random* to be convinced of the hardships, most of them needless and preventible, which shortened the career of many a sailor.[1] TOBIAS SMOLLETT (1721–71) had been a surgeon's mate, and knew his topic from sad personal experience.

It is true that James Lind had already brought about some improvement ; his name must remain pre-eminent in the annals of naval medicine. Two of his immediate followers are worthy of attention, Gilbert Blane and Thomas Trotter.

Sir GILBERT BLANE (1749–1834), a native of Ayrshire and of well-to-do parentage, studied in Edinburgh, graduated M.D. at Glasgow, and then, through the influence of William Hunter, whose lectures he attended in London, was appointed personal physician to Admiral Sir George Rodney.[2] Accompanying the Admiral to raise the siege of Gibraltar in 1779, Blane so distinguished himself that he was appointed Physician to the Fleet. After further active service in the West Indies, he returned to London in 1783, and setting up in practice as a physician, was appointed to the staff of St. Thomas's Hospital. Nevertheless, he had now so high a reputation in the navy that throughout his life he was frequently consulted by the Government on matters concerning public health, and in particular the health of the navy. Although James Lind had in 1753 (p. 233) advised the use of fresh fruit and vegetables for the prevention of scurvy, the system was not officially adopted until Blane was in a position to enforce

---

[1] E. Ashworth Underwood, " Medicine and Science in the Writings of Smollett," *Proc. Roy. Soc. Med.*, 1937, vol. xxx. p. 25 ; C. R. Drinker, " Doctor Smollett," *Ann. Med. Hist.*, 1925, vol. vii. p. 31
[2] Sir Humphry D. Rolleston, " Sir Gilbert Blane, M.D., F.R.S.," *Jour. Roy. Nav. Med. Ser.*, 1916, vol. ii. p. 72

it in 1796, and in doing so he gave Lind full credit for his efforts. When the new regulation came into force, scurvy at once disappeared from the official returns.[1] Previous to that date, the diseases of seamen appeared to fall into four categories : fever, fluxes, scurvy, and other complaints. This we learn from Sir Gilbert Blane's *Observations on the Diseases Incident to Seamen*, 1785. The navy of that time (1781) showed a sickness rate of one man in fifteen, and a death rate of one in seven among the sick.

Blane outlined a plan for the better ventilation and cleansing of ships. He advised, besides fruit and vegetables, the use of wine in place of rum, or " the diluted rum, known as grog " ; he urged that soap should be supplied to the men, " in the same manner as tobacco and slops," and that drugs and medical stores, which up to that time had been provided by the surgeon himself, should be supplied at public charge. He also favoured the use of hospital ships, to take the place of shore hospitals, which were apt to be dreadfully overcrowded. Blane was made a baronet in 1812, and he received many other honours for his public services. His manner was somewhat austere, which accounted for his nickname of " Chilblain " among flippant colleagues. He has been justly termed " The Father of Naval Medical Science."

Blane had a colleague and contemporary, a fellow Scot, whose energy in promoting reform was no less energetic than his own. No meteoric rise to power marked the career of THOMAS TROTTER (1760–1832).[2] Born at Melrose, he studied at Edinburgh, and entered the navy as surgeon's mate in 1779, gradually rising to become Physician to the Channel Fleet in 1794. He retired from the navy in 1802, and practised in Newcastle until a few years before his death.

Trotter was a prolific writer on many subjects, and he was a far-seeing and clear-headed reformer, although, according to Sir Humphry Rolleston, he was one of those "who have striven and deserved, but have not attained success as ordinarily estimated." His best known work is *Medicina Nautica*, 1797–1803, in three volumes, a sort of encyclopaedia of naval medicine. In dealing with scurvy Trotter took the view that crystallized citric acid was better than preserved lemon juice, a view which has been shared by others since his time. He urged that the war against scurvy,

---

[1] R. S. Allison, *Sea Diseases. The Story of a Great Natural Experiment in Preventive Medicine in the Royal Navy*, 1943, p. 192

[2] Sir Humphry D. Rolleston, " Thomas Trotter, M.D.," *Jour. Roy. Nav. Med. Serv.*, 1919, vol. v. p. 412

so successful in the navy, should be extended to the mercantile marine. He insistently demanded that the pay of seamen should be raised to a level corresponding to that of soldiers, and he proposed that seamen should be supplied with uniform. (This was not done until 1857.) On the introduction of vaccination in 1798 he urged its advantages to the navy, although his advice was not taken until 1858, and in 1801 he inspired a number of naval surgeons to present Edward Jenner with a gold medal. Trotter's advocacy of better hygienic conditions, higher pay, and better food for seamen should ever be remembered in the annals of naval medicine.

The first Medical Director-General of the Royal Navy was another Scotsman, Sir WILLIAM BURNETT (1779–1861).[1] Joining the navy at an early age, he served with distinction in a series of naval engagements, including the Battle of Trafalgar. His efficiency and zeal led to rapid promotion. After having been knighted in 1831, he became sole Medical Commissioner to the Admiralty, later he was appointed Physician-General, a title which was changed to Inspector-General of Hospitals and Fleets, and finally, in 1844, to Director-General of the Medical Department of the Navy. An able administrator, he founded the libraries and museums at the two great naval hospitals, Haslar and Plymouth. His chief contribution to medical literature was *A Practical Account of the Mediterranean Fever* (1814), a fever which he regarded as miasmic in origin, writing, as he did, long before the discovery of Micrococcus Melitensis. Burnett's name is also associated with a disinfecting fluid, of which zinc chloride was the main ingredient, which was used on a large scale even in recent years.

The greatest medical pioneer of the American Navy was EDWARD CUTBUSH (1772–1843), who was also the first American writer on naval medicine.[2] His *Observations on the Means of Preserving the Health of Soldiers and Sailors* appeared in 1808. It is a compact and common-sense little book, useful even to the naval surgeon to-day.

Medical Men as Explorers

Since early times a number of naval surgeons have distinguished themselves as naturalists and explorers.

[1] Sir Humphry D. Rolleston, " Sir William Burnett. The First Medical Director-General of the Royal Navy," *Jour. Roy. Nav. Med. Serv.*, 1922, vol. viii. p. 1
[2] L. H. Roddis, *A Short History of Nautical Medicine*, New York, 1941, p. 181

Sir JOHN RICHARDSON (1787–1865), who was born at Dumfries and who died at Grasmere, served in the naval medical service for forty-eight years.[1] He saw a good deal of active service afloat, but the chief interest of his career was in his close association with Sir John Franklin, the Arctic explorer.

As surgeon and naturalist he took part in three Arctic expeditions, twice with Franklin, and then in the futile search for Franklin. The assistant surgeon who had accompanied Franklin on his last voyage (in 1845) was Harry Goodsir, a brother of John Goodsir, the anatomist (p. 271). The zoological collections of the first two voyages formed the subject of Richardson's great four-volume work, *Fauna Boreali-Americana*. From 1838 to 1855 he was physician to Haslar Hospital. In 1848 he led the expedition which spent almost two years in a fruitless quest for Franklin. Richardson passed the last ten years of his life in retirement at Grasmere, steadily engaged in literary work and in scientific study. Among his pupils at Haslar were many distinguished men, including Sir JOSEPH DALTON HOOKER (1817–1911), who succeeded his father, Sir William Hooker, as Director of the Royal Gardens at Kew, and THOMAS HENRY HUXLEY (1825–95),[2] who commenced his distinguished career as a zoologist by acting as surgeon and naturalist aboard H.M.S. *Rattlesnake* (Captain Owen Stanley), on a three years' survey of the sea between Australia and the Great Barrier Reef.

Incidentally, it is of interest to note that CHARLES DARWIN (1809–82), whose views were strongly supported by Huxley, and who, though not himself a medical man, profoundly influenced the trend of medicine by his work, *The Origin of Species*, 1859, also inaugurated his life work by a voyage of five years in southern waters as naturalist to the expedition of H.M.S. *Beagle* (Captain Fitzroy.)[3]

Many other naval surgeons have distinguished themselves as explorers, especially of the polar regions. ELISHA KENT KANE (1820–57), an American naval surgeon, set sail in the *Advance*

[1] Rev. J. McIlraith, *Life of Sir John Richardson, C.B., LL.D., F.R.S.*, 1868 ; Sir Humphry D. Rolleston, " Sir John Richardson, C.B., M.D., LL.D., F.R.S.," *Jour. Roy. Nav. Med. Serv.*, 1924, vol. x. p. 161
[2] J. R. Ainsworth Davis, *Thomas H. Huxley* (English Men of Science), 1907 ; Julian Huxley, ed. of T. H. Huxley's *Diary of the Voyage of H.M.S. Rattlesnake*, 1935
[3] N. Barlow, ed. of Charles Darwin's *Diary of the Voyage of H.M.S. Beagle*, Cambridge, 1933

in 1853 in an attempt to find Franklin, returning thirty months later after terrible hardships. Kane had been farther north than any previous explorer, and had charted a thousand miles of new sea coast.

A British naval surgeon, GEORGE BASS (1771–1803), whose name is closely linked with that of his friend Matthew Flinders, both hailing from Lincolnshire, sailed to Australia aboard H.M.S. *Reliance*, explored part of the coast of New South Wales in the *Tom Thumb*, a tiny eight-foot craft, and then extended his survey southwards in a whale boat with a crew of six, mapping six hundred miles of coast, and proving that Tasmania was not part of Australia, but was separated by the strait now known as Bass Strait.[1] In a later voyage Bass and Flinders circumnavigated Tasmania. Bass then set off on a voyage to South America in a trading ship of his own, which disappeared with all hands.

In more recent times JEAN CHARCOT (1867–1936), son of the famous neurologist, and himself a neurologist for a time, became the leader of two expeditions to the Antarctic. He explored North Polar regions as well ; on the last voyage his vessel, the *Pourquoi Pas ?* sank near Iceland and all were drowned.

A final naval surgeon to be honoured as an explorer, although only a small selection has been made from the long list, is EDWARD ADRIAN WILSON (1872–1912), surgeon, naturalist, and artist, who accompanied Captain Scott in the *Discovery* in 1901, and in the *Terra Nova* in 1910. The epic story of the second and last expedition is familiar to everyone. *Edward Wilson of the Antarctic*, by George Seaver, is a fascinating work, which ranks high among medical biographies of modern times.[2] Wilson was a noble and saintly figure.

A few words may here be added regarding a few of the many medical men who have explored on land. It must suffice to select two, the scene of whose labours was " The Dark Continent," although the list might be widely extended to include medical explorers of nearly every part of the world.

MUNGO PARK (1771–1806), after a voyage to Sumatra as ship's surgeon, offered his services to the African Association, which had been formed to develop trade in West Africa. Accompanied

[1] Laurence Duncan, " Medical Men as Explorers," *Med. Jour. of Austral.*, 1938, vol. xxv. p. 875 ; H. M. Bowden, *George Bass, 1771–1803*, 1952
[2] G. Seaver, *Edward Wilson of the Antarctic*, 1933

only by two natives, he spent over two years in searching for the source of the River Niger.[1] Although he did not attain this object, he collected much valuable information, and in 1799 he published an account of his travels. On his return he practised medicine for six years at Peebles, where he was the friend of Sir Walter Scott, and he may have been the prototype of Gideon Gray in *The Surgeon's Daughter*. Nevertheless, the life of a country practitioner did not attract him, and in 1805 he sailed again for Africa with other forty-four Europeans in order to continue the exploration of the Niger. Only five of the party remained alive when the river was reached, and all were drowned in the rapids while escaping from hostile natives, news of the disaster reaching England some five years later.

Another medical explorer of undying fame was DAVID LIVING-STONE (1813–73), who commenced his working life as a mill worker in Blantyre, near Glasgow.[2] Being determined to become a medical missionary, he qualified in 1840 and offered his services to the London Missionary Society. His exploration of the Zambesi, his discovery of the Victoria Falls, his efforts to track the sources of the Nile, his disappearance for years in the heart of Africa, his meeting with H. M. Stanley, who had been sent to find him, his death at Chitambo's village, and his burial in Westminster Abbey, are facts which build up a familiar and inspiring story. In his *Missionary Travels and Researches in South Africa* (1857), Livingstone gives an account of the tsetse fly, and of the diseases of horses and cattle, resulting from its bite, although as yet the trypanosome carried by the fly was undiscovered. Livingstone was the first to administer arsenic to horses as a remedy for the disease known as " nagana."

No one has done more for African geography than this missionary explorer during his thirty years of service. His wonderful record inspired other explorers, but he was greater than any of them, almost worshipped by natives, and respected even by Arab slave traders. His simple motto was, " Fear God and work hard."

---

[1] Joseph Thomson, *Mungo Park and the Niger*, 1890 ; Lewis Grassic Gibbon, *Niger : The Life of Mungo Park*, 1934
[2] W. G. Blaikie, *The Personal Life of David Livingstone*, 1880

The Conquest of Tropical Disease

A century ago life in the tropics was full of danger. The diseases peculiar to warm countries were ill understood, and the means of preventing them, now familiar to all, were then unknown. The story of the gradual discovery of the cause and cure of certain tropical diseases is curious and romantic, fully proving the contention that truth is stranger than fiction.

It is, however, a lengthy and intricate tale, and it must suffice, for the purposes of the present work, to sketch in broad outline the main discoveries, and to glance at the lives of a few of the distinguished men who blazed the trail. It may also be advisable to confine our attention to three of the main scourges of the tropics—malaria, yellow fever, and sleeping sickness.

Malaria has been known since ancient times (p. 83), and was once much more widespread than it is to-day. It was prevalent in England in Sydenham's day, and even in the nineteenth century " marsh fever " was still to be found in the fens of Cambridgeshire and Lincolnshire, and in certain other districts. The name " malaria " is derived from the view of its origin which was held for centuries. A synonym was " paludism," which expressed the same idea, namely, that the disease was caused by noxious air arising from marshy land.

Various observers had noted " particles of pigment " in the blood of patients suffering from malaria, but it was not until 1880 that ALPHONSE LAVERAN (1845–1922), a young medical officer of the French Army stationed in Algeria, discovered the parasite in the blood corpuscles, and noted, first, the little circular body, then, the increase of pigment, and finally, the extrusion of wavy, thread-like flagellae, or " oscillaria " as he called them.[1] For centuries there had been a vague idea that insects played some part in transmitting malaria and other diseases. The first definite proof of a relationship between insects and tropical disease was supplied by Sir PATRICK MANSON [2] (1844–1922), a graduate of Aberdeen University who spent twenty-four years in China, first in Formosa and Amoy, and then in Hong Kong, where he demonstrated, in 1877, how the embryos of the minute worm known as filaria, the cause of elephantiasis and other lesions, were taken at night from human blood by the culex mosquito, developed within the body

[1] H. H. Scott, *A History of Tropical Medicine*, 2 vols., 1939, vol. i. p. 151
[2] P. Manson-Bahr and A. Alcock, *The Life and Work of Sir Patrick Manson*, 1927

of the insect, and were transmitted when another human subject was bitten. Manson's paper on the subject, published in the *Transactions* of the Linnean Society in 1879, was received with incredulity, but on his retirement from practice in Hong Kong a few years later he resumed his researches in London, where he was employed as Medical Adviser to the Colonial Office. He founded the London School of Tropical Medicine in 1897, and there he worked almost to the end of his life.

It was in 1894 that Manson met the young doctor who became Sir RONALD ROSS (1857–1932), then on leave from India, and showed him the parasite of malaria in the blood. By this time a number of observers, notably in Italy, had confirmed Laveran's discovery. CAMILLO GOLGI (1844–1926), who was also celebrated for his studies in the histology of the nervous system, had noted the difference between the parasites of tertian fever and those of quartan fever, and had observed that the stage of sporulation corresponded to that of the malarial rigor (p. 371).

Manson believed that the extrusion of flagellae, which took place after the blood had been withdrawn from the human body, was " a natural organic process in the life history of the parasite, with a view to its further development in some suctorial insect." He explained his views to Ross, who attacked the problem with enthusiasm.[1] Eventually, on August 20, 1897, Ross discovered the malarial parasite in the stomach of the spotted-winged mosquito, anopheles, which, as proved in the following year by another ardent worker, GIOVANNI GRASSI of Rome (1854–1925), was the only genus capable of transmitting malaria.

Gradually, the life cycle of the parasite in man and mosquito was clearly traced, and the conclusive evidence was supplied by Manson in 1900, when infected mosquitoes sent from Italy to London were allowed to bite a healthy young man, Manson's son, who developed malaria, and when three of Manson's assistants lived in perfect health throughout the malaria season in a mosquito-proof hut in the Roman Campagna.[2] Since that day, mosquito control, by the destruction of mosquitoes and mosquito larvae, the drainage of marshes, the screening of dwellings, and the distribution of quinine and specific synthetic drugs, has achieved wonderful results, although the problem of malaria is by no means fully solved.

[1] R. L. Megroz, *Ronald Ross, Discoverer and Creator*, 1931
[2] Sir W. Hale-White, *Great Doctors of the Nineteenth Century*, 1935, p. 290

CONQUEST OF TROPICAL DISEASES

Yellow Fever, another deadly disease of the tropics, was at one time very prevalent in West Africa, in the West Indies, and South America.[1] Coleridge, in his *Ancient Mariner*, describes a ship smitten by the disease, a tale often paralleled in actual history. Yellow fever is caused by an ultra-microscopic virus, of which the urban form is transmitted by the striped or tiger mosquito known as stegomyia or aëdes, the rural form by other mosquitoes. In former times it was confused with malaria.

In 1881 CARLOS FINLAY of Cuba (1833–1915), expressed his belief that yellow fever was transmitted by the stegomyia mosquito, although he had no definite evidence in support of his theory.[2]

Another noteworthy name in the history of yellow fever is that of WALTER REED (1851–1902).[3] Reed was a young army surgeon with a keen interest in bacteriology who had studied under Professor William H. Welch of Baltimore, and who was sent to Havana in 1900 as director of a Yellow Fever Commission. Along with two other bacteriologists from Baltimore, JAMES CARROLL (1854–1907), who was second in command under Reed, and JESSE LAZEAR (1866–1900), who had already been working in Cuba, the commission set to work with the co-operation of Carlos Finlay. Carroll acquired yellow fever after allowing himself to be bitten by an infected mosquito. He recovered, but Lazear, who was also bitten by a stegomyia mosquito, died of yellow fever after a few days' illness. Thus it became proved that infected mosquitoes could transmit yellow fever. Reed continued the work, and recommended preventive measures which were so successful that Havana was free from the scourge within a year.

Another name in the story of the campaign against yellow fever is that of HIDEYO NOGUCHI (1876–1928), who, like Lazear, fell a victim to the disease. This brilliant investigator, of Japanese birth and a pupil of Kitasato, who had already done good work at the Rockefeller Institute, was studying yellow fever at Accra, West Africa, when he succumbed,[4] as also did his colleagues, ADRIAN STOKES and W. A. YOUNG. A brilliant member of the Liverpool School of Tropical Medicine was WALTER MYERS (1872–1901), who died of yellow fever while investigating the disease at Pará.

No reference to the history of yellow fever is complete with-

[1] H. H. Scott, *A History of Tropical Medicine*, 2 vols., 1939, vol. i. p. 279
[2] F. Dominguez, *Docteur Carlos J. Finlay*, Paris, 1935
[3] Howard H. Kelly, *Walter Reed and Yellow Fever*, New York, 1906 ; A. E. Truby, *Memoir of Walter Reed : The Yellow Fever Episode*, New York, 1943
[4] G. Eckstein, *Noguchi*, New York, 1931

out some mention of the work of WILLIAM CRAWFORD GORGAS (1854–1920).[1] His introduction to yellow fever was personal, as he was himself attacked by the disease while acting as an army surgeon in Texas in the early days of his career. He became chief sanitary officer in Havana, where it was his duty to apply the means of prevention which had been recommended by Walter Reed, and which proved so highly successful. Part of the plan adopted by Gorgas was to isolate every case of yellow fever in a mosquito-proof room, and to institute a very thorough anti-stegomyia campaign. The name of Gorgas is chiefly remembered, however, for his work in rendering habitable the deadly Panama Canal zone.

Ferdinand de Lesseps, the great French diplomat, who had so successfully completed the Suez Canal, addressed himself to a similar task of canal construction at Panama in 1880. Nevertheless, after eight years, the work was abandoned, largely on account of the unhealthy conditions which prevailed. Malaria and yellow fever had produced a death rate of 176 per thousand. In 1904 the Americans assumed control, with Colonel Gorgas in charge of the medical department.[2] Even then Gorgas had a hard fight to convince the authorities that it was not filth, but the mosquito, which spread most of the disease. Undeterred, he applied the measures which had proved so effective in Cuba. Support was forthcoming ; sanitary brigades were organized on a large scale. Within a few years the death rate was greatly reduced. The last fatal case of yellow fever occurred in 1906, and by 1914, when the canal was completed, the Panama Canal Zone showed a general death rate of only six per thousand, as compared with fourteen per thousand in the United States, and fifteen per thousand in London.[3]

Gorgas did splendid work in organizing the army medical service of America during the Great War. He retained his energy to the end of his life, and even in 1920, at the age of sixty-six, when he attended an International Congress of Hygiene in London, he was preparing to sail for the Congo to investigate a yellow fever epidemic when he was taken ill, and died after a few days' illness.

[1] M. D. Gorgas and B. J. Hendrick, *William Crawford Gorgas : His Life and Work*, Philadelphia, 1924
[2] C. M. Wilson, *Ambassadors in White*, New York, 1942 (a history of the conquest of tropical disease and especially yellow fever)
[3] H. H. Scott, *A History of Tropical Medicine*, 2 vols., 1939, vol. ii. p. 979

Sleeping Sickness, or Trypanosomiasis, need only be briefly mentioned. The disease had been known in Africa for many years, and towards the end of the nineteenth century it reached epidemic proportions, apparently as the result of the extension of trade routes and increased facilities of travel. The fly disease of cattle, or nagana, was also well known and widespread. Livingstone, in his *Travels,* refers to a fly called tsetse (*Glossina morsitans*) which was very " fatal to horses and cattle, and a barrier to progress " (p. 356).

In 1894 Sir DAVID BRUCE (1855–1931), an army medical officer and an Edinburgh graduate who had already won a reputation for his investigations on Malta or Mediterranean fever, arrived in Natal to investigate nagana, and discovered in the blood of all the affected animals a protozoal parasite or trypanosome, which came to be known as *Trypanosoma brucei.*[1] Assisted in all his researches by his wife, to whose work he paid high tribute, Bruce showed that this trypanosome was conveyed by the bite of the tsetse fly. Next, a trypanosome was found in human blood in 1901 by JOSEPH EVERETT DUTTON (1874–1905), who was working in Gambia, and who named the parasite *Trypanosoma gambiense.* Dutton unfortunately died four years later, of tick-borne relapsing fever, which he was investigating on the Congo. To return to the story of Bruce, he and his wife arrived in Uganda in 1903 in order to assist in the solution of the sleeping sickness problem. Together with Aldo Castellani, E. D. W. Greig, D. Nabarro, and others, Bruce confirmed Castellani's discovery of trypanosomes in the cerebro-spinal fluid of sleeping sickness patients. Subsequently Bruce found trypanosomes also in the blood. Profiting by his studies and discoveries on nagana, he showed that the tsetse fly was the carrier, that Europeans as well as natives are susceptible to sleeping sickness, and that the spread of the disease might be limited by the destruction of flies and their breeding places, and by checking the movements of infected natives.

The fly, he concluded, was a simple carrier, and there was no complex life cycle of the parasite as in malaria. This view was modified later by the work of Klein.

Thanks to the labours of Bruce and his followers, and to chemotherapy, sleeping sickness is no longer a major scourge in Africa.

Into the further history of sleeping sickness, the means of

[1] H. H. Scott, *A History of Tropical Medicine,* 2 vols., 1939, vol. ii. p. 1018

treatment, the possibility of big game acting as a " reservoir " for the parasites, and other problems still unsolved, it is not proposed to enter. Nor need the story of tropical pathology be pursued further, as sufficient has been said to indicate its importance and its place in medical history.

BOOKS FOR FURTHER READING

ALLISON, R. S. *Sea Diseases. The Story of a Great Natural Experiment in Preventive Medicine in the Royal Navy*, 1943
BLAIKIE, W. B. *The Personal Life of David Livingstone*, 1880
BRERETON, Lt.-Col. F. S. *The Great War and the R.A.M.C.*, 1919
COOK, Sir E. T. *The Life of Florence Nightingale*, 2 vols., 1913
DAVIS, J. AINSWORTH. *Thomas H. Huxley* (English Men of Science), 1907
GORGAS, M. D., and HENDRICK, B. J. *William Crawford Gorgas : His Life and Work*, Philadelphia, 1924
KELLY, HOWARD H. *Walter Reed and Yellow Fever*, New York, 1906
LARREY, BARON. *Mémoires de Chirurgie militaire et Campagnes*, 3 vols., Paris, 1812
MAKINS, Sir GEORGE. *Surgical Experiences in South Africa*, 1901
MANSON-BAHR, P., and ALCOCK, A. *The Life and Work of Sir Patrick Manson*, 1927
MEGROZ, R. L. *Ronald Ross, Discoverer and Creator*, 1931
RODDIS, L. H. *A Short History of Nautical Medicine*, New York, 1941
SCOTT, Sir H. H. *A History of Tropical Medicine*, 2 vols., 1939
SEAVER, G. *Edward Wilson of the Antarctic*, 1933
SMITH, Col. FRED. *A Short History of the Royal Army Medical Corps*, Aldershot, 1929
THOMSON, JOSEPH. *Mungo Park and the Niger*, 1890

CHAPTER XIX

THE RISE OF SPECIALISM AND OF PREVENTIVE MEDICINE

THE field of the historian steadily extends from day to day. Deeds and discoveries of our time will be found in works on history, not yet written, which will be read by our children and our grandchildren. Nevertheless the events of to-day, and indeed all events within living memory, do not immediately fall into their places in the epic of history. Some are ephemeral, perhaps important to-day, yet forgotten to-morrow. Others, which appear to be of no moment in our eyes, may prove to be of supreme value to the next generation. Thus, one of the difficulties of presenting history is that of deciding at what point the narrative should cease, or rather should be allowed to merge into what may be termed present-day knowledge. Perhaps the most logical solution of the problem, so far, at least, as biography is concerned, is to refrain from mentioning the name of anyone, however distinguished, who is fortunately still with us. As for the spectacular medical discoveries of recent times, these are so well known that it would be superfluous to include them in this history.

The full story of hormones, vitamins, insulin, sulphonamides, viruses, penicillin, and a host of other familiar discoveries must be told in the future, when their integration into the general concept of medical science is complete.

In the meantime, however, our narrative of the march of medicine down the ages must include two important trends of recent years—Specialism and Preventive Medicine. Those two lines, along which modern medicine has advanced and is still advancing, are not divergent branches of progress. The need of rendering available to the public the benefits of specialized medicine has brought about an enlargement of all that is implied in the term, "preventive medicine," which is no longer merely public hygiene, still less sanitation, though it passed through those phases. Conversely, preventive medicine is itself a special branch of medicine, and it is now in the hands of specialists, who have accepted the enormous responsibility of guiding and directing the entire medical profession in its efforts to serve the community.

Specialization in Medicine

Medicine and surgery have become so highly specialized in recent years that the old-fashioned " general " physician or general surgeon may hardly be said to exist, although, of course, the general practitioner remains the backbone of the medical profession. Obstetrics pursues its even way, as it was a specialty from the first and remains so.

Whether the subdivisions of medicine and surgery are a sign of advance and evidence of progress need not be discussed here. There are some who deplore it as a decadent trait, and advise a return to Hippocratic methods, with the patient more definitely in the centre of the picture. In this chapter, however, it is proposed merely to record the appearance of specialism in the nineteenth century, and its growth up to the present time, taking as examples a few of the lines which it has followed.

The dividing of surgery into various sections has already been discussed in a previous chapter. In medicine this tendency was probably more gradual and less obvious. Nevertheless, it appeared among some of the greatest physicians during that period of intense activity about the middle of the nineteenth century. It was then that neurology became a distinct branch of medicine ; psychiatry received a powerful stimulus from the development of the new psychology ; cardiology arose out of physiology ; diseases of metabolism were elucidated by the growth of bio-chemistry ; pediatrics became no longer a mere side-line of general medicine.

Disorders of Metabolism

The special study of *Diseases of Metabolism* was greatly assisted by the researches of Liebig (p. 276) and others in what was called chemical physiology. One of the pioneers on the clinical side was BERNHARD NAUNYN (1839–1925), an assistant of Frerichs at Berlin, who eventually succeeded Kussmaul at Strassburg (p. 299). The history of diabetes may be traced back to the time of Aretaeus (p. 71), who first named the disease, and to Thomas Willis (p. 200), who noted the presence of sugar in the urine. Applying the new chemical knowledge, Naunyn carried the work a stage further, and published his results in 1898 in an important monograph, *Der Diabetes mellitus.* He was the first, in 1906, to note the formation of acid in diabetic coma, to which he applied the term

" acidosis," a word now so widely used. Naunyn wrote an attractive autobiography which appeared in the year he died.[1]

CARL VON NOORDEN (1858–1944), who succeeded Nothnagel at Vienna, devoted much attention to the study of diabetes and to the influence of diet on the condition.

In England the leading authority in the field was FREDERICK WILLIAM PAVY (1829–1911), of Guy's Hospital, a pupil of Claude Bernard (p. 279). He sought to show that the excess of sugar obtained by Bernard from the liver was a post-mortem change, and that the part played by the liver in producing sugar from glycogen might be questioned. The entire outlook in diabetes was altered by the discovery of insulin in 1922 by Sir FREDERICK BANTING of Toronto (1891–1941), in conjunction with CHARLES HERBERT BEST (1899–   ) and JOHN JAMES RICKARD MACLEOD (1876–1935). The story of Banting's achievement is admirably told by Professor Lloyd Stevenson (*Sir Frederick Banting*, 1947).

Endocrines and Vitamins

The discovery of "internal secretions," later known as hormones, by Claude Bernard (p. 280) was one of the first steps in the development of the new science of endocrinology, which received a strong stimulus from the work of Sir EDWARD SHARPEY-SCHAFER (1850–1935) of Edinburgh. A further important advance, this time in the science of nutrition, was made in 1906 by Sir FREDERICK GOWLAND HOPKINS (1861–1947), when he showed that nutrition was not merely a question of foods and calories in correct proportions. It was necessary for health that food should contain small quantities of the " necessary food factors," which later came to be known as vitamins.

Diseases of the Heart

Our modern knowledge of *cardiology* was largely the outcome of various researches in physiology and in pharmacology. Among the physiologists was WILHELM HIS (1863–1934), son of the distinguished embryologist of Basel, who became professor at Leipzig, and who noted the myogenic nature of the heart beat ; AUGUSTUS WALLER (1859–1922), a general practitioner of Kensington, London, who recorded the electrical impulses of the heart, an observation which led to the introduction of the electro-

[1] Bernhard Naunyn, *Erinnerungen, Gedanken, und Meinungen*, Munich, 1925

cardiograph ; and WALTER HOLBROOK GASKELL of Cambridge (1847–1914), who studied the nerves of the heart, who was the first to apply the term " heart-block," and who laid the foundation of our modern knowledge of the autonomic nervous system.[1]

The development of cardiology was facilitated also by the work of Sir LAUDER BRUNTON (1844–1916), physician to St. Bartholomew's Hospital, who noted the effect of nitrites in producing vaso-dilatation and in relieving the pain of angina pectoris. This discovery he made while he was a young house physician (1867). Brunton's lectures on *The Action of Medicines* (1897) are still worth reading, as he always sought to apply the lessons of the laboratory to clinical practice.

Sir THOMAS RICHARD FRASER (1841–1920), who succeeded Christison as Professor of Materia Medica in Edinburgh, studied the action of many drugs, including strophanthus, which he preferred to digitalis as a cardiac stimulant. Fraser's successor, ARTHUR ROBERTSON CUSHNY (1866–1926), also studied the action of drugs upon the heart.

The introduction of percussion by Auenbrugger in 1761, and of auscultation with the stethoscope by Laënnec in 1816, tended to focus attention upon such physical aids to diagnosis (p. 258).

A further step was taken when estimation of the blood pressure, with the aid of the sphygmomanometer, was undertaken as a routine procedure by PIERRE CARL POTAIN of Paris (1825–1901). In this country the method was introduced by Sir THOMAS CLIFFORD ALLBUTT (1836–1925), Regius Professor of Medicine at Cambridge, an authority on cardio-vascular disease.[2] He also edited a *System of Medicine*, which enjoyed a wide circulation. He was, moreover, a medical historian of distinction, as was shown by his Fitzpatrick Lectures on " Greek Medicine in Rome " (p. 407). His contemporary at Oxford, Sir William Osler (p. 408), also made original observations on cardiology.

Accurate instrumental methods of recording the pulse, such as the sphygmograph, were gradually applied to clinical practice, after having been mere laboratory apparatus for years. In 1902 Mackenzie invented his polygraph, and recording by its aid the arterial and jugular pulses simultaneously " brought order out of the chaos of cardiac irregularities," showing that certain

[1] F. H. Garrison, " Walter Holbrook Gaskell, 1847–1914," *Brit. Med. Jour.*, 1914, vol. ii. p. 559
[2] Sir Humphry D. Rolleston, *The Life of Sir Clifford Allbutt*, 1929

forms were of little significance, while others betokened grave disease.[1]

Sir JAMES MACKENZIE (1853–1925), founder of a new era in cardiology, was born at Scone, Perthshire, and studied medicine in Edinburgh.[2] For many years he was engaged in general practice in Burnley, Lancashire. Here he applied himself to such problems as the mechanism of pain and the significance of irregularities of the pulse. One of the results of his investigations was to alter the attitude towards abnormal heart sounds (murmurs) and abnormalities of the heart's action, neither of which, he submitted, need be viewed with alarm.[3] The important factor in prognosis was the ability of the heart to react to increased effort ; the condition of the myocardium should be the main guide in forming an opinion as to the outlook. He laid down definite rules for the use of digitalis. Mackenzie was fifty-four years of age when he left Burnley for London, but such was his reputation that he soon acquired a large practice, as well as appointment to the staff of the London Hospital. He died of angina pectoris, a disease which he had done much to elucidate.

In America one of the pioneers in cardiology was AUSTIN FLINT (1812–86) of New York.[4] He was one of the first to use the binaural stethoscope in the diagnosis of cardiac and pulmonary disease, and was the author of many valuable monographs.

Another American physician who, during the Civil War, made a study of functional disease of the heart in soldiers was JACOB DA COSTA of Philadelphia (1833–1900), who had studied under Trousseau in Paris. Da Costa was one of the best teachers of his time, and his treatise on diagnosis was widely appreciated.

Diseases of Children

Pediatrics,[5] as a special branch of medicine, arose from two sources—obstetrics, which comprised diseases of the new-born child, and general medicine, which included the diseases of children who were no longer infants. One of the first to devote his attention to pediatrics in London was CHARLES WEST (1816–1898), he having approached the subject by the gateway of

[1] Sir Humphry D. Rolleston, *Cardio-vascular Diseases since Harvey's Discovery* (Harveian Oration), 1928, p. 105
[2] R. McNair Wilson, *The Beloved Physician : The Life of Sir James Mackenzie*, 1926
[3] James Mackenzie, *Diseases of the Heart*, 1908
[4] J. B. Herrick, *A Short History of Cardiology*, Springfield, Ill., 1942, vol. iii. p. 102
[5] Or pædiatrics

obstetrics, which he continued to practise. His *Lectures on Diseases of Children* (1847) became a standard work, and the Hospital for Sick Children in Great Ormond Street was founded in 1852, largely as a result of his labours. In more recent times an eminent physician to that institution was Sir GEORGE FREDERICK STILL (1868-1941), who made many valuable contributions to pediatrics, including a history of the subject as far as the eighteenth century (*The History of Pædiatrics*, 1931).

Another pediatrician of world-wide fame was JOHN THOMSON of Edinburgh (1856-1926).[1] He greatly advanced the subject by his researches, his textbook being widely read in Britain and America ; the French and Spanish translations were also in great demand. His quiet and kindly manner, and his enthusiasm for his subject, made him a popular figure with colleagues and students alike.

In Germany the subject of children's diseases was developed by EDUARD HEINRICH HENOCH of Berlin (1820-1910), and by his successor in the chair, OTTO HEUBNER (1843-1926), whose work on infant feeding became the basis of all subsequent researches.

In America the study of diseases of children was promoted by ABRAHAM JACOBI of New York (1830-1919), a German who settled there in 1853, and who continued to teach the subject for forty-two years.[2] By his work and writings he rendered noteworthy service to American medicine as also did his contemporary, JOB LEWIS SMITH (1827-97), who published a *Treatise on the Diseases of Childhood* (1869) based on his original observations. The first to occupy the Chair of Pediatrics at Harvard (1888), was THOMAS MORGAN ROTCH (1849-1914), who rendered valuable public service by his advocacy of a pure milk supply.

Neurology

The study of nervous diseases became a specialized branch of medicine largely through the teaching and writings of the French school, although, as already noted, the subject had long engaged the attention of physicians. Robert Whytt of Edinburgh described tuberculous meningitis in 1768. Domenico Cotugno of Naples wrote a treatise on sciatica in 1770, and James Parkinson of London gave an account of paralysis agitans in 1817.

[1] J. D. Comrie, *History of Scottish Medicine*, 2 vols., 1932, vol. ii. p. 685
[2] F. H. Garrison, "Abraham Jacobi, 1830-1919," *Ann. Med. Hist.*, 1919, vol. ii. p. 194

The first modern treatise on nervous diseases was the *Lehrbuch der Nerven-Krankheiten* (1840–46), the work of MORITZ HEINRICH ROMBERG (1795–1873). It is based on personal observation, and gives the first clear account of the ataxies. Romberg's clinic at Berlin attracted many students. Another eminent German neurologist of later date was WILHELM HEINRICH ERB of Heidelberg (1840–1921), who made many original contributions to the subject, noting the significance of tendon reflexes, studying the relation of syphilis to tabes, and perfecting the technique of electro-diagnosis.

It is to France, however, that we must turn for the early history of modern neurology. This branch of medical science owes much to GUILLAUME BENJAMIN AMAND DUCHENNE (1806–1875), who was content to wander for over thirty years in the hospitals of Paris, with no thought of self-advancement, but seeking only to extend the knowledge of neurology. Sir Arthur Keith refers to him as " one of the most remarkable figures which has ever appeared on the medical stage." [1] Born in Boulogne, the son of a sea captain, he studied medicine in Paris and returned to practise in his native town. He had occasion to use the Faradic current, then something of a novelty, in treating the victims of chronic rheumatism who so frequently consult the youngest practitioner. He discovered that there was no need to puncture the skin in order to stimulate the muscles ; all that was necessary was to place a wet sponge on the terminals. There was thus revealed to him a new means of studying muscular action, and to this study he devoted himself with great patience and energy.

After twelve years in Boulogne, having acquired a modest competence, he set out for Paris at the age of thirty-six, carrying with him the beloved battery which was to bring him fame. From that time until his death he haunted the hospitals, following up the patients, and recording their progress, often at great personal inconvenience. Some of the physicians resented the intrusion of this unknown practitioner from the country, or at least viewed him with suspicion ; others, good-humouredly, regarded him as a harmless crank. His tact and perseverance won the day, and he addressed himself to the self-appointed task, which he continued almost to the date of his death.

He observed and described many diseases not then known to medical science, including locomotor ataxia, progressive muscular

[1] Sir A. Keith, *Menders of the Maimed*, 1919, p. 91

atrophy, and bulbar paralysis, but perhaps his greatest achievement was his great work, *Physiologie des Mouvements*, which appeared in 1867. He showed how muscles never act singly, but always in groups, and how the same muscle may subserve different functions. Duchenne did not attain fame during his lifetime ; indeed, some years elapsed before his views received the recognition they deserved. His contemporary, JEAN-MARTIN CHARCOT (1825–93) entered the field in more orthodox fashion and became one of the most famous teachers of the time.[1] Charcot's clinic at the Salpêtrière was the Mecca of neurologists the world over.[2] He was a gifted orator, a clear writer, and an inspiring leader.

One of Charcot's most distinguished disciples was PIERRE MARIE (1853–1940), who described many new diseases of the nervous system. He explained the cause of acromegaly, contributed to the knowledge of aphasia, and studied peripheral nerve injuries during the Great War.

Other pupils of Charcot were JOSEPH JULES DÉJERINE (1849–1917), who wrote an important work on the anatomy of the central nervous system as well as many clinical studies, and JOSEPH BABINSKI (1857–1932), known for his work on hysteria and for the reflex sign of toe movement which bears his name.

In Britain the pioneer of modern neurology was JOHN HUGHLINGS JACKSON (1834–1911).[3] Born near York, he spent his boyhood there, studied medicine in London, and became lecturer on Pathology, and later on Physiology, at the London Hospital, eventually becoming physician to that institution. Early in his career he turned his attention to neurology, and when the National Hospital for the Paralysed and Epileptic (now National Hospital, Queen Square) was founded in 1859 he became a member of the staff. For forty years he conducted a large consulting practice at 3 Manchester Square, in a house which bears a tablet to his memory. Jackson rendered great service to neurology, and he was held in high esteem by his contemporaries. Although he was never a successful lecturer, his writings were precise and logical. His fame has grown steadily since his death, and he is still regarded as the ultimate authority on many neurological problems. His

[1] M. Allen Starr, "Memorial of Professor Jean-Martin Charcot," *Internat. Clinics*, 1894, 4th series, vol. i ; Bernard Naunyn, "Jean Martin Charcot," *Arch. f. Exper. Pathol.*, 1893, vol. xxxiii. p. 1

[2] F. H. Garrison, "Charcot and the Salpêtrière," *Bull. N.Y. Acad. Med.*, 1926, vol. ii. p. 81

[3] Sir W. Hale-White, *Great Doctors of the Nineteenth Century*, 1935, p. 268

first researches concerned speech defects associated with lesions of the brain. He confirmed the discoveries of Broca (p. 333), by showing how, in right-handed persons, the seat of the trouble was in the left cerebral hemisphere.

Another problem which he solved was that of the localized epileptic movements, now known as Jacksonian epilepsy. Jackson correlated such movements with lesions of the motor area of the cerebral cortex. A third matter to which he devoted much attention was the classification of pathological muscular movements as high, middle, and low, according to the level of the causative lesion in the central nervous system. Hughlings Jackson was no mere theorist ; he illustrated his deductions by records of numerous cases, most carefully observed.

Scarcely less renowned was Jackson's contemporary, Sir WILLIAM RICHARD GOWERS (1845–1915), who described the tract in the spinal cord, and the syndrome known by his name. Gowers was one of the first to recognize the importance of the ophthalmoscope in neurology. His textbook on medical ophthalmology is illustrated by himself.[1] (See Supplement, page 462.) More recently British neurology has been well upheld by Sir HENRY HEAD (1861–1940), who made notable studies of aphasia, and who submitted to division of his own radial nerve in order to observe the resulting phenomena.

The pioneer neurologist of the United States was SILAS WEIR MITCHELL of Philadelphia (1829–1914), who introduced the " Weir Mitchell treatment " of certain types of nervous disease by rest in bed and strict isolation.[2] He made valuable contributions to neurology, and wrote a semi-popular treatise, *Fat and Blood* (1877) which had a large circle of readers and was translated into several languages. Earlier in his career, during the Civil War, he had written an account of injuries to nerves. Weir Mitchell also attained distinction as a poet and as a novelist.

The clinical study of neurology was greatly assisted by the researches of laboratory workers, who investigated the finer microscopic details of the nervous system, and who devised improved methods of staining nerve cells and fibres. The leaders of the movement were CAMILLO GOLGI (1844–1926), whose name has been mentioned in connection with malaria, and the Spanish

[1] Macdonald Critchley, *Sir William Gowers, 1845–1915,* 1949
[2] W. W. Keen and others, *S. Weir Mitchell, M.D., LL.D., F.R.S., 1829–1914,* Memorial Addresses, Philadelphia, 1914

scientist, SANTIAGO RAMON Y CAJAL of Madrid (1852–1934), who added so much to the knowledge of the histology of the central nervous system. The Nobel Prize was awarded, jointly, to Golgi and Ramon y Cajal in 1906.

Ramon y Cajal is the author of an interesting autobiography which is of special interest, as it gives a picture of the medical life of Spain, so little known and appreciated in other countries.[1] Among his other works is a collection of charming essays entitled *Charlas de Café* (Café Gossip), Madrid, 1921.

Psychiatry and Medical Psychology

Nothing is more impressive in medical history than the change of attitude towards mental disease which has taken place within the past hundred and fifty years.

It was in 1792 that the noble-minded PHILIPPE PINEL (1745–1826) boldly advised removal of the chains which restrained insane persons, at the Bicêtre hospital of Paris.[2] One had been chained for forty years, another for thirty-six years. Pinel affirmed that the mentally sick should not be treated as criminals. He introduced the idea of the mental hospital, in which mental disease would be treated like other forms of disease, and in which case-histories would be recorded and scientific investigations conducted. Pinel was a bold man to advise such reforms during the years of Revolution, and it is recorded that he was attacked by a mob, who accused him of harbouring refugees, and was rescued only by the intervention of a patient whom he had liberated.

The new outlook upon " insanity " and " madness " was but slowly adopted, and even in 1830 JOHN CONOLLY (1794–1866), physician to Hanwell Asylum, was conducting an energetic campaign in favour of non-restraint. It became a subject of heated argument in all circles of society. While Pinel was still at work in Paris in 1792, William Tuke, a Quaker philanthropist, who was not a medical man, formed the Retreat at York, an institution designed to mitigate the unhappy fate of mental patients. Here there was no restraint and no chains, and the success of the enterprise did much to alter public opinion, and to hasten the adoption of humane treatment. William Tuke's great-grandson,

[1] Santiago Ramon y Cajal, *Recollections of My Life*, trans. by E. H. Craigie, Philadelphia, 1937 ; Dorothy Cannon, *Explorer of the Human Brain*, 1949 ; Harley Williams, *Don Quixote of the Microscope*, 1953
[2] G. Zilboorg and G. W. Henry, *A History of Medical Psychology*, New York, 1941

DANIEL HACK TUKE (1827–95), studied medicine and became a psychiatrist. He also was associated with the York Retreat [1] (p. 249). An enlightened and scholarly man, he did much to raise the status of his specialty in Britain and America. His many contributions to the subject were published in the *Journal of Mental Science*, of which he was editor. Another editor of this journal, and also a Yorkshireman, was HENRY MAUDSLEY (1835–1918), who practised in London. [2] He wrote extensively on the mutual relationships of body and mind, and discussed the connection of insanity with crime.

Sir THOMAS SMITH CLOUSTON (1840–1915) of Edinburgh, was an excellent teacher of psychiatry. His *Textbook of Mental Diseases* was widely used, while his work on *The Hygiene of Mind* is full of salutary advice, and foreshadowed the present-day vogue for popular expositions of psychology.

In Germany the leading exponent of psychiatry was EMIL KRAEPELIN (1856–1926), most of whose work was done at Munich. [3] His monumental textbook describes the two major groups of mental diseases—the manic-depressive psychoses and dementia praecox, the former usually curable, the latter incurable. Kraepelin's system is no longer adopted, but he rendered good service by showing that mental disease follows a definite course, like many other diseases.

Meanwhile, in 1885 to be precise, there was working in Charcot's clinic in Paris a young man who was destined to revolutionize psychiatry, and indeed to change the outlook in the whole field of medicine. Darwin and Huxley, by viewing man from a zoological standpoint, had profoundly influenced the current of medical thought. In like manner Freud, by his discovery of the unconscious mind, altered the trend of medicine, and gave a salutary check to the materialistic tendencies of the age of specialism. SIGMUND FREUD (1856–1939), who revolutionized the entire field of psycho-pathology, lived most of his life in Vienna. [4] In his autobiography he tells us that in 1889 he realized that " there could be powerful mental processes which nevertheless remained hidden from the consciousness of men." [5]

[1] G. Zilboorg and G. W. Henry, *A History of Medical Psychology*, New York, 1941, p. 422
[2] G. T. Bettany, *Eminent Doctors : Their Lives and Work*, 1885, vol. ii. p. 232
[3] G. Zilboorg and G. W. Henry, *A History of Medical Psychology*, New York, 1941
[4] F. Wittels, *Sigmund Freud : His Personality, His Teaching, and His School*, 1924
[5] Sigmund Freud, *An Autobiographical Study* (Eng. trans. by J. Strachey), 1935, p. 450

From this idea Freud evolved his system of " psycho-analysis " and found that he could dispense with hypnotism, which he had been employing. Freud's principles, now so familiar, were only slowly adopted, and at first he was severely criticized on account of his preoccupation with sex psychology. Despite the opposition, his discovery of the unconscious mind was more important than any other in the whole history of mental disorders. He showed, moreover, that there was no clear borderline between normal and abnormal psychology, and his ideas have assumed importance in almost every field of human activity.

Freud lived long enough to see his views widely accepted, although the end of his life was clouded, and he died in London as a refugee. The importance of the Freudian revolution is not yet fully realized. To-day, medical psychology is permeating all branches of medicine, and it may prove to be the activating factor of a new era in medical science.

Ophthalmology

Although diseases of the eye had provided a field for specialism since the earliest days of medicine, the nineteenth century witnessed an immense advance in our knowledge of this branch of medicine. The invention of the ophthalmoscope by Helmholtz in 1851 was a strong impetus to the study of the eye. The work of Helmholtz has been already described, and we may therefore turn to another distinguished pioneer, whose name is often linked with that of Helmholtz. The Young-Helmholtz theory of colour vision is well known. THOMAS YOUNG (1773–1829) was undoubtedly the most versatile and learned physician of his day. A native of Taunton, Somerset, and of Quaker parentage, he was a precocious child with an insatiable thirst for knowledge.[1] It was during his student days at St. Bartholomew's Hospital that he discovered the effect of the ciliary muscle upon the shape of the lens of the eye. Previous to this time it had been believed that accommodation was effected by an elongation of the entire eyeball. Young's communication on the subject secured for him the Fellowship of the Royal Society at the early age of twenty-one.[2] After a further period of study at Edinburgh, Göttingen, and Cambridge, he succeeded his uncle,

[1] G. Peacock, Life of Thomas Young, M.D., F.R.S., 1855
[2] W. Stirling, Some Apostles of Physiology, 1902, p. 78

Dr. Brocklesby, in a fashionable London practice, and became physician to St. George's Hospital. A man of great energy and diligence, Young was a student of many subjects. His researches on the mechanism of the eye were followed by a series of lectures on Natural Philosophy at the Royal Institution, which contained many original ideas and afterwards appeared in print.[1] He took up the study of optics where Newton had left it, and contributed a number of papers on the subject to the Royal Society. He also wrote a number of articles on physics for the *Encyclopaedia Britannica*. Another of Thomas Young's achievements, which occupied the later years of his life, was his interpretation of the hieroglyphic inscriptions of the Rosetta Stone, a block of basalt discovered in Egypt in 1799 which was transferred to the British Museum after the French capitulation (*cf.* p. 274).

Worthy to stand beside Helmholtz and Young as a pioneer of ophthalmology was FRANS CORNELIS DONDERS (1818–89), the Professor of Physiology at Utrecht, whose great work, *The Anomalies of Refraction and Accommodation*, was published in English in 1864 and is the foundation of all subsequent studies. In this work he differentiated the various errors of refraction, and indicated how they might be corrected. From 1862 until his death, Donders devoted all his time to the practice and study of ophthalmology, and acquired an international reputation.

Another physiologist who turned his attention to ophthalmology was Sir WILLIAM BOWMAN (1816–92).[2] During the early part of his career, while he was Demonstrator of Anatomy at King's College, London, he made a number of important discoveries relating to the minute structure of muscle and to the physiology of the kidney ; indeed, Sir Michael Foster called him "the Father of the Kidney," so greatly did he extend the knowledge of the microscopic structure of that organ.[3] He also discovered the basement membrane of the cornea, which bears his name. In 1846 he joined the staff of the Royal Ophthalmic Hospital at Moorfields, and from that time devoted all his attention to diseases of the eye.[4] For many years he was the leader of ophthal-

[1] F. Oldham, *Thomas Young, F.R.S., Philosopher and Physician*, 1933
[2] B. Chance, " Sir William Bowman, Anatomist, Physiologist, and Ophthalmologist," *Ann. Med. Hist.*, 1924, vol. vi. p. 143
[3] Sir W. Hale-White, *Great Doctors of the Nineteenth Century*, 1935, p. 177 ; G. T. Bettany, *Eminent Doctors : Their Lives and Work*, 2 vols., 1885, vol. ii. p. 260
[4] E. Treacher Collins, *The History and Traditions of the Moorfields Eye Hospital*, 1929, p. 94

mic practice in London, where he was one of the first to employ the ophthalmoscope. A baronetcy was conferred on him in 1884. Bowman introduced the treatment of lachrymal obstruction by the use of graduated probes, and he perfected the operations of iridectomy and of removal of cataract.

A contemporary British ophthalmologist was WILLIAM MAC-KENZIE of Glasgow (1791–1868), a keen observer, who made careful notes of his cases, and wrote a *Practical Treatise on the Diseases of the Eye* in 1830.

In Edinburgh, at a slightly later period, there was an ophthalmologist of world-wide reputation, DOUGLAS ARGYLL ROBERTSON (1837–1909), the first to be appointed Lecturer on Diseases of the Eye at the University of Edinburgh.[1] He made many original observations, and his name is commemorated by the pupil reaction known as "Argyll Robertson pupil."

The modern surgery of the eye was largely developed by ALBERCHT VON GRAEFE (1828–70)[2] son of the surgeon (p. 342), who devised many operations, including iridectomy for glaucoma and the linear extraction of the lens for cataract, although the pioneer of the latter operation was JACQUES DAVIEL of Paris (1696–1762). The name of Von Graefe is familiar to every medical student in the "Von Graefe sign" in exophthalmic goitre and the Von Graefe cataract knife. Von Graefe spent all his short life at Berlin, becoming professor two years before his death from tuberculosis at the age of forty-two. As a teacher he acquired an international reputation, and he was the first to recognize the importance of the ophthalmoscope and to describe ophthalmoscopic findings. Along with Donders, Von Graefe founded the *Archiv für Ophthalmologie*, which did so much to raise the status of the specialty.

Later in the century the greatest teacher of ophthalmology was ERNST FUCHS of Vienna (1851–1930), to whose clinic came medical men from all countries, and who wrote an important textbook. He had an international practice, and was a great traveller, visiting Britain and America on several occasions. His attractive personality and charm of manner attracted many friends and patients.

[1] J. D. Comrie, *History of Scottish Medicine*, 2 vols., 1932, pp. 531, 708
[2] R. H. Major, *Classic Descriptions of Disease*, 1932, p. 244

SPECIALISM AND PREVENTIVE MEDICINE

Otology and Laryngology

Although otology has been recognized as a separate branch of medicine for little more than a century, the intricacies of aural anatomy attracted anatomists of every generation. Eustachius and Fallopius imprinted their names upon the organ of hearing, but the first monograph containing any reference to diseases of the ear was the little book, *Traité de l'organe de l'ouïe* (1683), by J. G. DUVERNEY (1648–1730), Professor of Anatomy in Paris.[1] It was translated into German (1732) and English (1748), and gave a clear account of the current knowledge, though treatment at that time was practically non-existent. Another name familiar to every otologist is that of ANTONIO VALSALVA (1666–1723), whose *Tractatus de aure humana* was published at Bologna in 1704. The treatment of deafness by " Valsalva " inflation was carried a step further when Guyot, a postmaster of Versailles, invented the Eustachian catheter and used it to relieve his own deafness.

Various efforts were made to establish otology on a scientific basis by such men as JOHN CUNNINGHAM SAUNDERS, who also practised ophthalmology, and founded in 1805 the " London Dispensary for Curing Diseases of the Eye and Ears," which later became the Royal Ophthalmic Hospital (Moorfields).[2] The first hospital exclusively devoted to diseases of the ear was established in 1816 by an unqualified practitioner, JOHN HARRISON CURTIS, and it eventually was named the Royal Ear Hospital.[3] Curtis deserves credit for the enterprise, although he appears to have been " profoundly ignorant even of the anatomy of the ear," and treated all cases by syringing, using an enormous instrument like a garden syringe.

Another pioneer of oto-laryngology was JAMES YEARSLEY (1805–1869), who deserves mention as the discoverer of the artificial tympanum, and as one of the first to point out that deafness may arise from affections of the nose and throat. Yearsley was the first qualified medical man to practice oto-laryngology as a specialist in London. In 1838 he founded the Metropolitan Ear and Throat Hospital in Fitzroy Square. He was the originator of the *Medical Circular* (1852) and one of the founders of the

[1] H. Haeser, *Geschichte der Medizin*, Jena, 1845, p. 772
[2] E. Treacher Collins, *The History and Traditions of the Moorfields Eye Hospital*, 1929, p. 17
[3] J. F. Clarke, *Autobiographical Recollections of the Medical Profession*, 1874, p. 358

Medical Directory (1845), a guide to the recognized medical profession and therefore a step towards the Medical Registration Act of 1858.

At the beginning of the nineteenth century otology was in danger of passing into unscrupulous hands, when there came upon the scene one who, at the Medical Society of London, vowed that he would "rescue aural surgery from the hands of quacks." This was JOSEPH TOYNBEE (1815–66),[1] a native of Lincolnshire, who began his career as assistant curator to Professor Owen at the Royal College of Surgeons. In his efforts to establish aural pathology as an exact science he made over two thousand dissections of the ear, many of which are described in his book on *Diseases of the Ear*, which must rank as a medical classic. He described ten cases of osseous tumour (exostosis) of the meatus, and also the "molluscous tumour," which we now recognize as cholesteatoma. His dissections proved that organic stricture of the Eustachian tube was a rare condition, and he was the first to demonstrate "ankylosis of the stapes" (otosclerosis) in 160 cases. He recognized that otitic infection could extend to the brain by way of the labyrinth, and though he never performed a mastoid operation, he mentioned that it might be considered.

In 1851 Toynbee was appointed aural surgeon to St. Mary's Hospital, the first general hospital to set aside beds for diseases of the ear. His death was the result of an experiment on himself. Believing that tinnitus might be reduced by inhalation of chloroform, and subsequent inflation of the ear, he subjected himself to the test. He was found dead in his consulting room, his notes and apparatus by his side. Toynbee was a keen observer and an original thinker. He may be regarded as the founder of modern otology.[3] Arnold Toynbee of Toynbee Hall was his second son.

Associated with Toynbee as assistant and successor in practice was JAMES HINTON (1822–75).[4] Hinton is remembered as a philosopher, and his little book on *The Mystery of Pain* is still read.[5] Nevertheless, his work on otology, *The Questions of Aural Surgery*,

[1] G. T. Bettany, *Eminent Doctors : Their Lives and Work*, 1885, vol. ii. p. 272
[2] Gertrude Toynbee, ed. of *Reminiscences and Letters of Joseph and Arnold Toynbee*, 1910
[1] D. Guthrie, "The Renaissance of Otology. Joseph Toynbee and his Contemporaries," *Jour. Laryng. and Otol.*, 1937, vol. lii. p. 163
[3] Ellice Hopkins, *The Life and Letters of James Hinton*, 1878 ; S. Wilks and G. T. Bettany, *History of Guy's Hospital*, 1892, p. 347
[5] G. T. Bettany, *Eminent Doctors : Their Lives and Work*, 1885, vol. ii. p. 277

is full of original ideas, and it must not be forgotten that it was he who in 1868 performed the first operation in England for mastoiditis, although the operation had been practised some years previously in Paris by JEAN LOUIS PETIT (p. 244). Mastoid surgery was placed upon a sound pathological basis by HERMANN SCHWARTZE (1837–1910), of Halle, who described it in his *Chirurgischen Krankheiten des Ohres* (1885).[1] Contemporary with Toynbee was Sir WILLIAM WILDE of Dublin (1815–76), the father of Oscar Wilde and a man of great energy and varied gifts. An authority on the history and archaeology of his country, he wrote several works on this subject. His first book, *Narrative of a Voyage to Madeira*, earned his reputation as a writer. Wilde also distinguished himself as Commissioner for the Irish Census, for which services he was awarded a knighthood. When he settled in Dublin as an aural surgeon in 1841 he established a dispensary in a disused stable, and in such humble quarters, and later in St. Mark's Hospital, he was the first to teach otology in the United Kingdom. His volume on *Aural Surgery* (1853) is the fruit of long and careful clinical observation, for Wilde was as essentially a clinician as Toynbee was a morbid anatomist. The case reports used by Wilde to illustrate his observations are models of clear reporting after the true Hippocratic tradition. Acute mastoiditis he treated by " Wilde's incision," an incision down to the bone, but with no bone operation. He realized the dangers of otitis, stating that " we can never tell how, when, or where it will end." A most interesting biography of Sir William Wilde has been written by Dr. T. G. Wilson of Dublin.[2]

On the Continent the pioneer of modern otology was JEAN MARIE GASPARD ITARD (1774–1838), a military surgeon of Paris who devoted special attention to the ear, and whose work, *Traité des maladies de l'oreille et de l'audition*, did much to establish otology on a scientific basis. He did good service by his efforts to improve facilities for the education of the deaf. The leading German otologist of the time was WILHELM KRAMER (1801–75), who wrote a well-known textbook on diseases of the ear, and was a strong advocate of the Eustachian catheter and bougie.

No one can write of the history of otology without mentioning ADAM POLITZER (1835–1920), who did so much for the specialty. For many years he occupied the Chair of Otology at Vienna, to

---

[1] Sir Charles Ballance, *The Surgery of the Temporal Bone*, 2 vols., 1919, vol. i. p. 51
[2] T. G. Wilson, *Victorian Doctor : The Life of Sir William Wilde*, 1942

which he had been appointed while still under thirty. He contributed to every department of otology, and as a teacher his influence and popularity were immense. He could teach with equal fluency in German, French, Italian, or English, and his clinic attracted medical men from all parts of the world. His *Lehrbuch der Ohrenheilkunde* (1878) continued through many editions, and remained the standard authority on otology for years. He lived to the ripe age of eighty-five, retaining to the end his interest in otology, as is shown by the publication a few years before his death of his *Geschichte der Ohrenheilkunde* (1913), which is a masterpiece of historical research.[1]

Modern laryngology may be said to date from the invention of the laryngoscope in 1855 by MANUEL GARCIA (1805–1906), a singing master of Paris (Plate LXIX). Garcia's report of his discovery to the Royal Society attracted little attention, but the possibilities of its value in clinical practice were envisaged by LUDWIG TÜRCK (1810–68) and JOHANN CZERMAK (1828–93) of Vienna, and before the end of his long life Garcia was acclaimed as the indirect founder of a new branch of medical science.[2]

Laryngology continued to advance in Vienna under such well-known men as OTTOKAR CHIARI (1853–1918) and MARKUS HAJEK (1861–1941), at whose clinics many students from other countries were trained in the art. One of the first in Britain to explore this field was Sir MORELL MACKENZIE (1837–92), who founded the Throat Hospital in Golden Square in 1863, and who wrote an excellent textbook (1884) which may still be consulted with profit. Mackenzie had studied under Czermak in Vienna, and on his return had been awarded the Jacksonian Prize of the Royal College of Surgeons for his essay on *Diseases of the Larynx*.[3] He conducted a large practice in London, although his career was clouded by the misunderstandings which followed his attendance on the German Emperor, Frederick III, the historic case of cancer of the larynx which focused attention on laryngology.[4] The details are given in a popular work by Mackenzie entitled,

[1] A. Politzer, *Geschichte der Ohrenheilkunde*, 2 vols., Stuttgart, 1907–13
[2] M. Neuburger, *British Medicine and the Vienna School*, 1943, p. 98 ; Gordon Holmes, "History of the Progress of Laryngology from the Earliest Times to the Present," *Med. Press*, 1885, Pt. ii. p. 49
[3] G. T. Bettany, *Eminent Doctors: Their Lives and Work*, 1885, vol. ii. p. 249; J. Donelan, "Morell Mackenzie, the Father of British Laryngology, Founder of the *Journal of Laryngology*," *Jour. of Laryng. and Otol.*, 1919, vol. xxxiv. p. 181
[4] H. R. Haweis, *Sir Morell Mackenzie*, 1893 ; R. Scott Stevenson, *Morell Mackenzie*, 1946

The Fatal Illness of Frederick the Noble, which naturally gives a one-sided account of the controversy.[1]

A prominent contemporary laryngologist of London was the German-born Sir FELIX SEMON (1849–1921), who did much to raise the status of the specialty, and whose autobiography is an interesting picture of consulting practice in those peaceful Victorian days.[2]

Laryngology was introduced into the United States by HORACE GREEN (1802–66), who had been a pupil of Trousseau.[3] Green was the first to describe laryngeal cysts and tumours before the introduction of the laryngoscope, and his *Treatise on Disease of the Air Passages* (1846) was one of the first monographs on the subject.[4]

A new off-shoot of laryngology, peroral endoscopy, was inaugurated by GUSTAV KILLIAN of Freiburg (1860–1921), who was the first to view the lower air passages and oesophagus by electrically illuminated tubes, introduced by the natural channels, a procedure which was modified and improved in America by CHEVALIER JACKSON of Philadelphia (1865–   ).

Dermatology and Venereal Diseases

The founder of British dermatology was ROBERT WILLAN (1757–1812).[5] The son of a physician at Sedbergh, he studied medicine at Edinburgh, and soon afterwards settled in London, where he practised as a general physician in Bloomsbury Square. He was a strong advocate of vaccination, and suggested that it should be made compulsory by law, a reform which was not introduced until forty-one years after his death. Willan did not confine his practice to diseases of the skin. His interest in this branch of medicine led to the publication in 1808 of his work, *On Cutaneous Diseases*, which was beautifully illustrated in colour. He classified and described many forms of skin disease, noting that certain of them were associated with definite trades or

---

[1] Sir M. Mackenzie, *The Fatal Illness of Frederick the Noble*, 1888
[2] Sir Felix Semon, *Autobiography*, 1926 ; P. McBride, " Sir Felix Semon : His Work and its Influence on Laryngology " (Semon Lecture), *Jour. of Laryng. and Otol.*, 1913, vol. xxviii. pp. 113, 169
[3] Jonathan Wright, *History of Laryngology and Rhinology*, St. Louis, 1893 ; R. Scott Stevenson and Douglas Guthrie, *A History of Otolaryngology*, 1949
[4] G. H. Bryan, " The History of Laryngology and Rhinology and the Influence of America in the Development of this Speciality," *Ann. Med. Hist.*, 1933, vol. v. p. 151
[5] H. MacCormac, " Robert Willan (1757–1812)," *Med. Press and Circ.*, 1935, xci.

occupations. His book was the first attempt to establish the subject on a scientific basis. Only the first volume of his great treatise appeared during his lifetime, but the scheme was continued by his pupil, THOMAS BATEMAN (1778-1821), whose *Delineations of Cutaneous Diseases* contained plates as admirable as those of Willan.

In France, dermatology was inaugurated by the work of ANNE CHARLES LORRY (1726-83) in the eighteenth century. His *Tractatus de morbis cutaneis*, published in Paris in 1777, is the first modern text on the subject. A more distinguished pioneer was JEAN LOUIS MARC ALIBERT (1768-1837), who was responsible for the foundation of that home of modern dermatology, the Hôpital Saint-Louis of Paris, and who became a baron of France.[1] His treatise on skin diseases (1829) contains his classification after the fashion of a family tree, *Arbre des dermatoses*, as well as original descriptions of mycosis fungoides and of keloid.

Among other distinguished dermatologists of the St. Louis Hospital were RAYMOND SABOURAUD (1864-1938), who made extensive studies of ringworm and other mycotic skin infections, and JEAN DARIER (1856-1938), the author of a comprehensive work, *Nouvelle pratique dermatologique*, in eight volumes (1936).

The most eminent British dermatologist of the nineteenth century was Sir ERASMUS WILSON (1809-84),[2] who founded a Chair of Dermatology at the Royal College of Surgeons, and who wrote extensively on the subject. Early in his career he had acted as sub-editor of *The Lancet* under the famous founder of that journal, Thomas Wakley. He also spent several years as a lecturer on anatomy, and wrote a *Dissector's Manual* (1838) and an *Anatomist's Vade-mecum* (1840). Having thus laid a sound foundation of general medical knowledge he turned his attention to the unexplored field of dermatology, and, as he remarked, he " never regretted the choice, as there was only one more beautiful thing than a fine healthy skin, and that was a rare skin disease." Wilson acquired a large practice, becoming a wealthy man and a philanthropist. His interest in Egyptology led him in 1877 to defray the expense, amounting to some £10,000, of transporting Cleopatra's Needle from Egypt to its present site on the Thames Embankment. His generosity was expressed in many other

[1] W. A. Pusey, *The History of Dermatology*. Springfield, U.S.A., 1933
[2] G. T. Bettany, *Eminent Doctors : Their Lives and Work*, 1885, vol. ii. p. 240

directions, and the extent of his benefactions to his poorer patients was considerable.

British dermatology continued to flourish in the hands of such men as TILBURY FOX (1836–79), HENRY RADCLIFFE CROCKER (1845–1909), and Sir JONATHAN HUTCHINSON (1828–1913), the last mentioned being a surgeon (p. 329) of encyclopaedic outlook who took a keen interest in skin diseases.[1]

In Edinburgh WILLIAM ALLAN JAMIESON (1839–1916) founded a school of dermatology, which was carried on by his successor, Sir NORMAN WALKER (1862–1942). Both wrote well-known textbooks on diseases of the skin.

The first work on dermatology to be published in America was *A Synopsis of Diseases of the Skin*, by NOAH WORCESTER (1812–1847) of Harvard. He had been a pupil of Laënnec in Paris, and like that great teacher, he died early of tuberculosis. Another Harvard man, JAMES WHITE (1833–1916) was the first in America to confine his practice to dermatology. He was the author of an important work on dermatitis venenata.

The picture of dermatological history is incomplete without reference to FERDINAND HEBRA (1816–80), who was regarded by some as the greatest dermatologist of the century.[2] He founded the great school of dermatology in Vienna, and was a brilliant teacher with a wide reputation. His classification of skin diseases was securely based upon pathology, and he laid stress upon the local causes, as opposed to the constitutional causes, which were favoured by the French school. He established the parasitic origin of many diseases, and made vast contributions to dermatology. Of equal importance to Hebra as an exponent of the pathology of skin diseases was PAUL GERSON UNNA of Hamburg (1850–1929).[3] A prolific writer, he published valuable works on the histo-pathology of the skin (1894) and on the treatment of skin diseases. His clinic attracted many visitors from other countries.

When dermatology first became a special branch of medicine it included syphilis, as the cutaneous manifestations of syphilis were then very prevalent. In the early years of the nineteenth century the leading authority on syphilis was PHILIPPE RICORD

[1] R. H. Major, *Classic Descriptions of Disease*, p. 43 ; Sir D'Arcy Power, " Hutchinson's Triad," *Brit. Jour. Surg.*, 1926, vol. xiv. p. 1
[2] F. H. Garrison, *An Introduction to the History of Medicine*, 3rd ed., 1924, p. 456
[3] W. A. Pusey, *The History of Dermatology*, Springfield, U.S.A., 1933, p. 159

of Paris (1800–1889). It was he who proved that John Hunter's conception of gonorrhoea and syphilis as phases of the same disease was erroneous. He was responsible for the grouping of syphilis into primary, secondary, and tertiary stages, a classification which met with general approval.[1]

A second Parisian syphilologist of note was JEAN-ALFRED FOURNIER (1832–1914), who was director of the Saint-Louis Hospital, and who wrote extensively on the clinical and social aspects of his subject.

The three leading contributions to the study of syphilis during the early part of the present century were made by laboratory workers. In 1905 FRITZ RICHARD SCHAUDINN (1871–1906) of Hamburg discovered Spirochaeta pallida, the causal organism of syphilis; in 1906 AUGUST VON WASSERMANN (1866–1925) of Berlin, who assisted Koch, discovered the blood test for syphilis known as the "Wassermann reaction"; and in 1909 PAUL EHRLICH of Frankfurt (1854–1915), also a pupil of Koch, after experimenting with a large variety of substances, discovered in "No. 606" a remedy for syphilis which he called salvarsan.[2] In 1912, he introduced the less toxic, and more easily administered, neo-salvarsan. Ehrlich created the new science of chemotherapy, in which so many discoveries have been made in recent times.

Radiology

Radiology was born when WILHELM CONRAD ROENTGEN of Wurzburg (1845–1923) discovered what he called "X-rays" in November, 1895.[3] He announced his discovery on January 23, 1896, at the Physical Society, University of Würzburg, in a paper, "Uber eine neue Art von Strahlen" (On a New Kind of Ray) (Plate LXX). Originally applied only in the diagnosis of fractures and of foreign bodies, the scope of the rays was soon extended to the recognition of calculi. The use of bismuth and later, barium, in the gastro-intestinal tract, and of various radio-opaque drugs which are excreted through the biliary and urinary tracts, further increased the usefulness of X-rays. Still later, the

[1] W. A. Pusey, The History and Epidemiology of Syphilis, Baltimore, 1933, p. 54
[2] C. L. Schleich, Besonnte Vergangenheit, Berlin, 1920, trans. by B. Miall under title "Those Were Good Days," 1935, p. 233   See foot-note to page 329.
[3] O. Glasser, Wilhelm Conrad Röntgen und die Geschichte der Röntgenstrahlen, Berlin, 1931. (Eng. trans., Boston, 1933)

PLATE LXIX THE INVENTOR OF THE LARYNGOSCOPE

Manuel Garcia in his hundredth year. Garcia was fifty years old when he invented the laryngoscope in 1855 (page 380). From a painting by John F. Sargent

PLATE LXX   A NEW KIND OF RAY

Radiogram of the hand of Professor Kölliker, taken by Professor Roentgen when he read his paper announcing the discovery of " A New Kind of Ray " (page 384)

method was applied in the diagnosis of lesions of the brain and of the lungs. The Nobel Prize was awarded to Roentgen in 1901. Unfortunately the Roentgen rays were in use for some years before their harmful effects, in producing cancer of the skin in the operators, were recognized, and many an X-ray martyr to science met his death owing to lack of that adequate protection which is now universally adopted.

The therapeutic value of X-rays in skin diseases was early recognized, and lately deep X-ray therapy has been largely applied in malignant disease.

NIELS RYBERG FINSEN (1860–1904) deserves mention, as he recognized the effect of ultra-violet light upon the skin and its therapeutic effect in cases of lupus, 1896. He was the founder of modern light therapy in the Finsen Institute of Copenhagen.

Another notable discovery, that of radium in 1898, by the Curies—(PIERRE CURIE (1859–1906) and MARIE SKLODOWSKA CURIE (1867–1934)—gave to the medical profession a powerful agent whose final place in treatment of cancer is not yet ascertained. The biography of Madame Curie by her daughter, Eve Curie, fully deserves its wide popularity.[1]

The list of special branches of medicine might be extended. Endocrinology, chemotherapy, nutrition, allergy, haematology, and other fresh sciences have afforded fresh fields for investigation and discovery. The results cannot yet be regarded as history, and therefore do not come within the scope of the present work.

Medicine as a Career for Women

An important development of the nineteenth century was the admission of women to the medical profession. From time to time, throughout the preceding centuries, women had been engaged in the practice of medicine and some of them, notably Trotula of Salerno, had assisted in medical teaching.[2] Nevertheless it was only within recent years that women came to be accepted as medical students and as practitioners on the same terms as men.

America can claim the first woman medical graduate, ELIZABETH BLACKWELL (1821–1910), a native of Bristol who had emi-

[1] Eve Curie, *Madame Curie*, 1938
[2] K. C. Hurd-Mead, *A History of Women in Medicine*, Haddam, Conn., 1938

grated with her parents and who received her degree at New York in 1849.[1] The following year marked the foundation in Philadelphia of the Women's Medical College of Pennsylvania, which still flourishes as the first school of medicine to be entirely reserved for women. In Britain, the first woman to qualify in medicine was ELIZABETH GARRETT (1836–1917), who later became Mrs. Garrett Anderson, and who encountered many difficulties before she eventually obtained the diploma of the Society of Apothecaries in 1865. She was the indefatigable pioneer for the admission of women to the profession of medicine, and it was as a result of her efforts, and those of Dr. Sophia Jex-Blake, that the London School of Medicine was established in 1874. Among the British universities, Edinburgh University was the first to admit women students, although for a time they received instruction in separate classes, and were not accorded the same status as men until the beginning of the present century.[2] Prominent among those Edinburgh students was SOPHIA JEX-BLAKE (1840–1913), who ultimately gained well-deserved recognition after years of hard effort in the face of much opposition. By the time she graduated in 1876, the General Medical Council had agreed to accept women as registered practitioners. Details of the controversy regarding the admission of women to medicine may be found in the *Life of Sophia Jex-Blake* (1918) by Margaret Todd.

The Growth of Preventive Medicine

While the practice of medicine and surgery was gradually becoming divided according to the various special branches, some of which have been mentioned in detail, there came into being another " specialty " more important than any other, that of preventive medicine.

Of course the hygienic needs of the community had been served long before the nineteenth century. In the days of the Roman Empire water supplies and sanitary arrangements were almost as good as those of modern times ; already the State had begun to assume responsibility for the health of the citizens. Nevertheless in Britain little attention was devoted to public health until the attention of humanitarians was attracted to the

---

[1] Elizabeth Blackwell, *Pioneer Work for Women*, 1895
[2] E. Moberley Bell, *Storming the Citadel : the rise of the woman doctor*

dreadful conditions prevailing among the poor, especially in industrial areas, and even in such State institutions as prisons and asylums. The glaring defects were accentuated by a series of epidemics of cholera.

Philosophy and Health

Stimulation of the public conscience during the early years of the century was largely the work of one man, and he was not a student of medicine, but of law, though he never practised. It was JEREMY BENTHAM (1748–1832), the utilitarian philosopher, who insistently preached the doctrine of " the greatest happiness of the greatest number," and advised the reconstruction or re-modelling of government with this end in view. Many of his suggestions, elaborated in his *Introduction to Principles of Morals and Legislation*, have now been legalized and adopted, although he was a man so far ahead of his time that many years elapsed before his views met with general acceptance. Indeed, like so many other pioneers, his work was better known abroad than at home during his lifetime. It was characteristic of Bentham that he requested in his will that his body should be dissected, "so that mankind may reap some small benefit in and by my decease." [1] This was done, and his skeleton, dressed in the clothes he wore, was preserved in the museum of University College Hospital, London. To Bentham belongs the credit for having drawn attention to the need for public health legislation ; he was indeed the Father of Modern Preventive Medicine.

Two other great reformers, Southwood Smith and Edwin Chadwick, carried Bentham's ideas a stage further.

THOMAS SOUTHWOOD SMITH (1788–1861), a graduate of Edinburgh and Physician to London Fever Hospital, carried out Bentham's request as to the disposal of his remains, and wrote a treatise on *The Use of the Dead to the Living*, a plea for the provision of anatomical material, which led eventually to the passing of the Anatomy Act in 1832. In another work, *The Philosophy of Health*, he emphasized the importance of national health. Southwood Smith strongly supported Chadwick (p. 388) as a member of the General Board of Health, while by his writings he drew attention to the prevalence of preventible sickness among the poor, and to the great need for improved sanitation.

[1] J. Timbs, *Doctors and Patients*, 2 vols., 1873, vol. i., p. 241

The Sanitary Idea

Closely associated with Southwood Smith, and perhaps better known to-day, was the lawyer EDWIN CHADWICK (1800–90), who became Sir Edwin Chadwick the year before his death.[1] Chadwick practised the humanitarian philosophy of his friend Jeremy Bentham, and by his continual insistence on what he called " the sanitary idea," he persuaded the government to appoint a Sanitary Commission in 1839. As a result of the report of this commission the General Board of Health came into being in 1848. Nevertheless the time was not ripe for radical reform, public opinion being insufficiently alive to the need, and the Board was dispersed ten years later. Such misfortune merely increased Chadwick's enthusiasm. He continued in face of opposition his advocacy of measures calculated to improve the health of the people, and before the end of his life he saw that his labour was coming to fruition.

Health as a National Problem

The importance of accurate statistical data was at this time emphasized by WILLIAM FARR (1807–83), a poor boy who became the greatest statistician of the period, and whose life was spent in the office of the Registrar General, although to begin with he engaged in medical practice in London. Farr's book on *Vital Statistics* was a valuable contribution to public health, and it was Farr who devised the classification and nomenclature of diseases, which, with some modifications, is still in use for registration purposes.

Another original thinker was JOHN SNOW (1813–58), who attained distinction as an anaesthetist (p. 305), and who, before the bacterial origin of disease became known, pointed out that cholera was water-borne, and that a certain outbreak in London would cease if the handle of the communal pump in Broad Street were removed, a suggestion which was adopted with excellent results.[2]

The next of the early sanitary reformers, and one of the foremost medical men of the nineteenth century, was Sir JOHN SIMON (1816–1904), who made such a valuable contribution to hygienic advance during his long life.[3] He was of a long-lived family,

[1] Sir A. Newsholme, *The Evolution of Preventive Medicine*, 1927, p. 116
[2] Sir B. W. Richardson, *Disciples of Aesculapius*, 2 vols., 1900, vol. i. p. 227
[3] Sir W. Hale-White, *Great Doctors of the Nineteenth Century*, 1935, p. 189

for his father, a London stockbroker, died at the age of ninety-seven, and his mother at the age of ninety-five. John was one of their fourteen children. After completing his medical studies at King's College, he became a lecturer on Pathology and a member of the surgical staff of St. Thomas's Hospital. Neither pathology nor surgery was to be his field, however, for we find him in 1848 appointed as the first Medical Officer of Health for the City of London.[1] The condition of the city with regard to water supply, sewage disposal, housing, and cleanliness afforded ample scope for improvement, and his reports are full of scathing and fearless comments upon the appalling conditions of the time.[2] The Government authorities, awaking to the need for action, invited Simon in 1855 to become Medical Officer to the General Board of Health, and when the Board ceased to exist three years later he became Medical Officer to the Privy Council. He demonstrated the danger of sewage-contaminated water by showing that when water was taken from an unpolluted part of the Thames the mortality from cholera during an epidemic was thirty-seven per thousand in the area supplied, as against a mortality of one hundred and thirty per thousand in an area supplied from a polluted part of the river. Thus did the public learn the advantage of pure water, although so many were the vested interests that a general distribution of pure water was secured only after years of delay. Simon also urged the value of vaccination, which was made compulsory in 1853. He had the satisfaction of seeing a steady advance of public opinion in the direction of better sanitation and improved health measures. His sanitary inspectors, or inspectors of nuisances as they were called, proved a great success. In each successive report Simon indicated some further glaring need for sanitary reform. In 1871 the Local Government Board assumed control, with Simon as Medical Officer. He retired in 1876.[3] His best known publication is *English Sanitary Institutions* (1890), which, despite its rather dull title, gives an interesting account of the progress of public health up to that time.

Bacteriology had not then become a science, yet he prophesied that living organisms would be found responsible for typhoid, cholera, diphtheria, and other infections.

[1] Liverpool had led the way in the previous year by appointing the first of all Medical Officers of Health, Dr. W. H. Duncan
[2] Sir G. Newman, *The Rise of Preventive Medicine*, 1932
[3] Sir Malcolm Morris, *The Story of English Public Health*, 1919, p. 54

Public Health in other Countries

Meantime one of the greatest pioneers of public hygiene was working on the Continent. MAX VON PETTENKOFER (1818–1901), a pupil of Justus von Liebig, for many years professor at Munich, commenced his professional career as a physiological chemist, and made noteworthy researches on bile salts and on other problems. Next, turning his attention to the broad aspects of public health, he investigated the relations of soil and atmosphere to health, noting the conditions which favoured the incidence of cholera epidemics so frequent at this time. In 1866 he founded the Institute of Hygiene at Munich, where his name is still commemorated in the university buildings, and he wrote a *Handbuch der Hygiene* (1882) which had a large circulation. Pettenkoffer did not accept the views of Koch, and was a sceptic regarding the rôle of organisms in disease. Indeed, he is said to have swallowed a culture of living cholera (some say typhoid) bacilli in order to disprove their effect, a foolhardy experiment which was, strangely and fortunately, without harmful result.[1] Pettenkoffer was highly esteemed in Munich, where his two popular lectures in 1873 on " The Value of Health to a City " exerted a powerful influence in the direction of sanitary reform, and helped to reduce the death rate, which at that time amounted to thirty-three per thousand.[2]

In the United States one of the most prominent authorities on public health was LEMUEL SHATTUCK (1793–1859), a bookseller and publisher with a keen interest in social welfare.[3] At the request of the city council he made a census of Boston in 1845. This work opened his eyes to the need for improvement in health and housing, and when he was nominated a member of the sanitary commission appointed to survey the entire State, he did most of the work, and wrote the Report of Massachusetts Sanitary Commission, 1850, which is one of the most remarkable documents in the annals of public health and might serve as an ideal even to-day. He pointed out the prevalence of preventible disease, and made certain suggestions, all of which were adopted in course of time. The Report went far towards awakening public interest.

[1] H. E. Sigerist, *Great Doctors*, New York, 1934
[2] H. E. Sigerist, trans. of Pettenkoffer's Lectures on " The Value of Health to a City," 1873, *Bull. Inst. Hist. Med.*, 1941, vol. x. p. 457
[3] G. C. Whipple, *State Sanitation: A Review of the Work of the Massachusetts State Board of Health*, 2 vols., Harvard Press, 1917, vol. i. p. 184

Boards of health were gradually established, the first in New Orleans in 1855, and eventually in all the other States. As bacteriology assumed importance, a State laboratory for Massachusetts was founded in 1895 under the control of THEOBALD SMITH (1859–1934), who was also the first to occupy the Chair of Comparative Pathology at Harvard.[1] Under his control diphtheria antitoxin and vaccine lymph were prepared in large quantities, and he supervised numerous bacteriological tests at a time when such tests were novelties. He demonstrated the parasite of Texas fever in cattle, and showed that it was transmitted by a tick. The differentiation of tubercle bacilli into human, bovine, and avian types was another of Theobald Smith's discoveries. The phenomenon of sensitivity to proteins, which became known as anaphylaxis, and later as allergy, was originally revealed by him. He was the foremost bacteriologist of America, one of whom his countrymen may well be proud (p. 288).

The Coming of Communal Medicine

During recent years public health has extended its scope very widely in Britain and elsewhere. The Public Health Act of 1875 imposed upon every urban or rural area the need to appoint a Medical Officer of Health, and at a later date it became essential that the M.O.H. should possess a special qualification in sanitary science. Public Health had become a specialty, and was no longer a mere appendage of medicine. Further legislation provided improvements in drainage and sewage disposal, pure water supplies, the isolation of infectious disease, better housing, improved ventilation, inspection of food supplies, medical inspection of school children, the control of syphilis and tuberculosis, and other reforms which are now accepted as the essentials of everyday life.

That, however, is only part of the story. Public Health is no longer an affair of plumbing and sanitation, important as such matters are. It has become Preventive Medicine in every sense of the term. The advent of specialism disturbed the easy relationship of doctor and patient. It became obvious that without outside assistance the doctor could no longer supply the needs of the patient when these included laboratory tests, vaccines, radiography, and many other specialized and " non-clinical " services.

[1] G. C. Whipple, *State Sanitation*, 2 vols., Harvard Press, 1917, vol. i. p. 96

Furthermore, it became obvious that there devolved upon the State the duty of providing medical attendance on a large scale. In Britain, the National Insurance Act of 1911 was the first step in this direction, and the Ministry of Health, set up in 1919, has interpreted still more widely the responsibility of a government for the health and well-being of the citizen. In 1946 the National Health Service Act was passed, and two years later the National Health Service was inaugurated to secure improvement in the mental and physical health of the people, and the prevention, diagnosis and treatment of illness. This development is still in progress and need not be considered here, although it will become history one day.

BOOKS FOR FURTHER READING

COLLINS, E. TREACHER. *The History and Traditions of the Moorfields Eye Hospital*, 1929

CURIE, EVE. *Madame Curie*, 1938

FRAZER, W. M. *A History of English Public Health, 1834–1939*, 1950

HALE-WHITE, Sir W. *Great Doctors of the Nineteenth Century*, 1935

HERRICK, J. B. *A Short History of Cardiology*, Springfield, Illinois, 1942

HOPKINS, E. *The Life and Letters of James Hinton*, 1878

KEITH, Sir A. *Menders of the Maimed*, 1919

MORRIS, Sir MALCOLM. *The Story of English Public Health*, 1919

NEEDHAM, J., and BALDWIN, E. (ed.). *Hopkins and Biochemistry*, 1949

NEWSHOLME, Sir A. *The Evolution of Preventive Medicine*, 1927

NEWSHOLME, A., and KINGSBURY, J. A. *Red Medicine*, 1933

OLDHAM, F. *Thomas Young, F.R.S., Philosopher and Physician*, 1933

POLITZER, A. *Geschichte der Ohrenheilkunde*, 2 vols., Stuttgart, 1907–13

PUSEY, W. A. *The History of Dermatology*, Springfield, U.S.A., 1933 ; *The History and Epidemiology of Syphilis*, Baltimore, 1933.

RAMON Y CAJAL, S. *Recollections of My Life*. Trans. by E. H. Craigie, Philadelphia, 1937

ROLLESTON, Sir HUMPHRY. *The Life of Sir Clifford Allbutt*, 1929

SEMON, Sir FELIX. *The Autobiography of Sir Felix Semon*, 1926

SIGERIST, H. E. *Great Doctors*, New York, 1934

STEVENSON, R. SCOTT, and GUTHRIE, DOUGLAS. *A History of Oto-laryngology*, 1949

WHIPPLE, G. C. *State Sanitation: A Review of the Work of the Massachusetts State Board of Health*, 2 vols., Harvard Press, 1917

WILSON, R. MCNAIR. *The Beloved Physician: The Life of Sir James Mackenzie*, 1926

WILSON, T. G. *Victorian Doctor: The Life of Sir William Wilde*, 1942

WITTELS, F. *Sigmund Freud: His Personality, His Teaching, and His School*, 1924

ZILBOORG, G., and HENRY, G. W. *A History of Medical Psychology*, New York, 1941

CHAPTER XX

JOURNALISM, BIBLIOGRAPHY, AND MEDICAL HISTORY

As a postcript to this survey of the history of medicine there may be added now a brief reference to the influence of journalism and bibliography upon the progress of medicine, as well as a tribute to a few eminent medical historians of recent times.

The Rise of Medical Journalism

Prior to the nineteenth century there were relatively few medical journals. Mention has been made of the first British medical journal, *Medicina Curiosa* (Plate LXXI), which appeared in two issues in 1684 but did not survive the year (p. 192). It would serve no useful purpose to name the thirty-seven medical periodicals which were published in Britain before the year 1800, as most of them had short lives and none now remain.[1]

Early in the nineteenth century the medical periodical assumed its present position as the most rapid and most suitable medium for the publication of original work, or for the dissemination of information relating to new medical discoveries.[2]

During the eighteenth century many important medical papers were read at the Royal Society, and appeared in the *Philosophical Transactions of the Royal Society*. At that period also a number of medical societies published transactions, but none continued to do so for very long. A publication of this nature, which endured until the turn of the century, was *Medical Transactions of the Royal College of Physicians of London* (1768–1820). *Transactions of the Medical Society of London*, founded in 1773, were first published in 1810, and have since continued in unbroken sequence, while the Medical and Chirurgical Society of London commenced the publication of *Medico-Chirurgical Transactions* in 1809, which continued as *Proceedings of the Royal Society of Medicine*

[1] F. H. Garrison, " The Medical and Scientific Periodicals of the Seventeenth and Eighteenth Centuries," *Bull. Inst. Hist. Med.*, 1934, vol. ii. p. 285
[2] W. R. Le Fanu, " British Periodicals of Medicine : A Chronological List " *Bull. Inst. Hist. Med.*, 1937, vol. v. pp. 735, 827 ; 1938, vol. vi. p. 614

when that new society was founded in 1907, and which still flourishes.[1]

The medical journal, as distinct from transactions of a society, was of late development, but it naturally had a wider range of usefulness, as it included not only original papers but also items of general medical interest such as reports of hospitals, abstracts of current medical literature, and reviews of books.

Among existing medical journals, the oldest in Britain is the *Edinburgh Medical Journal*, which, but for the slight change of title from *Edinburgh Medical and Surgical Journal* in 1855, has steadily continued publication since 1805. Next in seniority is *The Lancet*, which was founded in 1823 by the energetic THOMAS HENRY WAKLEY (1795–1862),[2] a general practitioner who took to journalism and set himself to report the lectures and even the operations of some of the most eminent teachers of medicine and surgery of the time. This practice was not always favoured by the lecturers, and on one occasion actually led to a law-suit, perhaps better now forgotten but mentioned here as it is described in detail by J. F. Clarke in a volume of reminiscences which gives a vivid picture of the medical life of London in his day.[3]

The *Glasgow Medical Journal* dates from 1828, and the *Dublin Medical Press*, founded 1839, joined the *Medical Circular*, dating from 1852, to form *The Medical Press and Circular* in 1866. *Guy's Hospital Reports* and *St. Thomas's Hospital Reports* have appeared regularly since 1836.

Meantime the British Medical Association, which had been founded in 1832 at Worcester Infirmary by Sir CHARLES HASTINGS (1794–1866), Physician to the Infirmary, published transactions of its meetings ; then in 1840 the *Provincial Medical and Surgical Journal* was produced, which became the *Association Medical Journal* in 1853, and eventually, in 1857, the *British Medical Journal*.[4]

The first of the specialist journals to appear, in 1853, was the *Asylum Journal of Mental Science*, which continued as the *Journal of Mental Science* after 1858. (See Supplement, page 462.)

Only the pioneers among medical journals have been mentioned. During the latter half of the century numerous new

[1] Reginald F. West, " A Chronological List of Medical Societies and Journals in the British Isles," *Med. Press and Circ.*, 1939, vol. ci. p. 117
[2] S. Squire Sprigge, *The Life and Times of Thomas Wakley*, 1899, p. 73
[3] J. F. Clarke, *Autobiographical Recollections of the Medical Profession*, 1874, p. 26
[4] E. M. Little, *History of the British Medical Association, 1832–1932*, 1932, p. 175

medical journals were founded, some of general scope, others devoted to a special branch of medicine. In an interesting paper on British periodicals of medicine, W. R. Le Fanu has given a list of 712 periodicals which were published between 1684 and 1899.[1] By 1938 the complete list for the years 1684 to 1938 had swollen to 1362, of which only 110 were surviving. F. H. Garrison states in his *Introduction to the History of Medicine*, 3rd ed., 1924, p. 807, that in 1913 there were 1,654 current medical periodicals in all languages. Of these 630 were American, 461 German, 268 French, 152 British, 75 Italian, and 29 Spanish. In 1925 1,927 periodicals were being supplied to the reading room of the Surgeon-General's library at Washington.

American Medical Journals

The first medical as well as the first scientific periodical to be published in America was a quarterly, the *Medical Repository*, which appeared in New York in 1797, and continued to flourish until 1824,[2] although some accord priority to *Mercurio Volante*, which appeared in Mexico City in 1773.[3] The early years of the nineteenth century produced a crop of American medical journals, eleven in all, only one of which lasted for more than a decade, and the majority for only a few years. The one exception was *The New England Medical Review and Journal*, founded in 1812, which became in 1827 the *Boston Medical and Surgical Journal*, and still exists under the name, *New England Journal of Medicine*.

In 1820, under the strong editorship of Nathaniel Chapman, said to be the most popular American physician of his time, there was launched the *Philadelphia Journal of the Medical and Physical Sciences*, which changed its name in 1827 to *American Journal of Medical Sciences*, and which still continues its long career. The first specialized journal to appear was the *American Journal of Obstetrics*, 1868 (since 1920 the *American Journal of Obstetrics and Gynaecology*); it was followed by others, including *Annals of Surgery*, 1885.

[1] W. R. Le Fanu, " British Periodicals of Medicine : A Chronological List," *Bull. Inst. Hist. Med.*, 1937, vol. v. p. 735, 827 ; 1938, vol. vi. p. 614
[2] John M. Armstrong, " The First American Medical Journals," in *Mayo Foundation Lectures*, Philadelphia, 1933
[3] A Chair of Medicine was founded in Mexico City as early as 1580.

Medical Journals of France

France can lay claim, not only to the first medical journal in the vernacular, but also to the first periodical of any kind. The latter is represented by *La Gazette de France*, a weekly paper first published in May 1631 by THÉOPHRASTE RENAUDOT (1586–1653), who thus earned the title, " The Father of Journalism." [1] Renaudot, having studied medicine at Montpellier, came to Paris in 1612, and became physician to the king and friend of Cardinal Richelieu.

Renaudot inaugurated a system of free medical treatment for poor persons reluctant to go to hospital, and as a further means of assisting the poor he founded the first pawnshop in Paris, the first of the *monts-de-piété* following the lead of the Italian *monte di pieta* of the fifteenth century. His most important work, however, was the publication, under government patronage, of the *Gazette*, which continued to appear until his death twenty-two years later. Renaudot's medical activities incurred the displeasure of the Faculty which, with Guy Patin at their head, took legal proceedings against him. The king was dead, Richelieu could no longer defend him, and eventually Renaudot, who had done so much for the poor, himself died a pauper.

The first medical journal of France was the creation of NICOLAS DE BLEGNY (1652–1722), who became physician to the king in 1687 [2] (see also p. 192). It was entitled *Nouvelles Descouvertes sur toutes les Parties de la Médecine*, although it underwent slight variations as to title after its first appearance in 1679, and eventually, on account of de Blegny's unpopularity with the Faculty, was transferred to Amsterdam in 1682, where for a short time it continued as *Le Mercure Savant*, the editor disguising his identity under the *nom de plume* of Gauthier. [3] Previous to this Latin and German translations of the journal had appeared at Geneva and Hamburg. According to recent authorities de Blegny was a mere charlatan, undeserving of the posthumous honour which has been given to him. They prefer to award the priority in medical journalism

---

[1] E. Forgue, " Théophraste Renaudot, médecin et père du journalisme," *Gaz. des Hôpitaux*, 1927, vol. c. p. 605 ; L. Böhmer, " Théophraste Renaudot, 1586–1653, der Bergründer der Pressein Arzt," *Deutsch. med. Woch.*, 1931, vol. lvii. p. 1076

[2] J. Lévy-Valensi, " Les Origines de la Presse médicale française," *La Presse médicale*, 1936, vol. xliv. p. 2125

[3] J. Lévy-Valensi, " Histoire de la Presse médicale française au XVIIᵉ siècle," *La Presse médicale*, 1938, vol. xlvi. p. 1229

to the Abbé de la Roque for his publication, the *Journal de Médecine*, which appeared in 1683, but did not survive the year. JEAN-PAUL DE LA ROQUE had been director of the *Journal des Sçavans* in 1665. This journal, as mentioned on page 192, was devoted to science, but it also accepted medical contributions, the first number containing a dissertation on sneezing, " De Sternutatione," by Martin Schooksis.

During the next hundred and fifty years, in France as in other countries, a number of short-lived medical periodicals had their day. The oldest still existing is the *Gazette des Hôpitaux civils et militaires*, which was founded in 1828, and which for a time bore the sub-title *La Lancette française*.

The *Bulletin de l'Académie de Médecine* commenced publication in 1836, *Le Progrès médical* in 1873, *Paris médical* in 1875, and *La Presse médicale* in 1880, and all exist to-day.

Among special journals one of the oldest is *Annales d'hygiène publique et de médecine légale*, which made its appearance in 1828, and still continues.

Medical Journalism in Germany and other Countries

Regarding the first German medical periodical to appear in the vernacular, there has been some difference of opinion among historians. According to Sudhoff the first medical journal published in Germany was *Acta medicorum Berolinensium*, Berlin, 1717.[1] This publication was in Latin, but the same year witnessed the appearance of *Sammlung von Natur und Medicin* in German. It thus seems that the latter journal is the pioneer German work.[2]

Another very early German medical journal was *Der patriotische Medicus*, published in Hamburg, 1724–26. At a slightly later date another weekly paper appeared, also at Hamburg, called *Der Arzt* (1759–64), soon to be followed by another short-lived weekly, *Der Landarzt* (1765–66).

The oldest surviving weekly medical publication in German may be the *Wiener medizinische Wochenschrift*, founded in 1851. It was followed in 1854 by the *Ärztliches Intelligenz-Blatt*, which, in 1885, became the *Münchener medizinische Wochenschrift*.[3] The

[1] K. Sudhoff, " Das medizinische Zeitschriftwesen in Deutschland bis zur Mitte des 19 Jahrhunderts," *Münch. med. Woch.*, 1903, vol. i. p. 455
[2] E. Runge, " Aus den Anfangen des deutschen medizinischen Zeitschriftenwesens," *Med. Welt.*, 1937, vol. xi. pp. 950, 984, 1019
[3] W. von Brunn, " Die Entwicklung des deutschen medizinischen Zeitschriften-wesens," *Deutsch. med. Woch.*, 1925, vol. li. p. 1077

Berliner klinische Wochenschrift began its career in 1864, the *Deutsche medizinische Wochenschrift* in 1875.

Germany also became noted for a number of "special" journals, the best known being the *Archiv für Anatomie und Physiologie* (since 1921 *Zeitschrift für Anatomie und Entwickelungsgeschichte*) founded by Johannes Müller in 1834, and Virchow's *Archiv für pathologische Anatomie und Physiologie und für klinische Medizin*, dating from 1847. Pflüger's *Archiv für gesamte Physiologie* was founded in 1868, and Langenbeck's *Archiv für klinische Chirurgie* in 1861.

The first Italian weekly medical journal was the *Giornale di Medicina*, which was produced in Venice by Pietro Orteschi in 1763 and continued until 1781.[1] The first Dutch medical periodical was *Collecteanea medico-physica oft Hollands Jaar Register*, Amsterdam, 1680,[2] while the first Russian journal was *Sankt Petersburgskoye Vrachevnie Vaidomosti*, St. Petersburg, 1792.[3] The first Spanish medical periodical, *Efemérides barométrico-médicas matritenses*, Madrid, 1734, dealt with medical meteorology.

Journals of Medical History

Among the numerous journals which were founded to represent the various special branches of medicine, there have been a number devoted to the history of medicine. The earliest periodical of this nature, as Garrison pointed out, was the *Archiv für Geschichte der Arzneykunde*, published at Nuremberg in 1790 by PHILIPP LUDWIG WITTWER (1752–92), a highly esteemed physician of that town.[4] Through lack of support, only one number of the journal appeared. In recent times there have been a number of journals of the history of medicine. A few may be mentioned, as they contain many references which are indispensable to the student of the subject. Although there is no British journal on the subject, the *Proceedings of the Historical Section of the Royal Society of Medicine* (inaugurated 1913) supply much interesting material.

[1] J. Lafont, "Les Débuts du Journalisme médical italien," *Progrès méd.*, 1926, vol. xli. p. 1947. E. Padovani, "Per la storia del giornalismo medico italiano," *Riv. di storia med. e nat.*, 1930, vol. xxi. p. 50
[2] C. C. Delprat, "History of Dutch Medical Journals, 1680–1857," *Neder. Tijdsch. v. Geneesk*, 1927, vol. i. p. 3
[3] B. S. Bessmertny, "History of the Russian Medical Press," *Sovet. vrach. zhur.*, 1940, vol. xliv. p. 859
[4] F. H. Garrison, "The First Periodical of Medical History," *Bull. N.Y. Acad. Med.*, 1932, vol. viii. p. 421

America has two publications, *Annals of Medical History* (Philadelphia, since 1918) and *Bulletin of the Institute of the History of
Medicine* (Johns Hopkins Institute, Baltimore, since 1933).

South America has two journals : *Revista Brasileira de Historia
da Medicina*, Rio de Janeiro (since 1949), and *Anales de la Sociedad
Peruana de Historia de la Medicina*, Lima (annually since 1939),
edited respectively by Professors Vasconellos and Lastres.

In Holland the publication in English, French, and German
known as *Janus* continued from 1896 to 1941 ; the sub-title
was *Archives internationales pour l'Histoire de la Médecine et pour
la Géographie médicale*, combining history and geography in an
interesting fashion. In France the *Bulletin de la Société française
d'Histoire de la Médecine*, founded 1906, was the periodical of
medical history ; in Germany the well-known *Archiv für Geschichte
der Medizin* was inaugurated by Sudhoff in 1907. Both of these
periodicals were current in 1939.

It is not easy to assign priority of publication in dealing with
medical periodicals. They arose partly as transactions of learned
societies and partly as scientific periodicals which accepted
medical papers, and did not spring forth as full-fledged medical
journals. Nevertheless, the above list, though by no means complete, may serve to illustrate the rise and progress of journalism
to the important place it holds to-day in medical science.

Medical Bibliography

During the nineteenth century the output of medical literature
increased to such an extent as to be almost beyond the control of
potential readers. In 1881 one-thirtieth of the entire world's
literature was medical. Anyone who has attempted to verify a
quotation from a lengthy novel, or to collect data on a given
subject by reading at random, must realize how futile and how
time-consuming such a task may become.

Books are useful tools in medicine, but the tool must have a
handle, and that handle is supplied by the index. There must be
an index to the entire literature, as well as to the individual book,
and it is the task of the bibliographer to supply such an index.

Even in the sixteenth century CONRAD GESNER of Zurich
(1516–65), the greatest naturalist and scholar of his day, had compiled a *Bibliotheca universalis*, three volumes (1543). ALBRECHT VON
HALLER (1708–77), two centuries later, published his *Bibliotheca*

Medicinae Practicae, four volumes (1776–78), in which he classified 52,000 publications on anatomy, botany, surgery, and medicine.

LUDWIG HAIN (1781–1836) produced his *Repertorium Biblio-graphicum* (1826–38), a list of incunabula, or books printed prior to the year 1500.

More ambitious than any previous achievement in medical bibliography was that of ADOLPH CARL PETER CALLISEN of Copenhagen (1787–1866). Callisen's *Medicinisches Schriftsteller Lexicon*, in thirty-three volumes, 1830–45, is one of the greatest tasks in bibliography ever accomplished by one man.[1] It is a complete index of all medical literature, 99,000 items in all, which had been published between the years 1750 and 1830.

All these bibliographic efforts, useful though they were, cannot compare in magnitude and usefulness with that of JOHN SHAW BILLINGS (1838–1913), to whom we owe the Index Catalogue of the Surgeon-General's Library, and the *Index Medicus*.[2] The son of a farmer in Indiana, Billings showed early promise of scholarship, taught himself Latin and Greek, and eventually became a graduate of the Medical College of Ohio, founded by Daniel Drake (p. 299), for whom Billings had ever a high regard. Billings was teaching anatomy in the college with a view to becoming a surgeon, when the Civil War broke out and he at once joined the army. He saw much active service during the next few years. His ability as a surgeon led to his frequent employment as a consultant in difficult cases, and he was the first surgeon in the war to perform excision of the ankle joint (1862), an unusual operation in those pre-antiseptic days.

In 1864 he was breveted Lieutenant-Colonel for his services, and transferred to the office of the Surgeon-General at Washington.

A survey of the marine hospital service which he undertook in 1869–74 focused his attention on problems of hospital construction and administration, on which he became the leading authority. His advice was eagerly sought in many quarters. It was he who planned the Johns Hopkins Hospital and Medical School at Baltimore, which was opened in 1889, and which has done so much to raise the standard of medical education in America. Later, Billings was Professor of Hygiene at Philadelphia

[1] A. C. P. Callisen, *Medicinisches Schriftsteller-Lexicon der jetzt lebenden Aerzte, Wundarzte, Geburtshelfer, Apotheker und Naturforscher aller gebildeten Völker*, Copenhagen, 1830–45
[2] F. H. Garrison, *John Shaw Billings: A Memoir*, New York, 1915. (The Index Catalogue is familiarly known as the "Surgeon-General's Catalogue.")

PLATE LXXI   THE EARLIEST MEDICAL JOURNAL
IN ENGLISH

Medicina Curiosa, 1684, the first medical periodical to be printed in English
(pages 192, 393)

PLATE LXXII   OSLER WRITING HIS TEXTBOOK

Partturit Osler   Nascitur Liber.

Osler devoted most of the year 1891 to this task. He had recently been appointed Professor of Medicine at Johns Hopkins University, Baltimore (page 409) from 1892 until 1896, when he accepted the post of director of the New York Public Library, which he retained until his death.

As one of the most eminent medical men of his generation, he was the recipient of honorary degrees from a number of universities in America and in Europe. Of all the manifold activities of this versatile man none ranks higher than his work as a bibliographer. Indeed, he was the greatest bibliographer in the history of medicine. When Billings assumed duty at the Surgeon-General's office in 1864 there was a small collection of some two thousand books for the benefit of the staff. From this small nucleus he built up the greatest medical library in the world, and supplied it with an index catalogue, thereby rendering a great service to medicine, a service which was regarded by Professor W. H. Welch as "America's greatest contribution to medical science."

The library grew steadily. The 2,000 volumes of 1864 became 13,000 in 1871. Billings continued his preparation of catalogues, and that of 1873 included 25,000 books and 15,000 pamphlets. In 1876 he published a specimen fasciculus of a catalogue of the National Medical Library, and submitted it for criticism and suggestions. A comprehensive index of the world's medical literature was envisaged, arranged alphabetically under authors and subjects, the classification being flexible so as to meet advances or changes in medicine. Billings believed that such a publication " would elevate the standard of medical education, literature, and scholarship, and would be for the benefit of the whole country." The fasciculus was well received, and a grant was made to enable the idea to be put into operation. The Surgeon-General's Library, as it was usually called, gradually became the greatest medical library of the world, and the index catalogue was therefore a guide to the world's medical literature from the earliest time to the present day. The first volume of the new *Index Catalogue* appeared in 1880, and the first series of sixteen volumes was completed in 1895. A second and a third series (1896–1916 and 1918–1932) followed, a fourth is now in process of publication, having in 1942 reached the letter H and volume vii.

In the colossal task of preparing the first index catalogue, Billings was fortunate in having the assistance of ROBERT FLETCHER (1823–1912), who joined him in 1876.[1] Fletcher, who had been

---

[1] Sir W. Osler, " Dr. Robert Fletcher, 1823–1912," *Bristol Med.-Chir. Jour.*, 1912, vol. xxx. p. 283

born and educated at Bristol, went to the United States at the age of twenty-four, and practised for some years in Cincinnati. Then, like Billings, he volunteered for service in the Civil War, and was eventually posted to the Surgeon-General's Library, where he spent the remainder of his long life. In addition to his bibliographic work, Fletcher was interested in medical juris-prudence, on which he lectured at Johns Hopkins Medical School, as well as anthropology and medical history.

While Billings and Fletcher were at work on the first volume of the index catalogue they conceived the idea of another publica-tion, which would keep the medical profession in touch with cur-rent literature. It had taken as long as fifteen years to work through the alphabet in the first series of the catalogue, so that while the information on zymotic diseases (Z), was up-to-date, that on abscess (A) was already fourteen years old. The additional index envisaged by Billings and Fletcher was a monthly index of the current medical literature of all countries. In 1879 the first number of the *Index Medicus* was published, Fletcher taking a leading part in its preparation, and continuing to do so for the next twenty-one years.[1] There was then a break in the con-tinuity for lack of financial support.

A praiseworthy attempt was made by Professor CHARLES RICHET of Paris (1850–1935), better known as the exponent of " anaphylaxis," to revive the idea by the preparation of *Biblio-graphia Medica*, of which three volumes appeared (1900–1902). In 1903 the *Index Medicus* resumed publication under the patron-age of the Carnegie Institution of Washington, with Fletcher as editor. After Fletcher's death the work was continued by Garrison, and in 1927 the *Quarterly Cumulative Index to Current Medical Literature*, which had been published for ten years by the American Medical Association, was amalagamated with the *Index Medicus* to form the *Quarterly Cumulative Index Medicus*, which continues to appear and is a complete and accurate guide to current medical literature. (See Supplement, page 462.)

Thus did the original idea of John S. Billings come to full fruition, a great ambition, nobly planned and amply fulfilled, " a world record of the scientific endeavour of physicians in all ages."

" I'll let you into the secret," said Billings to one who praised

[1] F. H. Garrison, " Dr. Robert Fletcher : An Appreciation," *Jour. Amer. Med. Assn.*, 1912, vol. lix. p. 1907

his work. "There's nothing really difficult if you only begin. There would be no coral islands if the first bug sat down and began to wonder how the job was to be done."

Medical Historians of Recent Times

A devoted pupil of Billings and Fletcher who became distinguished as a historian of medicine was FIELDING HUDSON GARRISON (1870–1935), author of the leading source-book to which every subsequent historian has turned for guidance.[1] The son of a government official whose ancestors had been planters in Virginia for generations, Garrison was born in Washington. He graduated in arts at Johns Hopkins University in 1890, and then entered the Surgeon-General's Library as a clerk, at the same time proceeding to the study of medicine. His medical training was completed at Georgetown University, Washington, but the practical side of medicine never attracted him. In the library he continued to work for the next forty years, with the exception of two years of military service in the Phillipine Islands (1922–24).[2] He had joined the army on a temporary basis during the Great War, and in 1920 had been awarded a permanent commission for his services. Ten years later he retired from the army with the rank of colonel, to spend the remaining five years of his life as librarian to the Welch Medical Library and Lecturer on the History of Medicine at Johns Hopkins University.

Garrison's life was dominated by two ruling passions, music and literature. Himself a gifted musician and a skilled pianist, he held that there was a correlation between medicine and music, since so many eminent physicians were lovers of music.[3] His favourite composers were Brahms and Schubert. An omnivorous and critical reader, he had a fine literary taste and a retentive memory. His extensive knowledge of literature was freely available to all who sought his assistance, and many a young author owed much to his wise and experienced guidance.

Much of his work at the Surgeon-General's Library, or Army Medical Library as it came to be called, was concerned with the preparation of the *Index Catalogue* and *Index Medicus*, under the

[1] S. R. Kagan, *Life and Letters of Fielding H. Garrison*, Boston, 1938
[2] Lt.-Col. E. E. Hume, "Garrison and the Army Medical Library," *Bull. Inst. Hist. Med.*, 1937, vol. v. p. 301
[3] F. H. Garrison, "Medical Men Who Have Loved Music," *Bull. Soc. Med. Hist.*, Chicago, 1920, vol. ii. p. 158

guidance of Billings and Fletcher. On the death of the latter in 1912, Garrison continued the work as editor of both publications.

He also published an abridged version of the great catalogue, entitled, *A Revised Students' Check-List of Texts Illustrating the History of Medicine* (*Bull. Inst. Hist. Med.*, 1933, vol. i., p. 333), and this proved so useful that it was revised and annotated by L. T. Morton.[1] It supplies in handy form a reference book giving data of the principal "classics" of medical literature, 5,506 in number.

Although he was a good linguist, a hard worker, and a scholar of high attainments, Garrison lacked the administrative ability which was so strongly developed in Billings. He hated publicity, and was a poor lecturer. Accordingly, he never rose beyond the position of assistant librarian. Garrison wrote many valuable books and articles, but his fame chiefly rests upon his *Introduction to the History of Medicine*, which was published in 1913, subsequent editions appearing in 1917, 1921, 1924, and 1929.[2]

Despite its modest title this work is a complete and concise history, accurate, thorough, and withal attractive to read. One half of the volume of 900 pages deals with the modern period, subsequent to 1800. It is not surprising that Garrison's *History* at once became the standard work, and that it still holds a leading position. It probably has done more than any other work to foster and promote an interest in medical history. Garrison was wise enough to see that no single volume could encompass the subject, yet his work is full of useful sign-posts, pointing the way for every inquiring investigator. Only a trained bibliographer could have produced such a work. The tradition of Billings and Fletcher had come to full fruition in Garrison.

On the continent of Europe the greatest medical historian of the modern period was KARL SUDHOFF (1853–1938). The background to his studies, which was provided by thirty years of general practice near Düsseldorf, partly accounted for Sudhoff's conspicuous success as a historian of medicine.[3] During those years he devoted all his spare time to the subject. In 1905 he was appointed the

---

[1] F. H. Garrison, compiler of, and L. T. Morton, reviser of, *A Medical Bibliography*, 1943
[2] F. H. Garrison, *An Introduction to the History of Medicine*, 1913
[3] W. von Brunn, "Nachruf auf Karl Sudhoff," *Arch. f. Gesch. Med.*, 1938, vol xxxi. p. 338 ; F. H. Garrison, "Professor Karl Sudhoff and the Institute of Medical History at Leipzig," *Bull. Soc. Med. Hist.*, Chicago, 1923, vol. iii. p. 1

first occupant of the Chair of History of Medicine in the University of Leipzig, a chair which had been endowed by Theodore Puschmann (p. 415), Professor of the History of Medicine at Vienna. Sudhoff founded an institute of medical history at Leipzig, and being now freed from the claims of practice he undertook a series of journeys to Italy in order to investigate the libraries and museums. A hard worker and a prolific writer, he published more than five hundred monographs during his lifetime. His researches dealt with many subjects—the history of dentistry, the School of Salerno, German medical incunabula, anatomical illustrations of the Middle Ages, the origin of syphilis, and above all, the place of Paracelsus in the history of medicine. His first edition of the works of Paracelsus, in fifteen volumes, appeared in 1933.

Sudhoff did much to emphasize the importance of the history of medicine, and to show that it is not merely a curious and interesting side-line but is in fact medicine itself. In his view history gave to medicine a broad general cutlture, and was the best school of medical ethics. A study of history tended to prevent that isolation which is a natural consequence of increasing specialism. Furthermore, the history of medicine was an essential link between medicine and the other sciences, and a link with theology, law, and philosophy. Sudhoff was a true disciple of Hippocrates in his endeavour to further the highest professional ideals.

In Great Britain the history of medicine has attracted many scholars, of whom several leaders may be specially mentioned. The work of others, still happily with us, is noted in the appendix dealing with bibliography.

One of the first in Britain to revive the study of the history of medicine at a time when it had come to be neglected was Sir NORMAN MOORE (1847–1922), Physician to St. Bartholomew's Hospital, and a man of strong personality and wide scholarship.[1] His *History of St. Bartholomew's Hospital* (1919), which occupied his leisure for many years, is a splendid memorial to his literary skill. Fluency and accuracy are also apparent in the biographies, some five hundred in all, which he contributed to the *Dictionary of National Biography*, and in his Fitzpatrick Lectures on *The History of the Study of Medicine in the British Isles* (1908). Those

[1] Sir Norman Moore, obituary notices in *Brit. Med. Jour.*, 1922, vol. ii. p. 1148 ; *Lancet*, 1922, vol. ii. p. 1250

lectures were among lecture courses in the history of medicine which still continue at the Royal College of Physicians in honour of Dr. THOMAS FITZPATRICK (1832–1900), a distinguished member of the college. Sir Norman Moore was especially interested in the mediaeval period, and his work is the fruit of much original research. He was distinguished as a clinical teacher as well as writer. " The three things he taught were, consideration of the patient, careful study of the signs of disease, and a precise statement of the facts observed." In alluding to the old books he loved so well he would say, " I do not want you to read these books because they are old, but because they are good."

Another distinguished member of the staff of St. Bartholomew's Hospital who was interested in the history of medicine, this time a surgeon, was Sir D'ARCY POWER (1855–1941), who made valuable contributions to the literature of surgery, in particular the surgery of the abdomen and of malignant disease.[1] His contributions to the *Dictionary of National Biography* were almost as numerous as those of Sir Norman Moore, and it was he who edited in 1930 Plarr's *Lives of the Fellows of the Royal College of Surgeons* (2 vols.), which had been completed at great pains by VICTOR GUSTAVE PLARR (1860–1929), who was librarian to the college for thirty-two years.

D'Arcy Power's first venture into the history of medicine was his edition of *Memorials of the Craft of Surgery in England* (1886), the material for which had been collected by JOHN FLINT SOUTH (1797–1882), Surgeon to St. Thomas's Hospital, as part of a history of surgery which he had intended to write. The *Memorials of John Flint South*, part biography, part autobiography, give an interesting account of the time.[2] The edition of John of Arderne's book on *Fistula in Ano*, published by the Early English Text Society, was edited by Sir D'Arcy Power. His literary work was by no means limited to editing. A volume of *Selected Writings* which appeared in 1931 contains essays on such varied subjects as the travels of William Harvey, how British surgery came to America, why Samuel Pepys discontinued his diary, surgery in England in the fourteenth century, and the education of a surgeon under Thomas Vicary.

[1] Sir D'Arcy Power, obituary notices in *Brit. Med. Jour.*, 1941, vol. i. p. 836 ; *Lancet*, 1941, vol. i. p. 709 ; *Brit. Jour. Surg.*, 1941, vol. xxix. p. 1
[2] Rev. C. L. Feltoe, *Memorials of John Flint South, twice President of the Royal College of Surgeons, and Surgeon of St. Thomas's Hospital (1841-63)*, 1884

Sir D'Arcy Power was not only an eminent scholar and bibliophile and a sound surgeon, he was endowed with a charm of manner and cheerful disposition which led him to be known to generations of students as " Sunny Jim."

London had no monopoly of historians of medicine. In Glasgow there was JAMES FINLAYSON (1840–1906), a leading physician of his time and a keen bibliophile.[1] His bibliographical demonstrations on medical classics in the library of the Faculty of Physicians and Surgeons of Glasgow proved a popular and interesting approach to the study of medical history. He did much to foster interest in the subject ; among his writings is an account of the founder of the Glasgow Faculty, *The Life and Works of Maister Peter Lowe* (*cf.* p. 154).

Edinburgh possessed an eminent historian of medicine in JOHN DIXON COMRIE (1875–1939), who lectured on the subject at the University of Edinburgh for over thirty years, and was the author of many original papers. His *History of Scottish Medicine*, 2 vols. (1932), is a noteworthy contribution to national medical history, well illustrated and carefully documented.

Oxford and Cambridge have also had their historians of medicine in recent times, both of them historians who were also eminent physicians. The services of Sir THOMAS CLIFFORD ALLBUTT (1836–1925) to cardiology have already been mentioned (p. 366). During his long life he witnessed many changes in medical science, the introduction of anaesthesia, the birth of bacteriology, the development of antiseptic surgery, the creation of the nursing profession, the progress of public health, the discovery of X-rays, radium, and vitamins, and the rise of specialization.

To those changes Allbutt freely contributed. In addition to his *System of Medicine* (six volumes), and his Fitzpatrick Lectures on *Greek Medicine in Rome*, he wrote a valuable little work on the composition of scientific papers, which every medical writer would do well to study. In his valuable contribution to the subject of medical education, he never tired of insisting on the value of a sound general education as a basis. As befitted a scholar and omnivorous reader, all his writing was careful, accurate, and well-phrased. Before he became professor at Cambridge he spent thirty years in practice at Leeds, and during this period he was well known to George Eliot, who is said to have depicted him as

[1] James Finlayson, obituary notice in *Glas. Med. Jour.*, 1906, vol. lxvi. p. 360

Dr. Tertius Lydgate in *Middlemarch*, that novel which Stephen Paget was wont to urge every medical student to read. It is interesting to note that Allbutt was the inventor, in 1867, of the short portable clinical thermometer, a great advance on Wunderlich's instrument, which was a foot long, and which took twenty minutes to register the temperature. A delightful biography of Sir Clifford Allbutt has been written by his successor in the Chair, Sir HUMPHRY DAVY ROLLESTON (1862–1944).[1]

Still more closely devoted to the history of medicine was Allbutt's contemporary at Oxford, Sir William Osler, a note of whose life and work may form a fitting conclusion to this volume.

Osler and Medical History

Sir WILLIAM OSLER (1849–1919)[2] probably did more than any other medical man to link the Old World with the New. Using the word " World " in its geographical sense, no one was more successful in promoting friendships between medical men and medical institutions on each side of the Atlantic, while, if the World of history be envisaged, Osler was the Janus who, looking back and looking forward, at the end of the nineteenth century, showed how important to the medicine of the present was an appreciation of the medicine of the past. In the words of his friend and colleague, Professor W. H. Welch, " Osler himself became part of the scheme which he laboured unceasingly to unfold during his lifetime." " His fame as a scholarly student of medical history is only second to his repute as a great clinical teacher."

Details of Osler's career may be found in the admirable biography of Harvey Cushing. A Canadian by birth, and Professor of Medicine successively at Montreal (1874), Philadelphia (1884), Baltimore (1889), and Oxford (1904), he left the stamp of his powerful personality in each of those centres of medical learning, and he achieved a truly international reputation. In his opinion, " our culture should be cosmopolitan, not national," and still less, the product of one school. " In-breeding," he wrote, " is as hurtful to colleges as to cattle," and he advised what he called

[1] Sir Humphry D. Rolleston, *Life of Sir Clifford Allbutt*, 1929
[2] H. Cushing, *The Life of Sir William Osler*, 2 vols., 1925 ; E. G. Reid, *The Great Physician : A Short Life of Sir William Osler*, 1931 ; M. E. Abbott, ed. of *Sir William Osler Memorial Volume*, Montreal, 1926

" a peripatetic professoriate," for he never could understand how some professors " have the hardihood to remain in the same position for twenty-five years." He favoured " a quinquennial brain dusting " as essential for all practitioners : " Every fifth year, back to hospital or laboratory for renovation, rehabilitation, rejuvenation and the like."

As a clinical teacher, he was unrivalled. " The Baby Pro-fessor," as he was affectionately called when he assumed the Chair at McGill at the age of twenty-five, was teacher, friend, and fellow-student, all combined. Although he always regarded the personality of the teacher as more important than his writings, and even suggested as his own epitaph, " I taught medicine at the bedside," his textbook, *The Principles and Practice of Medicine*, 1892, had an enormous circulation (Plate LXII). It was translated into French, German, Spanish, and Chinese, and is still a standard work, which has gone into many editions.[1] Osler drew his inspiration, not only from an extensive clinical and pathological experience, but from a wide knowledge of classical medical literature. When the textbook was criticized for a lack of detail regarding treatment, he replied that already there was far too much treatment, and that he had little faith in drugs. " Time, in divided doses," was a favourite prescription with Osler. He often told his class that Oliver Wendell Holmes learned three things in Paris—" not to take authority when he could take facts, not to guess when he could know, and not to think that a man must take physic because he is sick." [2]

Osler's keen interest in pathology is illustrated by the oft-quoted tale of the old and seedy individual who begged for alms on the street. He gave the man a coin, with the remark " There is only one thing of value about you, and that is your ' hobnailed liver,' referring to the appearance of the alcoholic liver, familiar to pathologists. Then, handing the beggar his overcoat, he added, " You may drink yourself to death, but I cannot allow you to freeze to death." The man inquired the name of his benefactor, and the reply came, " Dr. William Osler, and don't forget the liver." When the old fellow died a fortnight later it was found that he had made a will, leaving " to my friend Dr. William Osler, his overcoat and my hobnailed liver."

[1] H. E. MacDermot, " Notes on Osler's Textbook of Medicine," *Ann. Med. Hist.*, 1934, vol. vi. p. 224
[2] Sir W. Osler, *An Alabama Student, and Other Biographical Essays*, 1908, p. 55

The magnetic personality of Osler was apparent to his numerous friends and to generations of students, who all revered him. His delightful volumes of historical essays, *Aequanimitas* (1904) and *An Alabama Student* (1908), are full of wise counsel, and should be in the hands of every medical student. Such works reveal anew the value and importance of the cultural side of medicine. " A physician," we read, " needs culture as well as learning. He may possess the science of Harvey and the art of Sydenham, and yet there may be lacking in him those finer qualities of heart and head which count for so much in life." He pointed out that throughout the ages the medical man was, in turn, priest, philosopher and physician. Osler was himself an example of all three. Optimism and equanimity were his watchwords. Of the first of these qualities he wrote : " Hilarity and good humour . . . a nature sloping ' towards the southern side,' as Lowell has it, help enormously both in the study and in the practice of medicine " ; of the second, " Imperturbability means coolness and presence of mind under all circumstances. It is the quality which is most appreciated by the laity though it is apt to be misinterpreted as callousness. The first essential is to have your nerves well in hand."

Osler could never have undertaken his vast programme had he not worked to a time-table in which each duty had its allotted hour. Life was to be lived in " day-tight compartments," for " when the day's activities are properly directed and rightly balanced, work is not work, but pleasure." " Banish the future ; live only for the hour and its allotted work."

Ever a lover of books, he built up a valuable library, now the property of the McGill University, Montreal. His *Bibliographia Osleriana* is an indispensable guide to the medical literature of the past. Not that his reading was wholly medical. His net was cast wide, and he had his favourites, chief among them being Sir Thomas Browne's *Religio Medici*, which he knew so well. He counselled his students to " start a bedside library and spend the last half-hour of the day in communion with the saints."

He was also tireless in his advocacy of a more widespread interest in the history of medicine, affirming that " by the historical method alone can many problems of medicine be approached profitably," and that " it is a dry age when the great men of the past are held in light esteem."

Conclusion

There could be no more suitable note on which to conclude this review of the healing art down the ages than Sir William Osler's reflections upon our medical heritage.[1]

" We may indeed be justly proud of our apostolic succession. Schools and systems have flourished and gone . . . the philosophies of one age have become the absurdities of the next, and the foolishness of yesterday has become the wisdom of to-morrow ; through long ages which were slowly learning what we are hurrying to forget, amid all the changes and chances of twenty-five centuries, the profession has never lacked men who have lived up to the Greek ideals. They were those of Galen and Aretaeus, of men of the Alexandrian and Byzantine schools, of the best of the Arabians, of the men of the Renaissance, and they are ours to-day."

[1] W. Osler, *Aequanimitas and Other Addresses*, 1904, p. 281

BOOKS FOR FURTHER READING

CLARKE, G. F. *Autobiographical Recollections of the Medical Profession*, 1874
CUSHING, HARVEY. *The Life of Sir William Osler*, 2 vols., 1925
GARRISON, F. H. *John Shaw Billings : A Memoir*, New York, 1915
GARRISON, F. H., and MORTON, L. T. *A Medical Bibliography*, 2nd ed., 1954
KAGAN, S. R. *Life and Letters of Fielding H. Garrison*, Boston, 1938
LITTLE, E. MUIRHEAD. *History of the British Medical Association (1822–1932)*, 1932
OSLER, Sir W. *An Alabama Student, and Other Essays*, 1908
SPRIGGE, S. SQUIRE. *The Life and Times of Thomas Wakley*, 1899
THORNTON, JOHN L. *Medical Books, Libraries and Collectors*, 1949

APPENDIX

A CLASSIFIED BIBLIOGRAPHY OF MEDICAL HISTORY

i HISTORIES OF MEDICINE

While the following list is not to be regarded as a complete catalogue of all the available histories of medicine, it is hoped that it may serve as a useful guide to the student who wishes to pursue the subject. The scope and nature of the various works are indicated in the following notes.

PIONEER WORKS

CHAMPIER, SYMPHORIEN (1472–1539). *De Medicinae claris scriptoribus in quinque partibus tractatus*, Lyons, 1506

FREIND, JOHN (1675–1728). *The History of Physick from the Time of Galen to the Beginning of the Sixteenth Century*, 2 vols., 1725–27

LE CLERC, DANIEL (1652–1728). *Histoire de la Médecine*, La Haye, 1729

MIDDLETON, P. (–1781). *A Medical Discourse, or an Historical Inquiry into the Ancient and Present State of Medicine*, New York, 1769

SPRENGEL, KURT (1766–1833). *Versuch einer pragmatischen Geschichte der Arztneikunde*, 5 vols., Halle, 1792–1803

Notes

SYMPHORIEN CHAMPIER of Lyons may be regarded as the pioneer of modern medical historians, as his book was the first to be written on the subject since the time of Celsus, with the single exception of the historical chapter in Guy de Chauliac's *Chirurgia Magna*, written in 1363 and printed in French in 1478. Champier's history, published at Lyons in 1506, remained the authority for many years, although it is now of interest mainly to the bibliophile.

JOHN FREIND was the first to write a history of medicine in English. He began the work while he was a prisoner in the Tower of London on a charge of treason, of which he was afterwards acquitted, thanks to the intervention of his friend Richard Mead. Freind designed his work as a continuation of the history which had just appeared from the pen of Daniel Le Clerc of Geneva. Freind's *History of Physick from the Time of Galen to Beginning of the Sixteenth Century* may still be read with profit, the sections dealing with Byzantine, Arabic, and Early English medicine being specially noteworthy (p. 255).

LE CLERC's *Histoire* is a handsome volume containing much information on Greek Medicine which is still authoritative, as well as much which must now be regarded as fictitious. The account practically ends with the period of Galen.

MIDDLETON's little book is mentioned as the first American contribution to medical history.

KURT SPRENGEL of Pomerania wrote a massive five-volume history which comes next in chronological order. To collect information for such a history

412

APPENDIX

from original sources was an immense undertaking, but it was so well accomplished that the work, completed in 1803, has remained an indispensable quarry for later historians.

MORE RECENT WORKS

ENGLISH

BERDOE, E. *The Origin and Growth of the Healing Art*, 1893

WITHINGTON, E. T. *Medical History from the Earliest Times*, 1894

CUMSTON, C. G. *The History of Medicine from the Time of the Pharaohs to the End of Eighteenth Century*, 1896

PARK, R. *An Epitome of the History of Medicine*, 1898

GARRISON, F. H. *An Introduction to the History of Medicine*, 1913 ; trans. Sudhoff's *Essays in the History of Medicine*, New York, 1926

BUCK, A. H. *The Growth of Medicine from the Earliest Times to 1800*, Yale, 1917 ; *The Dawn of Modern Medicine (Eighteenth and Early Nineteenth Century)*, Yale, 1920

OSLER, Sir W. *The Evolution of Modern Medicine*, 1921

SINGER, C. *A Short History of Medicine*, 1928 ; *Studies in the History and Method of Science*, 2 vols., Oxford, 1917–21

STUBBS, S. G. B., and BLIGH, E. W. *Sixty Centuries of Health and Physick*, 1931

CASTIGLIONI, A. *History of Medicine*, 1941. (Trans. from Italian by E. B. Krumbhaar.)

THORNDIKE, L. *History of Magic and Experimental Science*, 6 vols., 1934–41

Notes

BERDOE'S work is of interest, especially those chapters dealing with Preventive Medicine, with the ancient civilizations of the East, and with the Greeks, though it is now somewhat outmoded.

WITHINGTON'S little volume, now becoming rare, is in some respects the best of all medical histories. It bears the unmistakable stamp of scholarship and original research. The author is no compiler, and his book is a stimulus and inspiration, although it does not take us beyond the eighteenth century.

CUMSTON adopts an unusual approach, dealing with trends and doctrines in medicine rather than with biographies of the great. He is most informative in his descriptions of the medical sects among the Greeks, though his volume cannot be classed as light reading.

ROSWELL PARK'S *Epitome* is a short survey, with special emphasis on American work.

GARRISON'S excellent and well-known history must receive priority of mention among the more modern works in English. No-one has done more than Garrison to deepen and extend interest in medical history on both sides of the Atlantic. His book is packed with information, and is liberally supplied with references and bibliographies. It is in fact the medical historian's Bible, and library copies are always in steady use. About one half of the volume deals with the nineteenth century and after.

BUCK, in his two books, one supplementary to the other, gives an interesting and flowing narrative which will attract readers. One wishes that he had given a larger bibliography as a guide to deeper study.

OSLER published his lectures on "The Evolution of Modern Medicine," a brief outline of the entire field, charmingly presented and illustrated, but intended merely as an introduction to wider study.

CHARLES SINGER is probably the most eminent living medical historian to-day. His *Short History of Medicine* is an account of the rise and progress of medicine which ought to be read by every medical student, as it will save him from becoming a mere technician in later practice.

STUBBS and BLIGH have traced the progress of healing through the centuries, with special reference to public health. Their story is fascinating, though it does not purport to be more than a semi-popular account of the history of medicine. The illustrations are unusual and informative.

FRENCH

DAREMBERG, C. *Histoire des Sciences médicales*, 2 vols., Paris, 1870
MEUNIER, L. *Histoire de la Médecine depuis ses origines jusqu'à nos jours*, Paris, 1911
LAIGNEL-LAVASTINE, M. *Histoire générale de la Médecine, de la Pharmacie, de l'Art dentaire et de l'Art vétérinaire*, vols. 1 and 2, Paris, 1934–38

Notes

Among French works that of DAREMBERG held the field for many years. His *Histoire* is still worthy of study, as he was the greatest medical historian of his time.

MEUNIER'S short book is well written ; naturally enough, French contributions to medicine are suitably stressed, but the general perspective is good.

LAIGNEL-LAVASTINE has embarked upon the ambitious project of editing a history of medicine and allied sciences, to be completed in three volumes, of which two have appeared.

GERMAN

HECKER, J. F. K. *Geschichte der Heilkunde*, 2 vols., Berlin, 1822–29
HAESER, H. *Geschichte der Medizin und der Volkskrankheiten*, Jena, 1845
BAAS, J. H. *Gründriss der Geschichte der Medizin*, Stuttgart, 1876 (Eng. trans., Handerson, 1889)
PUSCHMANN, T. *Handbuch der Geschichte der Medizin*, 3 vols., Leipzig, 1902–5
NEUBURGER, M. *Geschichte der Medizin*, 2 vols., Stuttgart, 1906–11. (Eng. trans., Playfair, 1910–25.)
MEYER-STEINEG, T., and SUDHOFF, K. F. J. *Geschichte der Medizin*, Jena, 1921
PAGEL, J. L., and SUDHOFF, K. *Einführung in die Geschichte der Medizin*, 3rded., Berlin, 1922

APPENDIX
Notes

Many good histories of medicine have been written in German. Mention may first be made of two works of which English editions have appeared.

BAAS produced a history which was very popular in Germany, and which, when translated into English, was the best-known work of its kind until Garrison's book appeared. Although not always completely reliable, it is liberally sprinkled with all manner of anecdotes and unusual information, and has been frequently quoted by other historians.

NEUBURGER'S *History*, a more recent publication, is also well known in its English version, although the complete work is not available. The first volume is especially useful as a guide to Greek and Roman Medicine, and is scholarly and convincing. Only part of the second volume was published; it deals with the Middle Ages. Unfortunately, the bibliography of the English edition is incomplete.

For those who can read German, a rich field of historical literature is available.

HECKER'S history is now rather out of date, though his history of the epidemics of the Middle Ages remains a useful work of reference which was translated into English for the Sydenham Society (p. 419)

HAESER'S work is still well known, and is continually read as a source book by historians. The account is concise and logical, and many references are given.

PUSCHMANN'S " handbook," in three volumes, which belie the name, gives a very complete account of the subject. It was written with the collaboration of many authorities, and is the most important book of its kind, ranking alongside the older work of Haeser.

SUDHOFF, who was the most eminent medical historian of his time and a tireless worker, collaborated with MEYER-STEINEG in writing a concise and clear history, which is attractive and easy to read. The illustrations are a noteworthy feature, but there is no bibliography.

PAGEL'S collection of lectures has been re-edited and improved by Sudhoff, and now contains a good bibliography.

Baas and Neuburger, whose works are included in the German list, have received mention in respect of the English translations.

SPANISH

MOREJON, A. H.   *Historia Bibliografica*, 7 vols., Madrid, 1842–52

ITALIAN

CASTIGLIONI, A.   *Storia della Medicina*, Milan, 1927.   (English trans., 1941.)

POLISH

SZUMOWSKI, W.   *Historja Medycynz*, Cracow, 1935

APPENDIX

2 COLLECTED MEDICAL BIOGRAPHIES

ELOY, N. F. J. *Dictionnaire historique de la Médecine ancienne et moderne*, 4 vols., Mons, 1778

WADD, W. *Nugae Chirurgicae ; A Biographical Miscellany*, 1824

MACMICHAEL, W. *The Gold-headed Cane*, 1827

THACHER, J. *American Medical Biography*, 2 vols., Boston, 1828

MACMICHAEL, W. *Lives of British Physicians*, 1830

PETTIGREW, T. J. *Medical Portrait Gallery*, 4 vols., 1840

GROSS, S. D. *Lives of American Physicians and Surgeons of the Nineteenth Century*, Philadelphia, 1861

MUNK, W. *The Roll of the Royal College of Physicians of London*, 2nd ed., 3 vols., 1878

BETTANY, G. T. *Eminent Doctors : Their Lives and Work*, 2 vols., 1885

RICHARDSON, Sir B. W. *Disciples of Aesculapius*, 2 vols., 1900

KELLY, HOWARD A. *A Cyclopaedia of American Medical Biography* (1610–1910), 2 vols., 1912

HALE-WHITE, Sir W. *Great Doctors of the Nineteenth Century*, 1935

PLARR, V. G. *Lives of the Fellows of the Royal College of Surgeons of England*, 2 vols., 1930

SIGERIST, H. E. *Great Doctors*, New York, 1933

POWER, D'ARCY. Ed. of *British Masters of Medicine*, 1936

GRAHAM, HARVEY. *Surgeons All*, 1939

Also numerous individual biographies, many of which have been mentioned in the text.

Note on Biographies

The chief collection of British biographies is the great *Dictionary of National Biography*, or *D.N.B.*, as it is familiarly called. When appropriate, the collected lives of Fellows of the Colleges of Physicians and of Surgeons may supply the required information. So far as America is concerned, the *Cyclopaedia* of Howard Kelly is complete, and has replaced the older work of Thacher. The volume edited by Gross deals only with a limited number of eminent Americans of the nineteenth century.

The works of Wadd and MacMichael are interesting and well written, and like the delightful volumes of G. T. Bettany and the more recent collection by D'Arcy Power, are concerned only with British physicians and surgeons. Pettigrew's *Medical Portrait Gallery* is a unique work, as it gives one or more portraits of the subject, as well as an excellent word-picture of each, dealing with sixty lives in all. It has become a relatively rare and valuable book, usually bound in two volumes. Richardson's *Disciples* is likewise attractive because, like Pettigrew, he selects from all countries and periods. A more recent work, which also recognizes no national boundaries, is the collection by Sigerist. Hale-White deals only with the nineteenth century in a work written in his usual clear style, and Harvey Graham confines his attention to surgeons.

APPENDIX

FURTHER WORKS ON MEDICAL HISTORY

The bibliographies which follow deal respectively with histories of periods and cultures, histories written from the national standpoint, histories of special branches of medicine and of special methods, and finally, works dealing with the relationship of medicine to art and literature.

It has not been thought necessary to annotate these lists : the titles are in most cases self-explanatory, and the majority of the books may be consulted in any large medical library, although many are now out of print.

3 HISTORIES OF PERIODS OR CULTURES IN MEDICINE

McKenzie, D.   *The Infancy of Medicine*, 1927
Rivers, W. H. R.   *Medicine, Magic, and Religion*, 1924
Moodie, R. L.   *The Antiquity of Disease*, Chicago, 1923
Black, W. G.   *Folk-Medicine, a Chapter in the History of Culture*, 1883
Hovorka, O., and Kronfeld, A.   *Vergleichende Volksmedizin*, Berlin, 1908–9
Brim, C. J.   *Medicine in the Bible*, New York, 1936
Dawson, W. R.   *Magician and Leech*, 1929 (Ancient Egypt)
Taylor, H. O.   *Greek Biology and Medicine*, 1923
Allbutt, Sir T. Clifford.   *Greek Medicine in Rome*, 1921
Hoernle, A. F. R.   *Studies in the Medicine of Ancient India*, 1907
Campbell, D.   *Arabian Medicine and its Influence on the Middle Ages*, 2 vols., 1926
Browne, E. G.   *Arabian Medicine*, 1921
Riesman, D.   *The Story of Medicine in the Middle Ages*, New York, 1935
Payne, J. F.   *English Medicine in Anglo-Saxon Times*, 1904
Walsh, J. J.   *Medieval Medicine*, 1920
Allbutt, Sir T. C.   *The Historical Relations of Medicine and Surgery to the End of the Sixteenth Century*, 1905

4 HISTORIES OF MEDICINE FROM THE NATIONAL STANDPOINT

Moore, Sir N.   *The History of the Teaching of Medicine in the British Isles*, 1908
Packard, F. R.   *History of Medicine in the United States*, 2nd ed., 2 vols., New York, 1931
Walsh, J. J.   *The History of Medicine in New York*, 5 vols., 1919
Heagerty, J. J.   *Four Centuries of Medical History in Canada*, 2 vols., Toronto, 1928
Comrie, J. D.   *History of Scottish Medicine*, 2 vols., 1932
Wickersheimer, C. A. E.   *La Médecine en France à l'époque de la Renaissance*, Paris, 1905
Rohlfs, H.   *Geschichte der deutschen Medicin*, 4 vols., Stuttgart, 1876
Renzi, S. De   *Storia della Medicina in Italia*, 5 vols., Naples, 1844–49
Garcia del Real, E.   *Historia de la Medicina en España*, Madrid, 1921
Lemos, M.   *Historia da Medicina em Portugal*, 2 vols., Lisbon, 1891
Laache, S. B.   *Norsk Medicin i hundrede aar*, Kristiania, 1911

APPENDIX

INGERSLEV, J. V. C. *Danmarks Laeger og Laegevesen fra de aeldste Tider indtil Aar 1800*, Copenhagen, 1873

WISTRAND, A. H. *Sveriges Lakare-historia ifran Konuh Gustaf I : till navarande tid*, Stockholm, 1873–76

RICHTER, W. M. *Geschichte der Medicin in Russland*, 3 vols., Moscow, 1813–17

FLORES, F. A. *Historia de la Medicina en Mexico*, 3 vols., Mexico, 1886–88

SCHIAFFINO, R. *Historia de la Medicina en el Uruguay*, 2 vols., Montevideo, 1927 and 1937

BELTRAN, J. R. *Historia del protomedicato de Buenos Aires*, Buenos Aires, 1937

BROECKX, C. *L'Histoire de la Médecine belge avant le XIXe siècle*, Ghent, 1837

SIGERIST, H. E. *Geschichte der Medicin in der Schweiz*, Zurich, 1924

MUKHOPADHYAYA, G. *History of Indian Medicine*, 2 vols., Calcutta, 1923

WONG, C. M. and WU, LIEN-TEH. *History of Chinese Medicine*, Tientsin, 1932

FUJIKAWA, Y. *Geschichte der Medizin in Japan*, Tokyo, 1911

Also small histories in Clio Medica series : British Isles (D'Arcy Power, 1930), Italy (Castiglioni, 1923), Russia (Gantt, 1937), Germany (Haberling), France (Laignel-Lavastine), Persia (Elgood), China (Morse), all 1934.

5 HISTORIES OF SPECIALTIES AND METHODS IN MEDICINE

ANATOMY

PORTAL, ANTOINE. *Histoire de l'Anatomie et de la Chirurgie*, 6 vols., Paris, 1770–73

KEEN, W. W. *The Early History of Practical Anatomy*, Philadelphia, 1874

SINGER, C. *The Evolution of Anatomy* (to the time of Harvey), 1925

DE LINT, J. G. *Atlas of the History of Medicine. I—Anatomy*, 1926

HUNTER, R. H. *A Short History of Anatomy*, 2nd ed., 1931

NEEDHAM, J. *The History of Embryology*, 1934

COLE, F. J. *A History of Comparative Anatomy*, 1944

PHYSIOLOGY

FOSTER, Sir M. *Lectures on the History of Physiology*, 1901

STIRLING, W. *Some Apostles of Physiology*, 1902

FULTON, J. T. *Selected Readings in the History of Physiology*, Springfield, 1930

PHARMACY

WOOTTON, A. C. *Chronicles of Pharmacy*, 2 vols., 1910

LEWIN, L. *Die Gifte in der Weltgeschichte*, Berlin, 1920 (Toxicology)

RHODE, E. S. *The Old English Herbals*, 1922

ARBER, A. R. *Herbals : their Origin and Evolution*, 2nd ed., 1938

SCHELENZ, H. *Geschichte der Pharmacie*, Berlin, 1903

LA WALL, C. H. *Four Thousand Years of Pharmacy*, Philadelphia, 1927

GRIER, J. A. *A History of Pharmacy*, 1937

PATHOLOGY AND BACTERIOLOGY

CROOKSHANK, E. M. *History and Pathology of Vaccination*, 2 vols., 1889

LONG, E. R. *A History of Pathology*, Baltimore, 1928

KRUMBHAAR, E. B. *History of Pathology* (Clio Medica series), New York, 1937

BULLOCH, W. *The History of Bacteriology*, 1938

APPENDIX

EPIDEMIOLOGY

HECKER, J. F. K.   *The Epidemics of the Middle Ages*, trans. by Babington, Sydenham Society, 1882

CREIGHTON, C.   *History of Epidemics in Great Britain*, 2 vols., 1891–94

MERCIER, C. A.   *Leper Houses and Mediaeval Hospitals*, 1915

PIÉRY, A. M., and ROSHEM, J.   *Histoire de la Tuberculose*, Paris, 1931

PUSEY, W. A.   *The History and Epidemiology of Syphilis*, Baltimore, 1933

ZINSSER, H.   *Rats, Lice, and History*, 1935.   (Deals especially with typhus fever.)

GEDDES SMITH.   *Plague On Us*, 1941.   (Semi-popular but well-documented history)

PUBLIC HEALTH

CLEMOW, F. G.   *The Geography of Disease*, 1903

DELAUNAY, H.   *L'Hygiène publique à travers les âges*, Paris, 1906

MORRIS, Sir M. A.   *The Story of British Public Health*, 1919

NEWSHOLME, Sir A.   *The Evolution of Preventive Medicine*, 1927

PETERSEN, W. F.   *The Patient and the Weather*, 4 vols., Ann Arbor, 1934–38

SURGERY

GURLT, E. J.   *Geschichte der Chirurgie und ihrer Ausübung*, 3 vols., Berlin, 1898

MILNE, J. S.   *Surgical Instruments in Greek and Roman Times*, Aberdeen, 1907

KEITH, Sir A.   *Menders of the Maimed*, 1919.   (History of orthopaedic surgery)

PARKER, G.   *The Early History of Surgery in Great Britain*, 1920

BALLANCE, Sir C. A.   *The History of Surgery of the Brain*, 1922

POWER, Sir D'ARCY.   *A Short History of Surgery*, 1933

LEONARDO, R. A.   *History of Surgery*, New York, 1942

THOMPSON, C. J. S.   *The History and Evolution of Surgical Instruments*, New York, 1942

OBSTETRICS AND GYNAECOLOGY

SIEBOLD, E. C. J. von.   *Versuch einer Geschichte der Geburtshulfe*, 2 vols., Berlin, 1839–45

AVELING, J. H.   *The Chamberlens and the Midwifery Forceps*, 1882

WITKOWSKI, G. J. A.   *Histoire des accouchements chez tous les peuples*, Paris, 1889

McKAY, W. J. S.   *The History of Ancient Gynaecology*, 1901

FASBENDER, H.   *Geschichte der Geburtshülfe*, Jena, 1906

SPENCER, H. R.   *History of British Midwifery*, 1927

JAMESON, E. M.   *A Short History of Gynaecology and Obstetrics*, New York, 1936

OPHTHALMOLOGY

HIRSCHBERG, J.   *Geschichte der Augenheilkunde*, 10 Pts., Leipzig, 1899–1911.   (In *Graefe-Saemisch Handbuch*)

PANSIER, P.   *Histoire des Lunettes*, Paris, 1901

JAMES, R. R.   *The History of Ophthalmology in England Prior to the Year 1800*, 1933

SORSBY, A.   *A Short History of Ophthalmology*, 1933

APPENDIX

LARYNGOLOGY AND OTOLOGY

POLITZER, A. *Geschichte der Ohrenheilkunde*, 2 vols., Stuttgart, 1907–13

WRIGHT, J. *History of Laryngology and Rhinology*, 2nd ed., Philadelphia, 1914

STEVENSON, R. S., and GUTHRIE, DOUGLAS. *A History of Otolaryngology*, 1949

DENTISTRY

SUDHOFF, K. F. J. *Geschichte der Zahnheilkunde*, Leipzig, 1921

LUFKIN, A. W. *A History of Dentistry*, Philadelphia, 1938

MISCELLANEOUS

BIGELOW, H. J. *Ether and Chloroform : A Compendium of Their History and Discovery*, Boston, 1848

NUTTING, M. A., and DOCK, L. L. *History of Nursing*, New York, 1907–12

CABANÈS, A. *Chirurgiens et Blessés à travers l'Histoire*, Paris, 1918

FABER, K. H. *Nosography in Modern Internal Medicine*, New York, 1923

STILL, G. F. *The History of Pediatrics*, 1931

CLAY, R. S., and COURT, T. H. *The History of the Microscope*, 1932

MAJOR, R. H. *Classic Descriptions of Disease*, 1932. (Quotes 179 writers ; biographical notes)

PUSEY, W. A. *The History of Dermatology*, Springfield, U.S.A., 1933

ROLLESTON, Sir H. *The Endocrine Glands in Health and Disease : With an Historical Review*, 1936

SCOTT, Sir H. H. *History of Tropical Medicine*, 2 vols., 1939

ZILBOORG, G., and HENRY, G. W. *A History of Medical Psychology*, New York, 1941

6 MEDICINE IN ART AND LITERATURE

KNOX, R. *Great Artists and Great Anatomists*, 1852

CHOULANT, L. *Geschichte und Bibliographie der anatomische Abbildung*, Leipzig, 1852. (Trans. by M. Frank, *History of Anatomic Illustrations*, Chicago, 1920)

MENIÈRE, P. *Etudes médicales sur les Poètes latins*, Paris, 1858

BUCKNILL, Sir J. C. *The Medical Knowledge of Shakespeare*, 1860

DAREMBERG, C. *La Médecine dans Homère*, Paris, 1865

CHARCOT, J. M., and RICHER, P. M. L. *Les Difformés et les Malades dans l'Art*, Paris, 1889

MOYES, J. *Medicine and Kindred Arts in the Plays of Shakespeare*, Glasgow, 1896

ANDREWS, W. *The Doctor in History, Literature, Folk-lore, etc.*, Hull, 1896

RICHER, P. M. L. *L'Art de la Médecine*, Paris, 1902

HOLLÄNDER, E. *Die Medizin in den klassischen Malerei*, Stuttgart, 1903

NASS, L. *Curiosités médico-artistiques*, 3 vols., Paris, 1907

STORER, H. R. *Medicina in nummis* (Medical History in Coins and Medals), Boston, 1911

ROBIN, P. A. *The Old Physiology in English Literature*, 1911

CRAWFURD, RAYMOND. *Plague and Pestilence in Literature and Art*, 1914

HAGGARD, H. W. *The Doctor in History*, Yale, 1934

INDEX

Authors referred to only in the footnotes and bibliographical appendix are not indexed

Abano, Peter of. *See* Peter of Abano
Abbott, Gilbert, 303
Abdomen, patron saint of, 99
Abdominal surgery, 328, 330–1, 332
Abella, one of " ladies of Salerno," 104
Aberdeen, family of Gregory at, 222–23 ; puerperal fever at, 318 ; McGrigor at, 341 ; Royal Infirmary, 288 ; University, surgery at, 288 ; graduates of, 343, 357
Abernethy, John, 241, 242–43, 312, 316
Aboriginal beliefs, 4, 5
Abortion, in Hippocratic Oath, 54
Abscess, 29, 113, 325, 333, Pl. VIII
Abú Alí al Hussein ibn Abdalláh ibn Síná. *See* Avicenna
Abú Bakr Muhammad ibn Zakariyya. *See* Rhazes
Abulcasis. *See* Albucasis
Académie des Sciences (Paris), 191
Acarus scabei, 94
Accademia dei Lincei (Rome), 191
Accra, West Africa, yellow fever at, 359
Acidosis, 365
Acoustics, physiological, 275
Acromegaly, 370
Acta medicorum Berolinensium, 397
Acupressure, 305
Acupuncture in ancient China, 35–36
Adale, the Arab, legendary founder of School of Salerno, 103
Adams, Francis, his editions of Hippocrates, 53 ; of Aretaeus, 71 ; of Paul of Ægina, 80
Adams, Robert, 296
Addison, Thomas, 291, 291-92
Addison's Disease, 291, 292
Ægidus Corboliensis. *See* Gilles de Corbeil
Ægina, Paul of. *See* Paul of Ægina
Aesculapius, 21, 29, 40, 43, 44, 45, 51 ; temples of. *See* Asklepieia
Aëtius of Amida, 70–71, 79–80
Africa, exploration of, by medical men, 355–56 ; sleeping sickness in, 361–62
Age-incidence of disease, 58, 59
Agrigentum, epidemic at, 50
Ague. *See* Malaria
Aiguières, trephined skull at, 6
Air pump, Robert Boyle's, 186
Albertus Magnus, 121
Albinus, Bernard Siegfried, 229, 238
Albucasis, 93, 124
Albuera, Battle of, 342
Albuminuria, 291
Alchemy, 87, 159, 160
Alcmæon of Croton, 49

Alderotti, Taddeo, 115
Alexander of Tralles, 80
Alexandria, medical school of, 63–64, 75
Algeria, native surgery in, 8, 9, 11 ; trephining in, 9, 11 ; malarial parasite discovered in, 357
Alibert, Jean Louis Marc, 382
Allbutt, Sir Thomas Clifford, 294, 366, 407–8
Allergy, 385
Alston, Charles, 230
Ambulances, Larrey's " ambulances volantes," 388, Pl. VIII
America. *See* United States
American Civil War, 349, 371
American Journal of Medical Sciences, 395
American Journal of Obstetrics, 395
American Medical Association, 402
Amida, Aëtius of. *See* Aëtius of Amida
Amputation, 146, 150, 239, 243, 244, 304, 307, 310, 339, 342, 344, 349
Amsterdam, Swammerdam of, 190 ; Tulp of, 194 ; early medical periodical at, 398
Amulets. *See* Charms
Anaemia, 204, 292
Anaesthesia, 301–6 ; in ancient China, 36 ; in Middle Ages, 73, 107–8, 116 ; local, 276, 327 ; spinal, 327
Anaphylaxis, 288, 391
Anatomical material, supply of, 122, 151, 153, 227–28, 270–71, 387
Anatomy, described in the Talmud, 31 ; Herophilus and, 64 ; Galen and, 76–77 ; in Middle Ages, 85, 92, 111, Pl. XXII ; at Salerno, 105 ; Salicet on, 117 ; restoration of, 122–23 ; Arab words in, 123 ; Guy de Chauliae on, 124 ; studied by artists, 135–36; Vesalius' work on, 136–42 ; English, 150–51 ; Paracelsus' contempt for, 159; at Leyden, 193–94, Pl. XXXIX ; Stahl and, 216 ; at Edinburgh under the Monros, 227–29 ; Windmill Street School of, 238 ; first to practise in, 269, 270 ; in nineteenth-century Europe, 271–72 ; study of, by frozen sections, 344. *See also* Dissection.
Anatomy (comparative), and Aristotle, 61 ; at Padua, 141 ; Harvey's studies in, 189 ; John Hunter's work on, 240 ; Müller and, 273
Anatomy (microscopic), 186, 271, 278
Anatomy (pathological), 245, 282
Anderson, Mrs. Elizabeth Garrett, 386
Anderson, Thomas, 323
Andromachus, inventor of theriac, 82

Aneurysm, 79, 147, 243, 301
Angelo, Michael, and dissection, 135
Angina pectoris, 250, 256, 296, 299, 365, 366, 367
Anima, Stahl's theory of, 216
Animal heat, 280
Animal magnetism, 262
Animal parasites, 317
Animal remedies, 25, 90
Animal spirit, 77
Animism, 11, 68, 216–17
Annales d'hygiène publique, 397
Annals of Medical History, 399
Annals of Surgery, 395
Anne, Queen, 210, 255, 264
Anodyne, Hoffmann's, 217
Antarctic exploration, 355
Anthony, St., 100–1
Anthrax, 284, 286
Anthropology, 138, 194, 270, 273, 282
Antimony, use of, 250
Antiseptic system, early use of, 116; first use of word, 233; antecedents of, 317–18; adoption of, 323–25, Pl. LXIV; criticism of, 326
Antyllus, 79
Aorta, disease of, 296; ligature of, 243
Apatosaurus, 2, Pl. I
Aphasia, 370, 371
Apollo, god of health, 40, 41–42, Pl. IX
Apollonia, St., 99
Apothecaries, of London, 192, 255; in British army, 347
Appendicitis, 29, 292, 330
Apuleius Platonicus, 117, 131
Apulia, tarantism in, 100
Aqua vitae, 113, 114, 153
Aqueduct of Fallopius, 141
Arabian :—medicine, 86–96; surgery, 9, 92–93, Pls. XV, XVII; translations of Greek texts, 88; words in medicine, 86, 123; influence at Salerno, 103, 105; blood-letting, 130; surgery today, 9
Arber, Agnes, 132
Archaeus, Paracelsus' theory of, 159, 199, 216
Archagathus, 66
Archiatri, 82, 101
Archigenes, 71
Archimatheus, 106
Archiv für Anatomie und Physiologie, 398
Archiv für gesamte Physiologie, 398
Archiv für Geschichte der Arzneykunde, 398
Archiv für Geschichte der Medizin, 399
Archiv für klinische Chirurgie, 343, 398
Archiv für pathologische Anatomie, etc., 398
Arctic exploration, 354, 355
Arderne, John, 125, 142, 150, 406
Aretaeus, 70–72, 364
Aristides, Ælius, 45
Aristophanes, account of incubation, 45
Aristotle, 60–61, 74, 91, 120, 121

Army. *See* Military hygiene, Military medicine, *and* Military surgery
Army Hospital Corps, 347
Arnold of Villanova, 92, 108, 112–13
Arteries, Galen on, 78 ; diseases of, 282 ; diseases and injuries of, 342 ; muscular coat of, 272 ; artery forceps, 147 ; arterial surgery, 301
Artificial respiration, 30, 250, 253, 277
Artists, dissection by, 135–36 ; medical subjects of, 130, 194, Pl. xxxv. *See also* Illustrations
Arzt, Der, 397
Arztliches Intelligenz-Blatt, 397
Ascaris, 80
Asclepiades, 67–68
Aselli, Gaspare, 185
Asepsis, 321, 329, 330
Asia Minor, incubation in, 46
Asia, origin of Black Death in, 126
Askew, Anthony, 255
Asklepieia, 43–46, 48, 51, 75
Asklepios. *See* Aesculapius
Aspirator, Dieulafoy's, 298
Asthma, 90, 162, 219
Astrology, 95, 107, 121, 132, 147, 159, 162, 255
Astronomy and medicine, 159, 178–79
Asylum Journal of Mental Science, 394
Atharva-Veda, 32
Athens, Asklepieion at, 43
Atrophy, acute yellow, 282 ; in the liver, 298
Auenbrugger, Leopold, 258, 259, 366
Aurelius Antoninus, Marcus, Emperor of Rome, 75, 79
Aures Mountains, native medicine in, 9 ; trephined skull from, 9, Pl. II
Aurignacian man, 1
Auscultation, 55, 257–59, 298, 366
Australia, aboriginals of, 4, 5 ; exploration in, 355
Avenzoar, 92, 93–94
Averroes, 94, 120
Avertin, St., 99
Avicenna, 67, 91–92, 157
Avignon, 123, 126

Babinski, Joseph, 370
Babylonia, medicine and surgery in, 17–19 ; seal of Babylonian physician, 17, Pl. V ; medical ethics in, 18–19
Bachtishua, Gabriel, 88
Bachtishua, George, 88
Bacilli, discoveries of, 286–88
Bacon, Francis, 177
Bacon, Roger, 120–21, 189
Bacteriology, 38, 272, 281–89 ; and public health, 388–91
Bado, Sebastian, quoted, 205
Baer, Ernst von, 273
Baghdad, 89, 96
Baglivi, Giorgio, 198

Baillie, Matthew, 235, 246, 254, 255, 277, 281
Baker, Sir George, 234
Ball, James Moores, quoted, 135
Ballantyne, John William, quoted, 175; 306
Ballingall, Sir George, 345-46, 349
Balsam, in wounds, 161
Baltimore, 330, 359 ; Osler at, 408
Banckes, Richard, 131
Banester, John, 151
Banks, Sir Joseph, 312
Banting, Sir Frederick, 365
Bantu legend of death, 3
Barbary ape, Galen's dissection of, 76, 77
Barber-surgeons, of Edinburgh, 153 ; of London, 150, 151, Pl. xxx ; of Paris, 119, 143, 144, 146
Barclay, John, 269-70, 308, 309
Barker, Arthur Edward James, 333
Barthez, Paul Joseph, 217
Bartholin, Thomas, 194
Bartholomeus Anglicus, 104
Basel, 141, 157, 365
Basil, St., of Caesarea, 85
Bass, George, 355
Bassini, Eduardo, 329
Bateman, Thomas, 382
Baths, public, of ancient Rome, 81 ; mediæval Italian, 81, Pl. xx
Beaulieu, Jacques de. See Jacques de Beaulieu
Beaumont, William, 300
Bedingfeld, Thomas, 164
Behring, Emil von, 287
Bell, Benjamin, 230, Pl. XLVII
Bell, Sir Charles, 230, 266-69, 270, 273, 277, 338, Pl. LV
Bell, John, 230, 231, 267, 269, 300
Bell, Joseph, 277, Pl. LVIII
Belladonna, homœopathic use of, 219
Benedict, St., of Nursia, 101
Bennett, John Hughes, 278, 294
Bentham, Jeremy, 387, 388
Bergmann, Ernst von, 287, 328-29
Beri-beri, 194, 346
Berkeley, Jenner at, 248-49
Berlin, Monro (secundus) at, 229 ; Henle at, 272 ; Müller professor at, 273 ; Helmholtz professor of physics at, 275 ; Physico-Technical Institute, 275 ; Virchow professor of pathology at, 282 ; Virchow Institute, 283 ; Institute for Infectious Diseases, 287 ; Fraenkel of, 288; Frerichs and Leyden professors at, 298 ; Langenbeck of, 316 ; Bergmann and Bier professors of surgery at, 328-29 ; Nitze and urology at, 334 ; Graefe, Dieffenbach, Langenbach, and military surgery at, 342-43 ; Pirogoff at, 344 ; Naunyn at, 364 ; Henoch, Heubner, and pediatrics at, 368 ; Romberg and neurology at, 369 ; Graefe and

ophthalmology at, 376 ; Wassermann and syphilology at, 384 ; medical periodicals at, 397
Berlin Papyri, 27
Berliner klinische Wochenschrift, 398
Bernard, Claude, 279-81, 365
Bernard de Gordon, 114
Bernardine, St., 98
Berne, 148, 150, 223, 224, 329
Berthelet, Thomas, 104
Best, Charles Herbert, 365
Bezoar stone, 13, 207
Bible, 3, 10, 14, 19, 29-31, 80, 116, 212
Bibliographia Medica, 402
Bibliography, medical, 171-73, 399-402
Bichat, François Xavier, 245-46, 272
Bidloo, Govert, 193
Bier, August, 329
Bigelow, Henry Jacob, 334
Bile salts, researches on, 390
Bilharzia in mummies, 29
Billings, John Shaw, 400-2
Billroth, Theodore, 328
Bingen, nunnery at, 102
Biochemistry, 298, 364
Birmingham, 257, 261, 330
Birth stool, 30, 69, 175
Black Death, 99, 100, 126-28, 164
Black, Joseph, 222, 261
Black wash, 201
Blackwater fever, 57
Blackwell, Elizabeth, 132, 385
Blaise, St., 98
Blane, Sir Gilbert, 351-52
Blas, Van Helmont's theory of, 199
Blast, injuries in modern warfare from, 350
Blegny, Nicolas de, 192, 396
Blindness, 238, 246
Blood, circulation of, in ancient Chinese writing, 35 ; Galen's theory, 77-78, 140 ; pulmonary, 139-41 ; Harvey and, 180, 181, 183-86, 226 ; change in colour of, 140, 187 ; coagulation of, 240, 323 ; red corpuscles, 189
Blood-letting, in Talmud, 31 ; Celsus on, 73 ; Bartholomeus Anglicus on, 104 ; influence of moon on, 110, 129 ; in Middle Ages, 111 ; Lanfranc on, 119 ; as cure for Black Death, 127 ; Arabian, 130 ; Brissot on, 130 ; Sydenham on, 204 ; criticism of, 277
Blood-pressure, 260, 276, 366
Blood-transfusion, 187, 350
Blue pill, 243
Boccaccio, Giovanni, 127
Bodleian Library, 71, 90, 98
Body-snatching, 137, 227-28. See also Resurrectionists
Boë, Franz de le. See Sylvius, Franciscus
Boerhaave, Hermann, 60, 80, 190, 203, 216, 217, 220-21, 226, 227, 228, 230, 231, Pl. XLIV

Bollstadt, Albert von. *See* Albertus Magnus
Bologna, University of, 104, 111, 112, 115–18 ; attended by Chauliac 123, Vesalius 137, Paracelsus 157, Cardan 162, Valsalva 244, Morgagni 245
Bone grafting by Arabs, 9
Bone setting, 263, 334
Bones, illustrations of, 239, Pl. XLVIII ; tuberculosis of, 211
Boniface VIII, Pope, 112, 122
Bonn, 273 ; University of, 275
Boorde (Borde), Andrew, 172–73, Pl. XXXIII
Borelli, Giovanni Alfonso, 197–98
Borgognoni, Ugo. *See* Hugh of Lucca
Borgognoni, Theodoric, Bishop of Cervia, 115–16, 117
Borneo, primitive beliefs in, 5, 11
Boston, Mass., 303, 330, 390
Boston Medical and Surgical Journal, 395
Boston Society of Medical Improvement, 319
Botanical gardens, at Edinburgh, 192 ; at Leyden, 194, 221 ; at London, 192 ; at Paris, 192 ; at Upsala, 215 ; at Upton, 250. *See also* Herb gardens
Botany, ancient, 61–62 ; mediæval and modern, 131–32 ; Fothergill and, 249–50 ; astrological, 132 ; microscopic, 190 ; Edinburgh Chair of, 230
Boulogne, Paré at, 145
Bowditch, Henry Pickering, 276
Bowman, Sir William, 375–76
Boyle, Robert, 186–87, 191, 202
Brachial plexus, injury to, 76
Brain, as seat of senses, 49 ; controlled by "red worm," 123 ; ventricles of, 135 ; anatomy of, 178, 200, Pl. XLI, 272 ; tumour of, 332 ; otitic abscess of, 333
Breast, diseases of, 243 ; removal of, 310, 331
Breasted, James Henry, quoted, 20, 22, 26
Breathing and combustion identical, 188
Breslau, 287, 298, 316, 328
Bretonneau, Pierre, 297
Bridget, St., 99
Bright, Richard, 290–91, Pl. LIX
Bright's Disease, 291, 294, Pl. LIX
Brissot, Pierre, 130
British Medical Association, 394
British Medical Journal, 394
British Museum, 22, 27, 131, 172, 174, 181, 192, 201, 375
Brittany, 6, 143
Broca, Paul, 6, 273, 333, 371
Brock, Arthur John, his edition of Galen, 78
Brodie, Sir Benjamin Collins, 312–13
Broussais, François Joseph Victor, 67, 297
Brown, John (founder of Brunonian system), 67, 218–19, 223

Brown, John (author of *Horae Subsecivae*), 53, 309
Browne, Edward Granville, quoted, 88, 90, 91
Browne, John, 210, Pl. XLIII
Browne, Sir Thomas, 120, 164, 176, 196, 211–14, 225
Browning, Robert, his *Grammarian* and Linacre, 167 ; his *Paracelsus*, 156, 161
Bruce, Sir David, 361
Brunfels, Otto, 131
Brunner, Johann Conrad, 194
Brunonian system. *See* Brown, John
Brunschwig, Hieronymus, 126, 337, Pl. XXVI
Brunton, Sir Lauder, 366
Brussels, Vesalius at, 136
Buckland, Frank, 242
Bulletin de l'Académie de Médecine, 397
Bulletin de la Société française et Histoire de la Médecine, 399
Bulletin of the Institute of the History of Medicine, 399
Bullets, extraction of, 126, 349
Burdon-Sanderson, Sir John, 278
Burke, William, 228, 270–71
Burnett, Sir William, 353
Bursae mucosae, 229
Burton, John, forceps of, Pl. L
Burton, Robert, his *Anatomy of Melancholy* quoted, 90, 164
Byrne, Patrick, an Irish giant, 241
Byzantine medicine, 79–80, 101

Cabbage as a remedy, 66
Cadwalader, Thomas, 250–51
Cæsar, Caius Julius, 65
Cæsarian section in ancient India, 33
Cairo, 27, 94, 95
Caius, John, 167–68, 169, 171
Calabria, monasteries in, 101
Calcar, Jan Stephan van, 137
Calculus, urinary, in mummies, 28
Caldwell, Richard, 181
Callisen, Adolph Carl Peter, 400
Calomel, 201, 243
Camarina, Lake, 42
Cambridge University Library, 172
Cambridge, University of, students or professors at :—Caius, 167–68 ; Harvey, 180 ; Glisson, 200 ; Woodhead, 288 ; Gaskell, 365 ; Allbutt, 366, 407 ; Young, 374 ; Caius College, 168, Pl. XXXII
Cancer, of the larynx, 380 ; of rectum, 125 ; of stomach, 328 ; radium and, 385 ; X-rays and, 385
Cannabis indica, 36
Canterbury Tales, doctor in, 114
Canton, hospital established at, 37
Capillaries, discovery of, 186
Caracalla, Emperor of Rome, 81
Carbolic acid, 324

Carbon dioxide, 261
Carcinoma of rectum, 329
Cardan, Jerome, 136, 161–64, Pl. xxxi
Cardanus, Hieronymus. *See* Cardan, Jerome
Cardiology, 365–67. *See also* Heart
Carnegie Institution of Washington, 402
Carrel-Dakin treatment of wounds, 350
Carrion, Daniel, 289
Carroll, James, 359
Cassanate, William, 162
Casserius, Julius, 141
Castellani, Aldo, 361
Castiglioni, Arturo, quoted, 108, 245, 266
Castor oil in ancient Egypt, 25
Casualty clearing stations, 349
Cataract, 73, 148, 244, 342, 376
Catgut ligature, 325
Catherine, Empress of Russia, 247
Catheter, Eustachian, 377, 379
Cato, Marcus Porcius, "The Censor," his *Præcepta ad Filium*, 65–66
Cautery, Arabian use of, 93 ; William of Salicet and, 117 ; Lanfranc and, 119 ; Guy de Chauliac and, 124 ; Paré on, 146 ; cauterisation by bullet, 152 ; Ballingall's use of, 345
Cell-theory, 190, 283
Celsus, Aurelius Cornelius, 64, 70, 72–74, 124
Cerebral function, localization of, 265, 273, 333
Cerebro-spinal fluid, 244
Cesalpino, Andrea, 140, 184
Cesi, Federigo, Duke of Acquasparta, 191
Chadwick, Sir Edwin, 387, 388
Chamberlen, family of, 235–37
Chapman, Edmund, 235, 237, Pl. L
Chapman, Nathaniel, 395
Charaka, 32
Charcot, Jean, 355
Charcot, Jean-Martin, 370
Chang Chung-King, 36
Charlemagne, 102, 103
Charles I, 181, 182, 183, 209
Charles II, 209, 210, 212, Pl. xliii
Charles IX, King of France, 147
Charms, 6, 13–14, 24, 125, Pls. iii–iv. *See also* Incantations
Chassaignac, Pierre Marie, 325
Chatham, hospital at, 341
Chaucer, Geoffrey, quoted, 114
Chauliac, Guy de. *See* Guy de Chauliac
Chelsea, Apothecaries Garden, 192 ; York Hospital, 341
Chemical physiology, 199, 364
Chemistry, 87, 199, 222 ; of Arabs, 87 ; of Van Helmont, 199 ; of Cullen, 222
Chemotherapy, 384, 385
Cheselden, William, 227, 235, 238–39, 240, Pl. xlviii
Chest, diseases of, 259, 296, 298
Cheyne, John, 296

Cheyne-Stokes respiration, 57, 296
Cheyne, Watson, 326
Chi Min Wong. *See* Wong, Chi Min
Chiari, Ottokar, 380
Chicago, surgery at, 330, 331
Chicken cholera, 284
Children, prehistoric trephining of, 6 ; diseases of, 367–68
China, folk-medicine in, 14, 15 ; ancient and modern medicine in, 34–37 ; inoculation for smallpox in, 36, 246 ; first ophthalmic hospital in, 37
Chinchon, Countess of, 205
Chloroform, 304–5
Cholera, vibrio of, discovered by Koch, 286 ; in Ireland, 296 ; in Britain, 387, 388, 389 ; mortality of, in London, 389 ; and water supply, 388, 389 ; Pettenkoffer and organisms of, 390
Cholesteatoma, 378
Chopart, François, 244
Chorea and St. Vitus, 100
Christison, Sir Robert, 294, 316, 366
Church, Christian, and medicine, 84–85, 117, 120, 120–21, 212 ; cures in, 46, 97 ; Galen approved by, 74 ; rhinoplasty opposed by, 149 ; Galileo censured by, 179. *See also* Monasteries
Ciliary action, discovery of, 278
Ciliary muscle, action of, 142, 374
Cinchona bark, 204, 205, 219, 250
Cincinnati, medical school of, 299
Circumcision, ritual, 30
Citric acid in scurvy, 352
Clarke, J. F., 394
Claviceps purpurea, 101
Clay used for fractured leg, 346
Clift, William, 314
Climate, influence of, 55
Clinical medicine, American, 299–301 ; Austrian, 244–45, 298, 299 ; Dutch, under Boerhaave, 220–21 ; English, 200–4, 290–94 ; French, 296–98 ; German, 298–99 ; Irish, 295–96 ; Scottish, 221–23, 225–26, 294
Clinical thermometer, 197, 257, 298, 408
Closed plaster method for compound fractures, 345, 350
Clouston, Sir Thomas Smith, 373
Clover, Joseph, 303, 305
Clovis I, King of France, 210
Clowes, William, 151–52, 337
Clysters, 125
Cnidos, school of, 56
Cockayne, Thomas Oswald, 131
Coction, 76
Cod liver oil, 278
Coffee, use of, 250
Coiter, Volcher, 141
Colchicum, 80
Cold baths, treatment by, 36, 258
Coleridge, Samuel Taylor, 359
Coles, William, 132

Collecteana medicophysica oft Hollands Jaar Register, 398
Colledge, Thomas Richardson, 37
Colmar, Paracelsus at, 158
Cologne, Albertus Magnus at, 121
Colombo, Realdo. *See* Columbus, R.
Colour, in folk-medicine, 14 ; in treatment of smallpox, 114 ; change of, in circulating blood, 187 ; theory of colour vision, 274, 374
Colton, Gardner Quincy, 302, 303
Columba, St., 98
Columbus, Realdus, 139–40, 151
Combe, Andrew, 264
Combe, George, 264
Comparative anatomy. *See* Anatomy (comparative)
Compound fractures. *See* Fractures (compound)
Comrie, John Dixon, 407 ; quoted, 99, 153
Conolly, John, 372
Consilia, introduction of, 115
Constantine the African, 105
Constantinople, plague in (542 A.D.), 83
Constanza, one of " ladies of Salerno," 104
Constellations and anatomy, 129
Cooper, Sir Astley Paston, 241, 243, 301, 311, 312, 339
Copeman, Monckton, 249
Copenhagen, 328, 400
Copernicus, Nicolaus, 135, 165
Copho. *See* Kopho
Coptic papyrus, 27
Corbeil, Gilles de. *See* Gilles de Corbeil
Cordova (Córdoba), 93, 94, 95, 96, Pl. XVI
Corpus Hippocraticum. See Hippocrates
Corrigan, Sir Dominic John, 296
Corrosion preparations, 272
Corvisart, Jean Nicholas, 258
Cos, Isle of, Asklepieia at, 43, 48 ; birthplace of Hippocrates, 51–52, Pls. XI–XII
Cosmas, St., 97, Pl. XVIII
Costerton, Charles, 314
Cotugno, Domenico, 244, 368
" Couching " for cataract, 73, 342
Cowper, William, 193, 238
Cowpox, 248
Crawford, James, 228
Crawford, Mrs. Jane Todd, 300
Creighton, Charles, quoted, 170
Crete, Minoan civilization of, 39–40
Crile, George Washington, 276, 331
Crime and insanity, 373
Crimean War, 344, 346, 347
Criminals, bodies of, for anatomical study, 122, 151, 153 ; inoculation of, 246
Crocker, Henry Radcliffe, 383
Croke, Sir Alexander, 109
Crump, J. A., quoted, 8
Crusaders, 94 ; at Salerno, 109 ; bones of, 122 ; and Knights of St. John, 128

Crystallography, Pasteur and, 284
Cuba, yellow fever in, 359, 360
Cullen, William, 218, 221–23, 231, 237, 261, Pl. XLV
Culloden, Battle of, 232
Culpeper, Nicholas, 132
Curie, Mme. Marie Sklodowska, 385
Curie, Pierre, 385
Currie, James, 257
Curtis, John Harrison, 377
Cushing, Harvey, 333, 408
Cushny, Arthur Robertson, 366
Cutbush, Edward, 353
Cuthbert, St., 98
Cyanide gauze, 324
Cyprian, St., 100
Cyprus, incubation in, 46
Cyst, sebaceous, 243
Cystoscope, invention of, 333–34
Czermak, Johann Nepomuk, 380

Da Costa, Jacob Mendez, 367
Damascus, hospital at, 95 ; Nicolas of. *See* Nicolas of Damascus
Damian, St., 97, Pl. XVIII
Dancing mania, 100
Dante Alighieri, 115
Danville, Kentucky, 300
Daremberg, Charles Victor, quoted, 65 ; editions of Galen, 78, of Oribasius, 79
Darier, Jean, 382
Darwin, Charles, 354
Darwin, Erasmus, 257
Daviel, Jacques, 376
Davy, Sir Humphry, 302
Dawson, Warren Royal, quoted, 28
Dead, disposal of, in plague of London (1665), 208
Deafness, 377, 379
Death, primitive idea of, 3
Deaver, John Blair, 330
Débridement, 350
Deil's Needle, Aberdeen, 13
Déjerine, Joseph Jules, 370
Delos, Isle of, 40, 41, Pl. IX
Delphi, Oracle of, 41–42 ; omphalos at, 41, Pl. IX
Dementia praecox, 373
Denmark, surgery in, 328
Dentistry, mediæval, 124–25 ; anaesthetic first used in, 303
Dephlogistigated air (*i.e.* oxygen), 261
Derivation in blood-letting, 130
Dermatitis venenata, 383
Dermatology, 381–84. *See also* Skin, diseases of
Derry, D. E., quoted, 28
Desault, Pierre-Joseph, 244, 245
Descartes, René, 177–78, 197, 216, Pl. XLI
Desegnettes, Baron René Nicolas Dufriche, 340
Dettingen, Battle of, 232
Deutsche medizinische Wochenschrift, 398

Deventer, Hendrik van, 195
Devonshire Colic, 234
Diabetes, 71–72, 200, 298, 299, 364–65
Dieffenbach, Johann Friedrich, 316, 343
Diet, Hippocrates on, 57–58; Asclepiades on, 67; Celsus on, 73; Isaac Judæus on, 90; Bartholomeus Anglicus on, 104; as advised at Salerno, 109; in British navy, 233, 351–53
Dieulafoy, Georges, 297–98
Digby, Sir Kenelm, 15, 160, 212
Digestion, 279, 298, 300
Digitalis, 257, 366, 367
Dimsdale, Thomas, 247, 343
Dinosaur, 2, Pl. I
Diocletian, Emperor of Rome, 81, 100
Dionis, Pierre, 209
Dioscorides, Pedacius, 62, 86, 88, 101, 116, 131
Diphtheria, described by Aretaeus, 71; epidemic of, in England in 16th century, 170; Whytt's description of, 231; bacillus of, 287; antitoxin for, 287, 391; tracheotomy for, 297; serum for, 286
Disease, and primitive man, 3–5, Pl. I; animistic view of, 11; cure of, by transference, 12–13; Chinese doctrines of, 35; Hippocrates on, 55; Aristotle's theory of, 61; Erasistratus' theory of, 64; Asclepiades' theory of, 67; Græco-Roman theories of, 68–69; Aretaeus on, 71–72; Galen on exciting and predisposing causes of, 76; Christian view of, in Middle Ages, 84–85, 97; named after saints, 100–1; Paracelsus' theory of, 159; Hoffmann's theory of "tonus" and, 217; Brown's theory of, 219; Cullen's classification of, 223; Abernethy's theory of, 243; and occupation, 260, 381–82; Broussais's theory of, 297; of the tropics, 357–62; nomenclature of, 388
Disinfecting fluid, Burnett's, 353
Dislocations, 9, 26, 58, 74, 93, 147, 243, 340
Dispensaries inaugurated in London by Lettsom, 253
Dissection (of human body), in ancient China, 35; by Herophilus, 64; forbidden by early Christians and Moslems, 77, 85; public, permitted, 122; illustration of Vesalius performing, 138; eighteenth-century Dutch paintings of, 130; public, by Lumleian lecturer, 181
Divination, practice of, 19, 65, Pl. VI
Doctor, first use of word, 107
Dogmatists (or Rationalists), 68
Dogs, as carriers of plague, 208; Caius' work on, 168

Domestic medicine, ancient, 11–13, 16; in Talmud, 31–32; in Rome, 65; at Salerno, 108–10; Boorde's work on, 173
Donders, Frans Cornelis, 375, 376
Doses, large and small, 218–20
Douglas, James, 237, 238
Douglas, John, 148, 239
Dover's powder, 203
Dover, Thomas, 203
Doyle, Sir Arthur Conan, 230
Drainage tube, rubber, 325
Drake, Daniel, 299–300, 400, Pl. LX
Dreams, 43, 163
Dressing, first field, 343
Dress, physician's, in Middle Ages, 130, 157; in eighteenth century, 253
Dropsy, described by Celsus, 73; William of Salicet on, 117; foxglove tea as remedy, 257; caused by kidney disease, 291
Drugs, in ancient Egypt, 24–25; in ancient China, 34–35; Celsus on, 73; Galen on, 76; Arabian, 86; Isaac Judæus on, 90; Avicenna on, 92; potency of, 219; in heart diseases, 366
Drummond, Adam, 227
Dublin Medical Press, 394
Dublin, School of Midwifery, 235; clinical medicine in Meath Hospital, 295–96; St. Mark's Hospital, 379; teaching of otology in, 379
Dubois, Eugène, 2
Dubois, Jacques. *See* Sylvius, Jacobus
Du Bois Reymond, Émil, 275–76
Duchenne, Guillaume Benjamin Armand, 369–70
Dum-dum fever (Kala-azar), 348
Dumas, J. B., 304
Dumb boy, cure of, 44
Dunant, Jean Henry, 232
Duncan, Andrew, 226, 294
Duodenal ulcer, 331
Duodenum, first named, 64
Dupuytren, Baron Guillaume, 258, 278, 309, 316
Durante, Francesco, 333
Dürer, Albrecht, and dissection, 135
Dusée, forceps of, Pl. L
Düsseldorf, Sudhoff's practice at, 404
Dutch, artists and medicine, 130, 194; anatomists, 194; ophthalmology, 375; early medical periodicals, 398, 399
Dutton, Joseph Everett, 361
Duverney, Joseph Guichard, 377
Dwarfs in ancient Egypt, 29
Dymphna, St., 99
Dysentery, in Hippocrates' *Epidemics*, 57; Ballingall on, 346

Ear, as organ of respiration, 25, 49; anatomy and physiology of, 141, 142, 186, 244; diseases of, 80, 377–80; foreign body in, 73; syringing of, 377

East India Company, 37, 152
Ebers, Georg, 24, 25, 26
Ebers Papyrus, 24–26
Eclectics, 68
Edessa (Urfa), 87
Edinburgh, Cardan at, 162 ; Harvey's visit to, 182 ; barber-surgeons. *See* Royal College of Surgeons of Edinburgh ; doctors, Pl. XLVII ; Extra-mural school, 322 ; Minto House, 310 ; physic garden, 192 ; Royal College of Physicians. *See* Royal College of Physicians of Edinburgh ; Royal College of Surgeons. *See* Royal College of Surgeons of Edinburgh
Edinburgh, Royal Infirmary, founded, 228 ; Cullen's clinical lectures at, 222 ; Wood at, 229 ; Benjamin and John Bell at, 230 ; first use of chloroform at, 305 ; Liston at, 308, 309 ; Syme at, 310 ; Fergusson at, 311 ; Lister at, 322, Pl. LXIII ; John Thomson at, 344
Edinburgh, University of, becomes centre of medical learning, 225 ; medical school founded, 228 ; anatomy, 227–28, 229, Pl. XLVI, 269–71 ; chemistry, 222 ; clinical medicine, 294 ; dermatology, 383 ; history of medicine, 407 ; materia medica, 366 ; medicine, 222, 225 ; military surgery, 344–46 ; obstetrics, 305–6 ; ophthalmology, 376 ; pathology, 345 ; pediatrics, 368 ; physiology, 222, 276, 278 ; surgery, 269, 308–11, 325, 331 ; students of, 218, 233, 249, 251, 252, 256, 278, 290, 291, 295, 296, 300, 311, 322, 330, 341, 344, 351, 352, 361, 374, 381, 387 ; first British university to admit women to medicine, 366 ; class cards, Pl. LIV
Edinburgh Medical Journal, 394
Edward the Confessor, 210
Edward IV, 14
Edward VI, 163, 168
Edward VII, 293, 330
Edwin Smith Papyrus, 26, Pl. V
Egypt, ancient, 19–29 ; modern, 339, 340, 341
Ehrlich, Paul, 384
Eiselberg, Anton von, 328
Electrical transmission of nerve impulse, 274
Electricity, derivation of the word ,179
Electro-cardiograph, 365
Electro-diagnosis, 369
Electro-physiology, 276
Elephantiasis, 357
Elf shot, 131
Elinus the Jew, legendary founder of School of Salerno, 103
Eliot, Robert, 227
Elixir of life, 87, 113

Elizabeth, Queen, 151, 152, 168, 179
Embalming, 27–29
Embryology, Aristotle and, 61 ; Harvey and, 183 ; Baer and, 273
Empedocles, 49–50
Emphysema of lung, 246
Empirics, 68
Endocrinology, 365, 385
Endoscopy, peroral, 381
Enemata, nutrient, 94
English Sweat. *See* Sweating sickness
Engravings. *See* Illustrations
Ephedrine, origin of, 35
Epidaurus, 43–45, Pl. X
Epidemics : Black Death, 126–28 ; Cholera in Ireland, 296 ; Cholera in London, 387, 388, 389 ; Dancing mania, 100 ; Ergotism, 101 ; Influenza, 350 ; Plague, bubonic, 101 ; Plague in modern Egypt, 340 ; Plague in London (1665), 206–9 ; Sore throat, 249 ; Sweating sickness, 169–71 ; Syphilis, 164 ; Typhus, 282 ; Typhus in Ireland, 296 ; Yellow fever, 243, 359, 360
Epidemiologist, the first, 165–66
Epilepsy, trephining as cure for, 8, 11 ; in Bible, 10 ; Hippocrates on, 55 ; patron saint of, 99 ; charm cures for, 6, 114, 125 ; Fothergill on, 250 ; Jacksonian, 371
Epsom, Mrs. Mapp of, 263
Erasistratus, 64
Erasmus, St., 99
Erb, Wilhelm Heinrich, 369
Ergotism, 101
Erichsen, Sir John Eric, 323
Erysipelas, 101, 323
Esmarch, Friedrich von, 343
Ether anaesthesia, first experiments in, 302–3 ; ether frolics, 302 ; controversy on discovery of, 303–4 ; first British use of, 304, 307, Pl. LXI ; in Russia, 344
Ethics, medical, in Babylonia, 18–19 ; in ancient Egypt, 23 ; in works of Hippocrates, 52, 53–54 ; in Middle Ages, 106, 117, 118, 124, 125
Etruscan medicine, 65
Eudamus, 76
Eustachian tube, 49, 142
Eustachius, Bartolomeus, 141–42, 377
Euthanasia, described by Paré, 145
Evolution, Aristotle and, 61
Exophthalmic goitre, 295, 376
Exostosis, in prehistoric man, 2 ; of the meatus, 378
Explorers, medical men as, 353–56
Eye, anatomy of, 272 ; care of, 110 ; diseases of, 25-26, 37, 80, 263, 264 ; patron saints of, 99 ; physiology of, 274–75, 375. *See also* Ophthalmology
Eye of Horus, as amulet, 20, Pl. IV

Fabricius, Hieronymus, of Acquapendente, 140–41, 149, 180, Pl. xxxvi
Fabricius Hildanus (Fabry of Hilden), 150
Faculty of Physicians and Surgeons of Glasgow. *See* Royal Faculty of Physicians and Surgeons of Glasgow
Fallopian tubes, 141
Fallopius, Gabriel, 141, 377
Faraday, Michael, 302
Farr, William, 388
Fee, of Arabian physician, 88 ; in Middle Ages, 118 ; in eighteenth century, 243
Fergusson, Sir William, 311–12, 315, 326
Fermentation, 199, 200, 284
Ferments of human body, 199
Fernel, Jean, 162
Feu sacré (St. Anthony's Fire), 101
Fevers, Chinese treatise on, 36 ; Celsus on, 73 ; Isaac Judæus on, 90 ; Sydenham on, 204 ; Jenner on, 294 ; Graves on, 295 ; Ballingall on, 346. *See also* Scarlet, Typhoid, etc.
Fiacre, St., 99
Fibrinogen, 240
Field hospitals, 349
Filaria, discovery of, 357
Finlay, Carlos, 359
Finlayson, James, 407
Finsen, Niels Ryberg, 385
First aid, 79, 343
Fistula in ano, treatment of, 125
Fitz, Reginald Heber, 330
Fitzpatrick Lectures, 405–6, 407
Fitzpatrick, Thomas, 406
Five figure series, 129
Fixed air, 261
Flavine, 350
Fletcher, Robert, 401–2
Flies and plague, 146
Flinders, Matthew, 355
Flint, Austin, 367
Flint surgical instruments, 1, 6, 7
Floyer, Sir John, 197, 257
Fludd, Robert, 158
Foetus, 135
Folk-medicine, 2, 11–15, 257
Fomites, 166
Foramen of Monro, 229
Forceps, obstetric, 235, 236, 237, Pls. xlix–l
Foster, Sir Michael, 278 ; quoted, 375
Fothergill, John, 235, 238, 249–50, 251, 252, 253, 254, 321
Fournier, Jean Alfred, 384
Fox, Tilbury, 383
Foxglove tea, as cure for dropsy, 257
Fracastorius, Hieronymus, 165–66, 189
Fractures (compound), amputation for, 239, 307, 339 ; Lister on, 324–25 ; Thomas's splint for, 334 ; closed plaster treatment of, 345–46, 350

Fractures, trephining skull for, 8, 9, 10–11, in ancient Egypt, 26 ; in Bible, 30 ; in ancient India, 33 ; Hippocrates on, 58 ; Celsus on, 74 ; Albucasis on, 93 ; Guy de Chauliac's treatment by extension for, 124 ; Paré and, 147 ; Pott's Fracture, 239 ; Sir Astley Cooper on, 243 ; Physick on, 244 ; Desault on, 244 ; Championnière's use of massage for, 327 ; Lane's plating of, 331 ; Thomas's treatment of, 334 ; Malgaigne on, 340 ; Ballingall on, 345
Fraenkel, Albert, 288
France. *See under* Montpellier *and* Paris
Francis II, King of France, 147
Francis, W. W., quoted, 213
Franco, Pierre, 148
Franco-Prussian War, 343
Frankfurt, Paul Ehrlich of, 384
Frank, Johann Peter, 260
Franklin, Benjamin, 250, 251
Franklin, Sir John, 354, 355
Fraser, Sir Thomas Richard, 366
Frederick II, 106, 107
Frederick III, 380
Freiburg, 329, 381
Freind, John, 255 ; his *History of Physick*, 80, 114
French Revolution, 338
Frerichs, Friedrich Theodor von, 298, 364
Freud, Sigmund, 373–4
Frost, Eben, 303
Fuchs, Ernst, 376
Fuchs, Leonhard, 132
Fumigation for plague, 128, 207
Furnivall, Frederick James, 173

Gaddesden, John of. *See* John of Gaddesden
Gaffky, Georg, 287
Gale, Thomas, 152, 337
Galen, 64, 68, 69, 70, 74–78, 84, 85, 88, 90, 91, 92, 95, 101, 111, 113, 122, 135, 136, 138, 140, 141, 157, 176, 185
Galiani, Alexandra, 123
Galilei, Galileo, 179, 191
Gall bladder, surgery of, 331
Gall, Franz Joseph, 264
Gallipoli, typhoid fever at, 348
Gall, St., 98
Gall-stones in mummies, 28
Gangrene, hospital, 307, 323, 345
Garcia, Manuel, 380, Pl. lxix
Gardens, botanical. *See* Botanical gardens ; herb. *See* Herb gardens
Garibaldi, Giuseppe, 341
Gariopontus, 104
Garrett Anderson. *See* Anderson
Garrick, David, 239
Garrison, Fielding Hudson, 402, 403–4, 414 ; quoted, 126, 156, 171, 266, 272, 343, 395, 398

Gas gangrene, 350 ; bacillus of, discovered, 289
Gas sylvestre, 199, 261
Gas warfare, 350
Gaskell, Walter Holbrook, 365
Gastric fistula, 300
Gastro-enteritis, 297
Gastroscopy, 299
Gazette de France, 396
Gazette des Hôpitaux, 397
General Board of Health, 387, 388, 389
General Medical Council, 155, 313
Geneva, Servetus martyred at, 140
Geneva Convention (1863), 232
Geography of disease, 300
George III, 233, 246, 256
George IV, 243, 313
Georgetown University, 403
Gerard, John, 132
Germany, bacteriology, 286–88 ; Black Death, 127 ; dermatology, 383 ; dancing mania, 100 ; herbalism, 131 ; journals, 397–98, 399 ; metabolism, 364–65 ; military surgery, 342–43 ; neurology, 369 ; ophthalmology, 376 ; otology, 379 ; pediatrics, 368 ; psychiatry, 373 ; public health, 390 ; surgery, 126, 149–50, 209, 244, 328–329 ; urology, 334. *See also* Berlin
Germs in atmosphere, 284
Gersdorff, Hans von, 126, Pl. xxvi
Gesner, Conrad, 163, 168, 399
Ghost-shooter, 5
Gibson, Joseph, 228
Giessen, Liebig's work at, 276
Giffard, William, 235
Gilbertus Anglicus, 113
Gilbert, William, 179
Gilles de Corbeil, 107
Giornale di Medicina, 398
Glanders, bacillus of, discovered by Loëffler, 287
Glanvilla, Bartholomæus Anglicus. *See* Bartholomeus Anglicus
Glasgow, control of practice in, 154 ; Royal Faculty of Physicians and Surgeons. *See* Royal Faculty, etc. ; Royal Infirmary, 323 ; University, founder of School of Medicine, 222, Pl. xlv ; lawsuits with Faculty of Physicians and Surgeons, 154–5 ; Boorde at, 173 ; Smellie at, 235 ; Lister at, 323–25 ; Thomson at, 344 ; Leishman at, 348 ; Blane at, 351 ; history of medicine, 407 ; medicine, 222 ; neuro-surgery, 333 ; ophthalmology, 376 ; ovariotomy, 301 ; surgery, 323
Glasgow Medical Journal, 394
Glaucoma, 376
Glisson, Francis, 191, 200–1, 224
Gloucestershire, cowpox in, 248
Glycogen, 279–80, 365
Glycosuria, 291

Godlee, Sir Rickman, 332, 333
Gods, in ancient Egypt, 20
Goitre, Celsus on, 73 ; exophthalmic, 295, 376 ; toxic, 331
Gold-headed Cane, 253–55
Gold, potable, 87
Golden Mirror of Medicine, 37
Golgi, Camillo, 358, 371
Gonococcus, 288
Gonorrhoea, 384
Goodsir, Harry, 354
Goodsir, John, 271, 283, 354
Gordon, Alexander, 318
Gordon, Bernard de. *See* Bernard de Gordon
Gorgas, William Crawford, 360
Göttingen, 218, 224, 272, 277, 286, 344, 374
Gourmelen, Estienne, 144
Gout, 28, 113, 114, 160, 203, 204
Gowers, Sir William Richard, 371
Graafian follicles, 195
Graaf, Regnier de, 195
Graefe, Albercht von, 376
Graefe, Karl Ferdinand von, 342–43
Graham, James, 263
Granada, conquest of, 96
Grassi, Giovanni, 358
Graves, Robert James, 295, 296
Gray, Henry, 272
Greatrakes, Valentine, 262
Great War, 348, 349–50, 360, 370
Greece, incubation in modern, 46
Greek medicine, 39–62 ; in Rome, 64–68
Greenhill, W. A., edition of Rhazes, 89
Green, Horace, 381
Gregory, James, 223, 230, 231, 344
Gregory, John, 222, 223, 231
Gregory's powder, 223, 231
Greig, E. D. W., 361
Gresham College, 191
Grew, Nehemiah, 190
Grieve, J., his edition of Celsus, 72
Grieve, Mrs. Maud, 132
Grog in navy, 352
Gröningen, 141
Gross, Samuel David, 301, 313
Gruner, O. C., his edition of Avicenna, 92
Guaiacum, 165, 169
Guidi, Guido (Vidius), 149
Guilds, barber-surgeon, in England, 150 ; union of barber-surgeons and surgeons in London (1540), 151
Guinea-worm, 346
Guinther (Gunter, Winter), Johannes, 137
Guiscard, Duke Robert, 104, 105, 109
Gull, Sir William Withey, 292–94
Gunpowder, invention of, and influence on surgery, 142 ; burns from, 337
Gunshot wounds. *See* Wounds (gunshot)
Gunter, Johannes. *See* Guinther
Guthrie, George James, 341–42, 349

Guthrie, Samuel, 304
Guy de Chauliac, 93, 114, 123–25, 142
Guyon, Felix, 334
Guyot, Edme Gilles, 377
Guy's Hospital (London), 290, 291, 292, 293, 335, 365
Guy's Hospital Reports, 394
Gynæcology, in ancient Egypt, 27 ; practised by Soranus, 69 ; in the United States, 301, 330

Haematology, 385
Haemolysis, 187
Haemorrhage, 106, 117, 119
Haemorrhoids, 125
Haemostasis, 305, 343
Haen, Anton de, 225
Haggis, A. W., quoted, 205
Hague, The, Van Deventer at, 195
Hahnemann, Samuel, 219
Hain, Ludwig, 400
Hajek, Markus, 380
Hakim, El, 94
Hale-White, Sir William, quoted, 295
Hales, Stephen, 260–61
Halford, Sir Henry, 254
Halket, James, 225, 227
Hall, Marshall, 276–77
Halle, Collegium Naturae Curiosorum, 191 ; University of, 216, 217, 287, 328, 379
Haller, Albrecht von, 200, 223–24, 399–400
Halsted, William Stewart, 331
Hamburg, 383, 384, 397
Hamilton, Alexander, 228, 231
Hamilton, Archibald, Archbishop, 162
Hamilton, Emma Lyon, Lady, 263
Hamilton, James, 231
Hamilton, Mary, on incubation, 46
Hamilton (Scotland), 221, 222, 237
Hammurabi, Code of, 18, 19
Hand, Bell's treatise on, 269
Hansen, Armauer, 288
Hanwell Asylum, 372
Hare-lip, operation for, 311
Hare, William, 228, 270–71
Harington, Sir John, 109
Harmony, and health, 49
Harrison, Benjamin, the Elder, 293
Hartford, Connecticut, 302
Hartshorn, in ancient Egyptian medicine, 25
Harvard University, 334, 368, 383, 391
Harvey, William, 138, 140, 141, 175, 180–85, 186, 188, 202, 226, 235, 266, 269, 337, 406, Pls. xxxvi–xxxvii
Haslar Hospital, 233, 234, 268, 353, 354
Hastings, Sir Charles, 394
Havana, yellow fever in, 359, 360
Headache, trephining as cure for, 8, 11 ; cured by incubation, 44
Head, Sir Henry, 371

Hearing, resonance theory of, 275
Hearst Papyrus, 26
Heart, in *Ebers Papyrus*, 25 ; Celsus on diseases of, 73 ; dropsy and disease of, 257 ; Rokitansky on diseases of, 282 ; Stokes on diseases of, 296 ; modern research on diseases of, 365–67 ; heart-block, 365 ; moderator band of, 135 ; motive power of, in circulation, 184 ; myogenic theory of action of, 224 ; septum of, 138 ; sounds of, 259
Heberden, William, 69, 235, 256
Hebra, Ferdinand, 383
Hebrew literature, 29–32
Hedgehogs, experiments on, 241
Heidelberg, University of, 201, 271, 275, 369
Heister, Lorenz, 244
Helmholtz, Hermann von, 274, 274–75, 374
Helmont, Jean Baptiste van, 68, 160, 199, 261
Henle, Jacob, 271–72, 273, 274, 286
Henoch, Eduard Heinrich, 368
Henri de Mondeville, 117, 118
Henry VIII, 150, 168, 172
Henry II, King of France, 147
Henry III, King of France, 147
Herb gardens, 96, 97, 98. *See also* Botanical gardens
Herbalism, 13, 116–17, 131–33 ; ancient Chinese, 34 ; Graeco-Roman, 62 ; Saxon, 102 ; at Salerno, 110 ; in Middle Ages, 111 ; modern, 131–33
Hermetic books of Thoth, 23
Hermodikes, stone of, 44, Pl. x
Hernia, 73, 124, 147, 148, 239, 243, 329, 331
Herodotus, quoted, 19, 27, 39
Herophilus, 64
Hertford, Dimsdale at, 247
Hertz, Heinrich, 275
Hertzian waves, 275
Heubner, Otto, 368
Hewson, William, 240
Hickman, Henry, 302
Hildegard of Bingen, 102
Hilton, John, 335
Hilton-Simpson, Melville William, quoted, 9, 10, 93
Hindus, medicine and surgery of, 32–34
Hinton, James, 378–9
Hippocrates, 21, 29, 39, 40, 42, 45, 48, 49, 51–60, 61, 62, 65, 67, 70, 71, 72, 74, 76, 78, 88, 90, 100, 101, 104, 130, 159, 196, 198, 221, 225, 259, Pls. xi–xii ; Aphorisms of, 52, 58–60
" Hippocrates, The English " (*i.e.* Sydenham). *See* Sydenham, Thomas
" Hippocrates, The, of chronic disease " (*i.e.* Asclepiades). *See* Asclepiades
Hippocratic facies, 56
Hippocratic Oath, 53–54

His, Wilhelm, 365
Histology, 245, 272, 278
Historians, recent medical, 403–10
History, journals of medical, 398–99
Hodges, Nathaniel, 207–8, 208
Hoffmann, Friedrich, 217
Hogarth, William, his cartoon of quacks, 264, Pl. LIII
Holbein, Hans, 151, 167, Pl. xxx
Holborn, Gerard's garden at, 131
Holland, Sir Henry, 290
Holmes, Oliver Wendell, 303, 319, 409
Holy Wood (guaiacum), 165, 169
Home, Francis, 230, Pl. XLVII
Home, Sir Everard, 312
Homer, medicine and surgery in, 46–48
Homœopathy, 219–20
Honain. See Hunayn ibn Isaq
Hong Kong, 37, 287, 357–58
Hooke, R., 187, 190, 191, 192, Pl. xxxviii
Hooker, Sir Joseph Dalton, 354
Hooker, Sir William, 354
Hooks, Malgaigne's, 340
Hopkins, Sir Frederick Gowland, 365
Horace, quoted, 66
Hormones, 280, 363, 365
Horoscope, Pl. xxxi
Horsley, Sir Victor, 333
Horus, Eye of, 20, Pl. IV
Hose, Charles, quoted, 5
Hospital gangrene, 307, 323, 345
Hospital ships, 352
Hospitals, of ancient Rome, 82–83 ; early Christian, 85 ; Rhazes' site for one at Baghdad, 89 ; in mediæval Cordova, 93 ; Moslem, 95–96 ; mediæval, 128–29, Pl. xxiii ; Geneva Convention, 232 ; Field, 349 ; Mental, 249, 372–73 ; Private, in ancient Rome, 82 ; at Berne, 150 ; at Edinburgh, 310 ; at Paris, 149. For separate hospitals, see under their names
Household medicine. See Domestic medicine
Housman, A. E., Shropshire Lad quoted, 70n
Houston, Robert, 301
Howard, John, 250
Hua Tu, 36
Hugh of Lucca (Ugo Borgognoni),111,115
Humanism and scholasticism, 134, 143
Humours, and disease, theory of, in ancient China, 35 ; in Greek medicine, 50 ; Aristotle on, 61 ; rejected by Erasistratus, 64 ; accepted by Galen, 76 ; at Salerno, 110 ; accepted by John of Gaddesden, 114 ; Caius on, 169 ; persistence of doctrine, 176 ; death-blow to, 283
Hunayn ibn Isaq (Honain or Johannitus), 88
Hunter, John, 121, 148, 164, 182, 235, 240–42, 243, 244, 247, 273, 277, 285, 329, 338, Pl. LI

Hunter, William, 222, 229, 237–38, 240, 351
Hunterian Museum (Glasgow), 151, 238
Hurry, Jamieson Boyd, quoted, 21
Husemann, T., 108
Huser, Johann, 158
Hutchinson, Sir Jonathan, 329–30, 383
Hutten, Ulrich von, 165
Huxham, John, 234
Huxley, Thomas Henry, 354
Hwang Ti, 35
Hydromel, 58
Hydrophobia, 250, 285, 326. See also Rabies
Hygiene, in Bible, 30–31 ; in Talmud, 31. See also Public Health
Hypnotism, 262, 302, 374
Hyrtl, Joseph, 272

Iatro-chemical theory, 197, 198–200, 204
Iatro-physical theory, 178, 196–98, 204, 226
Iceland, 290
Igneo-aerial particles, 188
Ignis sacer (St. Anthony's Fire), 101
Illustrations, medical, 126, 129–30, 131, 137, 141–42, 185. See also Artists
Imhotep (Imonthes),20, 21–23, 29, Pl. vii
Immortality, belief in, 3
Incantations, 24, 27, 80, 125. See also Charms
Incorporation of Barber-Surgeons, Edinburgh. See Royal College of Surgeons of Edinburgh
Incubation, 23, 43–46, 97
Index Medicus, 400, 402, 403
India, medicine of ancient, 32–34 ; health of troops in modern, 341, 348
Infant feeding, 368
Infectious disease, 272, 288
Inflammation, 73, 323, 345
Influenza, discovery of bacillus of, 287 ; world epidemic of, 350
Ingrassia, Giovanni Filippo, 141
Innes, John, 228
Inoculation, against smallpox, in ancient China, 36, 246 ; in England, 246–47 ; against typhoid, 349
Inquisition, Spanish, 139
Insanity, trephining as cure for, 8 ; Aretaeus on, 71 ; Celsus on, 73 ; patron saint of, 99 ; enlightened attitude to, 249 ; new outlook on, 372 ; and crime, 373
Insects and tropical disease, 357
Instruments, surgical, prehistoric, 1, 6, 7 ; primitive, 8 ; Arabian, 9, 93, Pl. xvii ; Sumerian, 17 ; ancient Indian, 33 ; Roman, 74, Pl. xiii ; German, 150, 209 ; English, 152 ; Lister's, 325 ; Scottish, Pl. xxix
Insulin, 363, 365
Intravenous medication, 200

Invisible perspiration, 197
Ipecacuanha, 219
Ireland, medical periodicals in, 394
  See also Dublin
Iridectomy, 376
Iridotomy, 238
Iris, contractile tissue of, 322
Iron in treatment of anaemia, 204
Isaac Judæus, 90
Italy, Black Death in, 127 ; Cardan, 161–62 ; Vesalius and anatomy, 137–142 ; bacteriology, 317–18 ; journal, 398 ; neurological surgery, 333 ; ophthalmology, 244 ; physiology, 197–98 ; surgery, 149, 244, 329. *See also* Bologna, Padua, Pisa, Rome, Salerno
Itard, Jean Marie Gaspard, 379

Jabir ibn Hayyan. *See* Jebir
Jackson, Charles Thomas, 303
Jackson, Chevalier, 381
Jackson, John Hughlings, 370–71
Jackson, Robert, 346
Jacobi, Abraham, 368
Jacobite Rebellion (1745), 232, 233
Jacques, Frère, 239
Jacques de Beaulieu, Frère, 149
James I, King of England, medical record of, 201 ; physicians to, 179, 181, 201
James III, King of Scotland, 153
James, John, 193
Jamieson, William Allan, 383
Jansen, Zacharias, 189
Janus, 399
Japan, medicine in, 37–38 ; Institute for Infectious Diseases, 287
Japan river fever, 289
Jaundice, described by Celsus, 73 ; Bright on, 291
Java man, prehistoric, 2
Jaw, dislocated, in papyrus, 26
Jean de Saint Côme, Frère, 149
Jebir (Jabir ibn Hayyan), 87
Jefferson, Georgia, 302
Jenner, Edward, 241, 247–49, 252, 257, 284, 353, Pl. LII
Jenner, Sir William, 294, 325
Jenner Institute. *See* Lister Institute
Jesuit's bark, 205
Jewish medicine, 29–32 ; greatest physician, 95
Jews, Black Death attributed to, 127
Jex-Blake, Sophia, 386
Johannitus. *See* Hunayn ibn Isaq
John XXI, Pope. *See* Petrus Hispanus
John of Arderne. *See* Arderne, John
John of Gaddesden, 113–14
John of Trevisa, 104
John Rylands Library (Manchester), 171
Johns Hopkins Hospital, 400
Johns Hopkins Institute, 399
Johns Hopkins Medical School, 400, 402
Johns Hopkins University, 288, 331, 403

Johnson, Samuel, 210, 239, 246, 255, 256, 263
Joints, diseases of, 312 ; tuberculous, 310
Jones, Sir Robert, 334–35
Jones, William Henry Samuel, his edition of Hippocrates, 53
Journal de Médecine, 397
Journal des Sçavans, 192, 397
Journal of Mental Science, 394
Journal of Pathology and Bacteriology, 288
Journals. *See* Periodicals
Judæus, Isaac. *See* Isaac Judæus
Juices of human body, 199, 279, 329
Julian, Emperor of Rome, 79
Jundi-shapur, 87
Jupille, Pasteur's patient, 284, Pl. LVII
Jurjis Bukht-Yishu. *See* Bachtishua, George

Kahun Papyrus, 27
Kala-azar, 348
Kane, Elisha Kent, 354–55
Kanutus, Benedictus, 171, 172
Kaye, John. *See* Caius
Keen, William Williams, 333
Keith, Sir Arthur, quoted, 335, 369
Kelly, Howard, 330, 331
Kelvin, William Thomson, Lord, 275
Kentucky, early medicine in, 299, 300
Kew Gardens, 250, 354
Keys, John. *See* Caius
Kharkoff, Metchnikoff born at, 285
Kidney, function of, 276 ; physiology of, 375 ; glomeruli of, first described, 186 ; Bright's Disease, 291, 294 ; tubules of, discovered by Henle, 272
Kiel, University of, Chair of Surgery, 343
Kien Lung, Emperor of China, 37
Killian, Gustav, 381
King's evil. *See* Scrofula
Kircher, Athanasius, 189, 317
Kirkes, William Senhouse, 314
Kitasato, Shibasaburo, 287, 359
Klein, Edward Emanuel, 361
Knee joint, osteo-arthritis in, of mummy, 29, Pl. VIII ; operation on, 326
Knox, Robert, 270–71, 311, 345
Knutsson, Bengt. *See* Kanutus, Benedictus
Knyveton, John, quoted, 234
Kocher, Theodore, 329
Koch, Robert, 286–87, 384, 390
Koch's postulates, 286
Kolletschka, Professor, 319
Kölliker, Rudolf Albert von, 322
Königsberg, 273, 274, 316
Kopho (Copho), 105
Kraepelin, Emil, 373
Kramer, Wilhelm, 379
Kraske, Paul, 329
Kussmaul, Adolf, 299, 364
Kyphosis, in mummies, 28

Lac plaster, Lister's, 324
Lacteals, discovery of, 185
Laënnec, René Théophile Hyacinthe, 258–59, 292, 296, 366, 383, Pl. LVI
"Lamb, Vegetable," 132
Lancet, The, 394
Lancisi, Giovanni Maria, 142
Landarzt, Der, 397
Lane, Sir Arbuthnot, 331
Lanercost, Priory of, 291
Lanfranchi, Guido, 117, 119
Lanfranc of Milan. *See* Lanfranchi
Langenbeck, Bernhard von, 316, 343, 398
Laparotomy in ancient China, 36
La Roque, Jean-Paul de, 397
Larrey, Baron Jean Dominique, 338–40, 342, 343, 345, 349, 350, Pl. LXVII
Laryngectomy, 328
Laryngology, 380–81
Laryngoscope, invention of, 380, Pl. LXIX
Larynx, cancer of, 380
Laudanum, 160, 204
Laughing gas (nitrous oxide), 302
Lausanne, Pierre Franco at, 148
Laveran, Alphonse, 357, 358
Lavoisier, Antoine Laurent, 188, 261, 262
Lawrence, St., 99
Lazear, Jesse, 359
Lead poisoning (Devonshire colic), 234
Leech Book of Bald, 102, 131
Leeches, 297, 345
"Leeches" or surgeons in the *Iliad*, 47–8
Leeds, 261, 331, 407
Lee Penny, 14, Pl. IV
Leeuwenhoek, Antony van, 189, 189–90, 317, Pl. XXXVIII
Le Fanu, W. R., 395
Leipzig, *Ebers Papyrus* in, 24 ; homœopathy at, 219 ; physiology at, 276 ; thermometry at, 298 ; surgery at, 328 ; embryology at, 365 ; history of medicine at, 405
Leishmaniasis (Kala-azar), 348
Leishman, Sir William Boog, 288,349
Lemaire, Jules, 324
Lembert, Antoine, 316
Lemon, cure for scurvy, 152, 234, 352
Leningrad, military hospital at, 344. *See also* St. Petersburg
Lenses, microscope, 189
Leontiasis ossea, 283
Leprosy, in Bible, 30 ; in Middle Ages, 129 ; discovery of bacillus of, 288 ; hospitals for, in Scotland, 305 ; research on, 329
Letheon, 303
Letts, Malcolm, quoted, 213
Lettsom, John Coakley, 235, 249, 251, 252–53, 254, Pl. LII
Leucin discovered in urine, 298
Leucocythemia, 278
Leucocytosis, 283

Levret, André, 237
Leyden, University of, foundation and fame of, 193–95 ; Sylvius professor at, 199–200 ; Sir T. Browne student at, 211, 225 ; Boerhaave professor at, 220–21, Pl. XLIV ; famous pupils of Boerhaave at, 223–25 ; Edinburgh professors students at, 225–31 ; Pitcairne professor at, 226; Sir J. Pringle student at, 232; W. Hunter student at, 238 ; Lettsom student at, 252 ; botanical gardens of, 194, 221
Leyden, Ernst von, 298, 299
Library, of Alexandria, 63, 85 ; of Mansur Hospital (Cairo), 96 ; Surgeon-General's (Washington), 401, 402 ; Welch Medical (Baltimore), 403 ; Osler's, 410
Liebig, Justus von, 276, 304, 364, 390
Ligature, 106, 119, 146
Lille University Chair of Chemistry, 283
Lima, quinine used in, 205 ; climate of, 223
Lime water, as remedy for scurvy, 152, 234 ; as remedy for stone, 231
Linacre, Thomas, 166–67
Lind, James, 152, 233–34, 351, 352
Linnaeus (Carl von Linné), 215
Lister, Agnes, Lady Lister, 322–23, 327
Lister Institute, 326
Listerism, 327
Lister, Joseph Jackson, 321
Lister, Joseph, Baron Lister, 285, 304, 306, 321–327, 328, 331, Pls. LXI, LXIII–LXIV
Liston, Robert, 304, 307–9, 310, 322, Pl. LXI
Liston's bone forceps, 309
Lithotrity, instead of lithotomy, 311 ; improved technique of, 334
Lithotomy, in ancient India, 33 ; in Hippocratic Oath, 54 ; Celsus on, 73 ; Arab surgeons and, 9, 93 ; Paracelsus on, 160 ; Cheselden's technique in, 238–39 ; Physick and, 244 ; Fergusson and, 311 ; Dupuytren and, 316 ; mortality of, 149, 239 ; rapidity of, 239, 308 ; lateral, 149, 239 ; suprapubic, 148, 239 ; itinerant lithotomists, 148–49
"Little animals" of Leeuwenhoek, 190
Littré, Émile, 53
Liver (of animal), divination by inspection of, 19, 65, Pl. VI
Liver (of human), anatomy of, 200 ; cirrhosis of, 245 ; diseases of, 298 ; function of, 279, 365
Liverpool, 258, 304, 334
Livingstone, David, 356
Lizars, John, 310
Locke, John, 202
Locomotor ataxia, 294, 369
Loeffler, Friedrich, 287

London, Black Death at, 126 ; Great Plague (1665) at, 206–9, Pl. XLII; control of medical practice in, 151, 167 ; mediæval hospitals of, 128 ; sanitation in, 206 ; sweating sickness in, 169 ; Apothecaries' Company, 192 ; barber-surgeons, 150–51 ; Hospital for Sick Children, 367–68 ; King's College, 326, 375 ; King's College Hospital, 311 ; London Dispensary for Curing Diseases of the Eye and Ears. *See* Royal London Ophthalmic Hospital ; London Fever Hospital, 387 ; London Hospital, 329, 367, 370 ; London School of Medicine for Women, 386 ; London School of Tropical Medicine, 358 ; Metropolitan Ear and Throat Hospital, 377 ; National Hospital, 370 ; Royal Samaritan Hospital, 320 ; St. Bartholomew's Hospital. *See* St. Bartholomew's Hospital ; St. George's Hospital. *See* St. George's Hospital ; St. Mary's Hospital. *See* St. Mary's Hospital ; St. Thomas's Hospital. *See* St. Thomas's Hospital ; Temple of Health, 263 ; Throat Hospital, 380 ; University College, 278, 309 ; University College Hospital, 304, 307, 321, 333, 387 ; Windmill Street School of Anatomy, 238, 267
London Medical Papyrus, 27
Long, Crawford Williamson, 302, 303, 304
Longmore, Sir Thomas, 349
Lorry, Anne Charles, 382
Louis XIV, King of France, 191, 210
Louis, Pierre Charles Alexandre, 297
Louvain, University of, Vesalius at, 136, 137 ; Guinther at, 137 ; Schevez student at, 153
Louvre Museum, 17, 18
Lowe, Peter, 154, 407, Pl. XXIX
Lower, Richard, 187–88, 191
" Lowsiness," in Boorde's *Breviarie*, 173
Loyalty Islands, trephining in, 8
Lucas-Championnière, Just, 327
Lucca, Hugh of. *See* Hugh of Lucca
Lucia, St., 99
Ludlow, Hickman's experiments at, 302
Ludwig, Carl, 276
Lumleian Lectures, 181, 200
Lumley, John, Baron Lumley, 181
Lunar Society of Birmingham, 257
Lungs, pneumonic consolidation of, 245 ; function of, 187 ; patron saint of, 98
Lupus, light treatment of, 385
Luz, bone called, in the Talmud, 31
Lydgate, Dr. Tertius, in *Middlemarch*, 408
Lymph vessels, 185, 240

Macao, hospital for diseases of the eye at, 37

McBurney, Charles, 330–1
McDowell, Ephraim, 300, Pl. LX
Macewen, Sir William, 333
McGill, John, 227
McGill University, Sir William Osler at, 409, 410
McGrigor, Sir James, 341, 346, Pl. LXVIII
Machaon, son of Aesculapius, 47
Machine, human body as, 178, 196–98
Mackenzie, Richard James, 322
Mackenzie, Sir George, 290
Mackenzie, Sir James, 56, 296, 366
Mackenzie, Sir Morell, 380–81
Mackenzie, William, 376
Macleod, John James Rickard, 365
MacMichael, William, 254
Mad dog, bite of, 113, 284, 285
Madrid, Vesalius at, 139 ; Ramón y Cajal at, 372
Magendie, François, 268, 279
Magnetism, Gilbert's work on, 179
Maimonides (Moses ben Maimon), 94–95
Mains de Palfyn, 237
Makins, Sir George, 349
Malaria, in ancient India, 32 ; in ancient Greece, 42 ; in Hippocrates' *Epidemics*, 57 ; and fall of Rome, 83 ; in England, 204, 357 ; use of cinchona for, 205, 219 ; Koch's study of, 286 ; discoveries in, 357–58 ; in Panama, 360
Mal des ardents, 101
Malgaigne, Joseph François, 124, 148, 316, 340
Malpighi, Marcello, 186, 188, 189, 198
Malta fever. *See* Mediterranean fever
Mammalian ovum, discovery of, 273
Manchester, 318, 324
Mandragora, 107, 116–17, Pl. XXI
Mandrake. *See* Mandragora
Mangold wurzel, 252
Man-midwife, 235
Manningham, Sir Richard, 235
Manson, Sir Patrick, 357–58
Mansur Hospital (Cairo), 95–96
Mapp, Mrs., 263, Pl. LIII
Marburg, 287
Margate, Royal Sea-bathing Hospital, 253
Marie, Pierre, 370
Markham, Sir Clements, quoted, 205
Marsh fever, 357
Martial, reference to doctors by, 66
Mary I, Queen of England, 168
Mary II, Queen of England, 254
Massachusetts General Hospital, 303
Massachusetts Sanitary Commission, 390
Massage, primitive use of, 11–12 ; in ancient China, 35–36
Mastoiditis, first operation for, in France, 244, 379 ; in England, 379 ; " Wilde's incision " for acute, 379

Materia Medica, in ancient China, 34–35 ; of Dioscorides, 62 ; Arab contribution to 86 ; Fothergill on, 250 ; Chair of, founded at Edinburgh, 230
Materia peccans, 130
Mathematics and medicine, 179
Maudsley, Henry, 373
Maxillary sinus, 135
Mayerne, Sir Theodore Turquet de, 176, 201, 207
Mayo, Charles Horace, 332
Mayo Clinic, 332, Pl. LXVI
Mayo, William James, 332, 334
Mayow, John, 187, 188, 191
Mead, Richard, 130, 226, 235, 238, 254, 254–55, 255
Measles, Rhazes on, 89 ; Ingrassia on, 141 ; epidemic of, in England, 170 ; Sydenham on, 203–4
Meath Hospital (Dublin), 295, 296
Meckel, Johann Friedrich, 229
Medical Act (1858), 155, 313
Medical Circular, 377, 394
Medical Directory, 378
Medical Officer of Health, First, 389*n*
Medical Press and Circular, 394
Medical Register, 154, 313
Medical Repository, 395
Medical Society of Aberdeen, 341
Medical Society of London, 252, Pl. LII
Medical Staff Corps, 347
Medical Transactions of the Royal College of Physicians of London, 393
Medicina Curiosa, 192, 393, Pl. LXXI
Medico-Chirurgical Transactions, 393
Mediterranean (or Malta) fever, 533, 361
Meibom, Heinrich, 194
Meister, Joseph, 284
Melanesia, 4–5, 8, 9, 11, Pl. II
Memphis, 23
Meningitis, described by Hippocrates, 57 ; otitic, 147 ; tuberculous, 231, 268
Mental disease, 372–74
Mental hospitals, 249, 372–73
Mercure Savant, 396
Mercurio Volante, 395
Mercury, in treatment of syphilis, 204
Mesmer, Franz Anton, 262, 302
Mesmerism, 262, 302
Metabolism, 197, 276, 364–65, Pl. XL
Metallic tractors, 263
Metchnikoff, Élie, 285
Metchnikoff, Mme. Olga, 285
Methodism, 67, 68, 69
Metoposcopy, Cardan's account of, 163
Mexico City, *Mercurio Volante* published at, 395
Meyerhof, Max, quoted, 91, 96
Miasmata, 286
Micrococcus catarrhalis, 287
Micrococcus Melitensis, 353

Microscope, inventors of, 121, 189 ; early medical research with, 188–90 ; Leeuwenhoek's discoveries with, 189–190, Pl. XXXVIII
Microscopic anatomy, 186, 271, 278
Middeldorpf, Albrecht Theodor von, 316
Middlesex Hospital, 268
Midwifery, first book in English on, 174 ; first original English work on, 183 ; first university chair of, 228 ; in eighteenth century, 235–238. *See also* Obstetrics
Midwives, Biblical mention of, 30
Migraine, trephining as cure for, 10 ; Hildegard and, 102
Mikulicz-Radecki, Johann von, 328
Miles, Alexander, quoted, 309, 311
Military hygiene, in Bible, 31 ; Pringle's work on, 233
Military medicine, 232–33
Military surgery, to eighteenth century, 337–38 ; nineteenth–twentieth centuries, 338–350 ; of modern warfare, 349–50 ; English, 151–52, 209, 337–38, 341–42 ; French, Paré's account of, 144–46 ; Larrey and nineteenth century, 338–341 ; German, mediæval, 126 ; Fabry of Hilden, 150 ; modern, 342–43 ; Greek (ancient), 47–48 ; Indian (ancient), 33 ; Roman, 81–82 ; Russian, 343–44 ; Scottish, 344–46
Milk, supply of pure, 368
Miller, James, 305
Millar, Margaret, 301
Mineral salts, used by Dioscorides, 62
Ministry of Health (Britain), 392
Minoan civilization, 39–40
Miracles of healing, 45, 85, 97, 102, 120
Mississippi Valley, diseases of, 300
Mitchell, Silas Weir, 371
Mithridates VI, King of Pontus, experiments by, 69, 70
Mithridaticum. *See* Theriac
Mohammed, the Prophet, 86, 87
Monasteries, medicine in, 85, 96–98, 101, 102, 103
Mondeville, Henri de. *See* Henri de Mondeville
Monks, influence of, 120–21
Monotheism, of Galen, 74, 84
Monro, Alexander (Primus), 226, 227–228, 249, 251, Pl. XLVI
Monro, Alexander (Secundus), 229
Monro, Alexander (Tertius), 229, 270
Monro, John, 227
Montagu, Lady Mary Wortley, 246
Monte Cassino, Monastery of, 101–2, 103, 105, 131
Monteith, Alexander, 227
Montpellier, University of, Arabic medicine at, 92 ; Medical School, 104, 112–15 ; Englishmen at, 113–14 ; Guy de Chauliac at, 123 ; John of

Arderne at, 125 ; Paracelsus at, 157 ; Boorde at, 172 ; Mayerne at, 201 ; Sydenham at, 203 ; Sir T. Browne at, 211 ; Barthez at, 217 ; Desgenettes at, 340 ; Renaudot at, 396
Montreal, Osler at, 408–10
Moodie, Roy M., quoted, 2
Moon, influence of, 110, 129
Moore, Sir Norman, 128, 201, 405–6, 406
Moorfields Eye Hospital. *See* Royal London Ophthalmic Hospital
Morgagni, Giovanni Battista, 245, 251, 281
Morgan, John, 251
Morley, Henry, quoted, 162
Mortality, of Hippocrates' cases, 56 ; Bills of, 206, 208 ; in British army, 348
Morton, L. T., 404
Morton, William Thomas Green, 303, 304
Moslems, medicine of, 86–96 ; Galen approved of by, 74 ; dissection prohibited by, 85
Mosquito, 357–60
Mott, Valentine, 301
" Mount Stuart " skull, 8, Pl. II
Moxa, Chinese origin of, 36
Moynihan, Berkeley George Andrew, Baron Moynihan, 331
Müllerian ducts, 273
Müller, Johannes, 61, 272–74, 278, 398
Münchener medizinische Wochenschrift, 398
Mummy, preparation of, 27–28 ; pathology of, 28–29, Pl. VIII ; powdered, as remedy, 144
Mundinus (Mondino de Luzzi), 122–23, 135
Munich, 328, 373, 390
Muniz, Manuel A., 7
Munk, William, 254
Munro, Robert, quoted, 8
Murmurs, heart, 367
Murphy, John Benjamin, 331
Murphy's button, 330
Musandinus, Petrus, 106
" Muscle man," in mediæval illustrations, 129
Muscles, stapes and tensor tympani, discovery of, 141 ; Haller and irritability of, 224 ; action of, 370
Museum, Harvey's, 183 ; Sir Charles Bell's, 268 ; Hunterian, of Glasgow, 238 ; John Hunter's, 241 ; Richard Mead's, 255 ; of Royal College of Surgeons of Edinburgh, 270
Music, therapeutic value of, 92, 96, 100, 118 ; and medical men, 403
Myers, Walter, 359
Myxœdema, 294

Nabarro, D., 361
Nagana, 356, 361

Naples, 46, 74, 141, 164, 244, 368
Napoleon, his physician, 258 ; military surgeons under, 297, 338–40
Nasal mucus, origin of, 188
National Insurance Act (1911), 392
Natural spirit, 77
Nature, healing power of, 57, 67, 75, 198, 297, 335
Naunyn, Bernhard, 364–65
Naval medicine, 233–34, 351–53
Necker Hospital (Paris), 258, 334
Needham, John Turberville, 318
Neisser, Albert, 287–88
Nélaton, Auguste, 316, 340–41
Nelmes, Sarah, 248
Neolithic Age. *See* Stone Age
Nepenthe, 48
Nephritis, Pl. LIX
Nerves, sensory and motor, 64, 77, 268 ; cranial, described by Galen, 77 ; sympathetic nervous system discovered by Galen, 77 ; Cullen on importance of, in disease, 223 ; Haller and sensibility of, 224 ; Sir C. Bell's experiments on, 268–69 ; vasomotor, 280 ; diseases of nervous system, 368–72 ; histology of, 371–72
Nervus acusticus, tumours of, 333
Nesperehan, mummy of, 28, Pl. VIII
Nestorian medicine, 87
Nestorius, 87
Netley, Army Medical College. *See* Royal Army Medical College
Nettle-sting, treatment of, 13
Neuburger, Max, 120
Neuralgia, 250, 269
Neurological surgery, 332–33
Neurology, 269, 299, 368–72
New Caledonia, trephining in, 8
New England Journal of Medicine, 395
New England Medical Review and Journal, 395
New Guinea, trephining in, 8
New Orleans, Board of Health, 391
New South Wales, exploration in, 355
New York, 330, 367, 368 ; *Medical Repository* of, 395 ; Medical School, foundation of, 301
Newark, John of Arderne at, 125
Newton, James, 132
Newton, Sir Isaac, 215, 238, 375
Nicaise, Édouard, 118
Nicholas V., Pope, MS. of Celsus' *De re medicina* found by, 72
Nicolas Myrepsos, 108
Nicolas of Damascus, 121
Nicolas of Salerno, 108
Niger, River, exploration of, 356
Nightingale, Florence, 344, 347
Nineveh, 18
Nitrites, effect of, for angina pectoris, 366
Nitro-aerial spirit, 188
Nitrous oxide, 302

Nitze, Max, 334
Nobel Prize, 285, 287, 372, 385
Noguchi, Hideyo, 38, 359
Nomenclature, medical, 86, 88, 100–1, 123
Noorden, Carl von, 365
Norwich, John Caius at, 167 ; plague at, 209 ; Sir Thomas Browne at, 211
Nose, diseases of, described by Aëtius, 80
Nothnagel, Hermann, 299, 365
Nottingham, 151, 277
Nourse, Edward, 239
Nouvelles Découvertes sur toutes les Parties de la Médecine, the first medical journal, 193, 396
Novaesium, Roman valetudinarium at, 83
Nuremberg, early medical periodical at, 398
Nursing, Sir W. Gull on, 294 ; schools for, 347 ; sick-room cookery, 106
Nussbaum, Johann von, 328
Nutrition, 365, 385

Oath, Hippocratic, 53–54
Oath of allegiance at Salerno, 107
Obstetric chair. *See* Birth stool
Obstetrics, 69, 174, 183, 195, 251, 305–6, Pl. xxxiv. *See also* Midwifery
Occupation, diseases of, 260, 381–82
Ogston, Sir Alexander, 288, Pl. lxv
Ohio, 299, 400
Oliver, William, 233
Omar Khayyám, 91
Omphalos of Delphi, 41, Pl. ix
Operation, without anaesthesia, 307 ; in private house, 308 ; by Ogston, Pl. lxv
Ophthalmologist, Queen Anne's, 264
Ophthalmology, Babylonian ophthalmic surgery, 18 ; in ancient Egypt, 25, 26 ; early textbook on, 88 ; Cheselden and, 238 ; quacks in, 263–64 ; medical, 371 ; nineteenth-century, 374–76. *See also* Eye
Ophthalmoscope, invention of, 274, 374 ; importance of, first recognized, 376 ; use of, in neurology, 371
Optics, study of, 375
Ordronaux, John, 109
Orfila, Matthieu Joseph Bonaventure, 294
Organisms, first observation of minute living, 189 ; and infection, 324
Organotherapy in ancient China, 36
Oribasius, 79, 80, 88
Orteschi, Pietro, 398
Orthopaedic surgery, 334–35, 343
Ortus sanitatis, 131
Osler, Sir William, 21, 156, 213, 288, 294, 331, 333, 366, 408–11, Pl. lxxii
Osteo-arthritis, 2, 28, 29, Pls. i, viii
Osteology, 272, Pl. xlviii
Osteomyelitis, 305

Otis, George Alexander, 349
Otitis, 57, 147, 245, 379
Oto-laryngology, first specialist in, 377
Otology, 377–80. *See also* Ear
Otosclerosis, 378
Ould, Sir Fielding, 235
Ovarian cyst, large, 301
Ovariotomy, 300–1, 320, 327, 330
Oxford, John of Gaddesden at, 114 ; Roger Bacon at, 121 ; Linacre at, 166, 167 ; controversy with Cambridge, 168 ; sweating sickness at, 169 ; Boorde at, 172 ; Harvey at, 183 ; scientists at, 186–88 ; Willis at, 200 ; Radcliffe's benefactions to, 254 ; Osler at, 366, 408 ; history of medicine at, 408
Oxygen, 188, 261
Oxymel, 58, 117
Oxyuris, 80

Paaw, Pieter, 194
Pacchioni, Antonio, 194
Padua, University of, Peter of Abano of, 119–20 ; anatomy at (Vesalius, Columbus, Fabricius, Casserius, Fallopius), 137–39, 141 ; Vicary at, 151 ; Paracelsus at, 157 ; Fracastorius at, 165 ; Caius at, 167 ; Harvey at, 180 ; Sanctorius of, 197 ; Sir T. Browne at, 211 ; Morgagni of, 245, 251 ; Ramazzini of, 260
Paget, Sir James, 312, 313–15
Paget, Stephen, 408
Pain, 120, 335, 378
Paine, W. H., 7
Palermo, incubation in, 46
Palfyn, Jean, 237, Pl. l
Palsy, described by Celsus, 73 ; John of Gaddesden on, 114
Paludism, 357
Panama Canal Zone, malaria and yellow fever in, 360
Pancreatic juice, 279
Papyri, 23–27
Paracelsists, 158
Paracelsus, 78, 100, 156–61, 199, 262
"Paracelsus of Scotland." *See* Brown, John (founder of Brunonian system)
Paraceutetes, 28
Paracusis of Willis, 200
Paralysis, bulbar, 299, 370 ; agitans, 368 ; as described by Aretaeus, 71 ; cure of, 44
Parasites, intestinal, 80
Parasitology, 317
Paratyphoid fever, 349
Paré, Ambroise, 78, 142–48, 337, 338, 340, 349, Pl. xxviii
Paris, Gilles de Corbeil at, 107 ; Lanfranc and surgery, 119 ; Roger Bacon at, 121 ; Albertus Magnus at, 111 ; Vesalius studies anatomy under Sylvius

and Guinther, 136–37 ; Paré at, 143, 144, 146–48 ; Frère Jacques, Frère Jean and lithotomy, 149 ; private hospital in, 149 ; Riolan, 185 ; Mayerne practises in, 201 ; J. L. Petit and surgery, 244 ; Bichat and pathological anatomy, 245–46 ; Lettsom at, 252 ; Laënnec's invention of stethoscope in, 258–59 ; Mesmer at, 262 ; Marshall Hall at, 276 ; Sharpey at, 278 ; Bernard and physiology, 280 ; Pasteur at, 283 ; Orfila and toxicology, 294 ; Broussais and Trousseau at, 297 ; Dupuytren at, 316 ; Velpeau at, 317 ; Larrey, 338, 339 ; Malgaigne at, 340 ; Potain at, 366 ; Charcot and neurology, 370 ; Pinel and insanity, 372 ; Daviel and ophthalmology, 376 ; Itard and otology, 379 ; Garcia's invention of laryngoscope in, 380 ; Alibert and dermatology, 382 ; Fournier and syphilology, 384 ; O. W. Holmes at, 409 ; Bicêtre Hospital, 372 ; Hôtel des Invalides, 339 ; Hôtel-Dieu, 143, 316, 338, Pl. xxviii ; Institût Pasteur, 283, 284, 286, Pl. lvii ; Jardin des Plantes, 192 ; Musée Dupuytren, 316 ; Necker Hospital, 258, 334 ; Saint-Louis Hospital, 340, 382, 384 ; Salpêtrière Hospital, 370
Paris médical, 397
Parker, Peter, 37
Parkinson, James, 368
Parkinson, John, 132
Park, Mungo, 355–56
Parliament, medical representation in, 342
Parr, Thomas, longevity of, 182
Parry, Thomas Wilson, 7
Passive congestion, Bier's, 329
Pasteurization, 284
Pasteur, Louis, 283–85, 323, 324, 325, 326, Pl. lvii
Patella, fracture of, 326, 340
Pater, Walter, his *Marius the Epicurean* referred to, 45
Pathology, earliest specimen in, 2 ; of mummies, 28–29 ; Plater's contribution to, 141 ; surgical, 241 ; applied, 245–46 ; as foundation of medicine, 281–82
Patin, Guy, 185, 396
Patrick, St., 98
Patriotische Medicus, Die, 397
Patron saints in medicine, 97, 98–101, Pl. xviii
Paul of Ægina, 80, 88, 93
Pavia, 162, 244, 260
Pavlov, Ivan Petrovich, 329
Pavy, Frederick William, 365
Pean, Julius, 327
Pecquet, Jean, 185
Pediatrics, 27, 69, 174, 367–68

Pelvis, deformities of female, 195
Pen Tsao (a Chinese herbal), 34
Penicillin, 350, 363
Pennsylvania, University of (Philadelphia), Medical School founded, 251 ; J. Morgan, 251 ; Physick and surgery, 243–44 ; D. Drake, 299 ; J. B. Deaver and surgery, 330 ; W. W. Keen and neurological surgery, 333 ; Da Costa and cardiology, 367 ; S. Weir Mitchell and neurology, 371 ; Jackson and peroral endoscopy, 381 ; Billings and hygiene, 400 ; Osler at, 408 ; Women's Medical College, 386
Pennsylvania Hospital, 243
Penn, William, 251, 274
Pepys, Samuel, 181, 191, 206, 208, 406
Percussion, 257–59, 298, 366
Pergamon Museum (Berlin), 75
Pergamos, 43, 75, 79
Periodicals, 191–92, 393–99, Pl. lxxi
Peritonitis, 330
Perkins, Elisha, 263
Perspiration, invisible, 197
Peru, trephined skulls found in, 7, 11, Pl. ii ; cinchona from, 205
Peruvian balsam, 205
Peruvian bark, 205
Peter of Abano, 119–20, 129
Peter the Great, Czar of Russia, 194
Petit, Jean Louis, 244, 379
Petrie, Sir Flinders, 27
Petrus Hispanus (Pope John XXI), 115
Pettenkofer, Max von, 390
Peyer, Johann Conrad, 194
Pfeiffer, Richard, 287
Pflüger, Eduard Friedrich Wilhelm, 398
Pfolspeundt, Heinrich von, 126
Phaer (Phayre), Thomas, 174
Phagocytosis, 285
Pharmacology, in ancient Egypt, 24–25 ; in ancient India, 33 ; in early Arabian medicine, 86–87 ; Gilbertus Anglicus and, 113. *See also* Drugs
Pharmacopœia, 69, 132n, 256 ; of Royal College of Physicians of London, 70, 132, 201, 207
Phayre, Thomas. *See* Phaer
Philadelphia Journal of the Medical and Physical Sciences, 395
Philae, Temple of, 23
Phillips, Professor Miles, quoted, 237
Philosopher-physicians of Greece, 48–50
Philosopher's stone, 160
Philosophical Transactions of the Royal Society, 191, 192, 393
Philosophy, 119, 120, 121, 159, 176–78, 211–13, 387
Phipps, James, 248
Phlogiston, 261
Phrenology, 264–65

Phthisis, 147; in ancient India, 32; Aretaeus on, 71; Sydenham on, 204; P. C. A. Louis on, 297
Phylactery, 14
Physical diagnosis, 298
Physical therapy, 67
Physician, in Old Testament, 30; need for surgical knowledge by, 118; dress, 130, 253; first American, 251
Physician's pulse watch, 257
Physick, Philip Syng, 241, 243
Physics and physiology, 273–76
Physiognomy, 107, 163
Physiological chemistry, 199–200, 276
Physiology, Erasistratus as founder of, 64; Galen's experimental, 76; in Middle Ages, 85, 92–93; Vesalius and, 138; Descartes and, 177–78; first textbook of, 177; Harvey, etc. and, 180–8; seventeenth-century Dutch, 195; seventeenth century theories of, 196–98; progress under Haller, 224; John Hunter and, 240; nineteenth-century, 273–81; British pioneers in, 276–78; at Edinburgh, 278; in France, 279–80; Brodie and experimental, 312; Lister on importance of, in surgery, 322
Piacenza, plague at, 99
Picardy sweat, 171
Pig, anatomy of, 105; Galen's experiments on, 76, 77
Pilomotor muscles, 322
Pineal gland as seat of soul, 178
Pinel, Philippe, 372
Pirogoff, Nikolai, 344
Pisa, Cesalpino of, 140; Galileo of, 179; Borelli of, 197–98
Pitcairne, Archibald, 226, 227, 255
Pithecanthropus, 2, Pl. 1
Pitt Rivers Museum (Oxford), 10
Pituitary body, 333
Plague, in Bible, 31; in ancient India, 32; in Rome, 75, 82; in Byzantine Empire, 83; patron saint of, 99–100; bubonic (mal des ardents), 101; in Middle Ages, 111; at Avignon, 123; the Black Death, 126–28; flies and, 146; sixteenth-century epidemic in England, 170; in London (1665), 206–9, Pl. XLII; in modern India, 286; bacillus of, discovered, 287; in Egypt under Napoleon, 340; self-inoculation with, 340
Plarr, Victor Gustave, 406
Plastic surgery, of ancient India, 33–34; mediæval, 126, 149; modern, 343
Platter, Felix, 141
Plethora, 64
Pleural effusion, 297
Pleurisy, Hippocrates on, 55, 259; Aretaeus on, 71; Alexander of Tralles on, 80

Pliny the Elder, 66
Plummer, Andrew, 228
Plymouth, Huxham of, 234; naval hospital at, 353
Pneuma, 50, 68, 77, 216
Pneumococcus, discovery of, 288
Pneumonia, described by Aretaeus, 71
Podalarius, son of Aesculapius, 47
Poisons, 69, 70, 80, 94, 113, 160, 255, 294
Polar exploration, 354–55
Police, medical, 260
Politzer, Adam, 379–80
Pollender, Franz Aloys Antoine, 286
Polygraph, Mackenzie's, 366
Polypharmacy, 70, 294
Pompeii, house of surgeon at, 74
Pontus, the Greek, legendary founder of School of Salerno, 103
Pope, a medical, 115
Pope, Alexander, quoted, 177, 238
Pores, Empedocles on breathing through, 50; disease and, 67; in septum of heart, 184
Post-mortem examinations, in ancient Egypt, 28; in Middle Ages, 122; of T. Parr, 182; Morgagni and, 245; Rokitansky and, 281; Bright and, 291; P. C. A. Louis and, 297; Semmelweiss and, 319
Potain, Pierre Carl, 366
Potato, introduction into England, 131
Pott, Percivall, 235, 239–40, 240, 242
Pott's disease, classic description of, 239
Pott's fracture, 239
Powder of sympathy, 15, 160
Power, Sir D'Arcy, 406–7; quoted, 125
Pregnancy, case of prolonged, 44
Prehistoric man, 1–2, 5–8
Prescriptions, recipe sign in, 20; in papyri, 24–25
Presse médicale, La, 397
Preston, Charles, 228
Preventive medicine, 386–92
Priestley, Joseph, 188, 261
Primitive man, 2–5, 8–11
Primrose (Prymross), Gilbert, 153–54
Pringle, Sir John, 232–33, 317, 338
Priscillian, 98
Probe, Nélaton's, 340–41
Proceedings of the Historical Section of the Royal Society of Medicine, 399
Proceedings of the Royal Society of Medicine, 393
Proctology, 125
Prognosis, by Oracle of Delphi, 42; in Hippocratic medicine, 56; in heart disease, 367
Progrès médical, Le, 397
Prostatectomy, 334
Provincial Medical and Surgical Journal, 394
Prunières, A., quoted, 5, 6
Psychiatry, 372–74
Psychoanalysis, 374

Psychology, 273
Psycho-pathology of Freud, 373, 374
Public Health, in Bible, 30–31 ; in Talmud, 31 ; in ancient Rome, 81–83, Pl. xiv ; mediæval hospitals, 128–29 ; during Great Plague of London (1665), 206–9 ; in eighteenth century, 259–62 ; first British diploma in, instituted, 296 ; modern, 386–92
Puerperal fever, the tragedy of, 318–20
Pugh, Benjamin, 237
Pulmonary tuberculosis. *See* Tuberculosis (pulmonary)
Pulse, in *Ebers Papyrus*, 25 ; in ancient China, 36 ; first counted by Herophilus, 64 ; importance of, in diagnosis, 104 ; Gilles de Corbeil's poem on, 107 ; Harvey on, 184 ; timed by Galileo, 179, by Sanctorius, 197, and by Floyer, 257 ; Stokes and Adams on slow, 296 ; modern study of, 366, 367
"Pupil, Argyll Robertson," 376
Purmann, Gottfried, 209
Pus, laudable, 76, 307
Puschmann, Theodore, 80, 405
Putrefaction and fermentation, 323
Pyaemia, 323, 328
Pyorrhoea alveolaris, in mummies, 29, Pl. viii
Pyrenees, Trois Frères Cave in, 1
Pythagoras, discoveries of, 49

Quackery in eighteenth century, 262–64, Pl. liii
Quain, Richard, 278
Quakers as physicians, 247, 249–53
Quarantine, first mention of, 127
Quartan fever, 55
Quarterly Cumulative Index Medicus, 402
Quina-quina, 205
Quincy, John, 197
Quinine, 205, 258

R sign in prescriptions, 20
" Rabbit woman." *See* Toft, Mary
Rabelais, François, 78
Rabies, Maimonides on, 95 ; Pasteur's experiments on, 284–85, Pl. lvii. *See also* Mad dog
Radcliffe, John, 235, 254
Radcliffe Infirmary (Oxford), 254
Radiology, 384–85
Radium, discovery of, 385 ; and cancer, 385 ; H. Kelly and, 330
Ragusa, quarantine at, 127
Rahere, 82
Rai, Persia, Rhazes born at, 89
Ramazzini, Bernardino, 260
Ramón y Cajal, Santiago, 372
Raphael and dissection, 135
Rashdall, Hastings, quoted, 103, 104, 112
Rationalists. *See* Dogmatists
Rats as carriers of plague, 208

Raynalde, Thomas, his *Byrth of Mankynde*, 69, 174
Read, William, 264
Rebecca, one of the " ladies of Salerno," 104
Reclus, Paul, 327
Rectum, patron saint of diseases of, 99 ; cancer of, 125 ; carcinoma of, 329
Red Cross, origin of, 232
Redi, Francesco, 317
Reed, Walter, 359, 360
Reflex action, discovery of, 277
Reflexes, conditioned, 329
Refraction, errors of, 375
Regimen Sanitatis Salernitanum, 108–10 ; commentary on, 112
Registrar General, 388
Registration, medical, 378 ; of births and deaths, 250
Religion and medicine reconciled, 95
Rembrandt, 194
Renaissance, influence of, 134
Renal cases in Guy's Hospital, 291
Renaudot, Théophraste, 396
Renzi, Salvatore de, 105 ; quoted, 104
Respiration, problems of, 186–88 ; chemistry of, 261–62 ; artificial. *See* Artificial respiration
" Restorer of Surgery, The " (*i.e.* Guy de Chauliac). *See* Guy de Chauliac
Resurrectionists, 270, 308. *See also* Body-snatching
Retreat, The (York), 249, 372–73
Revulsion, in blood-letting, 130
Reynolds, Sir Joshua, 241
Rhazes, 89–90
Rheims, University of, Pitcairne at, 226
Rheneia, Isle of, 40
Rheumatism, Sir W. Gull on acute, 294 ; Duchenne's treatment of, 369 ; charm for cure of, Pl. iv
Rheumatoid arthritis. See under Osteo-arthritis
Rhinoplasty, in ancient India, 33–34 ; in mediæval Europe, 149
Rhodes, incubation in, 46 ; mediæval hospital established at, 128, Pls. xxiii–xxiv
Rhubarb, 80
Richard I, Cœur de Lion, 94
Richardson, Sir John, 354
Richelieu, Armand Jean du Plessis, Cardinal Duke de, 192, 396
Richet, Charles, 402
Rickets, and mummies, 29 ; early reference to, by Soranus, 69 ; Glisson's description of, 200–1
Ricketts, Howard Taylor, 289
Ricord, Philippe, 383–84
Riggs, John Mankey, 303
Rig-Veda, 32
Rinderpest, 286
Ringworm, 382

Riolan, Jean, 185
Rivers, William Halse Rivers, quoted, 4
Robert, Duke of Normandy, 109
Robertson, Douglas Moray Cooper Lamb Argyll, 376
Rochester, Minnesota, Mayo Clinic, 332
Roch, St., 99, 100
Rockefeller Institute, 359
Rocky Mountain fever, 289
Rodney, Admiral Sir George, 351
Roentgen rays. See X-rays
Roentgen, W. C., 384–85, Pl. LXX
Roesslin, Eucharius, 69, 174
Roger II, King of Sicily, 106
Roger of Palermo, 105–6, Pl. XIX
Rohde, E. S. 133
Rokitansky, Carl, 281–82
Roland of Parma, 106
Rolleston, Sir Humphry Davy, 408 ; quoted, 352
Roman army, military surgeons of, 81–82
Roman medicine. See Rome (ancient)
Romberg, Moritz Heinrich, 369
Rome (ancient), Greek medicine in, 64–68, Pl. XIII ; Galen at, 75 ; public hygiene in, 81, Pl. XIV ; state medical service, 81–82 ; hospitals of, 82–83 ; fall of, 83
Rome (mediæval and modern), theories of pulmonary circulation of Columbus and Cesalpino at, 139–40 ; Eustachius and anatomy at, 141–42 ; Linacre at, 167 ; Baglivi's work at, 198 ; Bassini and abdominal surgery at, 329 ; Durante and neuro-surgery at, 333 ; Grassi's researches on malaria at, 358 ; Papal Library. See Vatican Library
Rondelles, 6, Pl. III
Rosencreuz, Christian, 158
Rosetta Stone, 375
Rosicrucians, 158
Ross, Sir Ronald, 358
Rotch, Thomas Morgan, 368
Roux, Émile, 269, 286
Royal Academy (London), Chair of Anatomy at, 267
Royal Army Medical College (Netley), 348–49
Royal Army Medical Corps, 346–48
Royal College of Physicians of Edinburgh, 226 ; founder of, 225 ; Pharmacopœia of, 132n. ; physic garden of, 192 ; President of, 233
Royal College of Physicians of London, 203 ; founded, 167 ; Fellows of, 180, 183, 201, 203 ; Fitzpatrick Lectures at, 405–6, 407 ; Library, 172, 183 ; Pharmacopœia of, 70, 132 ; Presidents of, 168, 179, 211
Royal College of Surgeons of Edinburgh, 236; foundation of, 153–54 ; anatomy in, 227 ; Chair of Surgery in, 344 ; Museum of, 268, 270

Royal College of Surgeons of England, 327 ; founded, 151, Pl. XXX ; Chair of Anatomy and Surgery, 268 ; Chair of Dermatology founded, 382 ; Lister at, 322 ; Hilton's lectures at, 335 ; Museum, 242, 314, 378 ; Presidents of, 311, 313, 342 ; Plarr's Lives of Fellows of, 406
Royal Ear Hospital(London),founded,377
Royal Faculty of Physicians and Surgeons of Glasgow, foundation of, 154 ; lawsuits with Glasgow University, 154–55; Finlayson's researches on, 407
Royal healers, 210
Royal Humane Society (London), 253
Royal London Ophthalmic Hospital (Moorfields), 375, 377
Royal Medical Society (Edinburgh), 218, 264
Royal Sea-bathing Hospital (Margate), 253
Royal Society of London, 186, 189, 190, 191, 233, 374
Royal Westminster Ophthalmic Hospital, 342
Royal touch. See Touch
Rudbeck, Olof, 185
Ruffer, Sir Marc Armand, 29
Rupture, in folk-medicine, 12 ; cured by rest, 94
Rush, Benjamin, 251
Rush Medical College (Philadelphia), 251
Russell, James, 310
Russia, Black Death in, 127 ; epidemics of ergotism in, 101 ; military surgery in, 343–44 ; first medical journal of, 398 ; nineteenth-century surgery in, 329
Rutherford, John, 228
Ruysch, Frederick, 194, Pl. XXXIX
Rye, disease of, 101

Sabouraud, Raymond, 382
Sacred disease (epilepsy?), Hippocrates on, 55, 100. See also Epilepsy
St. Andrews (Scotland), Schevez at, 153 ; Brown at, 218
St. Anthony's Fire, 100–1
St. Bartholomew Island, 82
St. Bartholomew, massacre of, Paré and, 147
St. Bartholomew's Hospital (London), founded, 82, 128 ; Clowes surgeon to, 151 ; Harvey physician to, 180 ; Pott surgeon to, 239 ; Abernethy surgeon to, 242 ; Paget surgeon to, 314, 315 ; Brunton physician to, 365 ; Young at, 374 ; Moore's history of, 405 ; Power surgeon to, 406 ; Rahere Ward in, Pl. LVIII
St. Clair, Andrew, 228
St. Côme, College of (Paris), Lanfranc at, 119 ; Paré and, 144, 146

St. Gallen, Paracelsus at, 158
St. George's Hospital (London), John Hunter surgeon to, 242 ; Baillie physician to, 246 ; Brodie surgeon to, 312 ; T. Young physician to, 375
St. John, Knights of, 128, Pls. XI, XXIII–XXIV
St. Mary's Hospital (London), 378
St. Petersburg, von Baer of, 273 ; Pirogoff of, 344 ; first medical periodical at, 398. *See also* Leningrad
St. Quentin, Battle of, Paré at, 146
St. Thomas's Hospital (London), founded, 128 ; Cheselden surgeon to, 238 ; lectures by Marshall Hall at, 277 ; school for nurses at, 347 ; Makins surgeon to, 349 ; Blane physician to, 351 ; Sir John Simon at, 389 ; South surgeon to, 406
St. Thomas's Hospital Reports, 394
St. Triduana's well (Edinburgh), 99
St. Vitus's Dance, 100
Saladin, 94
Salerno, School of, 80, 102–10 ; foundation of, 103 ; teachers at, 104–8 ; surgery at, 105–6, Pl. XIX ; curriculum at, 106–7 ; famous graduates of, 107–108 ; the *Regimen Sanitatis Salernitanum*, 108–10 ; Arabian influence on, 105 ; Constantine the African at, 105 ; Crusaders at, 109 ; " ladies of Salerno," 104
Salernus, the Latin, legendary founder of School of Salerno, 103
Saliceti, Gugliemo. *See* William of Salicet
Salivary calculus, 114
Salvarsan, discovery of, 384
Salzburg, Paracelsus at, 158
Sammlung von Natur und Medicin, 397
Sanatoria for tuberculosis, 298
Sanctorius, Sanctorius, 197, 258, Pl. XL
Sanderson, Burdon. *See* Burdon-Sanderson, Sir John
Sanitation. *See* Public Health
Sankt Petersburgskoye Vrachevnie Vaidomosti, 398
Sanskrit texts, medical, 32
Sardinia, incubation in, 46
Saunders, John Cunningham, 377
Saxon medical manuscripts, 102, 131
Saxtorph, Mathias Hieronymus, 328
Scarlet fever (scarlatina), 141, 219, 249
Scarpa, Antonio, 244
Schaudinn, Fritz Richard, 384
Schevez, William, 153
Schleiden, Jacob, 190
Schliemann, Heinrich, 46, 282
Schneider, Conrad Victor, 194
Schoolmen, 121, 179, 202
Schooskis, Martin, 397
Schwann, Theodor, 190, 274
Schwartze, Hermann, 244, 379
Sciatica, 244, 368

Scotland, medicine in :—mediæval, 152–154, seventeenth and eighteenth centuries, 221–23, 225–31, nineteenth century, 269–71 ; abdominal surgery in, 331 ; dermatology in, 383 ; medical historians of, 407 ; medical periodicals in, 394 ; neurological surgery in, 333 ; ophthalmology in, 376 ; psychiatry in, 373 ; visits to, by :—Boorde, 173, Cardan, 162, Harvey, 182. *See also* Aberdeen, Edinburgh, Glasgow
Scot, Michael, 107, 152
Scott, Sir Walter, *The Abbot*, 163 ; *The Surgeon's Daughter*, 356 ; *The Talisman*, 14, 94, Pl. IV
Scrofula (struma, King's Evil), 209–11, 262, Pl. XLIII
Scultetus, Johann, 150, 209
Scurvy, 152, 233–34, 351–52
Scutari, Florence Nightingale at, 347
Seamen, diseases of. *See under* Naval medicine
Seasonal incidence of disease, 59, 92
Seaver, George, his life of Edward Wilson, 355
Sebastian, St., 100
Sects in medicine, 68–69
Sekhet'enanach, 21
Selborne, folk-medicine at, 12
Seminaria, Fracastorius' theory of, 166
Semmelweiss, Ignaz Philipp, 319–20
Semon, Sir Felix, 381
Senn, Nicholas, 330
Sepsis, Theodoric Borgognoni on, 116 ; dangers of, 307 ; from dissecting room, 319 ; intestinal, 285–86 ; Lister's researches on, 324
Serum, anti-diphtheritic, 286, 287
Servetus, Michael, 140, 184
Shakespeare, William, on death of Falstaff, 56 ; and mandragora, 116 ; and " humours," 176
Sharpey, William, 277–8, 309, 322
Sharpey-Schafer, Sir Edward, 465
Shattuck, Lemuel, 390
Shen Nung, Emperor of China, 34
Shields, John, Pl. XLVII
Shippen, William, 251
Ships, hospital, 352
Shock, treatment of surgical, 331
Shrewsbury, Caius at, 168, 169 ; sweating sickness in (1551), 169, 170
Shropshire, folk-medicine in, 257
Sibbald, Sir Robert, 192, 225, 227
Sick-room cookery, 106. *See also* Nursing
Sign, Von Graefe, 376
Signatures, doctrine of, 160
Silesia, typhus epidemic in, 282
Silkworm disease, 284
Similia similibus curantur, 219
Simon, Sir John, 388–89
Simon, Max, his edition of Galen, 78
" Simpling," 132–33

Simpson, Sir James Young, 304–6, 321, 323, 330
Simpson Maternity Hospital (Edinburgh), 306
Sims, James Marion, 301
Singer, Charles, quoted, 102, 105, 121, 142
Sinus forceps, Lister's, 325
Skin diseases, 106, 381–83. *See also* Dermatology
Skin grafting, 328
Skin, layers of, first described, 186; muscular tissue of, 322
Skoda, Joseph, 298
Slaves, medical treatment of, in Babylonia, 18; as physicians in ancient Rome, 65, 72; hospitals for, in ancient Rome, 82
Sleeping sickness, 361–62
Sloane, Sir Hans, 192, 202
Smallpox, in ancient India, 32; inoculation against, in ancient China, 36, 246; Rhazes' work on, 89; treatment of, by colour, 114; Sydenham's treatment of, 203; inoculation against, introduced, 246–47
Smellie, William, 235–36, 237, Pls. XLIX–L
Smith, G. Elliot, quoted, 28
Smith, Job Lewis, 368
Smith, Theobald, 288, 291
Smith, Thomas Southwood, 387, 388
Smollett, Tobias, 351
Snakes, in Greek medicine, 43, 45
Sneezing, dissertation on, 397
Snow, John, 305, 388
Societies, scientific, 191–92
Soil, influence of, on health, 390
Soranus, 69
Sorbonne. *See* Paris
Soubeiran, Eugène, 304
Soul, and disease, 5, 15; Descartes on, 178; Sir T. Browne on, 212; Stahl's theory of body and, 216
South, John Flint, 406
South African War, 348, 349
South America, yellow fever in, 359
Spain, Arabian medicine in, 92–95; medicine in modern, 371–72; Harvey in, 182
Spallanzani, Lazzaro, 317–18
Specialism, in medicine, 363–85
Spectacles, first mentioned by Bernard de Gordon, 114; Roger Bacon and, 121, 189
Speech, disorders of, 299, 371; motor speech centre discovered, 273
Spencer, W. G., his edition of Celsus, 72
Sphygmograph, 366
Sphygmomanometer, 366
Spinal cord, Galen on effect of division of, 77; reflex action in, 231; tumour of, 333; tract in, described, 371
Spinal nerve roots, function of, 268, 273

Spine, tuberculous disease of, in mummies, 29, Pl. VIII; Pott's description of, 239
Spiritus, 140
Spirochaeta pallida, discovery of, 384
Spleen, Boorde on, 173; lymph nodes of, first described, 186
Splints, in ancient Egypt, 26; in Talmud, 31; Celsus on, 74; used by Guy de Chauliac, 124; Thomas's, 334
Spongia somnifera, 108
Spontaneous generation, 317–18
Spray, Lister's carbolic, 324, Pl. LXV
Spurzheim, J. C., 264
Squillace, 101
Squire, Peter, 304, Pl. LXI
Stafford, Withering at, 257
Stahl, Georg Ernst, 68, 216–17
Staphylococcus, 288
Stars, influence upon disease of, 176; and diagnosis, 111
Stasis, chronic intestinal, 331
State laboratory founded, 391
Statistics, medical, 297; vital, 388
Steen, Jan, 194, Pl. XXXV
Stensen, Nicolas, 194
Sterility, primitive cure for, 13; mandragora as cure for, 116
Sterilization by steam, 329
Stethoscope, invention of, 258–59; Laënnec's, Pl. LVI; Stokes's treatise on, 295–96; in diagnosis, 366; first use of binaural, 367
Stewart, John, 326
Still, Sir George Frederick, 368
Stimulation, doctrine of, 219
Stoddart, Mrs. Anna M., quoted, 161
Stokes, Adrian, 359
Stokes, Whitley, 295
Stokes, William, 295–96
Stone Age, 1–2, 5–8, 10
Stone, dissolving, 114, 231; Paracelsus on cause of, 160. *See also* Lithotomy *and* Lithotrity
Strassburg, Guinther at, 137; Pasteur at, 283; Kussmaul at, 299, 364
Streptococcus, 288
Stretcher bearers, 347
Stromeyer, Georg Frederick Louis, 328, 343
Strophanthus, 366
Struma. *See* Scrofula
Struthers, J., quoted, 228
Styria, incubation in, 46
Succus nervens, 198
Sudhoff, Karl, 399, 404–5; quoted, 108, 129, 156, 397
Sugar, in diabetic urine, 200; produced by liver, 280
Sulphonamides, 350, 363
Sumerian civilization, 17, 19
Sun Yat Sen, 37

Suppuration, bacteriology of, 288
Suprarenal capsules, 292
Surgeon, attributes of, defined by Hippocrates, 58, by Celsus, 74 ; status of, in Roman army, 81–82 ; Henri de Mondeville on the need for medical knowledge by, 118 ; an early itinerant, 125 ; status of, 209
Surgeon-General's Catalogue. See Washington, Surgeon-General's Library
Surgery, ancient, 26, 30, 33–34, 36, 73–74 ; mediæval, 111, 113, 115–17, 123–26, 142–54 ; modern, 307–35 ; early nineteenth-century, 307–20 ; Lister and his followers, 321–28 ; abdominal, 328–31, 332 ; specialism in, 332–35 ; patron saints of, 97, Pl. XVIII ; first work on, to be illustrated, 93 ; first English textbook of, 154 ; itinerant lithotomists, 148–49 ; American, 243–44, 331–32 ; Arabian, 92–93 ; Babylonian, 18 ; Biblical, 30 ; Byzantine, 80 ; Chinese (ancient), 36 ; Danish, 328 ; Egyptian (ancient), 26 ; English, 150–52, 209, 211, 238–40, 329–31 ; French, 113, 119, 142–48, Pl. XXVIII, 209, 244, 316–17, 327–28 ; German, 126, Pl. XXVI, 149–50, 209, 244, 328–29 ; Greek (ancient), 58 ; Indian (ancient), 33–34 ; Italian, 105–6, Pl. XIX, 115–17, 149, 329 ; Roman (ancient), 73–74 ; Russian, 329 ; Scottish, 152–54, 229–30, 269, 310, 331, Pl. XXIX ; Swiss, 329
Surgical Instruments. See Instruments
Susruta, 32, 33
Suture, the Lembert, 316
Swammerdam, Jan, 190
Sweating sickness, 164, 169–71
Sweat, measurement of, 197
Swieten, Gerhard van, 224–25, 264
Switzerland, St. Gall in, 98 ; Paracelsus in, 157 ; nineteenth-century surgery in, 329
Sydenham, Thomas, 60, 196, 202–4
Sylvius, Franciscus, 193, 199–200
Sylvius, Jacobus, 136–137, 162
Syme, Agnes. See Lister, Agnes
Syme, James, 278, 305, 308, 309–11, 322, 325, 346, Pl. LXII
Sympathy, powder of, 14–15, 160
Syndrome, Gowers's, 371 ; Stokes-Adams, 296
Syphilis, and mummies, 29 ; and aneurysm, 147 ; origin of, 164 ; Fracastorius' poem on, 165 ; mercurial treatment of, 204 ; inoculation of, 242, 286 ; Hutchinson's research on, 329 ; and tabes, 369 ; modern research on, 383–84. *See also* Gonorrhoea *and* Venereal diseases
Syriac translations of Greek texts, 88

Tabes, syphilis and, 369
Tagliacozzi, Gaspare, 149
Tait, Robert Lawson, 330
Talismans. *See* Charms
Talmud, medicine in, 31–32
Tamatetikwa, 5
Tapeworm, 80, 294
Tarantellas, 100
Tarantism, 100
Taricheutes, 28
Tarnier, Étienne Stéphane, 236
Tartaglia, 163
Tartar on teeth, Paracelsus' theory, 160
Tasmania, 355
Tasrif, by Albucasis, 93
Taylor, Chevalier, 263, Pl. LIII
Teeth, patron saint of, 99 ; Paracelsus' theory of tartar on, 160
Teething, advice on, 174
Telescope, 178, 179
Temperaments, 76, 110
Temperature chart, 298
Temple-sleep. *See* Incubation
Tenos, incubation in, 46
Tenotomy, 343
Tertian fever, 55
Tetanus, in *Edwin Smith Papyrus*, Pl. V ; Hippocrates on, 59 ; described by Aretaeus, 71 ; bacillus of, 287 ; Ballingall on, 345 ; inoculation against, 350
Texas fever, 288, 391
Texas, yellow fever in, 360
Thaddeus Florentinus. *See* Alderotti, Taddeo
" Thames " skull, 7, Pl. II
Thebes, 23, 24
Themison, 67, 68
Theodoric, King of the Ostrogoths, 101
Theodoric of Cervia. *See* Borgognoni, Theodoric, Bishop of Cervia
Theologians and animism, 216
Theophrastus, 61, 62
Theriac (mithridatium), 69–70, 82, 169, 176, 256
Thermometer, clinical, 197, 257, 298, 408
Thiersch, Karl, 328
Thirty Years' War, 150
Thomas, Hugh Owen, 334
Thompson, Sir Henry, 334
Thomson, Allen, 278
Thomson, George, 208, Pl. XLII
Thomson, John (pediatrician), 368
Thomson, John (surgeon), 344
Thomson-Walker, Sir John, 334
Thorndike, L., quoted, 105
Thoth, Hermetic books of, 23
Threipland, Sir Stuart, 233
Throat, diseases of, described by Aëtius, 80 ; patron saint of, 98
Throat Hospital (London), 380
Thyroidectomy, 329, 332
Tiberias, tomb of Maimonides at, 95

Tinctures, invention of, 113
Tissues, classification of, 245
Tobacco plant, 133
Toft, Mary, 235n
Tonsillectomy, Celsus on, 73
Tonus, doctrine of, 217
Toothache in folk-medicine, 12, Pl. IV
Torre, Marco Antonio della, 136
Tortola, island of, Lettsom at, 252
Touch, cure by, 12 ; Royal, 196, 210, Pl. XLIII ; imitators of Royal, 262
Toulouse, Larrey at, 338
Tourniquet, invention of, 244 ; used by Fabricius Hildanus, 150
Tours, Bretonneau's researches on diphtheria at, 297
Toxicology, 294
Toynbee, Joseph, 378
Tracheotomy, mentioned by Asclepiades, 68 ; described by Antyllus, 79 ; Sanctorius' invention for, 197 ; and laryngeal diphtheria, 297
Trajan's column, 82
Tralles, Alexander of. See Alexander of Tralles
Transactions of the Medical Society of London, 393
Transactions. See Periodicals
Trench fever, 289, 350
Trench foot, 350
Trench nephritis, 350
Trendelenburg, Friedrich, 329
Trendelenburg position, 124
Trephining, prehistoric, 2, 5–8, 11, 273, Pls. II–III ; by modern primitive man, 8–11, Pl. II ; by Hippocrates, 58
Treveris, Peter, 131
Treves, Sir Frederick, 330
Trevisa, John of. See John of Trevisa
Trichina spiralis, 314
Trichinosis, 283
Triduana, St., 99
Trois Frères Cave, 1
Tropical disease, conquest of, 357–62
Trotter, Thomas, 352–53
Trotter, Wilfred, 332
Trotula, one of the " ladies of Salerno," 104, 105, 385
Trousseau, Armand, 295, 296, 297, 298, 367, 381
Truss, first description of, 114 ; used by Guy de Chauliac, 124
Trypanosomiasis, 361–62
Tsetse fly, described by Livingstone, 356 ; and sleeping sickness, 361
Tubercle bacillus, discovery of, 286 ; bacilli classified, 391
Tuberculin, 287
Tuberculosis, prehistoric, 2 ; Koch's researches on, 286–87 ; in children, 253 ; human and bovine differentiated, 288 ; sanatorium treatment of, 253, 298

Tuberculosis (pulmonary), first regarded as contagious by Avicenna, 92 ; Laënnec's work on, 258, 259 ; Addison on, 292
Tuberculosis (spinal), in mummies, 29, Pl. VIII ; Pott's description of, 239
Tuberculosis (surgical). See Scrofula
Tübingen, 122, 165
Tuffier, Marin Théodore, 327
Tuke, Daniel Hack, 373
Tuke, William, 249, 372
Tulp, Nicolas, 194
Tumours, excision of, in ancient India, 33 ; Morgagni's discoveries about, 245 ; first microscopic classification, 273 ; abdominal, 291 ; of the brain, 332, 333 ; of spinal cord, 333
Türck, Ludwig, 380
Turin, Paré at, 144–45
Turner, William, 132
Turquet de Mayerne, Sir Theodore. See Mayerne
Tympanum, artificial, 377
Typhoid fever, 293 ; treated by cold baths, 258 ; sero-diagnostic test for, 286 ; discovery of bacillus of, 287 ; P. C. A. Louis's study of, 297 ; inoculation against, 348, 349, 350
Typhus fever, Fracastorius first to recognise, 166 ; cause of, 289 ; epidemics of, in Silesia, 282, in Ireland, 296
Tyrosin discovered in the urine, 298

Ultra-violet treatment, 385
Unanue, Hipolito, 223
Unicorn, 66 ; horn of, as remedy, 144, 207 ; liver of, as remedy, 102
United States, physicians in eighteenth-century, 250–51 ; foundation of medical education in, 251 ; Gall and Spurzheim in, 264 ; pioneers of early nineteenth-century, 299–301 ; history of anaesthesia in, 302–4 ; bacteriology, 288–89 ; cardiology, 367 ; dermatology, 383 ; gynaecology, 330 ; journals, 395, 399 ; laryngology, 381 ; military medicine, 251 ; naval medicine, 353 ; neurology, 371 ; neurological surgery, 333 ; pediatrics, 368 ; public health, 390–91 ; surgery, 243–244, 330, 331–32 ; urology, 334
Unna, Paul Gerson, 383
Upsala, botanical garden at, 215
Upton, Essex, 321 ; Fothergill's botanical gardens at, 250
Ur, city of, 17
Urine, 90, 107, 298 ; inspection of, in Middle Ages, 90, 104, 111, 130
Urology, 333–34
Uroscopy, or water-casting. See Urine
Utrecht, physiology at, 375

Vaccination, Jenner and, 241, 247–49 ; defended by Lettsom, 252 ; advocated by Trotter for navy, 353 ; compulsion urged by Willan, 381 ; made compulsory, 389 ; Lister and Vaccination Bill (1897), 327
Vaccine lymph, 391
Vaccine therapy, 288, 349
Valentine, Basil, 158
Valetudinaria in ancient Rome, 82
Valsalva, Antonio, 186, 244, 245, 377
Vasomotor mechanism, 280
Vatican Library, 71, 142
"Vegetable Lamb," 132
"Vein man " in mediæval illustrations, 130
Veins, valves in, 138, 140–41, 180, Pl. XXXVI
Velpeau, Alfred Armand Louis Marie, 316, 317
Venables, James, 302
Venereal diseases, described by Celsus, 72 ; Clowes's treatise on, 151 ; modern research on, 383–84. See also Syphilis
Venesection. See Blood-letting
Venice, early medical periodical at, 398
Venomous animals, 70
Ventilation, 260–61
Verona, home of Fracastorius, 165, 166
Vertigo, 11 ; patron saint of, 99
Vesalius, Andreas, 31, 78, 123, 135, 136–139, 141, 142, 147, 149, 167, 175, 184, 272, Pl. XXVII
Vesico-vaginal fistula, 301
Vespasian, Emperor of Rome, 81
Vicary, Thomas, 150–51, 406, Pl. XXX
Victoria, Queen, 305, 311, 313, 325
Vidius. See Guidi, Guido
Vienna, Imperial Library, 131 ; Maternity Hospital, Semmelweiss and puerperal fever in, 319 ; Military Hospital, Auenbrugger physician to, 258 ; University Medical School founded, 224–225 ; Mesmer at, 262 ; F. J. Gall at, 264 ; anatomy, 272 ; clinical medicine, 298, 299 ; dermatology, 383 ; history of medicine, 405 ; laryngology, 380 ; metabolism, 365 ; ophthalmology, 376 ; otology, 379–80 ; pathology, 281 ; physiology, 276 ; psychopathology, 373 ; public health, 260 ; surgery (abdominal), 328
Vieussens, Raymond, 194
Vigo, John de, 145
Vinci, Leonardo da, 135, 136
Virchow, Rudolf, 246, 274, 282–83, 398. See also Archiv für pathologische Anatomie
Virus infection, 170
Virus inoculators, 247
Viruses, 363
Vis Medicatrix Naturæ, 57
Vital spirit, of Erasistratus, 64 ; of Galen, 77

Vital principle, Barthez's theory of, 217
Vitamins, 363, 365
Vitus, St., 100
Vivisection, Lister and, 326 ; human, 64
Volkmann, Richard, 328

Wadd, W., quoted, 210
Wakley, Thomas, 382, 394
Waldie, David, 304
Walker, Sir Norman, 383
Waller, Augustus, 276, 365
Walton, Isaak, quoted, 177
War and surgery. See Military surgery
Ward, Joshua, 263, Pl. LIII
Warren, John Collins, 303
Warrington, Priestley at, 261
Warts in folk-medicine, 12, Pl. IV
Washington, Surgeon-General's office, catalogue of the library, 400–3
Wassermann, August von, 384
Wassermann reaction, 384
Water, supply of, in ancient Rome, 81 ; use of boiled, 230
Water-casting. See Urine
Waterloo, Battle of, Sir C. Bell at, 268 ; Robert Knox at, 270 ; Larrey at, 339 ; G. J. Guthrie and, 342 ; John Thomson at, 344
Weapon salve. See Powder of Sympathy
Weather and disease, 59, 250
Weighing machine of Sanctorius, 197, Pl. XL
Welch, William Henry, 288–89, 331, 359 ; quoted, 401, 408
Wellcome Historical Medical Museum (London), 17, 22
Wellington, Arthur Wellesley, Duke of, surgeons under, 341–42
Wells, Horace, 302–3
Wells, Sir Thomas Spencer, 320, 330
West Africa, yellow fever in, 359
West, Charles, 367–68
West Indies, syphilis acquired in, 164 ; yellow fever in, 359
Western Journal of Medical Science, 299
Westminster Hospital, 342
Whales, Knox's papers on, 271
Wharton, Thomas, 194
White, Charles, 318
White, Gilbert, quoted, 12
White, James, 383
White, Sir William Hale. See Hale-White
Whooping-cough in folk-medicine, 12
Whytt, Robert, 222, 231, 368
Widal, Fernand, 286
Widal test, 286
Wiener medizinische Wochenschrift, 397
Wigan, John, edition of Aretaeus, 71
Wilde, Sir William, 379
Wilde's incision, 379
Wilkie, Sir David Percival Dalbreck, 331
Wilks, Sir Samuel, 294

Willan, Robert, 381–82
William III, 210, 254
William IV, 313
William of Salicet, 117, 119
Willis, Thomas, 191, 200, 364, Pl. XLI
Willughby, Percivall, 183
Wilson, Edward Adrian, 355
Wilson, Sir Erasmus, 382–83
Wilson, T. G., 379
Windsor Castle, drawings by Leonardo da Vinci at, 136
Wine as wound dressing, 116
Winter, Johannes. *See* Guinther
Wirsung, Georg, 194
Wiseman, Richard, 196, 209–11, 337
Witch doctor, 1
Witches, Sir Thomas Browne and, 213-14
Withering, William, 235, 256–57
Withington, Edward Theodore, quoted, 21, 33, 86, 96, 141, 156
Wittwer, Philipp Ludwig, 398
Women in medicine, 385–86
Wong, Chi Min, quoted, 34
Wong Foon, 37
Wood, Alexander, 229–30, Pl. XLVII
Woodall, John, 152, 234
Woodham Mortimer Hall, 237
Woodhead, Sir German Sims, 288
Worcester, foundation of British Medical Association at, 394
Worcester, Noah, 383
Worde, Wynkyn de, 104
Worm, controlling brain, 123
"Wound man," in mediæval illustrations, 130
Wounds, treatment of, in ancient Egypt, 26 ; in the *Iliad*, 47-48 ; tar used by Hippocrates for, 58 ; Celsus on treatment of, 73 ; Theodoric Borgognoni on, 116 ; dry treatment of, by Henri de Mondeville, 117 ; early German treatises on, 126 ; Paré on, 145 ; Ballingall on, 345 ; suppuration of, regarded as essential, by Galen, 76, by Roger of Palermo, 106 ; theory opposed by Theodoric Borgognoni,
116 ; Lister and his followers on, 323–28
Wounds (arrow), 126
Wounds (broadsword), 232
Wounds (gunshot), first detailed account of, 126, 337 ; Paré on, 145, 146 ; Clowes on poison in, 152 ; Gale on, 152 ; Wiseman on, 211 ; at Waterloo, 268 ; in South African War, 349 ; in stomach, 300 ; leeching of, 345
Wounds (shell), 349–50
Wren, Sir Christopher, 191, 200
Wright, Sir Almroth, 288, 348
Wunderlich, Carl Reinhold August, 298, 408
Würzburg, Kircher of, 189 ; Virchow at, 282 ; Kölliker of, 322 ; Roentgen of, 384
Wylie, Sir James, 343-44

X-rays, Simpson's forecast of, 306 ; discovery of, 384, Pl. LXX ; effect of, on early operators, 385 ; deep X-ray therapy, 385

Yajur-Veda, 32
Yang and Yin, 35
Yearsley, James, 377-78
Yellow fever, 243, 359-60
Yersin, Alexandre, 287
York, the Retreat at, 249, 272-73
Young, Hugh Hampton, 334
Young, Thomas (obstetrician), 228
Young, Thomas (ophthalmologist), 274, 374-75
Young, W. A., 359
Young-Helmholtz theory, 274

Zayochek, General, 339
Zeitschrift für Anatomie, 398
Zodiac, influence of, on body, 98
"Zodiac man," in mediæval illustrations, 129, Pl. XXV
Zoser, King of Egypt, 22
Zurich, Paracelsus at, 157, 158 ; Cardan at, 163 ; Gesner of, 168, 399 ; Henle at, 271 ; Ludwig at, 276

SUPPLEMENT
TO THE REVISED EDITION

CONTENTS OF SUPPLEMENT

Peruvian Mummies   453

The Plague of Justinian   453

The Development of Pharmacopoeias   453

Vegetable Remedies   454

Mummy and Unicorn as Remedies   455

Jean Fernel   455

The Beginning of Pathology   456

The Lymphatics   456

" The Sceptical Chymist "   457

Early Blood Transfusion   457

The Microscope in Medicine   457

Early Danish Anatomists   457

Witches and Witch-hunting   458

The Red Cross   458

Early Medical Teaching in Aberdeen   459

Pieter Camper : Obstetrician and Artist   459

William Cumberland Cruikshank   459

Antonio de Gimbernat   459

The " other " Heberden   460

Mesmer and Mesmerism   460

Jan Evangelista Purkinje   461

The Rise of the Nursing Profession   461

Sir William Gowers   462

Adolf Meyer   462

Early Medical Journals   462

The " Index Medicus "   463

CONTENTS OF SUPPLEMENT

Egyptian Mummies ... 453
The Plague of Justinian ... 453
The Development of Pharmacopoeias ... 453
Vegetable Remedies ... 454
Mummy and Unicorn as Remedies ... 455
Jean Fernel ... 455
The Beginning of Pathology ... 456
The Lymphatics ... 456
The Serpical Obelisk ... 457
Early Blood Transfusion ... 457
The Microscope in Medicine ... 457
Early Dutch Anatomists ... 457
Witches and Witch-hunting ... 458
The Red Cross ... 458
Early Medical Teaching in Aberdeen ... 459
Pietro Camper: Obstetrician and Artist ... 459
William Cumberland Cruikshank ... 459
Antonio de Gimbernat ... 459
The "other" Héberden ... 460
Mesmer and Mesmerism ... 460
Jan Evangelista Purkinje ... 461
The Rise of the Nursing Profession ... 461
Sir William Gowers ... 462
Adolf Meyer ... 462
Early Medical Journals ... 462
The "Index Medicus" ... 463

SUPPLEMENT
TO THE REVISED EDITION

PERUVIAN MUMMIES (page 29)

The practice of mummification or embalming was not confined to Egypt, although that country may have been the original home of the technique. It spread to Africa and the Far East, and became a feature of the Inca Civilization of Peru. The Peruvian mummy differs markedly from the Egyptian in that the body, with the joints of all the limbs strongly flexed, is seated in a basket, and is painted with copal varnish or other preservatives, and wrapped in many yards of woven cloth so that a somewhat pear-shaped bundle is produced, about four feet in height. Large numbers of those mummy bundles have been found in the flask-shaped vaults which were dug in the earth to serve as catacombs.

THE PLAGUE OF JUSTINIAN (page 83)

Procopius, the historian who described this plague, which is sometimes named the Plague of Justinian, after the reigning Emperor, stated that " the whole human race was near being exterminated." All work in the city of Byzantium was at a standstill. There was no one to bury the dead, and the bodies were piled up to the roof in unoccupied buildings, a procedure which naturally favoured the spread of the epidemic. Rome shared in the pestilence, and the processions there to allay the scourge, led by Saint Gregory, have been the model for many artists.

THE DEVELOPMENT OF PHARMACOPŒIAS (page 132)

The word pharmacopœia, or the making of medicines, was first applied during the sixteenth century to any list of drugs or formulae, corresponding to the Antidotaria of earlier times, to which reference has been made on p. 108. In the seventeenth century, there were published various guides to drugs, such as René Pomet's *Histoire Générale des Drogues* in 1694, and in the same year there appeared another unofficial publication, *The London Dispensatory*, by John Pechey. Soon, however, the term pharmacopœia came to be restricted to those lists which conformed to a definite standard, and which met with official sanction.

The first pharmacopœia to be printed, in 1498, was the *Nuovo Receptario*, but its standards applied only to the city of Florence, and it was not until 1573 that it was adopted for the Grand Duchy of Tuscany, and thus became, in a sense, a national pharmacopœia, called the *Recettario Florentino*.

A *Dispensatorium* had been compiled for the city of Nuremberg in 1546 by Valerius Cordus, who is sometimes credited with the discovery of ether. Later, other cities, such as Barcelona, Augsburg, Cologne and Mantua, had their own lists and their own standards. None was officially applied

453

within a political unit, and accordingly the Florentine work of 1573 must be regarded as the pioneer of official pharmacopœias. The French pharmacopœia, or *Codex Medicamentarius*, was printed in 1638, while the *Pharmacopœia Matritensis* became official throughout Spain in 1739.

The *Dispensatorium Austriaco-Viennese* of 1729 was a combined effort, and by the end of the eighteenth century the majority of European countries had their own pharmacopœias.

In England, the Royal College of Physicians of London considered, in 1585, the idea of compiling a pharmacopœia, but the task was not completed until 1618, when the *Pharmacopœia Londonensis* was published under the direction of Sir Theodore Turquet of Mayerne (p. 201). The list includes 1,208 simples and 932 compounds, many of them containing more than ten ingredients. The fifth edition, dated 1746, still included bezoar stone, crabs' eyes and theriac, although mummy and unicorn had been discarded. The tenth and last edition of 1851 mentioned only 273 remedies.

In 1699, the Royal College of Physicians of Edinburgh published their *Pharmacopœia Edimburgensis*, the President being then Sir Robert Sibbald. Fourteen editions were printed, the last in 1841. Dublin also had its pharmacopœia between 1807 and 1830, sponsored by the Royal College of Physicians in Ireland.

All those pharmacopœias of Great Britain and Ireland were superseded by the *British Pharmacopœia*, first issued by the General Medical Council in 1864; revised editions every few years ensure its being up to date.

In addition, there were many pharmacopœias of local origin, such as the *Pharmacopœia Amstelredamensis* of 1701, describing the various medicaments then in use in Amsterdam.

Certain hospitals printed their own pharmacopœias : one of the earliest was the *Pharmacopœia Nosocomii Vigornensis* of Worcester Hospital, published in 1750, and there were many others in the hospitals of London, Edinburgh and elsewhere.

BOUSSEL, P. *Histoire Illustrée de la Pharmacie*, 1949
THOMPSON, C. J. S. *The Mystery and Romance of Alchemy and Pharmacy*, 1899

VEGETABLE REMEDIES (page 133)

The discovery of America led to the importation into Europe of a large number of new vegetable remedies. One of the earliest descriptions of those drugs, and of the plants from which they were derived, was written by NICOLAS MONARDES of Seville, and it appeared in 1569 under the title *Dos libros el veno que trata de todas las cosas que traen de nuestras Indies Occidentales*. Monardes never visited America, but in his capacity as a physician he set himself to experiment clinically with the drugs which were sent to him from the Spanish colonies of the West. In 1577, John Frampton of Dorset rendered the book into English under the quaint title *Joyfull Newes out of the Newe-founde Worlde*. It contains the first illustration of the tobacco plant to appear in a printed book, and it records the fact that tobacco was smoked by the Indians of that time as a remedy for " wearinesse."

454

SUPPLEMENT

Mummy and Unicorn as Remedies (page 144)

At this point it may be convenient to mention the two drugs against which Paré protested when he wrote his *Discours de la Momie et de la Licorne*, in 1528. Powdered mummy continued in use as a means of treating hæmorrhage long after the time of Paré : indeed, its virtues were extolled by Robert Boyle a century later. Originally, it was a product of Egyptian mummies, and its value may have been due to the resins and balsams used in embalming. When the real Egyptian product was not available, any dead body was used, and deception was frequent.

In his essay on *Urn Burial*, published in 1658, Sir Thomas Browne states that " Mummy is become merchandise and Pharaoh is sold for balsams."

As for the therapy of unicorn, mention has been made of unicorn's liver as a remedy (p. 102), but the horn of this mythical creature was the part more generally employed. The unicorn has been variously identified with the rhinoceros, the oryx and the narwhal. Certainly it was the narwhal tusk which was displayed in churches and museums as " the horn of a unicorn," but it is the horn of the rhinoceros, fashioned into the form of a cup, which is still vaunted in India and Africa as a protection against poisons, and as an aphrodisiac.

In medieval times it was said to cure " fluxes, consumptions, ulcers and all corruptions."

One of the principal contributions to the literature of the unicorn was *De Unicornu*, by Thomas Bartholin of Copenhagen. It is dated 1678. (See also p. 195.) A more modern study of unicorns is *The Lore of the Unicorn*, by O. Shepherd, published in 1930, and giving a scholarly account of the whole subject.

Jean Fernel (page 164)

A contemporary, whose views were even more enlightened than those of Cardan, was Jean Fernel (?1497–1588) of Paris, regarded by Fallopius as " the greatest physician and philosopher of this age." Even Guy Patin, whose pen was so caustic, wrote of Fernel, " He is one of my saints, along with Galen."

Fernel's was, indeed, a voice with a new message ! In 1542, there appeared his famous treatise, *De Naturalis Parte Medicinae*. In later editions he used the word *Physiologia*, and he was one of the first to employ this term. Of course Fernel's Physiology is long since outmoded : it was rendered obsolete by Harvey's discovery of the circulation of the blood about a century later. Fernel, although he retained the orthodox tradition of his time in regard to humours and temperaments, and the functions of the heart and liver, rejected astrology as an adjunct to medicine, and, unlike Cardan, he was strongly opposed to magic.

In Fernel's view, anatomy could reveal only the structure of the body, not its function. The bodily processes could be understood solely by observation of the body, in sickness as well as in health.

Moreover, Fernel infused humanism into his conception of medicine.

455

He regarded mental activity as an integral part of physiology, the product of the brain, and one third of his book deals with this theme. For him, body and soul are one.

The *Physiologia* was followed by a treatise on pathology, *Pathologia*, which was published in 1555, and which paved the way to the modern conception of disease.

Above all, as Sir Charles Sherrington wrote in his delightful study of Fernel, " he was one who never let himself forget that the sick man lay against the great background of living things in general, and the stars and a Deity beyond the stars."

SHERRINGTON, SIR CHARLES. *The Endeavour of Jean Fernel*, Cambridge, 1946

THE BEGINNING OF PATHOLOGY (pages 164 and 281)

One of the first to recognize the value of postmortem observations, half a century before Fernel coined the word " pathology," was ANTONIO BENIVIENI (1440–1502), of Florence. The records of his findings in twenty autopsies are embodied in a little posthumous work, entitled *De abditis nonnullis ac mirandis morborum et sanationum causis*, 1507, which was a praiseworthy effort to explain the hidden causes of disease. The notes are brief, but they represent the first step towards the correlation between disease and morbid anatomy. (See also pp. 211, 245.)

The first work devoted to surgical pathology appeared in 1632. It was written by MARCO AURELIO SEVERINO (1580–1656) of Naples, and was entitled *De Recondita Abscessum Natura*, and it dealt, not only with abscesses, as the name suggests, but with all manner of swellings. It was the first book of its kind to include illustrations.

A more ambitious treatise, and one which covered the entire field of medicine, based upon 3,000 postmortem examinations by many workers, was the *Sepulchretum sive Anatomia Practica ex cadaveribus morbo donatis*, dated 1679, the work of THEOPHILE BONET (1620–89) of Bologna. This ponderous book of 1,700 pages is a monument of industry, but Bonet was content merely to record. He lacked that critical faculty which was to be so well applied by his successor Morgagni (p. 245). No picture of seventeenth-century pathology is complete without some mention of the work of JOHANN JAKOB WEPFER (1620–95) of Schaffhausen, who in 1658 called attention to the fact that apoplexy or " stroke," a frequent cause of sudden death, was due to a cerebral hæmorrhage.

LONG, ESMOND R. *A History of Pathology*, 1928

THE LYMPHATICS (page 185)

It has been claimed that the priory for the discovery of the lymph vessels should be accorded to GEORGE JOYLIFFE (1621–58) who, when he was a student at Cambridge between 1650 and 1652, told Francis Glisson, then Professor of Physic, that, besides the arteries, veins and nerves, there existed a fourth set of vessels, the lymphatics, which contained a watery fluid. Joyliffe afterwards practised in London, and lectured to the Royal College of Physicians on what he called the *vasa lymphatica*.

" THE SCEPTICAL CHYMIST " (page 187)

Boyle proved that air was a substance which could be weighed and measured. In his view it was "not a simple body, but a confused aggregate of effluviums."

Boyle's principal work, *The Sceptical Chymist*, which appeared in 1661, gave a new impetus to chemistry, a subject which now came to be studied for its own sake, and not merely as an adjunct to alchemy or as an aid to medicine.

Thus did the mystery of respiration become gradually less mysterious, though much still remained obscure.

EARLY BLOOD TRANSFUSION (page 187)

Inspired by Robert Boyle and Sir Christopher Wren, Lower, in 1666, was the first to perform blood transfusion from one animal to another.

The pioneer experiment of Richard Lower was followed by JEAN BAPTISTE DENIS who, in 1667, transfused the blood of a lamb into the veins of a young man. Many failures and even fatalities followed, and the method fell into disrepute.

It was not until 1900 that Landsteiner discovered the various blood groups, which were further classified by Jansky in 1907.

The citrate method was introduced in 1914, and, now that recognition has been given to the blood bank, the use of plasma and the importance of the Rh factor, blood transfusion is widely employed as a therapeutic measure.

THE MICROSCOPE IN MEDICINE (page 189)

According to Professor Singer, the first medical work involving the use of the microscope was Pierre Borel's *Centuria Observatorum Microscopiarium*, dated 1655. Borel was Physician of Louis XIV of France. He described minute insects in the air, which caused plague, and worms in the blood of fever patients, so that he may well have been the first to produce evidence of the so-called germ theory of disease.

EARLY DANISH ANATOMISTS (page 195)

THOMAS BARTHOLIN (1616–80), professor of anatomy at Copenhagen, was a member of an anatomical dynasty comparable to that of the Monros of Edinburgh. To him we owe the discovery of the thoracic duct and the lymphatic system in man.

Another famous Dane, NIELS STEENSEN or NICOLAS STENO (1638–66), whose name is variously rendered, was an outstanding scholar of the seventeenth century who won distinction in geology and in theology, as well as in anatomy. His name is associated with the parotid duct, which he discovered in a calf, in 1661, and he was perhaps the first to show that while a muscle underwent a change in form during contraction, it remained

457

SUPPLEMENT

unaltered in volume. He also proved that the heart was a muscle which behaved like other muscles. One of Steno's most interesting works is *A Dissertation on the Anatomy of the Brain*, originally published in French in 1669. Recently it has been reprinted by Prof. Godfredson of Copenhagen. It was Steno who, by describing the lachrymal gland, showed that tear fluid did not come from the brain, as was stated by Wharton in his *Adenographia*, in 1656.

GARBOE, A. *Thomas Bartholin*, Copenhagen, 1950

WITCHES AND WITCH-HUNTING (page 214)

The persecution of witches was no new trend in the days of Sir Thomas Browne. Three hundred years earlier Pope Innocent VI, viewing with alarm this menace to religion, appointed Henry Kraemer and James Sprenger to deal with the problem. Those inquisitors produced their notorious book, *Malleus Maleficarum*, or *The Hammer of the Witches*, in 1487. Witch-hunting became a popular pastime, and thousands of innocent persons were executed or burned alive. Most of them were women, but a famous exception was Dr. Fian of North Berwick, who was executed at Edinburgh in 1591, after he had raised a storm by throwing cats into the sea while King James VI of Scotland was bringing home his bride, Anne of Denmark.

The King had already written a counterblast to witchcraft entitled *Daemonologie*, a book which, like *The Hammer of the Witches*, detailed the tests for a witch. Bound hand and foot, she was thrown into a pond or river. If she floated, she was guilty : if she sank, she was innocent, but usually drowned. Thus were innocent and guilty alike destroyed.

Only a few bold spirits dared to protest against the edict " Thou shalt not suffer a witch to live." One of the first was Johann Weyer, who wrote his *De Praestigiis Daemonorum* in 1563, and who is often acclaimed as the founder of modern psychiatry. Another who protested was Reginald Scot, a Kentish squire whose *Discoverie of Witchcraft* is dated 1584. Despite such efforts at reform, the belief in witchcraft died hard, and it was not until 1782 that the last execution for witchcraft was carried out, in Switzerland.

GUTHRIE, D. *From Witchcraft to Antisepsis*, Kansas, 1955
MAJOR, RALPH. *Faiths that healed*, 1940
ZILBOORG, G. *The Medical Man and the Witch*, 1935

THE RED CROSS (page 232)

The Red Cross idea was slow to reach Britain, where the Order of the Knights of St. John was the first to take action by incorporating the St. John Ambulance Brigade in 1888. It was not until 1905 that the British Red Cross Society came into being and it received a Royal Charter from King Edward VII in 1908. The World War of 1914–18 gave an immense impetus to the work, and vastly increased its significance.

SUPPLEMENT

EARLY MEDICAL TEACHING IN ABERDEEN (page 234)

Although it may be claimed with justice that the Monros led the way towards the establishment of a Faculty of Medicine in the University of Edinburgh, and that Cullen performed a similar service for Glasgow University, recognition had been accorded to medicine in Aberdeen at a much earlier date.

When the University of Aberdeen, originally named St. Mary's College, and later, King's College, was first established in 1494, provision was made for the teaching of medicine by a " Mediciner," but whether this implied the creation of a Chair of Medicine has been a matter of argument ever since.

If the claim is allowed, this would appear to be the first recognition of medical teaching in any British university. Cambridge followed in 1540, Oxford in 1546.

The third of the Aberdeen " mediciners," appointed in 1556, was Gilbert Skene, author of a little treatise on plague, *Ane breve description of the Pest*, dated 1568, the first medical book to be printed in Scotland, of which the only copy known to be extant is in the National Library of Scotland.

PIETER CAMPER : OBSTETRICIAN AND ARTIST (page 236)

When William Smellie was at the height of his fame in London, there came to visit him a young student from Leyden, named PIETER CAMPER (1722–89).

Camper, who became distinguished for his services to anatomy, to art and to obstetrics, made three successive journeys to Britain, and his *Travel Journals*, which have been published in English, give an excellent picture of the obstetrical teaching of the time, and especially of Smellie, for whose Treatise Camper drew a number of illustrations. Camper attained high eminence in his profession, as Professor at Amsterdam, and later at Groningen. He wielded a versatile pen and was a good artist.

Douglas Guthrie. " The Travel Journals of Pieter Camper," *Edin. Med. Journ.*, 1948, Vol. lv, p. 338

WILLIAM CUMBERLAND CRUIKSHANK (page 240)

William Cumberland Cruikshank (1745–1800), who succeeded Hewson, continued the Windmill Street School of anatomy after William Hunter's death, and was the first to demonstrate, in 1776, by experiments on dogs, the regeneration of divided nerves.[1]

[1] W. Holmes, " The repair of nerves by suture," *Jour. Hist. Med.*, Vol. vi, No. 7, 1951, p. 44.

ANTONIO DE GIMBERNAT (page 244)

A disciple of Hunter was the Spanish anatomist and surgeon ANTONIO DE GIMBERNAT (1734–1816). He was still under thirty when appointed professor of anatomy at Barcelona. Next, we hear of him attending John Hunter's lectures in London, and visiting William Cullen in Edinburgh, and Pieter Camper in Holland. Returning to Spain, he drew up plans for a Medical School in Madrid, where he became professor of surgery and where he spent the remainder of his long and useful life. His name survives, or did so until recently, in Gimbernat's ligament, the description of which was only one of his many contributions to anatomy. When asked to recommend a textbook of anatomy, Gimbernat would reply, " My favourite author is the human body." [1]

[1] N. M. Matheson, " Antonio Gimbernat, 1734–1816," *Proc. Roy. Soc. Med.* (*Sect. Hist.*), Vol. xiii, No. 6, June 1949.

THE " OTHER " HEBERDEN (page 256)

Heberden was twice married, and had seven children, but the only member of the family to survive him was his son WILLIAM HEBERDEN THE YOUNGER (1767–1845), who, though scarcely so eminent as his father, deserves also to be remembered. He was a Physician to St. George's Hospital, and author of several works, including an *Epitome of Diseases of Children*, but perhaps his chief claim to fame arose from the fact that he was physician to King George III during the long illness of that monarch.

MESMER AND MESMERISM (page 262)

Many of Mesmer's imitators were charlatans, but some were medical men of distinction ; among them was JOHN ELLIOTSON (1791–1868), who in 1831 became the first Professor of Medicine at University College, London, the so-called " Godless College," open to all students and not merely to members of the Church of England. Elliotson was an excellent clinical teacher, and his interest in neurology led him to study phrenology and mesmerism, which were enjoying a wide popularity. This aroused the antagonism of his colleagues and led to a heated controversy. As a result, Elliotson was obliged to resign from his Chair in 1838.

He emerged from the contest, however, without any stain on his personal character, and he continued to practise mesmerism and to give demonstrations at his house.

Elliotson's most capable follower was JAMES ESDAILE, a Scottish doctor of the East India Company. Elliotson had lessened or prevented the pain of surgical operations by mesmerism, or had claimed to have done so. Esdaile carried the experiments a stage further, and it was hoped that the problem of anaesthesia might be solved by mesmerism, or hypnotism, as it had been called by James Braid of Manchester, another worker in this field.

At this time, however, the discovery of ether anaesthesia in America diverted the attention of investigators towards the inhalation of various vapours, and hypnotic anaesthesia was forgotten.

JAN EVANGELISTA PURKINJE (page 274)

A contemporary pioneer of physiology, although not associated with Müller, was JAN EVANGELISTA PURKINJE (1787–1869), of Prague and Breslau. Purkinje is said to have been the first to employ the microtome, to coin the word " protoplasm," and to note the value of finger-prints as a means of identification. Being a Czech, he was not welcomed in Germany, but his friendship with Goethe was to his advantage, and by his own brilliance he achieved distinction and disarmed criticism.

THE RISE OF THE NURSING PROFESSION (pages 294, 347)

One of the first references to the profession of nursing is to be found in the writings of the surgeon of ancient India, Susruta, who advised that, in choosing a nurse for the sick, preference should be given to those who were cool-headed and strong. St. Jerome has described the work of one of the earliest pioneers of nursing, the noble Roman lady named Fabiola, who built a hospital and devoted her life to nursing the sick during the early part of the Christian era. Among the Christian abbesses who made nursing their chief duty was St. Radegund of Poitiers, who died in 589.

Some historians allege that the " Ladies of Salerno " were nurses, but they were more probably doctors ; and about this time, too, the Knights of St. John included in their order a female branch, the Sisters of St. John, who were certainly nurses.

Everyone is familiar with St. Francis of Assisi, the " poor little man of God," but not so many remember his chief disciple St. Clare, who established the Second Order of Franciscans, the " Poor Clares," in 1212, and who ministered to the afflicted, and especially to lepers. There was a third order, comprising those who continued their family life while devoting themselves to charity, and to this order of Tertiaries, as they were called, belonged Elizabeth of Hungary, who lived with her husband, a nobleman, in the Wartburg Castle in Thuringia. St. Francis had a great regard for Elizabeth, and he gave her his grey cloak, having nothing else to give. Thus the sisterhood of St. Elizabeth became the Grey Nuns. Another member of the Tertiaries was St. Catherine of Siena, who was born in 1347, and whose devotion to the profession of nursing was so deep that she is often regarded as the Patron Saint of Nursing.

More definitely organised was the order of the Béguines, founded about A.D. 1180 by Lambert de Bégue, Bishop of Liége. The Béguines took no vows, and were even free to marry and hold property. The movement spread to other countries, and the German Béguines adopted a blue uniform and were called the Blue Nuns, although of course they were not really nuns. By the year 1300, the Béguines numbered 300,000.

An older Order, and one of secular origin, was that of the Augustinian Nuns of the Hôtel Dieu of Paris, which imposed a strict discipline upon its members, and which continued to flourish until the beginning of the present century.

Of later Societies, the most important was that of the Sisters of Charity, founded by St. Vincent de Paul in 1617. Like the Béguines, no vows were demanded. Viñcent de Paul disapproved of any indiscriminate charity and of misplaced sacrifice : his work was always sensible and practical.

In Britain, before Florence Nightingale came on the scene, the standards of nursing were lower than on the Continent, and there was great need for the reform which she accomplished so thoroughly.[1]

[1] Cecil Woodham-Smith, *Florence Nightingale*, 1950

SIR WILLIAM GOWERS (page 371)

Gowers emphasised the value of shorthand in medical work, and founded the Society of Medical Phonographers, which flourished from 1894 to 1912. His *Manual of Diseases of the Nervous System*, of which the first volume appeared in 1886 is a clinical treasure trove, and to this day is regarded as the "Bible of Neurology."

Gowers' versatility is shown by his invention of a magnifying otoscope, a haemocytometer and a haemoglobinometer, and also by his skill as an artist and his interest in archaeology and botany, although he lacked the gracious personality of Hughlings Jackson.

ADOLF MEYER (page 374)

Perhaps the greatest figure in the domain of psychiatry during the early part of the present century was the Swiss-born ADOLF MEYER (1866–1950) whose work was done in America. Meyer laid stress upon "the total personality reaction in all its aspects, as the only basis for the proper understanding of the patient." [1]

[1] G. Zilboorg, *A History of Medical Psychology*, 1941, p. 503

EARLY MEDICAL JOURNALS (page 394)

It has been claimed that the pioneer of medical journals was *Acta Medica et Philosophica Hufniensis*, 1673–80, edited by Thomas Bartholin of Copenhagen.

Medicina Curiosa was the first British periodical denoted entirely to medicine, although it was preceded by the first English abstracting journal, a periodical entitled *Weekly Memorials for the Ingenious, or, An Account of Books lately set forth in various languages*, which first appeared in January 1682, and continued until the 29th number, maintaining a high standard.[1]

America may claim to have published the first dental journal, the *American Journal of Dental Science*, New York, 1839–1800, as well as the first periodical dealing with nursing, which was called *The Nightingale*, New York, 1886, but which did not outlive that year.

The first British periodical devoted to dentistry was the *British Quarterly Journal of Dental Science*, 1843, although only two numbers appeared.

[1] Poynter, F. L. N., "The First English Medical Journal," *Brit. Med. Journ.*, 1948, Vol. ii, p. 307

The " Index Medicus " (page 402)

The fact that the volumes which have already appeared contain nearly three million entries gives some indication of the magnitude of the task.

It is not easy to keep such a list fully up to date. In order to supply a more timely index, a *Current List of Medical Literature*, which has been a weekly publication since 1941, now appears monthly and is produced in conjunction with the *Quarterly Cumulative Index Medicus*, and it may be possible to fuse these two publications.

At the present time the *World List of Scientific Periodicals* mentions over 30,000 journals, of which about 5,000 are counted as exclusively medical. Obviously it is difficult to define the word "medical", as applied to literature, when there are numerous journals dealing with nutrition, technology, sanitary science, nursing, etc., but it is generally admitted that the strictly medical periodical now number more than 2,000. The Army Libraries List of the U.S.A. indexes 1,225 current journals : 526 of them (43 per cent) are in English, and 699 (57 per cent) in other languages.

Printed in Great Britain by
Thomas Nelson and Sons Ltd, Edinburgh